## SECOND EDITION
# NEONATAL RESPIRATORY CARE

──────── SECOND EDITION ────────

# NEONATAL RESPIRATORY CARE

**Waldemar A. Carlo, M.D.**
Assistant Professor of Pediatrics and Reproductive Biology
Case Western Reserve University
Associate Director
Newborn Intensive Care Nursery
Rainbow Babies and Childrens Hospital
Cleveland, Ohio

**Robert L. Chatburn, R.R.T.**
Technical Director of Respiratory Care
Rainbow Babies and Childrens Hospital
Cleveland, Ohio

**YEAR BOOK MEDICAL PUBLISHERS, INC.**
CHICAGO • LONDON • BOCA RATON

Copyright © 1979, 1988 by Year Book Medical Publishers, Inc. All rights reserved. No part of this publication may be reproduced, stored in a retrieval system, or transmitted, in any form or by any means—electronic, mechanical, photocopying, recording, or otherwise—without prior written permission from the publisher. Printed in the United States of America.

1  2  3  4  5  6  7  8  9  0  C R  92  91  90  89  88

**Library of Congress Cataloging-in-Publication Data**

Neonatal respiratory care.
   Rev. ed. of: Newborn respiratory care. c1979.
   Includes bibliographies and index.
   1. Respiratory insufficiency in children.  2. Infants (Newborn)—Diseases.  3. Neonatal intensive care.  I. Carlo, Waldemar A.  II. Chatburn, Robert L.  III. Newborn respiratory care.  [DNLM: 1. Infant, Newborn, Diseases—therapy.  2. Respiratory Tract Diseases—in infancy & childhood.  3. Respiratory Tract Diseases—therapy.     WS 280 N4385]
RJ312.N48   1988       618.92′2       88–148
ISBN 0–8151–5636–7

Sponsoring Editor: Richard H. Lampert
Associate Managing Editor, Manuscript Services: Deborah Thorp
Copyeditor: Sally J. Jansen
Production Project Manager: Nancy C. Baker
Proofroom Supervisor: Shirley E. Taylor

*This book is dedicated to neonatal patients, their parents, and caretakers; Eugenia, Wally, Enrique, Julian, and Maria Carlo, and DEE and Maya Chatburn for their support, understanding, and encouragement; and to Marvin Lough, R.R.T., and Doctors Avroy A. Fanaroff and Richard J. Martin, who taught us neonatal care.*

# CONTRIBUTORS

**Robert H. Bartlett, M.D.**
Professor of Surgery
University of Michigan Medical
  Center
University of Michigan
Ann Arbor, Michigan

**James B. Besunder, D.O.**
Fellow, Pediatric Critical Care and
  Clinical Pharmacology
Case Western Reserve University
  School of Medicine
Rainbow Babies and Childrens
  Hospital
Cleveland, Ohio

**Jeffrey L. Blumer, Ph.D., M.D.**
Associate Professor of Pediatrics
Assistant Professor of Pharmacology
Case Western Reserve University
Chief, Division of Pediatric
  Pharmacology and Critical Care
Rainbow Babies and Childrens
  Hospital
Cleveland, Ohio

**Waldemar A. Carlo, M.D.**
Assistant Professor of Pediatrics and
  Reproductive Biology
Case Western Reserve University
Associate Director
Newborn Intensive Care Nursery
Rainbow Babies and Childrens
  Hospital
Cleveland, Ohio

**Robert L. Chatburn, R.R.T.**
Technical Director of Respiratory
  Care
Rainbow Babies and Childrens
  Hospital
Cleveland, Ohio

**Avroy A. Fanaroff, M.D.,
F.R.C.P.E.**
Professor and Vice Chairman
Department of Pediatrics
Case Western Reserve University
Director of Nurseries
Rainbow Babies and Childrens
  Hospital
Cleveland, Ohio

**Tilo Gerhardt, M.D.**
Associate Professor of Pediatrics
University of Miami
Director of Pulmonary Laboratory
Jackson Memorial Hospital
Miami, Florida

**Mary Fran Hazinski, R.N.,
M.S.N.**
Clinical Specialist
Pediatric Intensive Care
Vanderbilt University Medical
  Center
Nashville, Tennessee

**Lars P. Jensen, M.D., M.B.,
Ch.B., M.Med.**
Assistant Professor of Obstetrics and
  Gynecology
University of Miami
Jackson Memorial Medical Center
Miami, Florida

**John H. Kennell, M.D.**
Professor of Pediatrics
Case Western Reserve University
  School of Medicine
Pediatrician, Rainbow Babies and
  Childrens Hospital
Cleveland, Ohio

**Marshall H. Klaus, M.D.**
Director, Academic Affairs
Childrens Hospital
Oakland, California

**Marvin D. Lough, R.R.T.**
Technical Director
Pediatric Pulmonary Function
  Laboratory
Rainbow Babies and Childrens
  Hospital
Case Western Reserve University
Cleveland, Ohio

**Richard J. Martin, M.D.**
Associate Professor of Pediatrics
Case Western Reserve University
Co-Director, Division of Neonatology
Rainbow Babies and Childrens
  Hospital
Cleveland, Ohio

**Martha J. Miller, M.D., Ph.D.**
Assistant Professor
Case Western Reserve University
Assistant Professor of Pediatrics
Rainbow Babies and Childrens
  Hospital
Cleveland, Ohio

**Stuart C. Morrison, M.B., Ch.B., M.R.C.P.**
Assistant Professor of Radiology
Case Western Reserve University
Rainbow Babies and Childrens
  Hospital
University Hospitals of Cleveland
Cleveland, Ohio

**Joanne J. Nicks, R.R.T.**
Respiratory Therapy Clinical
  Specialist
Department of Pediatric Respiratory
  Therapy
University of Michigan Medical
  Center
Ann Arbor, Michigan

**Annette Simpson Pacetti, R.N., B.S.N., M.S.N.**
Adjunct Faculty
Vanderbilt University School of
  Nursing
Neonatal Nurse Practitioner
Neonatal Nurse Educator
Vanderbilt University Medical
  Center
Nashville, Tennessee

**Michael D. Reed, Pharm.D., F.C.C.P.**
Assistant Professor of Pediatrics
Case Western Reserve University
  School of Medicine
Rainbow Babies and Childrens
  Hospital
Cleveland, Ohio

**Bradford J. Richmond, M.D., C.R.T.T.**
Staff, Diagnostic Radiology
Cleveland Clinic Foundation
Cleveland, Ohio

**Huda K. Rosen, R.R.T., M.S.**
Supervisor, Clinical Sup. II
University of Michigan Medical
  Center
Ann Arbor, Michigan

**James M. Sherman, Jr., M.D.**
Associate Professor of Pediatrics
Director, Pulmonary Division
Department of Pediatrics
University of South Florida
Vice Chief of Pediatrics
Tampa General Hospital
Tampa, Florida

**Bonnie Siner, R.N.**
Research Nurse
Rainbow Babies and Childrens
  Hospital
Cleveland, Ohio

**R. Brian Smith, M.D.**
Professor and Chairman
Department of Anesthesiology
University of Texas Medical School
Anesthesiologist-in-Chief
Medical Center and Audie L.
    Murphy Memorial Veterans
    Hospital
San Antonio, Texas

**Joseph F. Tomashefski, Jr., M.D.**
Assistant Professor of Pathology
Case Western Reserve University
    and Cleveland Metropolitan
    General Hospital
Cleveland, Ohio

**William E. Truog, III, M.D.**
Professor of Pediatrics
University of Washington School of
    Medicine
Medical Director
Infant Intensive Care Unit
Children's Hospital Medical Center
Seattle, Washington

**Michele C. Walsh, M.D.**
Senior Instructor
Case Western Reserve University
Neonatologist, Assistant Director of
    Extracorporeal Membrane
    Oxygenation
University Hospitals of Cleveland
Cleveland, Ohio

**Robert E. Wood, Ph.D., M.D.**
Professor of Pediatrics
University of North Carolina at
    Chapel Hill
The North Carolina Memorial
    Hospital
Chapel Hill, North Carolina

# PREFACE

In the 9 years since the first edition there have been tremendous changes in the field of neonatal respiratory care. This book has been revised and updated to reflect this evolution, and every effort has been made to include the latest developments. Sections on high-frequency ventilation, extracorporeal membrane oxygenation, pulmonary function, gas exchange, and complications of assisted ventilation have been added to reflect the enhanced perspective gained from extensive research and experience.

Advances in respiratory care have led to the increased survival of critically ill neonates. Unfortunately, there has been an associated increased incidence of complications. The intent of this book is to guide postgraduate health care professionals and students, including respiratory therapists, nurses, and physicians, in the care of critically ill neonates. It is our firm hope that the information provided in this text will improve neonatal respiratory care and continue to further reduce both morbidity and mortality in this patient population. With thoughtful care, these ill neonates will survive to lead full and productive lives.

*Waldemar A. Carlo, M.D.*
*Robert L. Chatburn, R.R.T.*

# CONTENTS

*Preface*   xi

1 / Development of the Respiratory System   1
   by Joseph F. Tomashefski, Jr., and Bradford J. Richmond

2 / Assessment of Neonatal Gas Exchange   40
   by Robert L. Chatburn and Waldemar A. Carlo

3 / Physiologic Monitoring and Pulmonary Function   61
   by Tilo Gerhardt and Lars P. Jensen

4 / The Airways   91
   by Robert E. Wood and James M. Sherman, Jr.

5 / Clinical Care Techniques   107
   by Marvin D. Lough and Waldemar A. Carlo

6 / Delivery Room Management and Resuscitation of the Newborn   130
   by William E. Truog, III

7 / Nursing Care of the Infant With Respiratory Disease   154
   by Mary Fran Hazinski and Annette Simpson Pacetti

8 / Care of the Parents   212
   by John H. Kennell and Marshall H. Klaus

9 / Neonatal Clinical Pharmacology: Principles and Practice   236
   by Michael D. Reed, James B. Besunder, and Jeffrey L. Blumer

10 / Respiratory Diseases of the Newborn   260
   by Michele C. Walsh, Waldemar A. Carlo, and Martha J. Miller

11 / Radiologic Findings of Newborn Respiratory Diseases   289
   by Stuart C. Morrison

12 / Assisted Ventilation of the Newborn   320
   by Waldemar A. Carlo and Robert L. Chatburn

13 / Complications of Neonatal Respiratory Care   347
   by Richard J. Martin and Avroy A. Fanaroff

14 / High-Frequency Ventilation    366
   by Waldemar A. Carlo and Robert L. Chatburn

15 / Extracorporeal Membrane Oxygenation and Other New Modes of Gas Exchange    394

   15A / Extracorporeal Membrane Oxygenation    394
       by Joanne J. Nicks and Robert H. Bartlett

   15B / Continuous-Flow Apneic Ventilation    409
       by R. Brian Smith

   15C / Liquid Ventilation    419
       by Huda K. Rosen

Appendix    424
   by Bonnie Siner and Waldemar A. Carlo

Index    455

# 1

# Development of the Respiratory System

Joseph F. Tomashefski, Jr., M.D.
Bradford J. Richmond, M.D., C.R.T.T.

For those involved in the care of the neonate, the newborn lung represents the dynamic interaction of two simultaneous processes: adaptation to extrauterine life and response to injury. The lung in utero develops according to a relatively fixed schedule. After birth, alveolar multiplication continues for at least 8 years. Knowledge of the intrauterine and extrauterine timetables of lung development is essential for an understanding of normal and abnormal neonatal respiratory physiology. It is also fundamental to an understanding of the response of the lung to various interventions to support respiratory function or stimulate lung growth. The selection of respiratory support modalities and the type of equipment used is often dependent on the gestational age of the neonate. It is unlikely that the lungs of the infant born prematurely maintain the intrauterine schedule of development, but the extent to which this schedule is modified in adapting to a new and often hostile environment is unknown. The spectrum of congenital abnormalities of the lung is likewise best understood in terms of the developmental stage at which interference with growth occurs.

In this chapter, we will review the anatomical and biochemical development of the upper and lower fetal respiratory tracts. Since pulmonary development and function are intimately associated with that of the heart, we will also briefly consider cardiac development. Finally, we will discuss the dramatic structural and functional remodeling of the cardiorespiratory system that occurs in the newborn period as the infant adapts to extrauterine life.

## EMBRYOLOGICAL GERM CELL LAYERS

It is not our intention to discuss embryogenesis in detail; for this the reader is referred to standard texts.[1-4] To understand lung development, however, it is important to be familiar with the embryonic germ cell layers and their derivatives. Shortly after conception, the fertilized ovum undergoes rapid cellular proliferation and subsequent internal cavitation to form the *blastocyst*. The cells of the blastocyst reorganize to form a bilaminar germ disk, which is converted to a trilaminar germ disk by the third week of embryonic life. The three germ layers, *endoderm, ectoderm,* and *mesoderm*, each give rise to specific body parts. The endoderm ultimately evolves into the lining epithelium of the entire digestive tract and lung, as well as the parenchyma of the liver and pancreas. The ectoderm gives rise to the central and peripheral nervous systems; sensory epithelium of the nose, ears, and eyes; and the skin and its appendages. The mesoderm, the last germ layer to form, establishes the cardiovascular, genitourinary, and lymphoid systems and also develops into a primitive form of connective tissue called *mesenchyme*. Mesenchymal cells have the potential to differentiate into fibrous tissue (fibroblasts), smooth and skeletal muscle (myoblasts), bone (osteoblasts), cartilage (chondroblasts), and blood vessels (angioblasts). The mesoderm also gives rise to *mesothelial cells* that line the serous cavities, i.e., pleura, peritoneum, and pericardium.

## DEVELOPMENT OF THE RESPIRATORY TRACT

In humans, completion of the development of the respiratory system occurs late in fetal life, and as a result, the lung is considered a nonfunctional organ until near term. Thus, in utero, the respiratory system develops independently of the functional demands of the growing embryo and fetus. Physiologic lung activity prior to birth is limited to some respiratory movements, growth, and secretion of various substances during specific times in development. At birth, the fetus is expelled from its aquatic surroundings, and the partially collapsed, fluid-filled lung must be prepared to adapt immediately to air breathing, thus facilitating the oxygen and carbon dioxide diffusion necessary for extrauterine life. The schedule of intrauterine respiratory tract development is summarized in Table 1–1. A list of important congenital malformations of the tracheobronchial tree is provided in Table 1–2. Congenital malformations of the respiratory tract are further discussed in Chapters 4 and 10.

Development of the Respiratory System    3

**TABLE 1-1.**
Summary of Respiratory Tract Development

| Approximate Time of Occurrence | Developmental Event |
|---|---|
| 20 days | Foregut established |
| 24 days | Laryngotracheal groove develops |
| 26-28 days | Bronchial buds form |
| 2 wk | Intraembryonic coeloms form |
| 3 wk | Diaphragm development begins |
| 4 wk | Primitive nasal cavities develop; tongue develops; pharynx formation begins; phrenic nerves originate |
| 5 wk | Pseudoglandular phase begins; lobar bronchi are present; pulmonary artery develops; pulmonary vein develops; lung bud migrates into pleural canals |
| 6 wk | Arytenoid swellings (lead to formation of larynx) develop |
| 7 wk | Oropharynx develops; tracheal cartilage is present; smooth muscle of bronchi develops |
| 8 wk | Vocal cords develop |
| 9 wk | Bronchial arteries develop |
| 10 wk | Secondary palate forms; cilia develop; mucous glands appear; cartilaginous rings of trachea develop |
| 11 wk | Lymphatic tissue appears |
| 13 wk | Goblet cells are present |
| 16 wk | Canalicular phase begins; preacinar bronchial branches are complete |
| 22 wk | Methyltransferase system for lecithin synthesis is present; lecithin appears |
| 24 wk | Terminal saccular (alveolar) phase begins; respiratory bronchioles develop; terminal sacs develop |
| 26-28 wk | Alveolar-capillary surface area of respiratory system developed sufficiently to support extrauterine life |
| 35 wk | Phosphocholine transferase system for lecithin synthesis is present |
| 36 wk | Mature alveoli are present |

**TABLE 1-2.**
Congenital Malformations of the Lower Respiratory Tract

| Congenital Malformation | Embryological Origin | Remarks |
|---|---|---|
| Tracheoesophageal fistula (four different varieties) | Results from incomplete division of the foregut into respiratory and digestive portions during the fourth and fifth weeks | Occurs in about 1 of 2,500 births, predominantly in males |
| Tracheal stenosis; tracheal atresia | Probably results from unequal partitioning of the foregut into the esophagus and trachea | Rare |
| Laryngeal web | A membranous web forms around the vocal cords, causing airway obstruction; results from the incomplete | Rare |

(*Continued.*)

**TABLE 1–2 (cont.).**

| | | |
|---|---|---|
| | recanalization of the larynx during the tenth week | |
| Congenital bronchial cysts | Cysts may develop when abnormal saccular enlargements occur in the terminal bronchioles | Rare |
| Agenesis of the lung (absence of the lung) | Results from failure of the lung bud(s) to develop | Unilateral more frequent than bilateral; however, both are rare |
| Hypoplasia of the lung | Lungs unable to develop normally because they are compressed by abnormally positioned abdominal viscera | Rare; seen in infants with posterolateral diaphragmatic hernia |

**The Upper Respiratory Tract**

In the fourth week of gestation, the buccopharyngeal (oropharyngeal) membrane ruptures, allowing communication between the ectoderm of the primitive oral cavity and the endoderm of the foregut. The primitive nasal cavities (nasal sacs) originate in the fourth week as two ectodermal thickenings (Fig 1–1) separated by mesenchymal cells destined to become the nasal septum and primary palate. An oronasal membrane separates the growing nasal sacs from the oropharynx. The disintegration of this membrane occurs during the seventh week, allowing the primitive nasal choana to form. Connection of the nasal cavities to the anterior oropharynx then is complete. At this time, lateral sheets of tissue begin to form the secondary palate while the nasal septum develops in continuity with the primary palate. The secondary palate is completed at 10 to 12 weeks of gestation. The anterior palate undergoes membranous ossification; the posterior portions do not become ossified but extend beyond the nasal septum as the soft palate and uvula. The nasopharynx is the region that communicates with bilateral nasal cavities and is roughly separated inferiorly from the oropharynx by the soft palate. Posteriorly the nasopharynx communicates with the oropharynx via the choana. Occasionally, the choana becomes sealed by membranous tissue that occludes the nasal passage. This condition, known as choanal atresia, can result in death of the nose-breathing neonate if medical intervention is not prompt. The tongue grows along the floor of the oral cavity during the fourth to seventh week.

The pharynx arises from the proximal foregut at 4 weeks. The laryngotracheal groove along the floor of the pharynx will give rise to the lower respiratory tract (Fig 1–2). The cranial portion of the tube forming

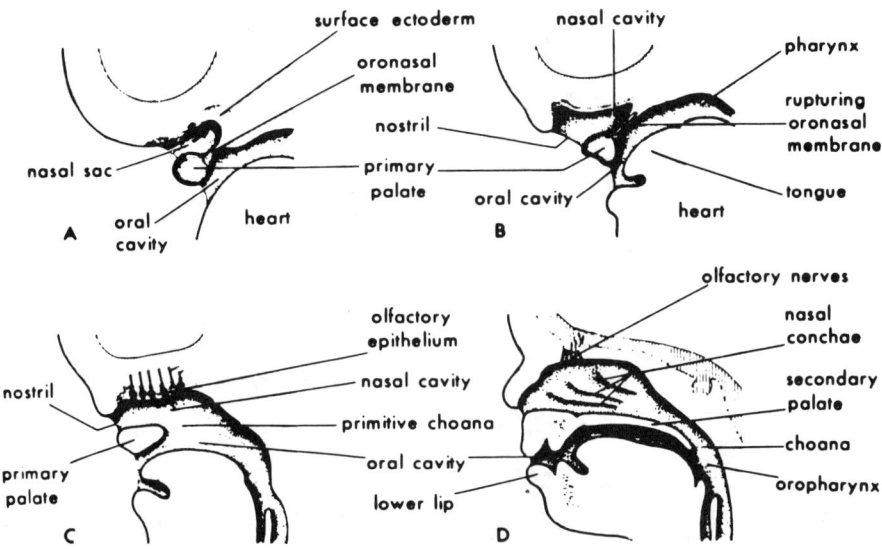

**FIG 1–1.**
Development of the nose. **A,** buccopharyngeal membrane separating nasal sac and oral cavity. **B** and **C,** buccopharyngeal membrane disintegrates, forming communication between oral and nasal cavities. **D,** nasal development at 12 weeks. (From Moore KL: *The Developing Human,* ed 2. Philadelphia, WB Saunders Co, 1977. Used by permission.)

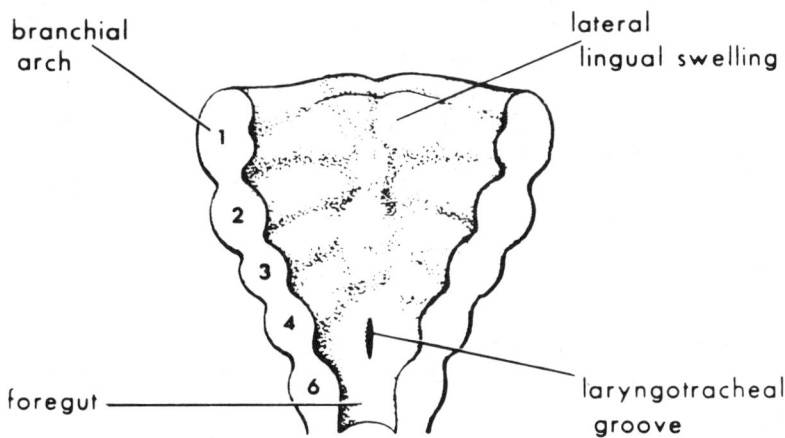

**FIG 1–2.**
The laryngotracheal groove. Precursor of the respiratory tract. (Modified from Moore KL: *The Developing Human,* ed 2. Philadelphia, WB Saunders Co, 1977.)

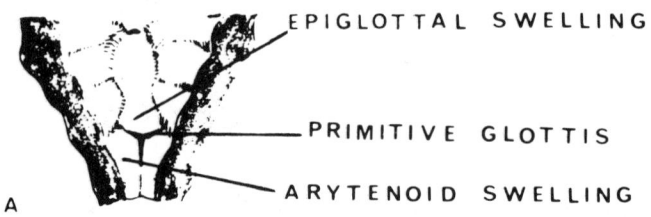
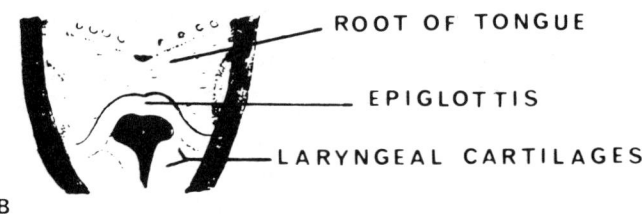

**FIG 1–3.**
Formation of the laryngeal orifice by arytenoid swellings. **A**, laryngeal orifice occluded by epithelial tissue at 6 weeks. **B**, epithelial tissue disintegrates, forming patent laryngeal orifice.

the primordial respiratory tract will become the larynx. At approximately the sixth week, epiglottal tissue has formed, with arytenoid swellings developing toward the tongue. These swellings will form the laryngeal orifice (Fig 1–3). Until the tenth week of gestation, the orifice is occluded by epithelial tissue. At 10 weeks, the epithelium disintegrates. The vocal cords appear as folds of connective tissue during the eighth week. The vocal cords act as a sphincter for normal breathing, cough, Valsalva maneuvering, and intonation.

## The Lower Respiratory Tract

### General Considerations

The key concepts of intrauterine lung growth are summarized in Reid's "laws of lung development"[5]:

*Law 1:* The number of preacinar airway branches is complete by the 16th week of intrauterine life.

*Law 2:* Alveolar development begins only after airway development is complete and occurs mainly after birth. Alveoli increase in number until about the age of 8 years and increase in size until growth of the chest wall ceases in early adulthood.

*Law 3*: The preacinar pulmonary vessels (arteries and veins) follow the development of the airways, whereas the intra-acinar vessels develop as alveoli multiply.

The basic subunits of lung anatomy referred to in this chapter are the *acinus, lobule, segment,* and *lobe*. The acinus, considered the basic respiratory unit of the lung, is defined as the terminal bronchiole and its distal branches (respiratory bronchioles, alveolar ducts, and alveolar sacs) with their attached alveoli. Throughout the neonatal and the adult lung there is a complex interdigitation of acini and extensive collateral ventilation between acini through the alveolar pores of Kohn and the bronchiolar canals of Lambert. The lobule is a larger subunit composed of five to ten acini. In certain regions of the lung, lobules, that are located immediately beneath the visceral pleura are bordered by connective tissue (interlobular) septa. The preacinar pulmonary artery and conductive airway run together in the central portion of the lobule, while the larger pulmonary vein branches travel in the periphery within the interlobular septa. The lung lobes are divided into large units, bronchopulmonary segments, each of which is supplied by a separate segmental bronchus. Adjacent intralobar bronchopulmonary segments are normally not separated by septa or fissures, thus allowing for additional collateral air drift within the lung lobes.

### *Early Lung Development—The Embryonic Period*

Lung growth can be considered to occur in four broad periods of time: embryonic (0 to 8 weeks gestation), fetal (9 weeks to term), perinatal, and childhood and adolescence. In the embryonic period, the foregut is established from the endodermal cell layer about the 20th day of gestation.[6] On day 24 the laryngotracheal groove begins to separate the primordial larynx and trachea from the pharynx and esophagus (see Fig 1–2). On day 26, a rounded cellular structure, the lung bud, arises from the anterior foregut near the laryngotracheal groove (Fig 1–4). By day 28 the lung bud has subdivided into right and left lung (bronchial) buds, which will mature into the mainstem bronchi. Subsequently, successive divisions of the bronchial buds give rise to lobar, segmental, and subsegmental airways. While the bronchial buds are dividing, the trachea is formed by concurrent elongation of the cranial portion of the lung bud (see Fig 1–4). The tracheoesophageal septum forms to separate the esophagus from the developing trachea. The elongation of the trachea moves the developing lung into its permanent position within the thorax.

From the onset, the developing lung bud is invested in mesenchyme, which serves to modulate lung development at the subcellular

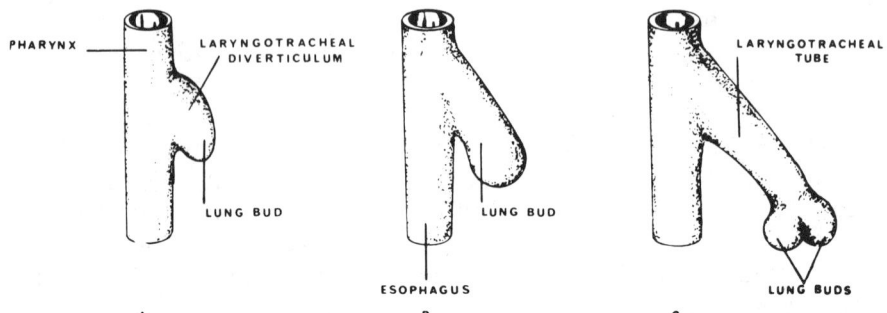

**FIG 1–4.**
Lung bud (laryngotracheal diverticulum). **A,** the beginning of the respiratory tract. **B** and **C,** elongation of the lung bud, with development of buds of the major bronchi.

level. A lung bud that has been experimentally divested of its mesenchyme will not develop normal bronchial branches.[7] The endoderm of the foregut provides the epithelial lining of the lung from the trachea to the alveolar surface; mesenchyme differentiates into the vasculature, pleura, and supportive framework, e.g., muscle, elastin, cartilage, and fibrous tissue.

### *Stages of Intrauterine Lung Growth in the Fetal Period*

In the fetal period, lung development is further characterized by three distinctive morphological stages: *pseudoglandular, canalicular,* and *terminal saccular.* In the pseudoglandular stage (5 to 16 weeks' gestation) the preacinar pattern of airway branching is established. The lung resembles an acinar gland—the airways are hollow, blind-ended tubules—lined by cuboidal epithelium and surrounded by mesenchyme (Fig 1–5). Capillaries are sparse and respiration is not possible.

In the canalicular stage (16 to 24 weeks), a rapid expansion of the vasculature of the lung occurs as capillaries project into the epithelial-lined tubules (Fig 1–6). The tubules themselves develop a more complex branching pattern and become lined by flattened epithelium. There is a marked reduction of the intertubular mesenchymal stroma. Many of the tubules at this stage represent primitive respiratory bronchioles and alveolar ducts, and the acinus is structurally defined. Near the end of this stage, respiration is theoretically possible.

During the terminal saccular ("alveolar") stage of development (24 weeks until term) structures resembling adult alveoli are formed (Fig 1–7). There is further hypertrophy of the capillary bed and reduction in mesenchyme, thus increasing the alveolar respiratory surface. At this stage, saccules become lined by type I and II pneumocytes structurally identical to those seen in the adult. According to Langston et al.,[8]

Development of the Respiratory System    9

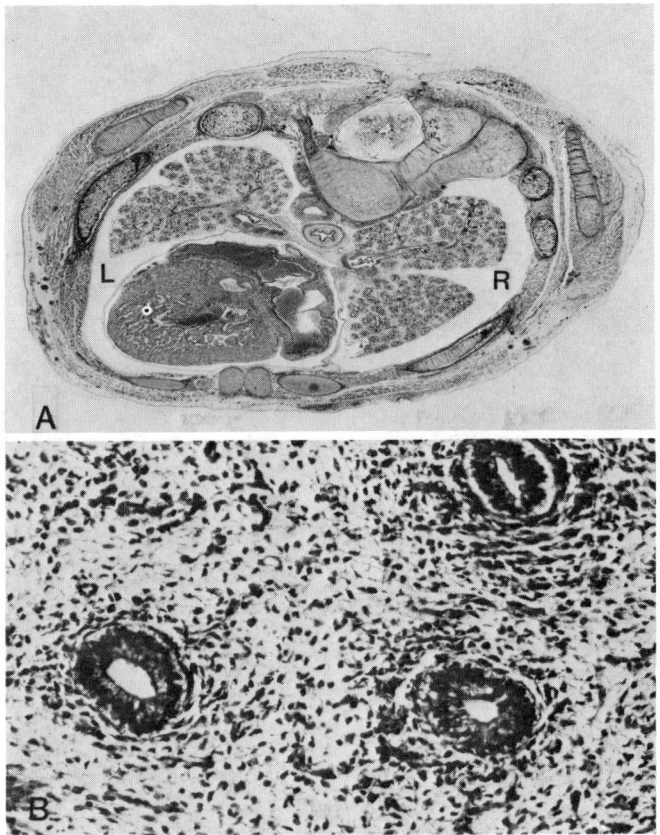

**FIG 1–5.**
Pseudoglandular stage. **A,** cross section of thorax from 10-week fetus. The right *(R)* and left *(L)* lungs are separated by the heart and mediastinal structures. Located dorsal to the heart are the esophagus, aorta, and spinal cord, respectively. The lungs do not fill the pleural spaces (hematoxylin-eosin; total magnification, ×10). **B,** Primitive bronchial tubules are surrounded by mesenchymal cells, which are densest in the peritubular area. Blood vessels are inconspicuous (hematoxylin-eosin, ×230).

definitive alveoli can be identified between 36 weeks' gestation and term.

### Trachea

The lung bud elongates in the caudal direction while beginning to form the trachea. Almost from the onset of elongation, the buds of the major bronchi are present on the most caudal end of the trachea (see Fig 1–4). During this elongation, the endodermal outgrowth forms the epithelial lining of the trachea and its glands. Early in the development

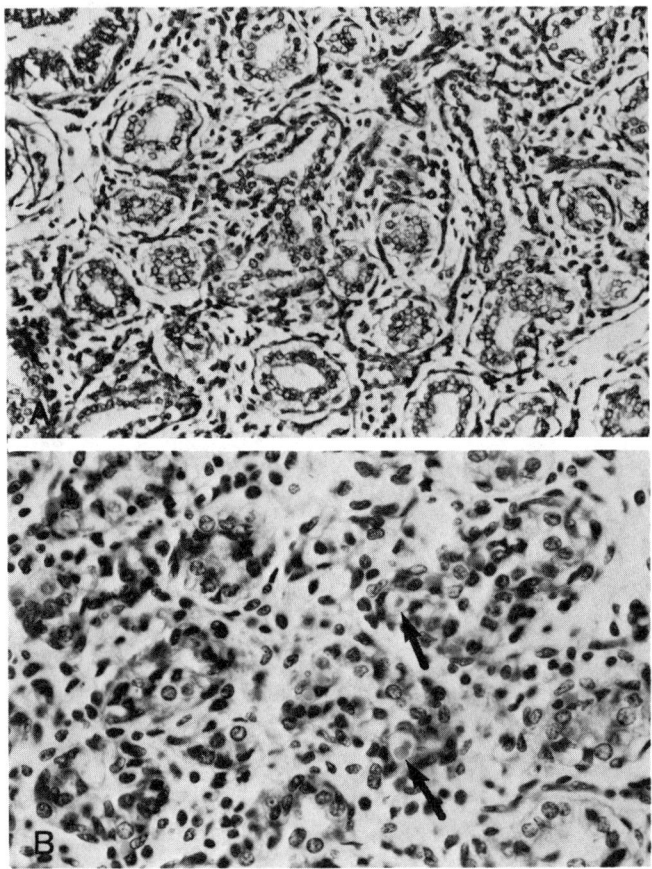

**FIG 1–6.**
Canalicular stage. **A,** lung from 16-week fetus. Respiratory tubules have a complex branching pattern. The mesenchymal stroma is markedly reduced (hematoxylin-eosin, ×230). **B,** lung from 20-week fetus. The glandular epithelium is beginning to flatten. Capillaries containing red blood cells protrude into the epithelial lining *(arrows)* (hematoxylin-eosin, ×474).

of the trachea, the epithelial lining consists of columnar cells that later undergo transformation into pseudostratified columnar epithelial cells. By 10 weeks of gestation, ciliary development has begun in these cells.

Mesenchyme that surrounds the trachea forms the cartilage, connective tissue, muscle, and vascular system. During the fourth week of gestation, the anlage of cartilage appears as cellular aggregates in the tracheal wall. Fully recognizable cartilage, however, is not seen until the seventh week of gestation. From the 10th to the 20th week, most of the glands of the trachea are formed, and by 13 weeks, the mucosal goblet cells are well developed.

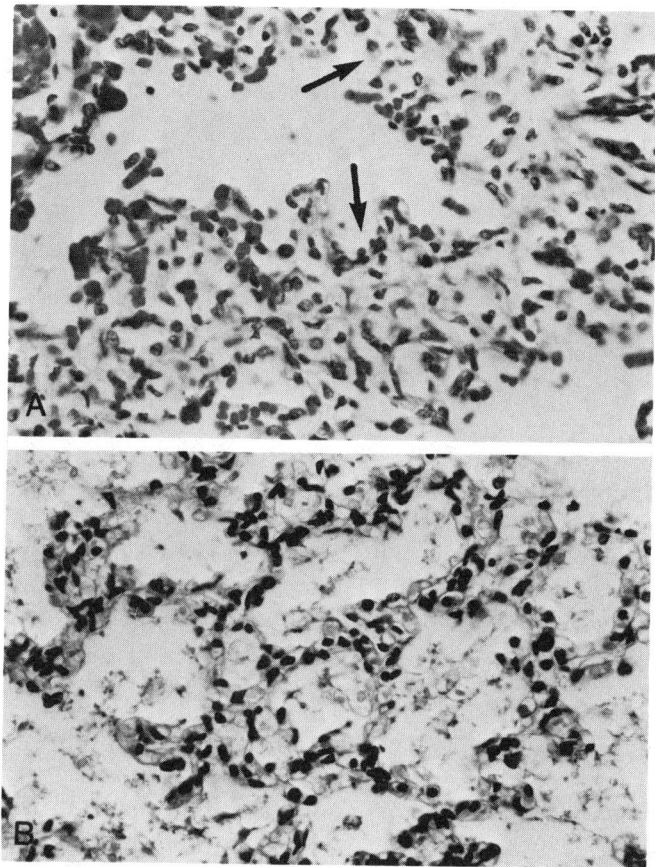

**FIG 1–7.**
Terminal saccular stage. **A,** lung from 27-week fetus. Primitive alveoli *(arrows)* are present as outpouchings from a larger saccule. Numerous capillaries are present (hematoxylin-eosin, ×474). **B,** lung from 33-week fetus. Alveolar septa resemble those of the adult. Alveolar capillaries are dilated and contain nucleated red blood cells. The precipitate within alveolar spaces represents postmortem artifact (hematoxylin-eosin, ×474).

## *Bronchi*

The conducting airways of the lung form a system of branching tubes that progressively narrow toward the periphery. Within each pulmonary segment, the number of preacinar airway branches varies from 15 to 25.[9] The proximal airways contain cartilage, while the distal branches are morphologically classified as bronchioles and have no mural cartilage. Preacinar bronchioles, as well as the terminal bronchiole, are circumferentially lined by respiratory epithelium, while the intra-acinar respiratory bronchioles in the adult have an incomplete

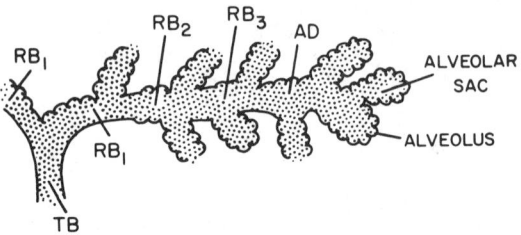

**FIG 1–8.**
Respiratory section of lung (acinus) demonstrating the terminal bronchiole *(TB)* giving rise to three orders of respiratory bronchioles *(RB)*, the alveolar ducts *(AD)*, alveolar sacs and alveoli in early alveolar stage. (From Lough MD, Doershuk CF, and Stern RC (eds): *Pediatric Respiratory Therapy*. Chicago, Year Book Medical Publishers, 1974. Used by permission.)

epithelium interrupted by alveolar outpouchings. Within the acinus are roughly three generations of respiratory bronchioles from which branch alveolar ducts, which are air channels completely lined by alveoli (Fig 1–8).

In the developing lung, lobar bronchi are present at 5 weeks, and by 16 weeks, all preacinar branching is complete. Between the 10th and 14th weeks a bronchial growth spurt occurs during which most of the conductive airways are formed (Fig 1–9). Beyond 16 weeks, the intra-acinar airways continue to develop, and during this latter period, there may be a slight reduction in preacinar airway number as one or two branches become alveolarized and incorporated into the acinus.

**Mucous Glands.**—Mucous glands are first observed in the bronchial wall at 13 weeks' gestation. Glands originate as solid cellular buds extending beneath the bronchial basement membrane. The cellular bud is converted to a hollow tubule that ultimately gives rise to a cohesive nest of mucous glands (acinus) that communicates with the bronchial lumen by an epithelial-lined duct (Fig 1–10). Glands are composed entirely of mucous cells until the 26th week when serous cells appear in the proximal airways. All glands are formed by term. During the first year of postnatal life, there is a reduction in the density of glands due to the relatively slower growth of glands compared to growth of the bronchial wall. The biochemical composition of mucus also undergoes a rapid transition in the newborn period from a highly sulfated fetal mucin to a mucin low in sulfate but rich in sialic acid.[10]

**Epithelium.**—The tubules of the pseudoglandular stage are lined by ciliated and nonciliated cells that contain abundant cytoplasmic glycogen, the main source of energy in the developing lung.[11] Both ciliated and mucus-secreting cells line the primitive bronchi by 13

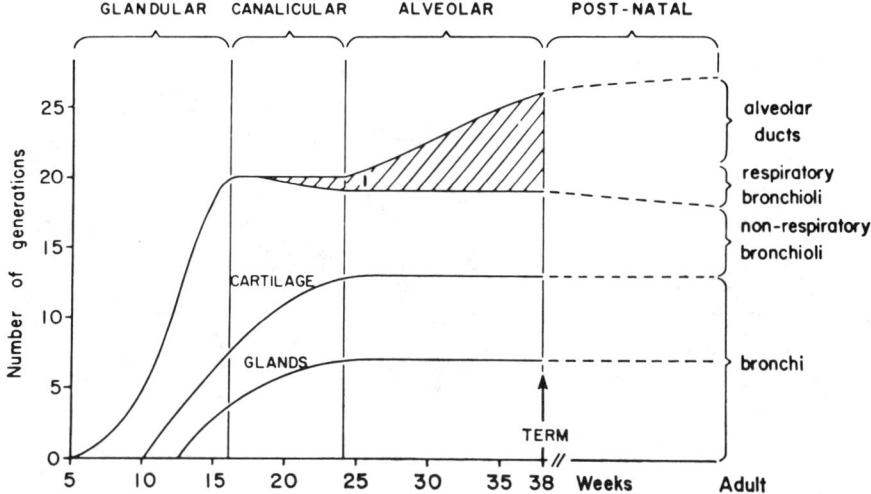

**FIG 1-9.**
Diagrammatic representation of the development of the bronchial tree. Lobar bronchi appear at the fifth week of gestation and by 16 weeks all nonrespiratory airways are present. Most respiratory airways appear between 16 weeks and birth; some appear in infancy. Cartilage and glands appear later and their extension is complete by 24 weeks' gestation. (From Hislop A, Reid L: Growth of the respiratory system, in Davis JA, Dobbing J (eds): *Scientific Foundations of Paediatrics,* ed 2. London, Heinemann Medical Books, Ltd, 1981. Used by permission.)

weeks' gestation, although ciliated cells are not found in the terminal bronchioles until near term. Goblet cells do not extend as far as the last plate of cartilage during fetal life. Mucus secreted by the surface epithelium is a relatively minor component of the total quantity of bronchial mucus, most of which is secreted by the bronchial glands.

**Cartilage, Smooth Muscle, Connective Tissue.**—Cartilage, muscle, and connective tissue, as well as the bronchial glands, form first in the proximal airways and extend peripherally in a centrifugal fashion. Mural cartilage appears around the tenth week of intrauterine life. Cartilaginous plates extend to their adult levels by the 25th week, although further maturation of cartilage occurs even after birth.

From the seventh week, smooth muscle cells, derived from the mesenchyme, appear in the bronchi and bronchioles. By 12 weeks' gestation, the smooth muscle aids in the support of the posterior wall of the larger proximal bronchi.

Mature collagen, the main connective tissue protein in the respiratory tract, is present histologically as fibrous tissue bundles by the 12th week. Collagen is considered to be an important protein in the subcellular regulation of bronchial development.[12]

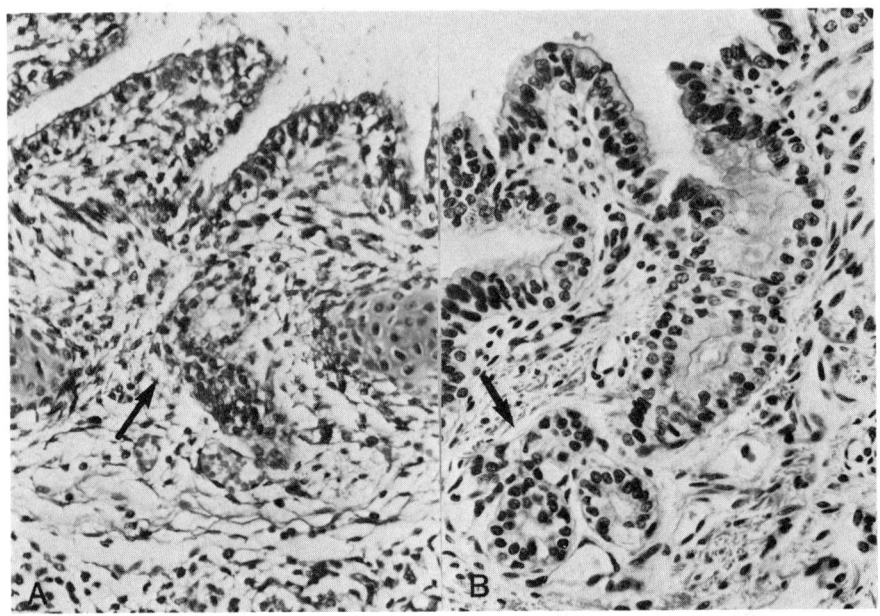

**FIG 1–10.**
Bronchial gland development. **A,** 16-week fetus. A tubule *(arrow)* extends deep to the bronchial mucosa between two plates of immature cartilage (hematoxylin-eosin, ×290). **B,** 20-week fetus. A duct extending from the bronchial mucosa terminates in a nest of coiled tubules *(arrows)* that represents the primitive glandular acinus. The bronchial mucosa is composed predominantly of ciliated cells (hematoxylin-eosin, ×370).

### *Alveoli*

In the canalicular stage, alveolar differentiation is heralded by a proliferation of capillaries and accompanied by a reduction of mesenchyme and thinning of epithelium overlying the capillary sprouts. The biochemical signal for capillary proliferation during this period is unknown. Two types of endodermally derived epithelial cells line the alveolar membrane of the infant and adult. Most of the respiratory surface is covered by type I cells with their flat expanse of cytoplasm readily penetrable by oxygen and carbon dioxide. Type II cells, the source of surfactant, also first appear in the canalicular period as cuboidal cells with surface microvilli, complex cytoplasmic organelles, a relatively decreased glycogen content, and osmiophilic lamellar bodies thought to represent surfactant. It is presumed that type I cells are derived from a primitive undifferentiated stem cell. In the developing lung of some animal species, and in the human lung following injury, type II cells have also been shown to differentiate into type I cells.

In the terminal saccular stage of development, alveolar epithelium is morphologically identical to that seen in the adult. While collagen

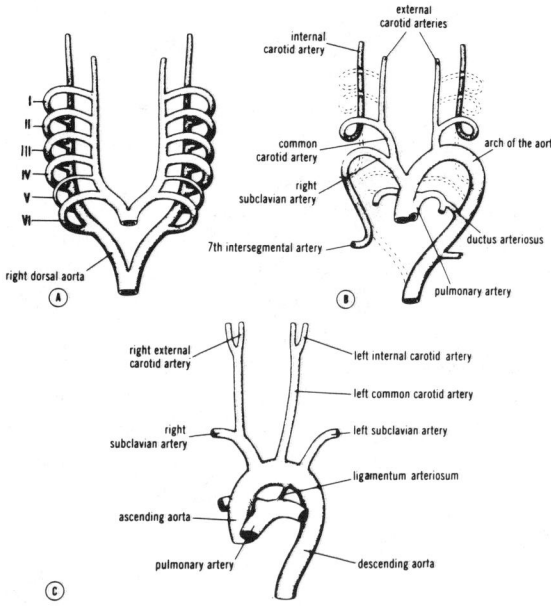

**FIG 1-11.**
**A,** diagram of the aortic arches and dorsal aortas before transformation into the definitive vascular pattern. **B,** diagram of the dorsal aortas after the transformation. The obliterated components are indicated by broken lines. Note the position of the ductus arteriosus. **C,** the great arteries in the adult. (From Langman J, *Medical Embryology,* ed 3. Baltimore, Williams & Wilkins Co, 1975. Used by permission.)

modulates the development of bronchi, it is the structural protein elastin that assumes prime importance in directing the formation of alveoli.[13] At 26 to 32 weeks' gestation, small crests with dense elastin fibers at their tips form shallow depressions in the walls of terminal saccules. As the crests lengthen, alveolus-like structures are formed. The number of so-called alveoli present at birth[14, 15] ranges from $24 \times 10^6$ to $71 \times 10^6$, compared to approximately $600 \times 10^6$ alveoli in the adult.[15]

### Blood Vessels

**Embryonic Period.**—In the embryonic period, the developing circulatory system consists of six pairs of aortic arches that join the dorsal and ventral aortas that arise from the primitive heart (Fig 1–11). The right and left pulmonary arteries are derived from the sixth aortic arch, which is formed by the 36th day of development. The dorsolateral portion of the right sixth aortic arch ultimately disappears; the ventral part persists as the proximal right pulmonary artery. The dorsal portion of the left sixth arch persists as the ductus arteriosus joining the pulmonary artery and aorta, while the ventral left sixth aortic arch becomes the proximal portion of the left main pulmonary artery. The right and left pulmonary arteries, by day 50, have joined the vascular plexus that surrounds the lung buds. The pulmonary trunk is formed as the aorticopulmonary septum divides the truncus arteriosus into two major channels, aorta and pulmonary artery.

A single main pulmonary vein initially arises from the cardiac atrium and is connected with the venous plexus around the esophagus and developing lungs. As the left atrium enlarges, it absorbs the main and then the right and left branches to just beyond the entry of their main tributaries. Ultimately, four separate venous openings are found in the dorsal wall of the left atrium. Even in the adult, small connections persist between the pulmonary and esophageal veins near the lung hilum. During fetal life, the pulmonary veins carry little blood and are largely free of muscle. A continuous smooth muscle coat is only present near term.

**Anatomy of Intrapulmonary Arteries.**—Branches of the pulmonary artery can be classified into two types based on their location within the lung.[16] *Conventional arteries* are those which branch with their accompanying airway. *Supernumerary arteries* are not associated with an airway branch but extend directly into the lung parenchyma and capillary bed from the vascular axial pathway. The proportion of supernumerary to conventional arteries increases in the periphery of the lung, and overall, supernumerary branches comprise 20% to 45% of the arterial cross-sectional area of the side branches. Supernumerary arteries develop definitively in utero and are present in the same proportion to conventional arteries in the fetus as in the adult.

In the child and adult, the histologic structure of a pulmonary artery branch varies with its diameter. Elastic arteries persist to a diameter of approximately 3,000 µm at which point there is a transition to a muscular artery that possesses only an internal and external elastic lamina separated by a concentric smooth muscle coat. Muscular arteries comprise the majority of arteries to a diameter of about 150 µm. Here the muscle coat gives rise to a spiral of muscle that finally disappears completely. In the region of the muscular spiral, arteries are said to be "partially muscular." All arteries less than 35 µm in diameter are nonmuscular[16] (Fig 1–12).

In the fetus, thin wisps of elastin are first observed in arteries at 12 weeks' gestation. The staining intensity of arterial elastin increases throughout fetal life. The main pulmonary artery of the fetus is structurally similar to the aorta, with concentric rings of continuous elastin fibers within its wall. Conversion to the adult pattern of interrupted

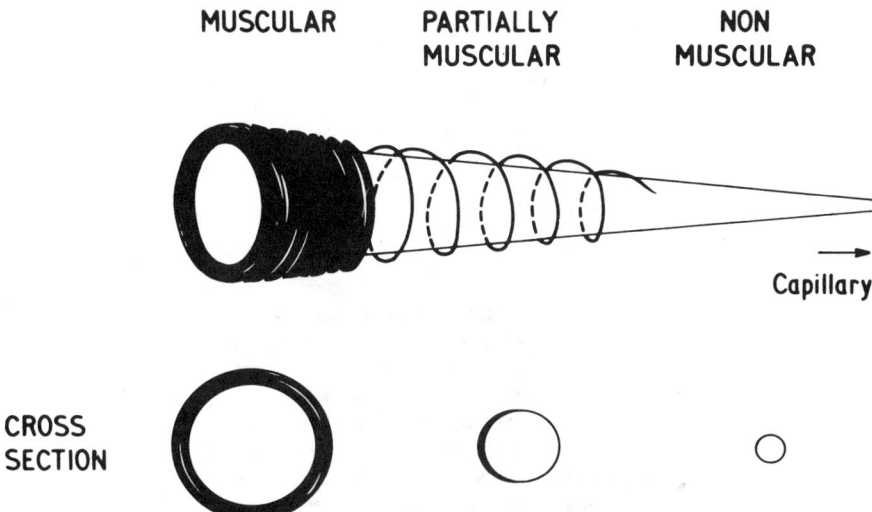

**FIG 1–12.**
Diagram representing the structure of a pulmonary artery at its distal end. The complete muscle coat gives way to a spiral of muscle before it completely disappears leaving a "nonmuscular artery." In cross sections, vessels within the spiral region have a crescent of muscle and are termed "partially muscular." (From Hislop A, Reid L: Growth of the respiratory system, in Davis JA, Dobbing J (eds): *Scientific Foundations of Paediatrics,* ed 2. London, Heinemann Medical Books, Ltd, 1981. Used by permission.)

elastin fibers takes place in the pulmonary artery only after birth, except in conditions where pulmonary hypertension is present from birth, in which case the aortic pattern of elastin is maintained even into adulthood.[17] Elastic arteries are present up to the seventh bronchial generation by 19 weeks' gestation, and this level is maintained in the adult.

The external diameter of the muscular and partially muscular pulmonary arteries is about the same in the fetus as in the adult; however, the transition from a muscular to a nonmuscular vessel occurs at the level of the terminal bronchiole in the fetus vs. the alveolar wall in the adult[18] (Fig 1–13). In fetal muscular arteries, muscle thickness is greater relative to the arterial external diameter than in the adult. In the first 2 weeks of extrauterine life, there is a sudden drop in muscular wall thickness followed by a more gradual reduction over the next 18 months. Abnormal extension of smooth muscle into normally nonmuscularized vessels is an anatomical hallmark of pulmonary hypertension.[19] In certain neonatal conditions such as persistent fetal circulation and meconium aspiration syndrome, abnormal extension of muscle apparently occurs in utero, probably in response to an as yet unidentified stress or insult.[20]

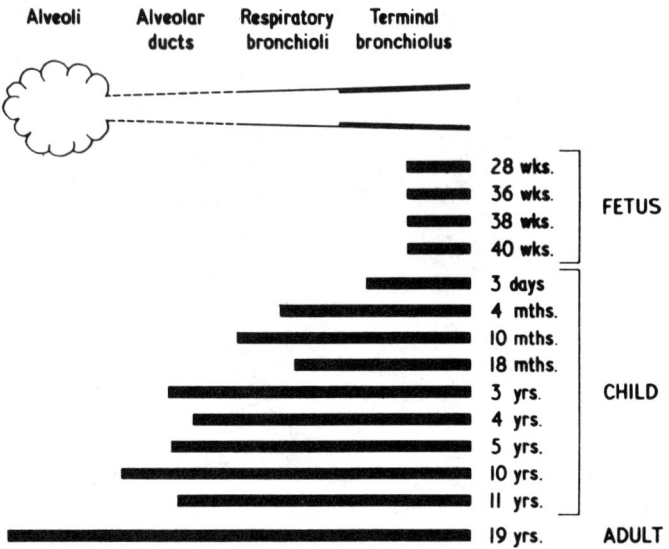

**FIG 1–13.**
The distance or "extension" within the acinus of muscular arteries. In the fetus, muscular arteries are not found with the respiratory bronchiole or beyond. During childhood, they extend further until, in the adult, they reach the pleural level. The acinus is the respiratory unit supplied by a terminal bronchiole. (From Hislop A, Reid L: Growth of the respiratory system, in Davis JA, Dobbing J (eds): *Scientific Foundations of Paediatrics,* ed 2. London, Heinemann Medical Books, Ltd, 1981. Used by permission.)

**Bronchial Arteries.**—During the embryonic period, transient feeding vessels extend directly from the dorsal aorta to the developing lung buds. Persistence of these vascular sprouts may result in aberrant systemic blood supply to the lung. Definitive bronchial arteries, which nourish the bronchi, pleura, and walls of vessels, arise from the aorta in the 9th to 12th week of gestation.[21] In the normal fetus, patent precapillary anastomoses between bronchial and pulmonary circulations are infrequently observed. There is, however, free communication between the two circulations at the capillary level, and both systems drain into the pulmonary veins.[5] Drainage from the bronchial arteries thus contributes to the normal anatomical shunt of the lung. In conditions where there is either obstruction of pulmonary arterial flow or intrinsic lung disease, blood flow through the bronchial circulation increases, and collateral channels develop between the bronchial and pulmonary circuits.

### Pleural Cavities and Diaphragm

The pleural cavities originate as two lateral tubes, the *pericardioperitoneal canals,* connecting the primitive pericardial and peritoneal

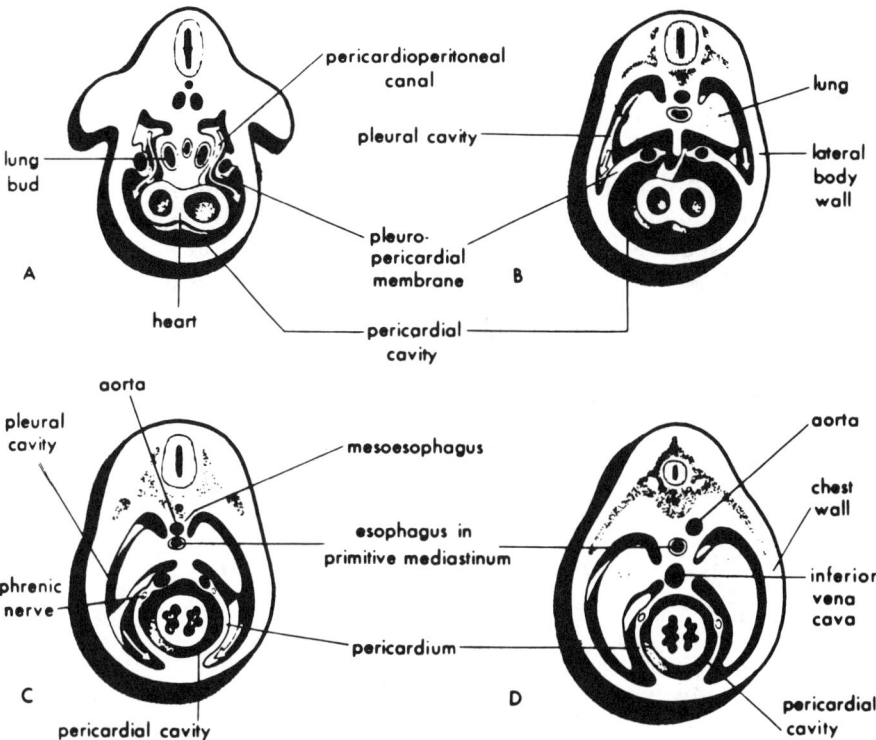

**FIG 1–14.**
Drawings of transverse sections through an embryo illustrating successive stages in the separation of the pleural cavities from the pericardial cavity. Also shown are the growth and development of the lungs and the expansion of the pleural cavities. **A**, the communications between the pericardial cavity and the pericardioperitoneal canals are indicated by the arrows in a 5-week embryo. **B**, at 6 weeks, the arrows show the development of the pleural cavities as extensions of the pericardioperitoneal canals and the expansion of the pleural cavities into the body wall. **C**, at 7 weeks, the pleuropericardial membranes are fused in the midline and the pleural cavities have expanded ventrally around the heart. **D** illustrates the continued expansion of the lungs and pleural cavities and the formation of the chest wall in an 8-week embryo. (From Moore KL: *The Developing Human,* ed 2. Philadelphia, WB Saunders Co, 1977. Used by permission.)

cavities (Fig 1–14). The pericardial cavity is bordered caudally by the *septum transversum*. By the fourth week, the lung buds, lined by splanchnic mesoderm, bulge into the pericardioperitoneal canals. As the lung buds grow, the primitive pleural cavity enlarges by extending into the chest wall. During development of the lung buds, the descent of the heart causes the lateral margins of the septum transversum to be raised as folds, the *pleuropericardial membrane*, which encloses the heart as the pericardial sac, thus separating the pericardial from the pleural cavities.

The communication between the primitive pleural and peritoneal cavities is closed by the ingrowth of a ridge of mesodermal tissue, the *pleuroperitoneal membrane*, which projects from the chest wall into the dorsolateral caudal portion of the pleural space. Eventually this membrane fuses medially with the mesenchyme anterior to the esophagus, thus completing the paired lateral leaves of the primitive diaphragm. The anterior, central portion of the diaphragm to which the pleuroperitoneal membrane fuses is termed the central tendon and is derived from the septum transversum. Failure of fusion results in congenital diaphragmatic hernia and entry of abdominal contents into the pleural space. Innervation of the diaphragm is via the phrenic nerve, which is derived from the anterior rami of the third, fourth, and fifth cervical nerves. Skeletal muscle migrates into the primitive diaphragm at an early stage. During fetal life, there is progressive caudal migration of the diaphragm.

## CIRCULATION—FETAL AND TRANSITIONAL

### The Placenta

The placenta serves two main functions: (1) exchange of gases and metabolites between the maternal and fetal circulation and (2) production of hormones to maintain pregnancy. Development of the placenta begins shortly after implantation of the zygote in the uterine wall. By the fourth week, lacunar spaces and villi have developed, and fetal blood flow through the villi is possible. Maternal uterine spiral arteries open into the intervillous spaces, while fetal arteries enter the placenta at the chorionic plate and undergo extensive branching to provide a large surface area for diffusion of oxygen and metabolites between the maternal and fetal blood. Figure 1–15 illustrates the structure of the placenta.

In the fetal placental circulation, deoxygenated blood enters the placenta through two umbilical arteries within the umbilical cord. The umbilical arteries divide into radial branches within the chorionic plate. These branches subsequently enter the chorionic villi where they establish an extensive capillary plexus, bringing fetal and maternal blood into very close proximity. Ordinarily there is no direct mixing of the two circulations. Oxygenated fetal blood passes into veins that converge to form the umbilical vein, which reenters the fetus.

In the maternal side of the placental circulation, oxygenated blood enters the intervillous space through the endometrial spiral arterioles (see Fig 1–15). The flow from these vessels is pulsatile and propelled at systemic arterial pressure toward the chorionic plate of the intervil-

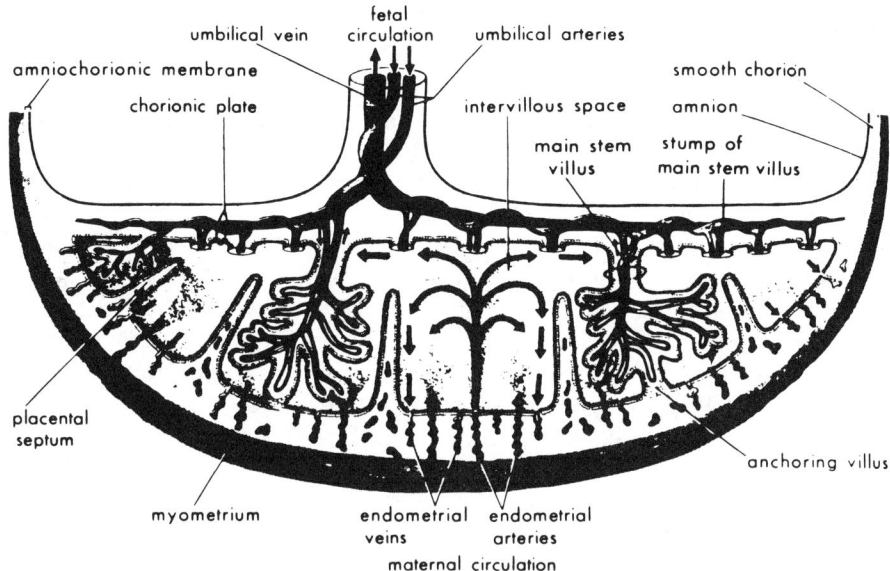

**FIG 1–15.**
Placental blood flow. Fetal blood enters the placenta through arteries, circulates in the villi and returns to the fetus via the vein. (From Moore KL: *The Developing Human,* ed 2. Philadelphia, WB Saunders Co, 1977. Used by permission.)

lous space. As the pressure subsides, blood flows over the surface of the villi where gas exchange between mother and fetus takes place. Maternal blood then flows toward the decidual plate, enters the endometrial veins, and returns to the maternal heart.

Oxygen and carbon dioxide move between the two circulations by simple diffusion. Gas diffusion is affected by both maternal and fetal blood pressure and by the rate of blood flow. The higher oxygen tension of the maternal side results in oxygen diffusion into fetal blood. Fetal blood has a higher affinity for oxygen and thus carries more oxygen at a given oxygen tension than does maternal blood. Carbon dioxide diffuses from fetal to maternal blood. Regulation of acid-base balance in the fetus is dependent on diffusion of carbon dioxide; the fetal kidneys have little role in acid-base regulation. Besides its function as an organ of gas exchange, the placenta, through various transport mechanisms, which include facilitated diffusion, active transport, and pinocytosis, supplies nutrients and allows electrolytes to pass freely to the fetus.

## Fetal Circulation

Early development of a functional circulatory system is paramount to the establishment of a means of nutritional support and waste disposal for the rapidly enlarging fetus. The heart is formed by the fusion of two endocardial tubes about the 21st day of gestation. Within the primitive pericardial sac, the heart takes a sigmoid form (bulboventricular loop) around the 25th day of gestation (Fig 1–16). By the eighth week of gestation, the four chambers are complete except for a patent interatrial foramen ovale. During fetal life, the right ventricle approaches the weight of the left, and the ratio of right ventricular muscle mass to left ventricular plus septal mass is much greater than in the adult.[22] In the fetus, the right ventricle pumps two thirds of the combined ventricular output at systemic pressure, which is equivalent to the pressure in the left ventricle (65 to 70 mm Hg, systolic).[23]

The placenta is the fetal organ of respiration—only 10% to 15% of the right ventricular output passes through the lungs. Oxygenated blood returning from the placenta via the umbilical vein enters the ductus venosus near the fetal liver. The majority of blood flow passes from the ductus venosus into the inferior vena cava. A variable portion of blood flows from the ductus directly into the hepatic sinusoids where it mixes with blood from the hepatic portal system. The amount of blood entering the liver parenchyma is regulated by a sphincter mechanism in the ductus venosus. Flow from the inferior vena cava is directed by the valve of the inferior vena cava into the right atrium and preferentially through the patent foramen ovale to the left atrium. Only a small amount of oxygenated blood enters the right ventricle. The blood in the left ventricle is pumped into the ascending aorta and immediately supplies the heart and brain via the coronary and carotid arteries, respectively. In this manner, these two vital organs receive the most highly oxygenated blood.

Desaturated blood returning to the heart from the superior vena cava is channeled into the right atrium and ventricle and exits the heart through the pulmonary trunk. Because of the high pulmonary vascular resistance, however, most of the right ventricular outflow is diverted into the descending aorta through the ductus arteriosus. The desaturated stream from the right heart then mixes with the oxygenated blood from the left. About 60% of the blood flow in the descending aorta is redirected to the placenta, the remainder goes to the abdomen and lower extremities and returns to the heart through the inferior vena cava. A schematic representation of the fetal circulation is seen in Figure 1–17.

The oxygen tension of fetal blood is significantly lower than in the adult. According to Rudolph,[23] oxygenated umbilical venous blood has a $Po_2$ of 30 to 35 mm Hg. Umbilical venous blood is admixed with desaturated blood from the distal inferior vena cava and, in the left ventricle, is also mixed with a small amount of venous return from the

Development of the Respiratory System    23

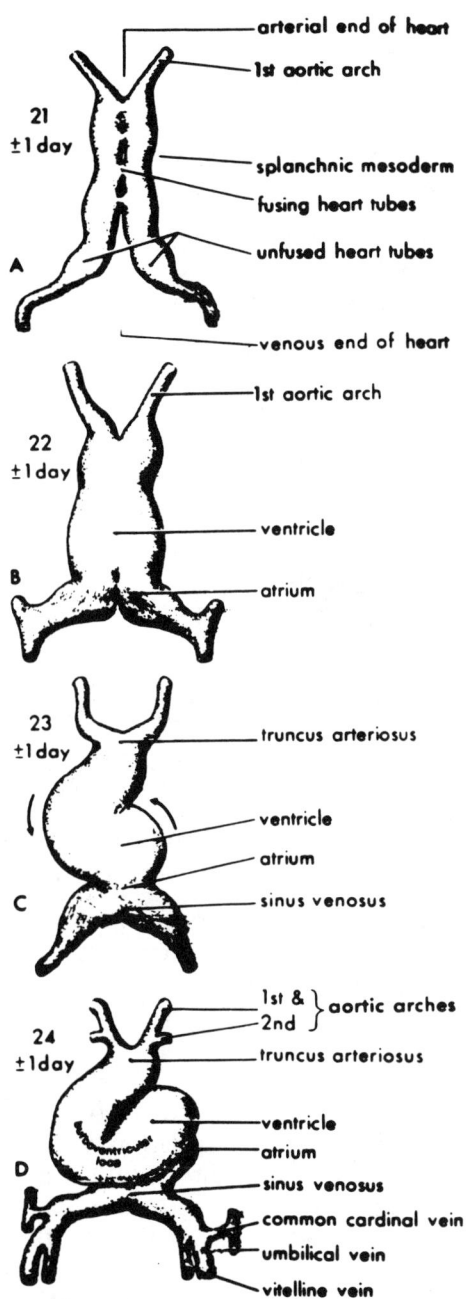

**FIG 1-16.**
Development of the fetal heart schematically demonstrated. Refer to text for description. (From Moore, KL: *The Developing Human*, ed 2. Philadelphia, WB Saunders Co, 1977. Used by permission.)

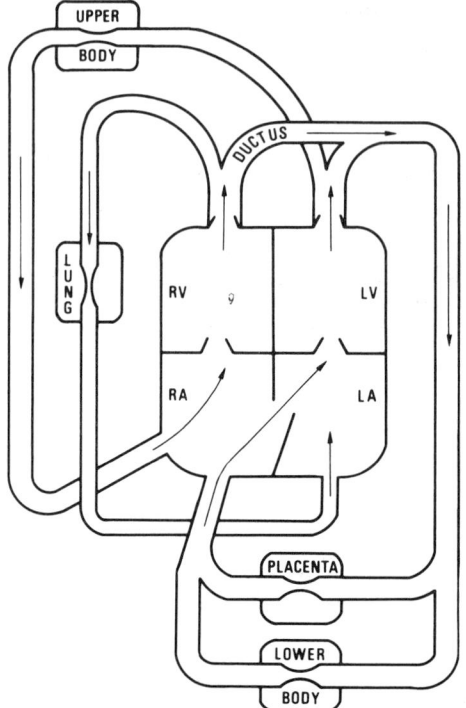

**FIG 1–17.**
Fetal circulation. *RV* = right ventricle; *LV* = left ventricle; *LA* = left atrium; *RA* = right atrium; the foramen ovale between RA and LA; ductus arteriosus shunts blood from high-resistance lung vessels. (From Lough MD, Doershuk CF, Stern RC (eds): *Pediatric Respiratory Therapy,* ed 3. Chicago, Year Book Medical Publishers, 1985. Used by permission.)

lungs, such that blood in the left ventricle has a $Po_2$ of 23 to 25 mm Hg. The right ventricular output, on the other hand, has a $Po_2$ of only 18 to 19 mm Hg.

## Transitional and Neonatal Circulations

At the time of birth there is a dramatic readjustment of the fetal circulation caused by two important events: (1) cessation of the placental circulation and (2) the first breath. When the umbilical cord is clamped, there is a marked reduction in venous return to the right heart. Eventually, anatomical closure of the ductus venosus by fibrous tissue forms the ligamentum venosum, while the obliterated umbilical vein ultimately becomes the ligamentum teres. Decreased systemic venous return results in a slight reduction of right atrial pressure. With the first breath, alveoli are expanded as the lungs fill with air. Shortly thereafter there is a marked increase in arterial oxygen saturation as oxygen diffuses into the pulmonary capillaries. In response to increased oxygen tension, the pulmonary vasculature dilates resulting in decreased pulmonary vascular resistance, increased pulmonary blood flow, and further reduction in right heart pressure. Within the first 15 minutes of extrauterine life, the increased oxygen tension also causes vasoconstriction and functional closure of the ductus arteriosus (bradykinin may act as a mediator of ductal closure). Incomplete closure of the ductus frequently results in a small left to right shunt for several weeks after birth, while total fibrous obliteration of the ductus to form the ligamentum arteriosum is achieved in 1 to 3 months. Postnatal hypoxia, however, will preserve patency of the ductus arteriosus and maintain the left to right anatomical shunt.

Complete separation of the right- and left-sided circulations is achieved by closure of the foramen ovale. Left atrial pressure becomes elevated above that on the right due to increased pulmonary venous return, as well as increased peripheral vascular resistance with secondary increase in left ventricular systolic and diastolic pressure. The unequal pressure gradient closes the flap valve covering the foramen ovale. A small left to right shunt may continue for several weeks due to incomplete closure of the foramen. Probe patency of the foramen ovale may even persist into adulthood in up to 20% of individuals. Diagrams of the transitional and adult type circulatory systems are depicted in Figures 1–18 and 1–19.

## FETAL BIOCHEMISTRY AND PHYSIOLOGY

### Surfactant and Biochemical Aspects of Lung Development

Avery and Mead[24] demonstrated a high surface tension in the lung extract of premature infants and a lower surface tension in that of larger, more mature infants. Absence of the surface active agent, surfactant, is the main contributing factor to the development of respiratory insufficiency in premature infants with respiratory distress syndrome (RDS). Surfactant has been extensively investigated since its role in RDS was first hypothesized. Adsorption of surfactant to the alveolar-air interface lowers surface tension in alveoli (to less than 10 dynes/cm) and reduces inspiratory effort by preventing complete collapse of alveoli at end expiration, thereby promoting alveolar stability.[25] In different species, between 80% to 90% of gestation must be completed before mature surfactant is synthesized.[26, 27] This event occurs at about 35 weeks in the human fetus.

Before surfactant is synthesized by type II pneumocytes in the fetal

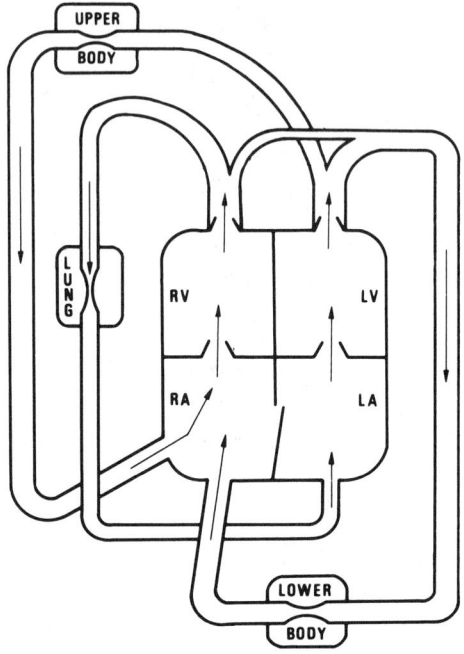

**FIG 1–18.**
Transitional circulation at birth. The ductus arteriosus begins to close. The foramen ovale closes from rising left atrial pressure. (From Lough MD, Doershuk CF, Stern RC (eds): *Pediatric Respiratory Therapy,* ed 3. Chicago, Year Book Medical Publishers, 1985. Used by permission.)

lung, these cells contain abundant intracytoplasmic glycogen. A precipitous drop in lung glycogen concentration occurs at the time of mature surfactant synthesis. Triacylglycerol, lactate, and choline in the fetal serum are used in the synthesis of surfactant.[27]

Lipids comprise approximately 90% of the dry weight of surfactant.[26] The relative proportion of lipids in surfactant is illustrated in Figure 1–20. Glycerophospholipids constitute the largest fraction of the lipids in surfactant. The most abundant glycerophospholipid, 1,2-dipalmitoyl-sn-glycero-3-phosphatidylcholine (DPPC or lecithin), is also the most surface active component. Other glycerophospholipids have varying degrees of surface activity. Immature lung surfactant has a higher percentage of phosphatidylinositol (PI), which contains desaturated fatty acids and has weak surface-active properties. In mature lung surfactant, PI is replaced by phosphatidylglycerol (PG), which is composed of saturated fatty acids and has a greater surface active potential.

Ten percent of surfactant is protein, half of which is apoprotein (molecular weight 35,000 to 40,000). Jobe[28] first detected apoprotein of surfactant in the human fetus of 30 to 32 weeks' gestational age. The

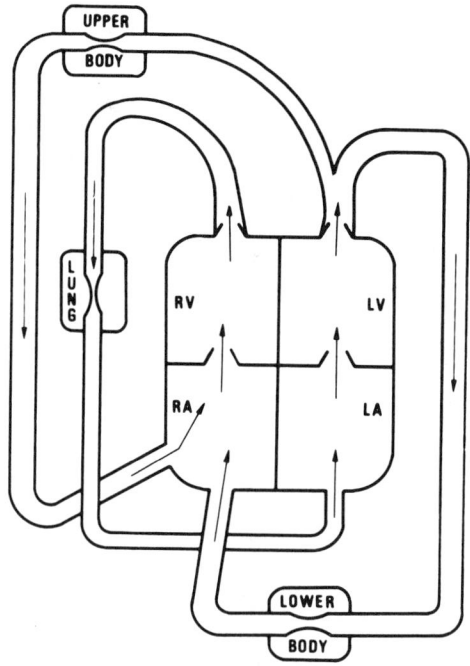

**FIG 1–19.**
Adult circulation after the ductus arteriosus closes functionally. The foramen ovale functionally closes immediately after the first breath, with a drop in pulmonary resistance. (From Lough MD, Doershuk CF, Stern RC (eds):*Pediatric Respiratory Therapy,* ed 3. Chicago, Year Book Medical Publishers, 1985. Used by permission.)

concentration of apoproteins parallels that of phospholipids and increases to a maximum at 37 weeks' gestation. The time at which apoproteins are initially synthesized is variable among fetuses. Apoproteins may aid in adsorption and spreading of surfactant along the alveolar surface.

Probable sites of synthesis of different components of surfactant in the type II pneumocyte are listed in Table 1–3. The major surface-active components of surfactant are DPPC, PG, and to a lesser extent PI. Surfactant glycerophospholipids are synthesized in the cytidine diphosphate (CDP)-choline pathway (Fig 1–21) and are dependent on the biosynthesis of phosphatidic acid that occurs late in gestation. Phosphatidic acid biosynthesis is regulated by cytidine triphosphate (CTP), cytidyltransferase and phophatidate phosphohydrolase (PAPase) in the adult.[26] Cytidine monophosphate (CMP) increases in concentration throughout gestation and may play an important role in the CDP-choline pathway by decreasing the concentration of PI and increasing the synthesis of PG.

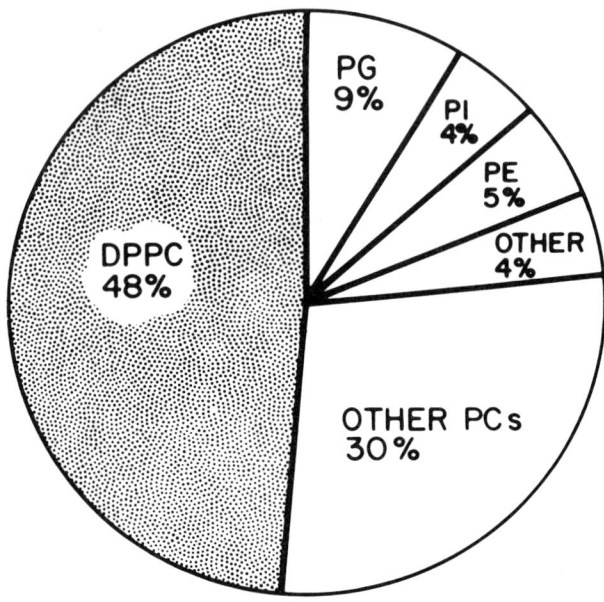

**FIG 1–20.**
The glycerophospholipid composition of a typical mammalian lung surfactant. PC = phosphatidylcholine; DPPC = dipalmitoylphosphatidylcholine (1,2-dipalmitoyl-sn-glycero-3-phosphatidylcholine); PG = phosphatidylglycerol; PI = phosphatidylinositol; PE = phosphatidylethanolamine. (From Bleasdale JE, Johnston JM: Developmental biochemistry of lung surfactant, in Nelson GH (ed): *Pulmonary Development: Transition from Intrauterine to Extrauterine Life.* New York, Marcel Dekker, Inc, 1985, pp 47–74. Used by permission.)

Myoinositol normally decreases in the fetal serum with increasing gestational age.[29] The mildly diabetic mother, however, is myoinositol intolerant. Maternal urinary myoinositol excretion increases and intracellular uptake is decreased in the diabetic mother resulting in increased concentrations of maternal and fetal serum myoinositol, which

**TABLE 1–3.**
Sites of Synthesis of Surfactant Components*

| Organelle | Surfactant Component |
|---|---|
| Rough endoplasmic reticulum | Apoprotein |
| Smooth endoplasmic reticulum | Most glycerophospholipids |
| Golgi apparatus | Glycosylation and processing of apoprotein |
| Lysosomes | Acid hydrolase-stored secreted surfactant |
| Mitochondria | ? Phosphatidylglycerol |
| Vesicles | ? Transport of surfactant |

*From Bleasdale JE, Johnston JM: Developmental biochemistry of lung surfactant, in Nelson GH (ed): Pulmonary Development: Transition From Intrauterine to Extrauterine Life. New York, Marcel Dekker Inc, 1986, pp 47–74. Used by permission.

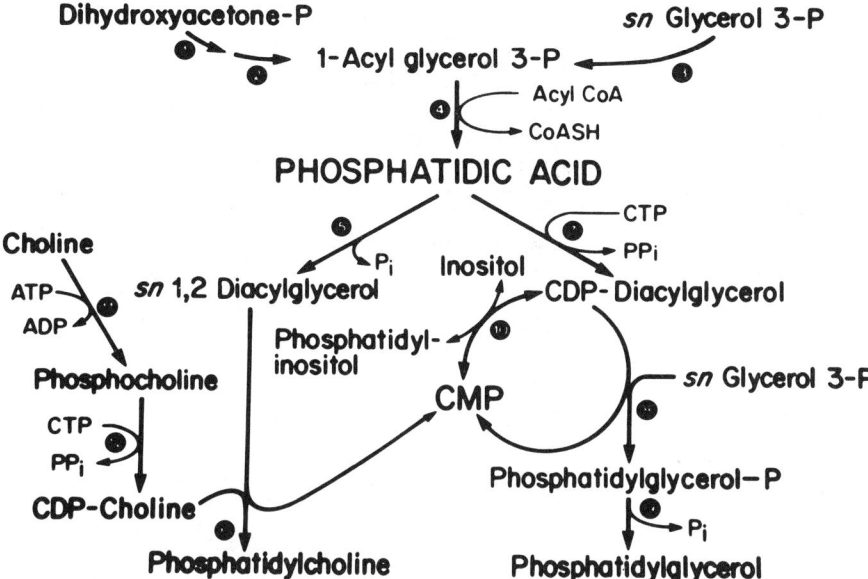

**FIG 1–21.**
Integration of the biosynthesis of phosphatidylcholine, phosphatidylinositol, and phosphatidylglycerol for lung surfactant. The enzymes that catalyze the individual reactions are (1) dihydroxyacetone phosphate acyltransferase; (2) 1-acyl dihydroxyacetone phosphate reductase; (3) glycerol 3-phosphate acyltransferase; (4) 1-acyl glycerol 3-phosphate acyltransferase; (5) phosphatidate phosphohydrolase (PAPase); (6) choline phosphotransferase; (7) CTP:phosphatidate cytidylyltransferase; (8) CDP-diacylglycerol:glycerol 3-phosphate phosphatidyltransferase; (9) phosphatidylglycerol phosphatase; (10) CDP-diacylglycerol:inositol phosphatidyltransferase; (11) choline kinase; and (12) CTP:phosphocholine cytidylyltransferase. (From Bleasdale JE, Johnston JM: Developmental biochemistry of lung surfactant, in Nelson GE (ed): *Pulmonary Development: Transition from Intrauterine to Extrauterine Life.* New York, Marcel Dekker, Inc, 1985, pp 47–74. Used by permission.)

delay synthesis of PG by promoting PI synthesis.[30] As a result, surfactant in infants of diabetic mothers is not mature relative to gestational age, and these infants are prone to develop RDS.

Hormonal effects on the secretion and synthesis of surfactant are listed in Table 1–4. Of the listed hormones, glucocorticoids (e.g., cortisol) are the most clinically important. Their mechanism of action is not entirely understood; however, endogenous glucocorticoid released during fetal stress, and exogenous cortisol administered to the mother prior to delivery, stimulate mature surfactant production in the fetus via increased glycerophospholipid synthesis. Glucocorticoids also produce glycogen depletion in the fetal liver and increased synthesis of phosphatidylcholine (PC) from choline. For a detailed discussion of hormones and lung maturation, the reader is referred to the treatise by Ballard.[31]

**TABLE 1-4.**
Hormonal Effects on Secretion and Synthesis of Surfactant

| Hormone | Effect on Surfactant | Further Reading* |
|---|---|---|
| Cholinergic antagonists | Increased secretion secondary to increased ventilation | Oyarzun and Clements (1977) |
| Prostaglandins $E_1$, $E_2$, $F_2$ | Increased secretion | Oyarzun and Clements (1978) |
| β adrenergics (catecholamines) | Increased secretion probably via c-AMP | Oyarzun and Clements (1978); Sommer-Smith and Giannopoules (1981); Brown and Longmore (1981) |
| Glucocorticoids | Increased synthesis; increased number of type II pneumocytes and lamellar bodies | Snyder et al. (1985)[11] |
| Adrenocorticotropic hormone | Increased choline to PC | Bleasdale and Johnston (1985)[26] |
| Thyroid hormone | Increased choline to PC; increased numbers of type II pneumocytes and lamellar bodies | Snyder et al. (1985);[11] Bleasdale and Johnston (1985)[26] |
| Thyrotropin-releasing hormone | Increased choline to PC | Bleasdale and Johnston (1985)[26] |
| Estrogens | Increased total glycerophospholipids, specifically PC; increased number of type II pneumocytes and lamellar bodies | Snyder et al. (1985);[11] Bleasdale and Johnston (1985) |
| Epidermal growth factor | Increased PC; increased number of type II pneumocytes and lamellar bodies | Snyder et al. (1985);[11] Bleasdale and Johnston (1985)[26] |
| Fibroblast pneumonocyte factor | Increased PC and PG | |

*For more extensive review of subject, refer to "Suggested Readings" or listed references.

Jacobs et al.[32] utilizing lung lavage in premature, near-term, and newborn monkeys concluded that migration of macrophages to the alveoli may be secondary to the presence of surface active material in the lung, since the macrophages increased in number in alveoli after mature surfactant was produced. The number of alveolar macrophages was reduced in animals that subsequently developed RDS. Alveolar macrophages catabolize apoproteins of surfactant; however, much of the surfactant may be recycled.

## Determination of Lung Maturation

Amniotic fluid, which contains secreted fetal lung fluid, is a mirror that reflects fetal lung maturation. The lecithin to sphingomyelin (L:S) ratio is an important index of lung development. Amniotic fluid lecithin concentration increases slowly until 34 to 35 weeks' gestation when it suddenly rises. In the late gestational period, lecithin accounts for 70% to 75% of amniotic fluid phospholipids. Gluck et al.[33] demonstrated the concentration of sphingomyelin to be equal to that of lecithin until 35 weeks' gestation. After 35 weeks, lecithin concentration increases to an L:S ratio of 2.0 or greater correlating with lung maturity (i.e., the presence of mature surfactant in quantities sufficient to support respiration). Phosphatidylglycerol first appears at this time, and PI concentration decreases.[34] Females achieve L:S ratios that are consistent with lung maturity $1^1/_2$ to $2^1/_2$ weeks earlier than males.[35] In infants of diabetic mothers (IDM), an L:S ratio of 3.5 or greater indicates lung maturity. Abnormally low sphingomyelin due to a defect in regulation may give a spuriously elevated L:S ratio in the IDM. The palmitic acid/stearic acid ratio may, therefore, be a more useful determinant of fetal lung maturity in the IDM.

Lecithin phophatase is also a good indicator of lung maturity, as is total phospholipid phosphorous (TPP) in a concentration of greater than 0.140 mg/100 ml of amniotic fluid.[36] A fraction of TPP, PG, is an indicator of mature surfactant and does not appear until about 36 weeks' gestation.

Physical methods to determine the presence of surfactant in amniotic fluid include the classical shake test, in which ethanol and amniotic fluid are mixed and agitated. The appearance of bubbles after 15 minutes is indicative of the presence of surfactant.[37] The tap test and, more recently, the fluorescence polarization of amniotic fluid may also be used for determining the presence or absence of surfactant.[36]

## Fetal Lung Fluid

The fetal lung is a metabolically active organ that secretes fluid into the amniotic cavity at various rates. Jobe[28] determined that in the term fetal lamb lung, fluid is present in a concentration of approximately 30 ml/kg of body weight. This is roughly equal to the functional residual capacity of the newborn lamb lung. This fluid is probably important for the development of the fetal lung. Fetal lamb lung fluid contains no protein and is higher in chloride and has a lower pH and bicarbonate concentration than fetal serum. Chloride is actively transported until shortly before birth when there is catecholamine-mediated cessation of the chloride pump. Fluid secretion from fetal lamb lung increases with gestational age from 1 to 2 ml/kg/day to 100 ml/kg/day. During this period, there may be transient bursts of up to 40 ml of fluid expelled into the amniotic space. At birth, fluid secretion abruptly ceases secondary to increased fetal tracheal pressure. The thyroarytenoid muscle of the larynx may play a role in regulating the flow of lung fluid into the amniotic space.[38] Neuropeptides, vasopressin and vasotocin may help decrease lung fluid production.[39] The relatively increased protein concentration in serum and lymph produces an osmotic pressure gradient that facilitates flow of fluid from the alveolar to the vascular compartment in the postpartum period. There is also expression of lung fluid during normal vaginal delivery. Following caesarean section, however, fluid removal from the lung is slower. At birth, upon aeration of the lung, there is a sudden reduction in alveolar epithelial permeability coupled with increased interstitial hydrostatic pressure, which restricts further diffusion of fluid into the alveolar space.

**Fetal Breathing Movements**

Fetal chest wall movement has been extensively evaluated by real-time ultrasound (Fig 1–22,A and B). Fetal breathing movements (FBMs) may be seen as early as 10 to 12 weeks' gestation. Dawes and Patrick[40] found that chest wall movement in FBMs varies from 0.5 to 5.0 mm, and paradoxical abdominal wall movements vary from 0.5 to 8.0 mm. Trudinger and Knight[41] demonstrated a decrease in FBM rate from 20 weeks' gestation to term. Fetuses less than 32 weeks' gestational age have short breathing times; those between 32 to 36 weeks have a long inspiratory phase; in fetuses older than 36 weeks, FBMs are more uniform. In the last 2 weeks of gestation FBMs are more regular and shallow with a variable pattern. Defining apnea as a cessation of FBM for greater than 6 seconds, Patrick et al.[42] found a progressive increase in both the incidence and duration of apnea as gestation progresses.

At 34 to 35 weeks' gestation, FBMs increase between 1 A.M. and 7 A.M.[43] probably representing a circadian rhythm related to maternal estriol and cortisol effects on fetal adrenal glands. At 38 to 39 weeks' gestation, this circadian rhythm ceases as the maternal estriol level increases and the fetus is better able to modify the effects of estriol on the adrenal gland.[44]

Maternal hypercapnia following the inhalation of 5% $CO_2$[45] causes increased FBMs except in small-for-gestational-age fetuses.[40] In sheep, hypocapnia decreases FBMs. Increased maternal oxygenation and hypoxia do not change FBMs. The effects on the fetus of changes in oxygen and carbon dioxide in maternal blood are thought to be mediated by fetal central chemoreceptors.

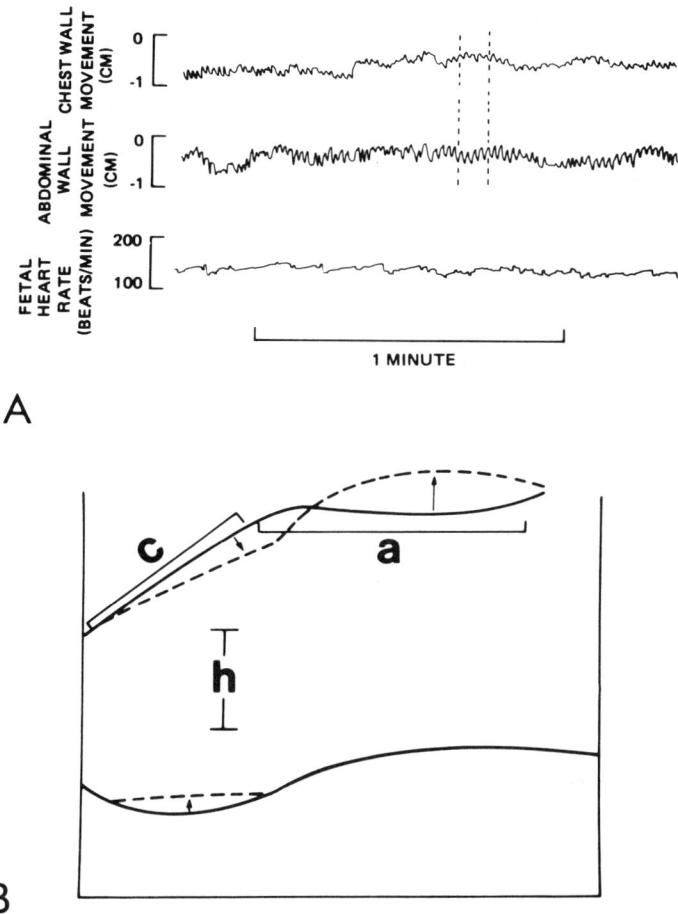

**FIG 1–22.**
**A,** chart recording of simultaneous measurements of chest and abdominal wall diameters during an episode of fetal breathing in a healthy fetus near term. Note that as chest wall moves inward (downward deflection), the abdominal wall moves outward in the opposite direction. (From Dawes GS, Patrick JE: Fetal breathing activity, in Nelson H (ed): *Pulmonary Development: Transition from Intrauterine to Extrauterine Life.* New York, Marcel Dekker, Inc, 1985, pp 75–100. Used by permission.)
**B,** representation of movement observed on real-time scanners during each fetal breath. Anterior and posterior fetal chest wall echoes move inward by about 2 to 5 mm, and anterior abdominal wall echoes move outward about 3 to 8 mm. $c$ = anterior chest wall; $a$ = anterior abdominal wall; $h$ = fetal heart. (From Patrick J, Fetherson W, Vick H, et al: Human fetal breathing movements and gross fetal body movements at weeks 34–35 of gestation. *Am J Obstet Gynecol* 1978; 130:693. Used by permission.)

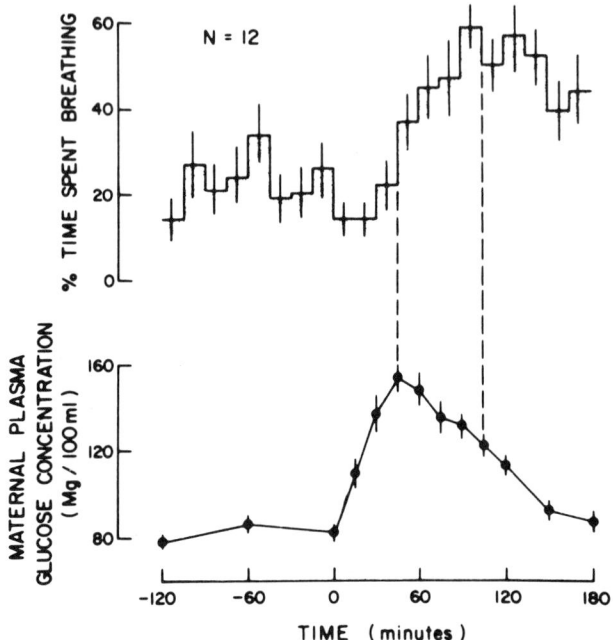

**FIG 1–23.**
The relationship between maternal plasma glucose concentration and fetal breathing activity. Peak maternal plasma glucose concentrations occurred at time (t) + 45 minutes. Fetal breathing activity began to increase at t + 60 minutes but did not reach a maximum until t + 105 minutes which was 60 minutes after the peak maternal plasma glucose concentration. (From Natale R, Patrick J, Richardson B: Effects of human maternal venous plasma glucose concentrations on fetal breathing movements. *Am J Obstet Gynecol* 1978; 132:36. Used by permission.)

An elevated 2- to 3-hour postprandial maternal glucose results in increased FBMs in the human fetus[46, 47, 48] (Fig 1–23). No change in FBM is seen following a meal high in fat or protein. Many other factors also appear to influence fetal breathing movements in man and experimental animals. Both cigarette smoking and catecholamines increase FBM. Slightly elevated levels of maternal serum ethanol decrease FBM probably by a central effect.[49] Methadone decreases FBM and reduces fetal $CO_2$ response.[45] In ewes, pentobarbital decreases both FBM and electrocortical activity.

Fetal breathing movements also vary with the maternal sleep-wake cycle. During rapid eye movement (REM) sleep in the last month of gestation, FBMs are rapid and regular. Upon maternal waking, FBMs are rhythmic, shallow, rapid, and variable in frequency. At parturition, FBMs decrease from 25.6% to 8.5% of a time interval during the latent phase of labor and to 0.8% of a given time interval during active labor[50] (Fig 1–24).

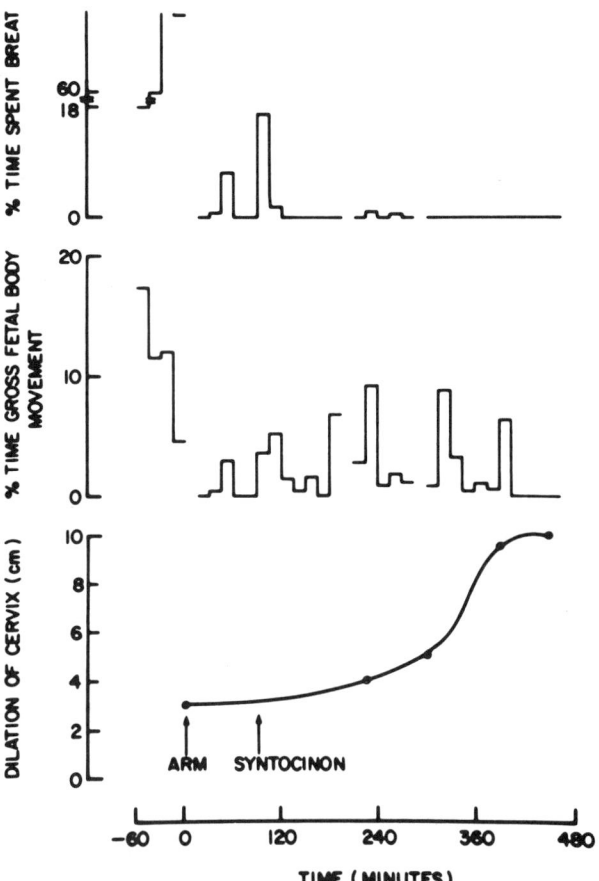

**FIG 1–24.**
The incidence of fetal breathing and gross body movements in one fetus were plotted in 15-minute intervals. During the control period before induction of labor with a solution of oxytocin (Syntocinon) and during prelatent-phase labor, episodes of breathing activity occurred during episodes of increased gross fetal body movements. During latent and active-phase labor, episodes of gross fetal body movements continued every 60 to 90 minutes, but fetal breathing movements were absent. ARM = artificial rupture of membranes. (From Richardson B, Natale R, Patrick J: Human fetal breathing activity during electively induced labor at term. *Am J Obstet Gynecol* 1979; 133:247. Reprinted with permission.)

## REFERENCES

1. Hamilton WJ, Boyd JD, Mossman HW: *Human Embryology (Prenatal Development of Form and Function)*, ed 3. Baltimore, Williams & Wilkins Co, 1962.
2. Langman J: *Medical Embryology*, ed 3. Baltimore, Williams & Wilkins Co, 1975.
3. Moore KL: *The Developing Human*, ed 2. Philadelphia, WB Saunders Co, 1977.
4. Boyden EA, Development of the human lung, in Kelley VC, (ed): *Practice of Pediatrics*, revised ed. Philadelphia, Harper & Row, 1986, Chapter 34.
5. Hislop A, Reid L: Growth and development of the respiratory system—anatomical development, in Davis JA, Dobbing J (eds): Scientific Foundations of Paediatrics, ed 2. London, Wm Heinemann Medical Books, Ltd, 1981, pp 214–254.
6. O'Rahilly R, Boyden EA: The timing and sequence of events in the development of the human respiratory system during the embryonic period proper. *Z Anat Entwicklungsgesch* 1973; 141:237.
7. Rudnik D: Developmental capacities of the chick lung in chorioallantoic grafts. *J Exp Zool* 1933; 66:125.
8. Langston C, Keda K, Reed M, et al: Human lung growth in late gestation and in the neonate. *Am Rev Respir Dis* 1984; 129:607.
9. Bucher W, Reid L: Development of the intrasegmental bronchial tree: The pattern of branching and development of cartilage at various stages of intrauterine life. *Thorax* 1961; 16:207.
10. Lamb D, Reid L: Acidic glycoproteins produced by the mucous cells of the bronchial submucosal glands in the fetus and child: A histochemical autoradiographic study. *Br J Dis Chest* 1972; 66:248.
11. Snyder M, Mendelson CR, Johnston JM: The morphology of lung development in the human fetus, in Nelson H (ed): *Pulmonary Development: Transition for Intrauterine to Extrauterine Life*. New York, Marcel Dekker, Inc, 1985, pp 19–46.
12. Spooner BS, Faubian JM: Collagen involvement in branching morphogenesis of embryonic lung and salivary gland. *Dev Biol* 1980; 77:84.
13. Loosli CG, Potter EL: Pre- and postnatal development of the respiratory portion of the human lung. *Am Rev Respir Dis* 1959; 80:5.
14. Dunnill MS: Postnatal growth of the lung. *Thorax* 1962; 17:329.
15. Thurlbeck WM, Angus GE: Growth and development of the normal human lung. *Chest* 1975; 67 (suppl):35.
16. Hislop A, Reid L: Intrapulmonary arterial development during fetal life-branching pattern and structure. *J Anat* 1972; 113:35.
17. Heath D, Wood EH, Dushane JW, et al: The structure of the pulmonary trunk at different ages in cases of pulmonary hypertension and pulmonary stenosis, *J Pathol* 1959; 77:443.
18. Hislop A, Reid L: Pulmonary arterial development during childhood: Branching pattern and structure. *Thorax* 1973; 28:129.

19. Reid L: The pulmonary circulation: Remodeling in growth and disease. Am Rev Respir Dis 1979; 119:531.
20. Murphy JD, Rabinovitch M, Goldstein JD, et al: The structural basis of persistent pulmonary hypertension in the newborn infant. Pediatr 1981; 98:962.
21. Boyden EA: The developing bronchial arteries in a fetus of the twelfth week. Am J Anat 1970; 129:357.
22. Hislop A, Reid L: Weight of the left and right ventricle of the heart during fetal life. J Clin Pathol 1972; 534.
23. Rudolph AM: Fetal circulation and cardiovascular adjustments after birth, in Rudolph A (ed): Pediatrics, ed 17. Norwalk, Conn, Appleton Century Crofts, 1982, pp 1231–1235.
24. Avery ME, Mead J: Surface properties in relation to atelectasis and hyaline membrane disease, Am J Dis Child 1959; 97:517.
25. King RJ; The surfactant system of the lung. Fed Proc 1974; 33:2238.
26. Bleasdale JE, Johnston JM: Developmental biochemistry of lung surfactant, in Nelson GH (ed): *Pulmonary Development: Transition From Intrauterine to Extrauterine Life*. New York, Marcel Dekker, Inc, 1985, pp 47–74.
27. Perelman RH, Farrell PM, Engle MJ, et al: Developmental aspects of lung lipids, Annu Rev Physiol 1985; 47:803.
28. Jobe A: Fetal lung maturation and the respiratory distress syndrome, in Beard RW, Nathanielsz PW, (eds): *Fetal Physiology and Medicine*. New York, Marcel Dekker, Inc, 1984, pp 317–351.
29. Quirk JG, Bleasdale JE: Myoinositol homeostasis in the human fetus. Obstet Gynecol 1983; 62:41.
30. Clements RS, Reynertson R: Myoinositol metabolism in diabetes mellitus. Diabetes 1977; 26:215.
31. Ballard PI: *Hormone and Lung Maturation*. Berlin, Springer-Verlag, 1986.
32. Jacobs RF, Wilson CB, Palmer S, et al: Factors related to the appearance of alveolar macrophages in the developing lung. Am Rev Respir Dis 1985; 131:548.
33. Gluck L, Kulovich M, Kirkpatrick E, et al: Diagnosis of the respiratory distress syndrome by amniocentesis. Am J Obstet Gynecol 1971; 109:440.
34. Hallman M, Kulovich M, Kirkpatrick E, et al: Phosphatidylinositol and phosphatidylglycerol in amniotic fluid: Indices of lung maturity. Am J Obstet Gynecol 1976; 125:613.
35. Torday JS, Nielson HC, Fencl M, et al: Sex differences in fetal lung maturation. Am Rev Respir Dis 1981; 123:205.
36. Nelson GH, Fadel HE, McPherson JC: Methods of amniotic fluid analysis for evaluation of fetal maturity, in Nelson GH (ed): *Pulmonary Development: Transition From Intrauterine to Extrauterine Life*. New York, Marcel Dekker, Inc, 1985, pp 127–142.
37. Clements JA, Platzker ACG, Tierney DF, et al: Assessment of the risk of

the respiratory distress syndrome by a rapid test for surfactant in amniotic fluid. N Engl J Med 1972; 286:1077.
38. Harding R: Function of the larynx in the fetus and newborn. Annu Rev Physiol 1984; 46:645.
39. Ross MG, Ervin G, Leake RD, et al: Fetal lung liquid regulation by neuropeptides. Am J Obstet Gynecol 1984; 150:421.
40. Dawes GS, Patrick JE: Fetal breathing activity, in Nelson GH (ed): *Pulmonary Development: Transition From Intrauterine to Extrauterine Life.* New York, Marcel Dekker, Inc, 1985, pp 75–100.
41. Trudinger BJ, Knight PC: Fetal age and patterns of human fetal breathing movements. Am J Obstet Gynecol 1980; 137:724.
42. Patrick J, Campbell K, Carmichael L, et al: A definition of the human fetal apnea and the distribution of fetal apneic intervals during the last 10 weeks of pregnancy. Am J Obstet Gynecol 1980; 136:471.
43. Patrick J: Fetal breathing movements. Clin Obstet Gynecol 1982; 25:787.
44. Patrick J, Challis J, Campbell K, et al: Circadian rhythms in maternal plasma cortisol and estriol concentrations at 30 to 31, 34 to 35, and 38 to 39 weeks gestational age. Am J Obstet Gynecol 1980; 136:325.
45. Richardson BS, O'Grady JP, Olsen GD: Fetal breathing movements and the response to $CO_2$ in patients on methadone maintenance. Am J Obstet Gynecol 1984; 150:400.
46. Lewis PJ, Trudinger BJ, Mangel J: Effect of maternal glucose ingestion on fetal breathing and body movements in late pregnancy. Br J Obstet Gynaecol 1978; 85:86.
47. Natale R, Patrick J, Richardson B: Effects of maternal venous plasma glucose on fetal breathing movements. Am J Obstet Gynecol 1978; 132:36.
48. Bocking A, Adamson L, Cousin K, et al: Effects of intravenous glucose injections on human fetal breathing movements and gross fetal body movements at 38–40 weeks gestational age. Am J Obstet Gynecol 1982; 142:606.
49. Fox HE, Steinbrucher M, Pessle D, et al: Maternal ethanol ingestion and the occurrence of human fetal breathing movements. Am J Obstet Gynecol 1978; 132:354.
50. Richardson B, Natale R, Patrick J: Human fetal breathing activity during induced labor at term. Am J Obstet Gynecol 1979; 133:247.

## SUGGESTED READINGS

Brown LS, Longmore WJ: Adrenergic and cholinergic regulation of lung surfactant secretion in the isolated perfused rat lung and the alveolar type II cell in culture. J Biol Chem 1981; 256:66.

Hislop A, Reid L: Development of the acinus in the human lung. Thorax 1974; 29:90.

Hislop A, Reid L: Fetal and childhood development of the intrapulmonary veins in man-branching pattern and structure. Thorax 1973; 28:313.

King RJ, Ruch J, Gikas EG, et al: Appearance of apoproteins of pulmonary surfactant in human amniotic fluid. *J Appl. Physiol.* 1975; 39:735.

Nelson GH (ed): *Pulmonary Development: Transition From Intrauterine to Extrauterine Life.* New York, Marcel Dekker, Inc, 1985.

O'Rahilly R: The early prenatal development of the respiratory system, in Nelson GH (ed): *Pulmonary Development: Transition From Intrauterine to Extrauterine Life.* New York, Marcel Dekker, Inc, 1985, pp 3–18.

Oyarzun MJ, Clements JA: Ventilatory and cholinergic control of pulmonary surfactant in the rabbit. *J Appl Physiol* 1977; 43:39.

Oyarzun MJ, Clements JA: Control of lung surfactant by ventilation, adrenergic mediators and prostaglandins in the rabbit. *Am Rev Respir Dis* 1978; 117:879.

Reid L, Rubino M: The connective tissue septa in the foetal human lung. *Thorax* 1959; 14:3.

Sommer-Smith SK, Giannopoulos G: Beta-adrenergic receptor binding in isolated fetal, neonatal and adult alveolar type II cells. *Fed Proc* 1981; 40:407.

# 2

# Assessment of Neonatal Gas Exchange

Robert L. Chatburn, R.R.T.
Waldemar A. Carlo, M.D.

The subject of neonatal gas exchange assessment has received little recognition in either textbooks or journal articles. There are many differences between neonatal and adult blood gas interpretation, and with the lack of universally accepted guidelines, controversies abound. Our goal in this chapter is to develop a rational approach to the subject and suggest clinically useful procedures. We begin with a brief review of gas exchange and acid-base physiology. This lays the foundation for a practical classification system. Finally, the techniques for obtaining blood gas data are explained. We will assume that the reader has a basic understanding of adult blood gas interpretation.

## GAS EXCHANGE PHYSIOLOGY

### Oxygen Transport

The transport of oxygen from the airway opening to the tissues can be conveniently divided into four phases, each associated with a characteristic oxygen tension ($P_{O_2}$): inspired $P_{O_2}$, alveolar $P_{O_2}$, blood (arterial) $P_{O_2}$, and tissue $P_{O_2}$. Each phase is affected by a number of variables, only some of which can be manipulated in the clinical setting. Thus, oxygenation of the sick neonate is often difficult and sometimes impossible to control. When it cannot be controlled, either by natural homeostatic mechanisms or by artificial means, severe hypoxemia and ultimately death result.

### Inspired Oxygen

The process of oxygen transport begins at the airway opening. Fortunately, the fraction of oxygen in dry inspired gas ($F_{I_{O_2}}$) is an easily controlled variable. This was not always the case, however. The use of enriched oxygen environments for the treatment of neonates with respiratory failure was not common until the 1940s.[1] Despite the dramatic improvement in survival that oxygen administration provided, guidelines for its proper usage were not developed until many years later. The modern concept of "oxygen as a drug" is the result of the recognition of oxygen toxicity and such oxygen-related disorders as retrolental fibroplasia.

In practice, $F_{I_{O_2}}$ is usually controlled by a commercial air-oxygen blender or, perhaps, by combining flows of pure oxygen and air into an enclosed environment (e.g., an oxygen hood or tent). Clinically, $F_{I_{O_2}}$ is easily measured using either polarographic or galvanic transducers incorporated in portable oxygen analyzers. These devices[2] actually measure $P_{O_2}$ but are calibrated to read $F_{I_{O_2}}$. Thus, the $F_{I_{O_2}}$ measured at the outlet of a blender (dry gas) will be different from the $F_{I_{O_2}}$ of gas at the outlet of a humidifier. The difference can be as much as 8% of the measured value depending on the barometric pressure and the characteristics of the humidifier. This is because the partial pressure of the oxygen is less due to the addition of water vapor. For example, suppose we are interested in measuring the $F_{I_{O_2}}$ delivered to a patient during mechanical ventilation. If an $O_2$ analyzer calibrated in 100% dry $O_2$ measures an $F_{I_{O_2}}$ of 0.80 at the outlet of the blender, the $F_{I_{O_2}}$ at the patient's airway opening will be 0.76 (assuming a barometric pressure of 760 torr and that the humidifier delivers 100% relative humidity at 34°C). The partial pressure of inspired oxygen ($P_{I_{O_2}}$) is given by

$$P_{I_{O_2}} = F_{I_{O_2}} \times (P_B - P_{H_2O}) \tag{1}$$

where

$P_B$ = barometric pressure

$P_{H_2O}$ = partial pressure of water vapor

The water vapor pressure of gas in contact and equilibrium with liquid water is a function only of the gas temperature. As inspired gas travels down the airways, it picks up heat and humidity. By the time it reaches the alveoli, it is saturated with water vapor at body temperature (37°C), which has a partial pressure ($P_{H_2O}$) of 47 torr.

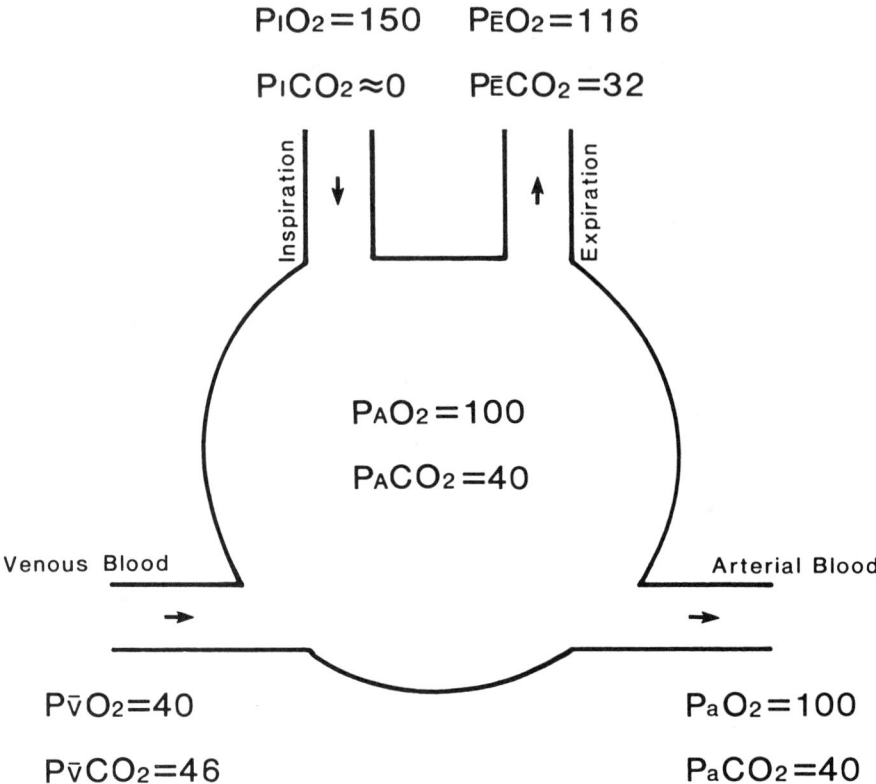

**FIG 2–1.**
An idealized alveolus at sea level. The alveolar gas partial pressures ($P_{A_{O_2}}$ and $P_{A_{CO_2}}$) are determined by the relative flows of $O_2$ and $CO_2$ entering and leaving the system. If the ventilating gases are blocked, diffusion will continue until alveolar gas pressures are equal to gas pressures of mixed venous blood ($P\bar{v}_{O_2}$ and $P\bar{v}_{CO_2}$). In the process, the volume of the alveolus decreases. If the process continues long enough, a critical volume will be reached at which time the alveolus will collapse from surface tension forces. If blood flow is blocked, ventilating gases will flush the alveolus, and alveolar gas partial pressures will approach inspired gas values. Because diffusion is negligible, alveolar volume remains constant. $P_{I_{O_2}}$ and $P_{I_{CO_2}}$ = partial pressure of inspired gases; $P\bar{E}_{O_2}$ and $P\bar{E}_{CO_2}$ = partial pressure of mixed expired gases; $Pa_{O_2}$ and $Pa_{CO_2}$ = partial pressure of gases in arterial blood.)

### *Alveolar Oxygen Tension*

Lung volume is predominantly composed of the space within alveoli and alveolar ducts. As such, it can be thought of as a reservoir normally containing nitrogen, oxygen, and carbon dioxide. Extending this analogy, we can visualize a single alveolus as an elastic container whose average volume and gas concentrations are determined by the relative flows input from two sources and output from two sources (Fig 2–1). The input represents gas flows from the airway opening (inspiration) and from the venous blood. The output represents gas traveling to the airway opening (expiration) and to the arterial blood. The concentration of oxygen in the alveolus, and hence the $P_{A_{O_2}}$, is determined by the balance between the input of oxygen from inspired gas and its output to exhaled gas and arterial blood. The situation is analogous, for example, to a bucket of water being continuously filled by one pipe and continuously drained by two others. Oxygen diffuses from areas of high concentration or partial pressure to areas of lower pressure. Thus, in our analogy, a relatively large flow of oxygen passes into and out of the alveolus while a portion of that flow is diverted to the arterial blood and ultimately the tissues. The flow of oxygen into the alveolar region of the lungs is about 13 to 20 ml/kg/minute, whereas the tissue oxygen consumption of the normal newborn is approximately 6 to 8 ml/kg/minute. Carbon dioxide also enters the alveolus from venous blood, diluting the oxygen concentration and reducing the average $P_{A_{O_2}}$. The interrelationship of these variables is summarized in the alveolar gas equation

$$P_{A_{O_2}} = P_{I_{O_2}} - P_{A_{CO_2}}/R + P_{A_{CO_2}} \times F_{I_{O_2}} \times (1 - R)/R \qquad (2)$$

where $P_{A_{CO_2}}$ is the alveolar carbon dioxide tension (often assumed to equal arterial $CO_2$ tension), and R is the respiratory exchange ratio (the ratio of carbon dioxide output to oxygen uptake as determined by the analysis of respiratory gases). This equation is sometimes simplified to

$$P_{A_{O_2}} = P_{I_{O_2}} - P_{A_{CO_2}}/R \qquad (3)$$

If the blood flow to an alveolus is cut off, its oxygen consumption is eliminated, and the $P_{A_{O_2}}$ will approach that of inspired gas. On the other hand, if the flow of gas from the airway opening is cut off, the $P_{A_{O_2}}$ will decrease as it approaches venous oxygen tension. In addition, since no fresh gas is entering the alveolus, its volume will decrease as alveolar oxygen is consumed. If this process continues long enough, a critical volume is reached, below which the alveolus will collapse. The presence of nitrogen in the alveolar gas greatly decreases the rate at which alveolar volume shrinks under these conditions,[3] which is one of the arguments for using the lowest $F_{I_{O_2}}$ possible to obtain acceptable arterial oxygen tension.

### *Oxygen Tension of the Blood*

Blood can be thought of as being a two-sectioned container of oxygen, one large and one very small. The largest section represents the oxygen-carrying capacity of hemoglobin; the smaller section represents the capacity of plasma. With a normal hemoglobin of 15 gm/100 ml, arterial blood transports approximately 20.8 ml of oxygen (1.39 ml $O_2$ per gram of hemoglobin) per 100 ml of blood (vol% is often used in place of milliliters of gas per 100 ml blood). Of this, 19.7 ml of oxygen per 100 ml of blood is carried by hemoglobin, the rest by plasma. It is the oxygen-carrying capacity of hemoglobin that sustains the oxygen consumption of the tissues. However, the force that loads hemoglobin with oxygen is the difference in oxygen partial pressure between the alveolus and the capillary blood. A $Po_2$ difference also unloads oxygen from the hemoglobin to the tissues. It is therefore important to understand the relationship between the oxygen content and partial pressure, which is most conveniently represented by the oxyhemoglobin dissociation curve (Fig 2–2).

There are several factors that can shift the curve either to the left or to the right. High blood pH, hypothermia, hypocapnia, and decreased 2,3-diphosphoglycerate (DPG) will shift the curve to the left indicating

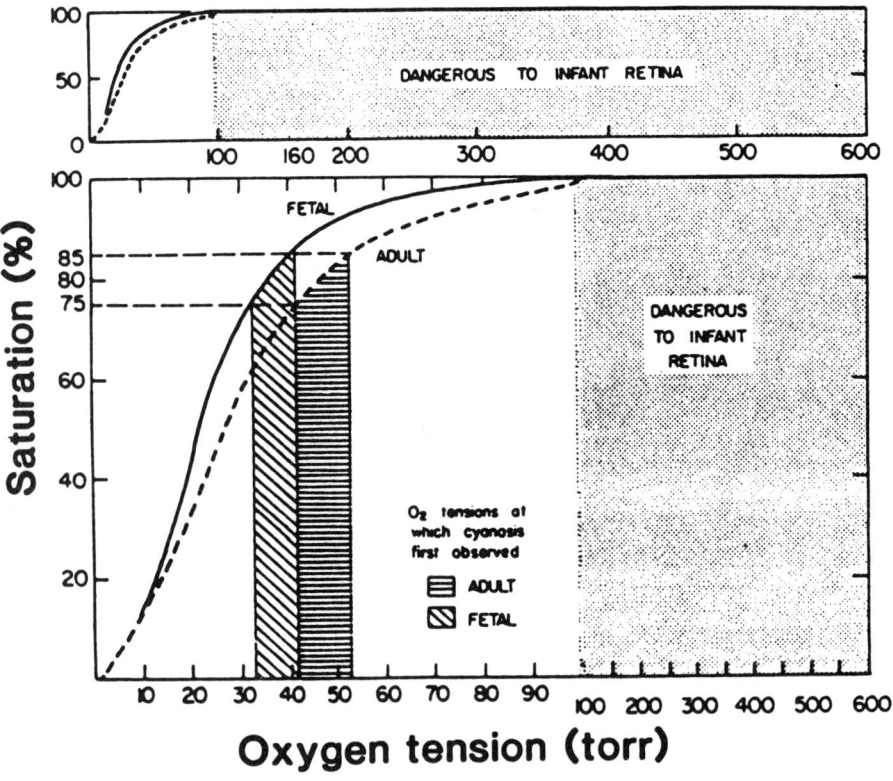

**FIG 2–2.**
The oxyhemoglobin dissociation curve. (From Klaus MH, Fanaroff AA: *Care of the High Risk Neonate.* Philadelphia, WB Saunders Co, 1986, p 173. Used by permission.)

an increased affinity between oxygen and hemoglobin. Low blood pH, hyperthermia, hypercapnia, and increased 2,3-DPG will shift the curve to the right as the blood exhibits a decreased affinity for oxygen. Normally, these factors facilitate oxygen loading of hemoglobin in the lungs and release to the tissues. Sudden severe shifts of the oxyhemoglobin curve can potentially decrease oxygen availability to the tissues.

As oxygen diffuses across the alveolar-capillary membrane, it is bound by hemoglobin. As the oxygen content of the capillary blood increases, the partial pressure of oxygen in the blood plasma increases. It is this pressure that is measured clinically as arterial oxygen tension ($Pa_{O_2}$). Thus, $Pa_{O_2}$ is an indirect index of the amount of oxygen available to the tissues, which is the variable we are most interested in optimizing.

The key point here is that the clinical utility of $Pa_{O_2}$ as an index of tissue oxygenation is entirely dependent on the amount of hemoglobin in the blood. For example, if pure plasma was injected into the pulmonary arteries, its $P_{O_2}$ as it emerged from the lungs would be the same as blood. However, because its oxygen content is less than 2% of what normal blood would be, its ability to oxygenate the body's tissues is nil. Infants with respiratory distress frequently have reduced hemoglobin levels for a variety of reasons. Thus, the $Pa_{O_2}$ must be interpreted with caution. A more precise index can be calculated using information about the patient's hemoglobin and arterial oxygen saturation (usually calculated from $Pa_{O_2}$).

$$Ca_{O_2} = (Hb \times 1.34 \times O_2 \text{ sat}) + (0.0031 \times Pa_{O_2}) \qquad (4)$$

where

$Ca_{O_2}$ = oxygen content of arterial blood in ml/100 ml of blood
Hb = hemoglobin content in gm/100 ml of blood
1.34 = a constant describing the amount of oxygen (ml at STPD) that can be carried by 1 gm of hemoglobin when it is fully saturated
$O_2$ sat = hemoglobin saturation expressed in decimal form
0.0031 = solubility coefficient of plasma

The above equation assumes a normal oxyhemoglobin dissociation curve.

### Oxygen Tension of Tissue

The delivery of molecular oxygen to the cellular mitochondria is essential for oxidative metabolism to occur. This process results in the release of the energy required for biochemical processes. Mitochondria can function at cellular oxygen tensions as low as 5 torr. Below this level, metabolic energy is produced by anaerobic mechanisms that are less efficient and produce by-products that can alter acid-base balance (e.g., lactic acid).

Tissue $PO_2$ provides an important feedback signal for the control of ventilation through the mechanism of the central and peripheral chemoreceptors. In particular, the carotid bodies are sensitive to both blood $PO_2$ and content. A reduction of either stimulates ventilation. However, premature infants often hypoventilate in response to hypoxia.

## Carbon Dioxide Transport

As with oxygen, the transport of carbon dioxide can be divided into four phases, each associated with a characteristic carbon dioxide tension ($PCO_2$). In this case, the $CO_2$ content is highest in the tissues and decreases as the gas travels from the venous blood to the alveoli. If the elimination of carbon dioxide from the tissues is blocked either through ventilatory or circulatory disorders, acidosis, cellular enzyme deactivation, and death ensue.

### *Tissue Carbon Dioxide*

Because of its relatively high solubility coefficient, the cellular diffusion of $CO_2$ is so efficient that no significant partial pressure gradient exists between venous blood and the tissues, provided that circulation is adequate.

Cellular $PCO_2$ plays an important role in the physiologic control of ventilation. Dissolved $CO_2$ moves much more rapidly across the membranes of peripheral chemoreceptors than hydrogen or bicarbonate ions. This makes the chemoreceptors sensitive to changes in ventilation. Increased cellular $PCO_2$ (e.g., as a result of hypoventilation) elevates cellular hydrogen ion concentration as $CO_2$ combines with cellular water to form carbonic acid. The increase in cellular hydrogen ion concentration stimulates neural impulses to the medullary center, which in turn stimulates ventilation. However, excessively high $PCO_2$ levels can depress ventilation.

### *Carbon Dioxide Tension of the Blood*

Carbon dioxide transport in the blood is more complicated than that of oxygen. There are three plasma compartments (bound to protein, as bicarbonate, and in physical solution) and three erythrocyte compartments (dissolved in erythrocyte water, combined with hemoglobin, and as carbonic acid). Normally, venous blood carries about 64 vol% of $CO_2$ and arterial blood about 56 vol%. Overall, 5% of the $CO_2$ in blood exists as dissolved gas or as carbonic acid; 10% is carried by

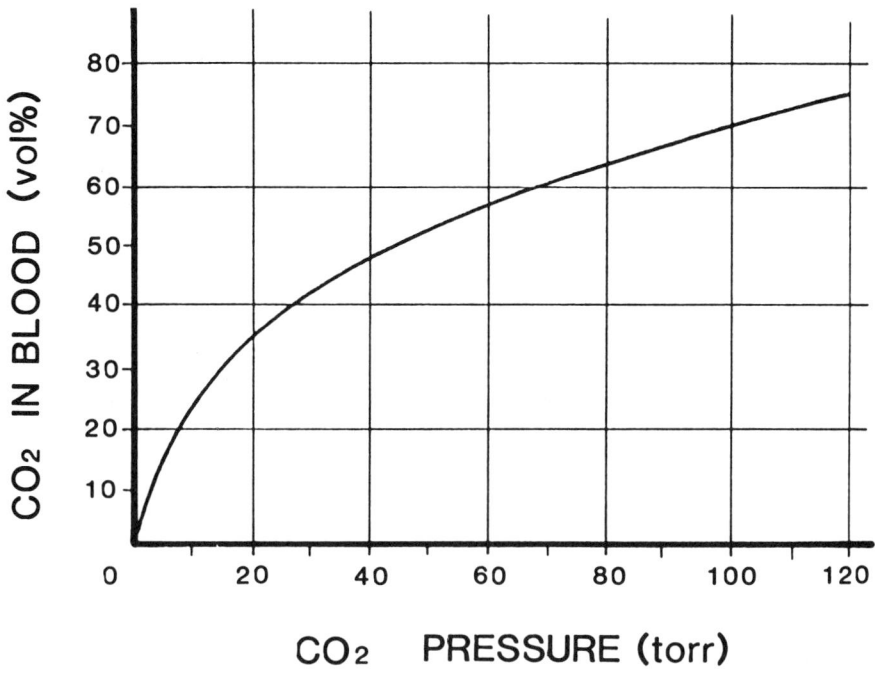

**FIG 2–3.**
The $CO_2$ dissociation curve for whole blood. (Adapted from Guyton AC: *Textbook of Medical Physiology,* ed 5. Philadelphia , WB Saunders Co, 1976.)

hemoglobin as carbamino compounds; and 85% is transported as bicarbonate ion.

The $CO_2$ dissociation curve for blood is shown in Figure 2–3. Note that it is more linear than that of oxygen, indicating that as $P_{CO_2}$ rises, more carbon dioxide is transported. In contrast, once hemoglobin is saturated with oxygen, an increasing $P_{O_2}$ will not significantly increase oxygen transport. Note also that the $CO_2$ dissociation curve is steeper than that for $O_2$. Thus, the small change between venous and arterial $P_{CO_2}$ (46 vs. 40 torr) results in a change in $CO_2$ content of about 4 vol%, whereas the same magnitude of change in $P_{O_2}$ would result in a difference of about 1 vol%.

### *Alveolar Carbon Dioxide Tension*

The normal alveolar-capillary interface is such that blood is exposed to alveolar gas long enough for the two to attain equal partial pressures of gases (i.e., nitrogen, oxygen, and carbon dioxide). Since arterial blood has a normal carbon dioxide tension of 40 torr, we infer that the "average" partial pressure of alveolar gas is the same as the arterial carbon dioxide tension ($Pa_{CO_2}$) for normal lungs. Then by definition, the fraction of carbon dioxide in alveolar gas ($FA_{CO_2}$) is

$$FA_{CO_2} = PA_{CO_2} / (PB - PH_2O) \qquad (5)$$

where, for computational purposes, $PA_{CO_2}$ is assumed to equal $Pa_{CO_2}$.

Under steady-state conditions, the rate of metabolic $CO_2$ production equals the rate of $CO_2$ elimination. Since virtually all of the $CO_2$ comes from the alveolar region of the lungs, $CO_2$ elimination ($\dot{V}CO_2$) is a product of the $FA_{CO_2}$ times the alveolar ventilation ($\dot{V}A$). In terms of the analogy illustrated in Figure 2–1, the alveolar ventilation "washes away" $CO_2$ from the alveoli. If the metabolic production of $CO_2$ increases, the $PCO_2$ of the blood will rise, which in turn increases the $FA_{CO_2}$ temporarily. The increased tension of $CO_2$ in the blood stimulates an increase in ventilation, decreasing $FA_{CO_2}$ and reestablishing a normal $Pa_{CO_2}$. Conversely, if ventilation is reduced, $FA_{CO_2}$ and, consequently, $Pa_{CO_2}$ increase. From a practical standpoint, these concepts can be summarized in mathematical form:

$$Pa_{CO_2} = \frac{\dot{V}CO_2}{\dot{V}A} \times (PB - PH_2O) \qquad (6)$$

where $\dot{V}A$ for the normal infant is about 100 to 150 ml/kg/minute. The utility of this equation is that it clearly shows the inverse relation between arterial carbon dioxide tension and alveolar ventilation. Since the expression ($PB - PH_2O$) is relatively constant and we can control $\dot{V}A$ with mechanical ventilation, $Pa_{CO_2}$ is usually not difficult to normalize unless lung function is extremely compromised.

### *Inspired Carbon Dioxide*

Atmospheric air contains negligible amounts of $CO_2$ that has no significant effect on $FA_{CO_2}$ and $Pa_{CO_2}$. However, endotracheal tubes and ventilator circuits can increase the volume of dead space and add exhaled $CO_2$ to inspired gas. The $PI_{CO_2}$ can be calculated in a manner analogous to equation 1. If the volume of artificial dead space is not too large, we can assume that it is flushed with alveolar gas at end exhalation. Thus, the next inspired tidal volume will contribute an alveolar volume that is less by an amount equal to the added dead space. Since alveolar ventilation is alveolar volume (tidal volume minus dead space) times respiratory frequency, the effect on $Pa_{CO_2}$ can be estimated from equation 6. For example, suppose an alveolar ventilation of 150 ml/kg/minute results in a $Pa_{CO_2}$ of 40 torr. If the addition of dead space reduces this to 120 ml/kg/minute, the $Pa_{CO_2}$ should rise to 50 torr.

In this case, a 20% reduction in alveolar ventilation resulted in a 25% increase in $P_{A_{CO_2}}$. However, due to the inverse relation between $P_{CO_2}$ and $\dot{V}_A$, the rate of change of one variable relative to the other is not constant. For example, if the ventilation is reduced by 40% to 72 ml/kg/minute, the $Pa_{CO_2}$ will rise 108% to 83 torr. If the rate of change was constant, we would expect only a 50% increase in $Pa_{CO_2}$. This relation has a tendency to make the effects of ventilator changes less intuitively obvious.

## ACID-BASE PHYSIOLOGY

Control of blood pH is one of the most important of the body's homeostatic activities. Fluctuations of pH above and below the normal range disrupts cellular metabolism, and extreme deviations can cause necrosis. When pH drops below 7.0 for extended periods of time, survival is unlikely. In neonates with respiratory distress syndrome, a low pH can contribute to intrapulmonary shunting that results in hypoxemia, lactic acidosis, and if severe enough, hypercapnia. These effects lead to an even lower pH and a vicious cycle is established that is life threatening. Breaking this cycle requires the judicious use of mechanical ventilation and bicarbonate. The interaction of these two variables is defined by the Henderson-Hasselbalch equation.

### The Henderson-Hasselbalch Equation

The acid-base status of the blood is most commonly assessed by measuring its pH. The term pH is defined as the negative logarithm of the hydrogen ion concentration. As it applies to the carbonic acid/sodium bicarbonate blood buffer system, the Henderson-Hasselbalch equation expresses pH as a function of bicarbonate ion and dissolved $CO_2$:

$$pH = 6.1 + \log \frac{HCO_3^-}{0.03 \times P_{CO_2}} \qquad (7)$$

where $HCO_3^-$ is bicarbonate ion concentration in mEq/L, and 0.03 is the factor to convert torr to the same units. Use of this equation is simplified by the Siggaard-Andersen alignment nomogram (see Appendix, Fig A–1).

Under normal circumstances, the body maintains a pH of 7.4, which results in a ratio of bicarbonate ion to dissolved $CO_2$ of 20:1. Since both the numerator and the denominator of this ratio can vary, there arise two ways that pH can be abnormally high (i.e., high $HCO_3^-$ or low

$PCO_2$) and two ways it can be low (i.e., low $HCO_3^-$ or high $PCO_2$). These combinations provide a basis for the classification of acid-base disorders. Bicarbonate ion concentration is primarily controlled by tissue metabolism and kidney function. $PCO_2$ is controlled by the respiratory centers that adjust the level of ventilation. Thus, acid-base disorders are said to be of either metabolic or respiratory origin. In addition, because the body compensates for bicarbonate ion concentration derangements by altering the blood $PCO_2$ and vice versa, the classification scheme can be expanded by detailing the nature and degree of compensation for a chronic acid-base disorder.

## Blood Gas Classification

The basis of any blood gas classification system is the notion of a "normal" value. Once this is established for a given variable, values above and below normal define categories of abnormality. For blood pH, values above normal designate alkalemia, while those below represent acidemia. The terms alkalemia and acidemia refer to measurements of blood pH whereas the terms alkalosis and acidosis are used to describe the underlying acid-base imbalance. The distinction here is that the suffix "-emia" refers to conditions of the blood, and the suffix "-osis" refers to a pathologic process.[4,5] As mentioned previously, there are four possible classifications for uncompensated disorders: respiratory acidosis, respiratory alkalosis, metabolic acidosis, and metabolic alkalosis. These disorders and their compensatory states are listed in Table 2–1.

### *Respiratory Acidosis*

Respiratory acidosis is defined as a low pH, high $PCO_2$, and a normal $HCO_3^-$. It is the result of an insufficient alveolar ventilation (see equation 6). Compensation occurs as the kidney decreases bicarbonate ion excretion in the urine along with sodium so that additional amounts of sodium bicarbonate are available to buffer the elevated hydrogen ion concentration. Increased renal excretion of hydrogen ions in the form of hydrochloric acid and ammonium chloride reduces the acidity of the blood. Complete renal compensation for acute respiratory acidosis may take 3 to 4 days. Bicarbonate administration is not recommended as it will react with acid in the blood to produce $CO_2$, increasing the effects of hypercapnia.

In addition to the response by the kidney, the high $PCO_2$ stimulates pulmonary and peripheral *vasoconstriction* along with cerebral and coronary *vasodilation*.

**TABLE 2–1.**
Blood Gas Classifications*

| Classification | pH | $Pa_{CO_2}$ | $HCO_3^-$ | BE |
|---|---|---|---|---|
| Respiratory disorder | | | | |
|   Uncompensated acidosis | ↓ | ↑ | N | N |
|   Partly compensated acidosis | ↓ | ↑ | ↑ | ↑ |
|   Compensated acidosis | N | ↑ | ↑ | ↑ |
|   Uncompensated alkalosis | ↑ | ↓ | N | N |
|   Partly compensated alkalosis | ↑ | ↓ | ↓ | ↓ |
|   Compensated alkalosis | N | ↓ | ↓ | ↓ |
| Metabolic disorder | | | | |
|   Uncompensated acidosis | ↓ | N | ↓ | ↓ |
|   Partly compensated acidosis | ↓ | ↓ | ↓ | ↓ |
|   Compensated acidosis | N | ↓ | ↓ | ↓ |
|   Uncompensated alkalosis | ↑ | N | ↑ | ↑ |
|   Partly compensated alkalosis | ↑ | ↑ | ↑ | ↑ |
|   Compensated alkalosis | N | ↑ | ↑ | ↑ |

*Arrows = elevated or depressed values; N = normal; BE = base excess.

### *Respiratory Alkalosis*

Respiratory alkalosis is defined as a high pH, low $P_{CO_2}$, and a normal $HCO_3^-$. It is the direct result of alveolar hyperventilation. Renal compensation is accomplished by an increased excretion of bicarbonate, retention of chloride, and reduction in both the excretion of acid salts and the formation of ammonia.

A low $P_{CO_2}$ stimulates pulmonary and peripheral *vasodilation* along with cerebral and coronary *vasoconstriction*. Because of its pulmonary vasodilatory effect, mechanical hyperventilation is sometimes used to decrease cerebral edema (for closed head trauma or postanoxic encephalopathy) and to increase pulmonary perfusion (for persistent pulmonary hypertension).[6,7]

### *Metabolic Acidosis*

Metabolic acidosis is defined as a low pH, normal $P_{CO_2}$, and a low $HCO_3^-$. It can be caused by any systemic disorder that increases the production of abnormal acids in the blood or the retention of acids (or excretion of bicarbonate ion) through kidney disease. Hypoxia can result in the production of lactic acid, which may lead to a metabolic acidosis. The low pH stimulates compensation by the respiratory system, which increases alveolar ventilation and decreases $P_{CO_2}$. Frequently, however, the neonate cannot hyperventilate because of prematurity, lung disease, or central nervous system depression. In this case, the metabolic acidosis can be corrected by administration of bicarbonate.

To treat metabolic acidosis, 1 to 2 mEq/kg of sodium bicarbonate (0.5 mEq/ml) should be administered no faster than 0.5 mEq/kg/minute. Rapid administration can cause hyperosmolarity of the blood, which may lead to intraventricular hemorrhage.[8] Therefore, administration over 30 to 60 minutes is preferable.[9] If the base deficit is known, the total amount of bicarbonate necessary to correct a metabolic acidosis can be estimated[10] as follows:

$$\text{NaHCO}_3 \text{ dose(mEq)} = \text{base deficit(mEq/L)} \times \text{weight(kg)} \times 0.3 \quad (8)$$

where base deficit of blood (i.e., a negative base excess) is defined as the amount of strong alkali required to titrate a sample of 1 L of blood with a $P\text{CO}_2$ of 40 torr to a pH of 7.40. Base deficit is provided by most modern blood gas analyzers, or can be found using the Siggaard-Andersen nomogram. The bicarbonate dose calculated in the above equation should be divided into convenient portions (e.g., in half) and its administration monitored with blood gas analyses.

### Metabolic Alkalosis

Metabolic alkalosis is defined as a high pH, normal $P\text{CO}_2$, and a high $\text{HCO}_3^-$. Although rare in neonates, it can be caused by administering too much bicarbonate. Other causes include diuretic therapy and loss of potassium and chloride from drainage of gastric secretions. Theoretically, the compensatory mechanism for a metabolic alkalosis is hypoventilation, which elevates the $P\text{CO}_2$ and carbonic acid content of the blood. However, at some point this mechanism is self-limiting because an increased $P\text{CO}_2$ is a stimulus for ventilation.

## CLASSIFICATION SYSTEMS

After the major types of blood gas disorders have been defined, it is useful to relate them with a system that facilitates the clinical interpretation of blood gas analyses.

One of the earliest attempts at blood gas classification[11] is illustrated in Figure 2–4. This graphical aid is based on a plot of plasma bicarbonate ion concentration vs. arterial pH. On this graph are drawn curves connecting values of $\text{HCO}_3^-$ and pH, which exist at equal arterial $P\text{CO}_2$ values (isobars) as determined by the Henderson-Hasselbalch equation. The $P\text{CO}_2$ isobars are plotted for an arbitrary range of 20 to 80 torr. The point corresponding to pH = 7.40, $P\text{CO}_2$ = 40 and $\text{HCO}_3^-$ = 24.5 is designated as "normal." Specific points (A–H) on the isobars around

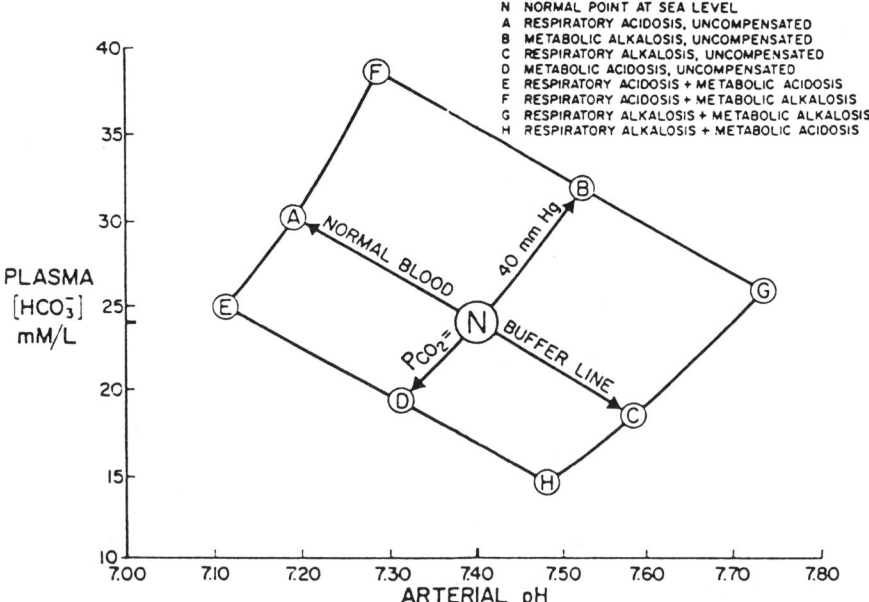

**FIG 2–4.**
A graphical approach to acid-base interpretation. (Redrawn with permission from Davenport WH: *The ABC of Acid-Base Chemistry,* ed 4. Chicago, University of Chicago Press, 1958, p 50.)

the normal values are designated with the various terms associated with blood gas abnormalities. For example, if a patient was found to have a pH = 7.20, $P_{CO_2}$ = 80 and $HCO_3^-$ = 30, the interpretation would be "uncompensated respiratory acidosis."

While useful as a way of visualizing the implications of the Henderson-Hasselbalch equation, this approach has two weaknesses. First, there is no obvious demarcation separating the points on the graph. For example, suppose a patient's blood gas analysis revealed a pH = 7.41, $P_{CO_2}$ = 48, and $HCO_3^-$ = 30, would it be classified as normal, uncompensated metabolic alkalosis, or something else? The other problem is that a particular point, such as respiratory acidosis plus metabolic alkalosis gives no clue as to which is the primary disorder and which is the compensatory reaction. The first problem is dealt with by establishing "normal ranges" for pH, $P_{CO_2}$ and $HCO_3^-$. The second involves the consideration of other factors associated with the patient's history and care that would help to discriminate the chronological order of blood gas derangements.

Before describing other classification schemes, it is instructive to first examine the philosophical foundation of the "normal range" and consider its relevance to neonatal blood gas interpretation.

## The Meaning of Normal

The concept of "normal" in modern medicine is often ambiguous and inconsistently applied. One author[12] has identified at least seven different meanings of the word *normal*. Before deciding if a patient is normal or abnormal, based on the value of a particular laboratory measurement, the clinician will often consider other correlated findings such as morphological and clinical observations. Because these other elements are not quantifiable, a subjective judgmental component makes the diagnosis about normality ambiguous. Even if the decision is restricted to just the value of a particular measurement, say pH, problems arise with demarcating the upper and lower limits of normal.

In the early 1800s, the German mathematician Johann Gauss proposed the "law of errors." This law states that if repeated measurements are made on the *same* physical object (e.g., the length of a desk), the values will vary about a mean value in a distribution that has come to be known as the gaussian or "normal" distribution. The shape of this distribution is such that 95% of all measurements will be within two standard deviations of the mean. This distribution is the basis of many commonly used statistical tests including the estimation of confidence intervals. It is important to note that the same measurements made on *different* objects (i.e., lengths of similar desks) may have any distribution, with the normal distribution as only one possibility. However, the widespread use of the normal distribution has led to its use to describe measurements of biologic variables on sick and healthy patients. It is assumed, often arbitrarily and erroneously,[13] that the results for a large enough number of people can be described by the normal distribution. Hence, calculations of a mean and standard deviation for the data are used to determine the upper and lower limits, which encompass 95% of "normal" values (i.e., the 95% confidence interval). Values outside of these limits are considered abnormal.

Besides the fact that data for a particular measurement may not be normally distributed, this approach ignores three other sources of variability.[14] These include the epidemiologic characteristics of the people selected to define the normal range (i.e., were they patients or staff volunteers?), the physiologic variability within particular individuals (i.e., due to sex, age, diet, or time of day), and the variability of the measurement device itself. Strictly speaking, a patient should not be classified as "normal" or "abnormal" unless provision has been made for the additional variability of these factors.

Nevertheless, a confidence interval based on the normal distribution is often encountered in the medical literature and, in particular, is used to define normal blood gas values.[15] For example, the normal laboratory range (mean plus or minus two standard deviations) for pH is said to be 7.35 to 7.45. In applying this strategy to neonatal blood gas interpretation, we encounter two difficulties. First, there are very little published data that can be used to determine an appropriate normal range for pH, $P_{CO_2}$, and $HCO_3^-$. Second, sick neonates, for whom a blood gas interpretation is most needed, are often supported by mechanical ventilation. Thus, normal homeostatic mechanisms are bypassed so that the resultant "normal range" of blood gas values is determined by the style of mechanical ventilation practiced by a particular institution. For example, some institutions prefer to allow high $P_{CO_2}$ values to minimize the effects of ventilating pressures and reduce the risk of pulmonary barotrauma.

For practical purposes, the designation of a normal (i.e., acceptable) range of pH, $P_{CO_2}$, and $HCO_3^-$ in our nursery and others is an arbitrary decision based on the values most frequently seen as a result of the current treatment practices.

### An Approach to Blood Gas Interpretation

Given the definition of the simple blood gas disorders, their compensatory mechanisms, normal values, and normal ranges, the interpretation of specific blood gas data is relatively straightforward. First, assume that the body will not compensate to a pH above or below the normal range. (Artificial compensatory maneuvers such as mechanical ventilation and bicarbonate administration may cause the pH to be out of the normal range and must be considered for an accurate interpretation.) Then, if the measured pH is abnormal, determine whether acidosis or alkalosis is present. Next, use the $P_{CO_2}$ and the $HCO_3^-$ to determine whether the disorder is primarily respiratory or metabolic. The mental decision-making process that might be used is illustrated in Figure 2–5. This type of flowchart is also helpful in creating computerized interpretation programs.[16] Note that if both $P_{CO_2}$ and $HCO_3^-$ are out of the normal limits, other patient information must be considered to distinguish which variable became deranged first. Hence, the disorder is simply classified as having both respiratory and metabolic components. Also, the flowchart shown in Figure 2–5 does not cover every possible combination of blood gas values. A more specific and detailed interpretation can be illustrated using a blood gas "map."

### The Blood Gas Map

In 1973, Goldberg et al.[17] described a computer-based approach for instruction about and diagnosis of acid-base disorders. By reviewing the published data on the various simple disturbances (i.e., respiratory

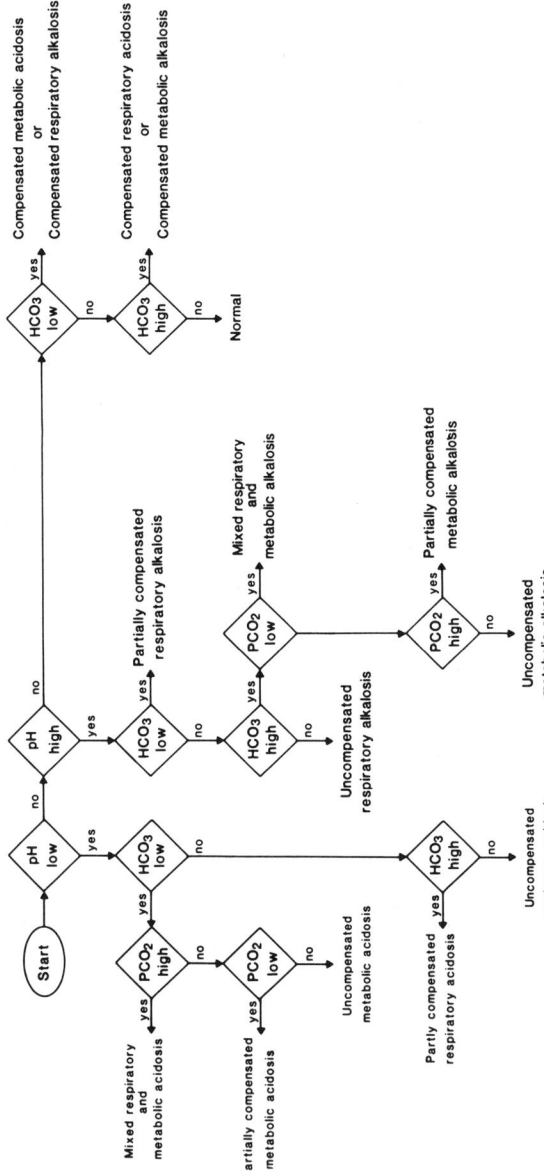

**FIG 2-5.**
A flowchart illustrating the mental process by which a set of blood gas values may be interpreted. (Modified from Hess D: The hand-held computer as a teaching tool for acid-base interpretation. *Respir Care* 1984; 29:375.)

acidosis, etc.) along with their own data, they were able to construct 95% confidence intervals along with normal values for pH, $P_{CO_2}$, and $HCO_3^-$. As a visual aid, they created a "map" or graph of pH vs. $P_{CO_2}$ along with isobars for $HCO_3^-$. Linear approximations of the confidence bands for the simple blood gas disturbances were plotted on this map (Fig 2–6). The map was used as the basis for a computer program that also considered ancillary clinical and laboratory information about the patient to arrive at the most likely differential diagnosis. As such, the program was one of the first computerized "expert systems" applied to the field of respiratory care.

We have taken a similar approach to develop an acid-base map applicable to neonatal intensive care. As mentioned previously, clinical blood gas values for infants often have different ranges than adult values. For example, pH values for sick premature infants frequently range from 7.25 to 7.40. Lower pH values are often tolerated because of the hazards associated with bicarbonate administration and because of the concern that increasing alveolar ventilation will increase the risk of pulmonary barotrauma. Figure 2–7 illustrates the neonatal acid-base map that results from these arbitrary ranges. In the absence of statistical data such as Goldberg et al.[17] used, the areas on the map demarcating

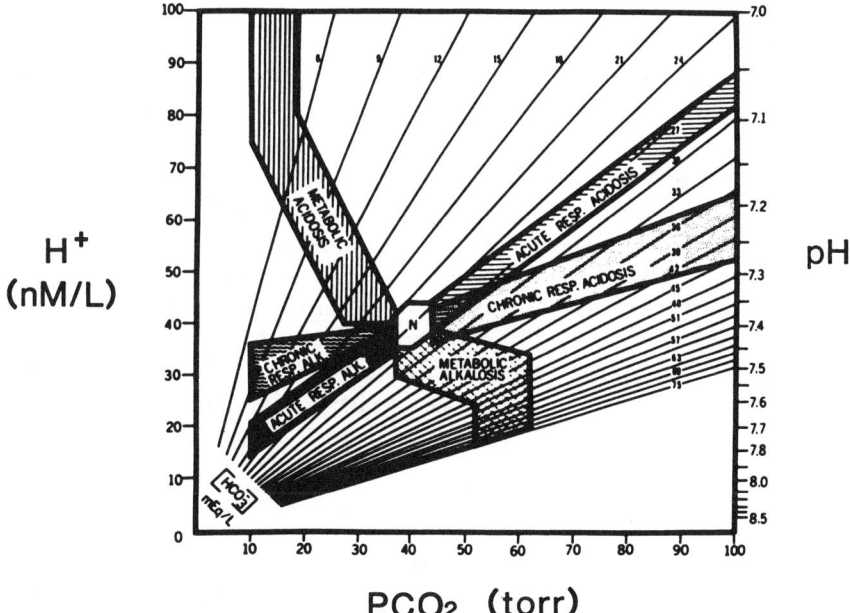

**FIG 2–6.**
An adult acid-base map. (From Goldberg M, Green SB, Moss MV, et al: Computer-based instruction and diagnosis of acid-base disorders. *JAMA* 1973; 223:269. Used by permission.)

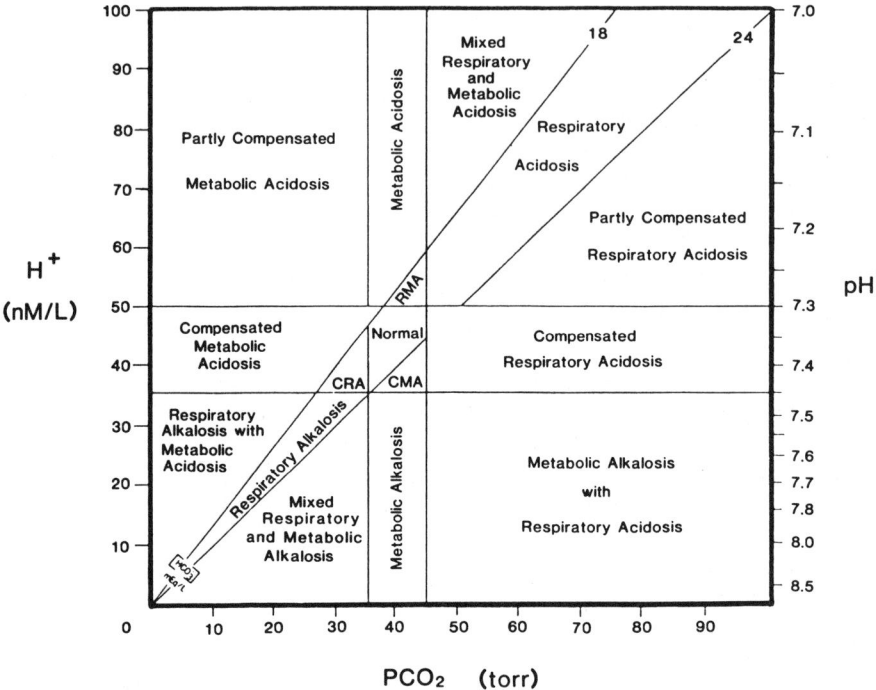

**FIG 2–7.**
A neonatal acid-base map. *CRA* = compensated respiratory alkalosis; *CMA* = compensated metabolic alkalosis; and *RMA* = mixed respiratory and metabolic acidosis.

the various disorder classifications are based entirely on the given ranges and the Henderson-Hasselbalch equation. When either a respiratory or metabolic process could be the cause of the disturbance, the most likely clinical diagnosis is given. For example, in a very premature infant a high $P_{CO_2}$ along with a high $HCO_3^-$ would most likely be the result of administering too much bicarbonate to an infant that already had respiratory acidosis. Thus, the differential diagnosis of "metabolic alkalosis with a component of respiratory acidosis" is proposed. This map has been successfully used as the basis of a computerized expert system for the management of neonatal mechanical ventilation.[18]

## Assessing Oxygenation

Normal newborns have a relatively high shunt fraction compared to older children due to both intrapulmonary and extrapulmonary shunts. These shunts decrease with age so that arterial $P_{O_2}$ increases from about 50 torr at birth to over 80 torr (in room air) at 1 week. The level at which $Pa_{O_2}$ should be kept during mechanical ventilation is a matter of controversy, but the consensus appears to be 50 to 80 torr. Arterial $P_{O_2}$ values above 100 torr in premature infants should be avoided because hyperoxemia has been associated with blindness caused by retrolental fibroplasia.

As mentioned previously, a complete evaluation of an infant's oxygenation requires knowledge of both arterial $P_{O_2}$ and the hemoglobin content. In addition, clinical observations such as skin color and capillary refill provide useful information for making clinical decisions.

If simultaneously drawn samples of arterial and mixed-venous blood are available, venous-admixture (shunt) can be estimated from the equation

$$\text{shunt (\%)} = \frac{Cc_{O_2} - Ca_{O_2}}{Cc_{O_2} - C\bar{v}_{O_2}} \tag{9}$$

where $Cc_{O_2}$ is pulmonary capillary oxygen content (from equation 4 assuming 100% saturation) and $C\bar{v}_{O_2}$ is mixed venous oxygen content. Unfortunately, relatively few infants have catheters placed that would allow true mixed-venous blood samples. As an alternative, various indices have been proposed[19] that are intended to relate inspired oxygen concentrations to the resultant $Pa_{O_2}$. Such indicators are meant to quantitate the degree of lung disease and, conversely, to assess the relative risk of oxygen toxicity. Perhaps the simplest index is the $Pa_{O_2}/F_{I_{O_2}}$ ratio. Although easy to calculate at the bedside, it does not take into account the effect of different levels of $Pa_{CO_2}$. Other popular indices include the $P_{A_{O_2}} - Pa_{O_2}$ gradient, i.e., the alveolar-arterial difference in partial pressure of $O_2$ (sometimes written as $A - aDO_2$ or $P(A-a)O_2$), and the $Pa_{O_2}/P_{A_{O_2}}$ ratio, the latter being comparatively more constant in the face of a changing $F_{I_{O_2}}$.[20]

One of the primary complications of prolonged mechanical ventilation is the chronic lung disease known as bronchopulmonary dysplasia. Although its exact etiology has not been described, it is commonly believed that high ventilating pressures along with high inspired oxygen concentrations are chiefly responsible. A useful index that takes into account both of these variables along with the level of ventilation (i.e., $Pa_{CO_2}$) is the *pressure cost of oxygenation* (PCO):

$$\text{PCO (cm } H_2O) = \frac{\bar{P}aw \text{ (cm } H_2O)}{Pa_{O_2}/P_{A_{O_2}}} \tag{10}$$

where $\bar{P}aw$ is mean airway pressure.

## REFERENCES

1. Silverman WA: *Retrolental Fibroplasia: A Modern Parable.* New York, Grune & Stratton, 1980.
2. McPherson SP, Spearman CB: *Respiratory Therapy Equipment,* ed 3. St Louis, CV Mosby Co, 1985, p 205.
3. Slonim NB, Hamilton LH: *Respiratory Physiology,* ed 2. St Louis, CV Mosby Co, 1976.
4. Egan DF: *Fundamentals of Respiratory Therapy,* ed 3. St Louis, CV Mosby Co, 1977.
5. Shapiro BA, Harrison RA, Trout CA: *Clinical Application of Respiratory Care.* Chicago, Year Book Medical Publishers, 1975.
6. Branson RD, Hurst JM, DeHaven CB: Use of high frequency jet ventilation during mechanical ventilation for control of elevated cranial pressure: A case report. *Respir Care* 1984; 29:1221.
7. Peckham GJ, Fox WW: Physiologic factors affecting pulmonary artery pressure in infants with persistent pulmonary hypertension. *J Pediatr* 1978; 93:105.
8. Papile L, Burstein J, Burstein R, et al: Relationship of intravenous sodium bicarbonate infusions and cerebral intraventricular hemorrhage. *J Pediatr* 1978; 93:834.
9. Goldsmith JP, Karotkin EH (eds): *Assisted Ventilation of the Neonate.* Philadelphia, WB Saunders Co, 1981.
10. Grodins FS, Yamashiro SM: *Respiratory Function of the Lung and its Control.* New York, Macmillan Publishing Co, 1978.
11. Davenport HW: *The ABC of Acid-Base Chemistry,* ed 4. Chicago, University of Chicago Press, 1958.
12. Murphy EA: The normal. *Am J Epidemiol.* 1973; 98:403.
13. Elveback LR, Guillier CL, Keating FR: Health, normality and the ghost of Gauss. *JAMA* 1970; 211:69.
14. Feinstein AR: The derangement of the "normal range," in Feinstein AR. *Clinical Biostatistics.* St Louis, CV Mosby Co, 1977.
15. Shapiro BA, Harrison RA, Walton JR: *Clinical Application of Blood Gases.* Chicago, Year Book Medical Publishers, 1977.
16. Hess D: The hand-held computer as a teaching tool for acid-base interpretation. *Respir Care* 1984; 29:375.
17. Goldberg M, Green SB, Moss MV, et al: Computer-based instruction and diagnosis of acid-base disorders. *JAMA* 1973; 223:269.
18. Carlo WA, Pacifico L, Chatburn RL, et al: Efficacy of computer-assisted management of respiratory failure in neonates. *Pediatrics* 1986; 78:139.
19. Hess, D, Maxwell C: Which is the best index of oxygenation—$P(A-a)_{O_2}$, $Pa_{O_2}/PA_{O_2}$ or $Pa_{O_2}/FI_{O_2}$? *Respir Care* 1985; 30:961.
20. Gilbert R, Keighley JF: The arterial-alveolar oxygen tension ratio: An index of gas exchange applicable to varying inspired oxygen concentrations. *Am Rev Respir Dis* 1974; 109:142.

# 3

# Physiologic Monitoring and Pulmonary Function

Tilo Gerhardt, M.D.
Lars P. Jensen, M.D., M.B., Ch.B., M.Med.

## PRENATAL MONITORING

### Characteristics of Fetal Heart Rate Patterns

Electronic monitoring of the fetus, initially developed to evaluate fetal status during labor, has now largely replaced biochemical tests (e.g., estriol levels) used to monitor the fetus before birth. The *cardiotocograph* or *fetal heart rate (FHR) monitor* has two components, one to recognize and process fetal heart rate, and the other to recognize uterine contractions.[1,2] Direct, internal, or invasive monitoring refers to devices attached directly to the fetus and placed within the uterine cavity, while external or noninvasive monitoring depends on recordings obtained from equipment applied to the maternal abdominal wall. Both heart rate and uterine contractions may be recorded with invasive or noninvasive devices.

### Baseline Fetal Heart Rate

A baseline fetal heart rate of 120 to 160 beats per minute is regarded as normal. Rates above 160 beats per minute are described as *tachycardia* and lower than 120 beats per minute as *bradycardia*. Tachycardia may occur in some cases of fetal hypoxia. Other causes of fetal tachycardia include maternal tachycardia, maternal treatment with β-agonists to halt premature labor, fetal infection, and extreme prematurity. Bradycardia is the initial and most frequent response of the fetus to acute hypoxia or asphyxia. A continued fetal heart rate below 100 beats per minute, not associated with heart block, will eventually lead to decompensation. Other nonasphyxial causes of bradycardia include heart block and drugs such as local anesthetic agents and β-blockers.

## Fetal Heart Rate Variability

Two types of fetal heart rate variability are described. *Short-term variability*, also known as beat-to-beat variability is the difference between adjacent beats or several beats. *Long-term variability* consists of irregular crude sine waves of 3 to 6 per minute of the fetal heart tracing. The pattern of variability of fetal heart rate may be classified as follows: (1) *normal*, with an amplitude range of six beats per minute; (2) *decreased*, with an amplitude range of less than six beats per minute; (3) *saltatory*, where the amplitude is greater than 25 beats per minute. A decreased or absent fetal heart rate variability may be due to hypoxia and may precede any abnormal types of decelerations. Other nonasphyxial causes of decreased variability in the fetal heart rate include anencephaly; drugs such as morphine, meperidine (Demerol), diazepam, magnesium sulphate, and atropine; and complete heart block. A saltatory pattern has been associated with cord complication and is considered a sign of increased fetal distress when accompanied by other fetal heart rate abnormalities.

## Basic Fetal Heart Rate Patterns

Four basic fetal heart rate patterns may occur in association with uterine contractions: (1) *early or type 1 decelerations*; (2) *late or type 2 decelerations*; (3) *variable decelerations*; and (4) *accelerations*.

### *Early (Type 1) Decelerations*
Early decelerations are due to head compression and on a recording appear as a mirror image of the contraction itself (Fig 3–1). The decelerations begin with the onset of contraction, rarely fall below 100 beats per minute, and return to baseline at the completion of the contraction. Early decelerations are most commonly seen in the second stage of labor and are believed to be caused by vagal discharge due to increased intracranial pressure. These decelerations are not associated with fetal distress or poor fetal outcome.

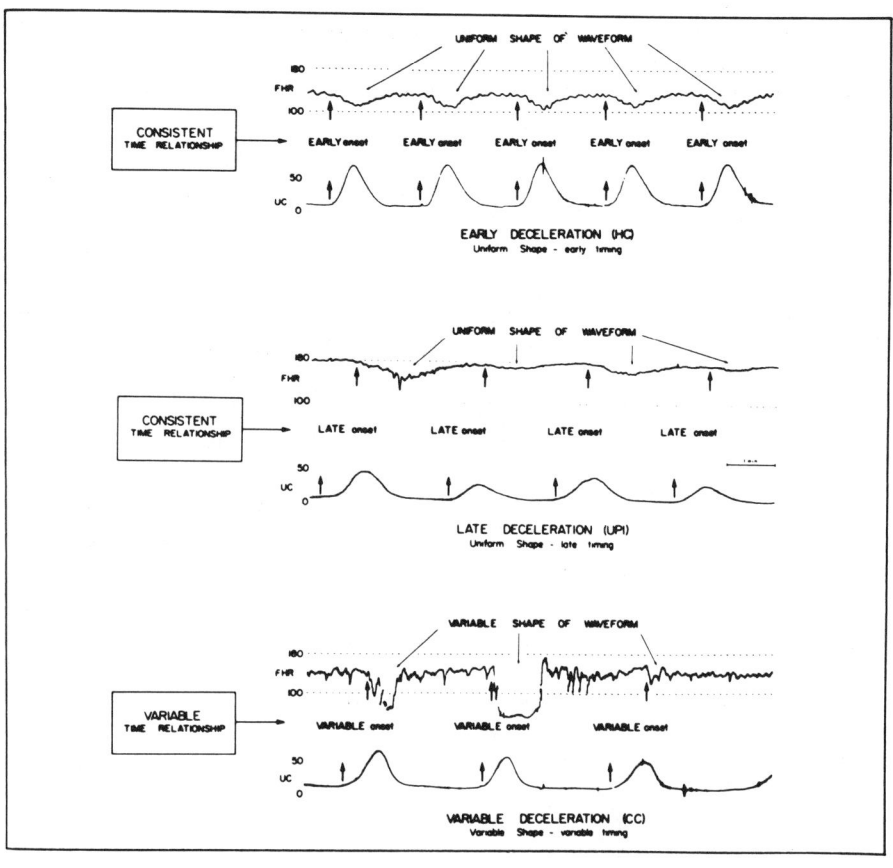

**FIG 3–1.**
Fetal heart rate decelerations in relation to the time of onset of uterine contractions. HC = head compression; UPI = uteroplacental insufficiency; CC = cord compression. (From Hon EG: *An Atlas of Fetal Heart Rate Patterns.* New Haven, Conn, Harty Press, 1968. Used by permission.)

### Late (Type 2) Decelerations

The onset, trough, and recovery of late decelerations are delayed 10 to 30 seconds beyond the onset, apex, and resolution of the contractions and are usually found in association with acute or chronic fetoplacental vascular insufficiency (see Fig 3–1). Late decelerations are always a cause of concern and should be dealt with immediately.[3, 4] Two types of late decelerations are described by Creasy[5]: (1) *reflex late decelerations* associated with a sudden acute insult such as maternal hypotension and (2) *myocardial hypoxia late decelerations* due to an insufficient bolus of oxygenated blood from the placenta to support myocardial action. When late decelerations occur, maternal position change and oxygen administration may improve oxygen delivery to the fetus.

The following tentative conclusions with regard to late decelerations in labor can be made[6]:

1. When late decelerations develop, there is an increased incidence of low Apgar scores and asphyxia.
2. Associated fetal heart rate baseline alterations (saltatory, fixed tachycardia) often develop.
3. About 50% of late decelerations will indicate fetal distress during labor, and one third of the infants will be born neurologically depressed.
4. Among late deceleration cases, small fetuses more often have low Apgar scores, preceded by tachycardia, fixed baseline, and clinical distress.
5. One half of small infants with late decelerations may be born neurologically depressed and have a very high incidence of neonatal morbidity and death.
6. Premature infants seem to respond differently and recover faster than term and postmature infants subjected to similar stresses.
7. The unfavorable conditions seem to accumulate in this sequence: small fetus from a pathologic gestation and subsequent development of late decelerations. These fetuses will have intrapartum distress terminating in cesarean section, a low Apgar score, and high incidence of neonatal complications. Appropriate intervention by the obstetrician may prevent the above sequence of events.
8. There is an extremely low likelihood of neonatal problems (0.5%) when there are no late decelerations of the fetal heart rate.

### Variable Decelerations

These decelerations are inconsistent in configuration, with variable relationship to the onset of the contraction (see Fig 3–1). They are generally of short duration with an abrupt onset and resolution. Variable decelerations appear to be caused by cord compression with variable impact on the fetus depending on the duration and completeness of the cord occlusion. Again, as with late decelerations, efforts should be made to abolish them.

### Accelerations

Accelerations with contractions appear to have no particular prognostic significance, as opposed to the accelerations seen with fetal movement in the antenatal period.

## Other Patterns

Other patterns such as *prolonged bradycardia* and *sinusoidal patterns* are not common and do not fit into the classifications above. Prolonged bradycardia indicates fetal distress. The sinusoidal pattern is rare but appears to be associated with fetal anemia as seen with severe Rh isoimmunization and fetal-maternal hemorrhage.[7]

## Fetal Scalp Blood Sampling in Labor

Acid-base evaluation by *fetal scalp sampling* is an essential part of monitoring of labor in any large center. All clinicians involved with labor and delivery should be familiar with the indications, technique, and interpretation of the results obtained. The following are indications for acid-base determination in the fetus[8]:

A. Fetal distress as indicated by
   1. Bradycardia
   2. Fetal heart rate decelerations
      a. Late decelerations
      b. Moderate to severe variable decelerations
   3. Tachycardia
   4. Diminished variability
      a. Progressive loss of variability without clinical explanation
      b. Persistent, diminished, or absent variability
   5. Meconium-stained amniotic fluid with vertex presentation
B. Clinical situations
   1. Maternal acidosis
   2. Evaluation of fetal status
   3. Evaluation of the effect of obstetric analgesia and/or anesthesia

The technique of fetal scalp blood sampling requires a skill that is easily mastered. Equipment should be complete before attempting the sampling and the blood gas analyzer adequately calibrated. Several sources may lead to error in fetal blood sampling. Severe fetal caput formation, contamination of the sample with amniotic fluid, bubbles in the capillary collection tube, clotting of samples, and/or a delay in blood gas analysis may give a false result.

Complications from fetal scalp sampling are rare but do occur. The major complication is laceration of the fetal scalp, which in some cases requires suturing. Prolonged bleeding from the scalp may be due to a coagulation disorder. Other complications are infection or leakage of cerebrospinal fluid.

Lauersen has described the following clinical application of intrapartum fetal pH values.[8]

| | |
|---|---|
| Normal pH | ≥7.25, repeat as indicated by fetal condition |
| Prepathologic pH | 7.20–7.24, repeat within 15 minutes |
| Acidotic pH | ≤7.19, repeat immediately and obtain concomitant maternal venous pH |

Fetal blood sampling for acid-base measurement during labor can aid the clinician in making adequate decisions and hopefully avoiding unnecessary cesarean sections. The limitations of this valuable diagnostic tool should be placed in perspective, taking the whole clinical picture into account.

## Antepartum Monitoring

Monitoring of the fetus in the antepartum period is presently achieved by a combination of clinical evaluation (high-risk patient), ultrasound imaging, and electronic monitoring. The latter is divided into two categories, nonstress testing (NST) and contraction stress testing (CST). Contraction can be induced by intravenous oxytocin administration or nipple stimulation.

### *Nonstress Test*

Nonstress testing involves an external cardiotocograph with the patient in the semi-Fowler's position. Fetal heart rate, uterine activity, and fetal movements are graphically recorded. Nonstress testing varies between centers, but the following is widely accepted[9-11]: (1) *reactive* NST: at least two fetal movements associated with acceleration of fetal heart rate of at least 15 beats per minute in a period of 20 minutes of observation and (2) nonreactive NST: no fetal movements or less than two accelerations of heart rate with movement in a period of 20 minutes of observation (Fig 3–2).

### *Contraction Stress Test*

Three 60-second contractions in a 10-minute period are necessary to simulate labor. Fetal heart rate and contraction patterns are monitored by means of external cardiotocography. Late decelerations associated with more than 50% of the contractions are regarded as a positive contraction stress test, even if less than three contractions occur in a 10-minute period (Fig 3–3). A positive CST has been associated with fetal compromise in 50% to 80% of the cases. Conditions that may contraindicate the use of contraction stress test include: (1) threatened preterm labor or history of preterm labor; (2) placenta previa; (3) polyhydramnios; (4) premature rupture of the membranes; (5) previous classical cesarean section or other uterine scar; and (6) incompetent cervix.

The contraction stress can have the following outcomes:

1. Negative CST: no late decelerations and normal baseline fetal heart rate.

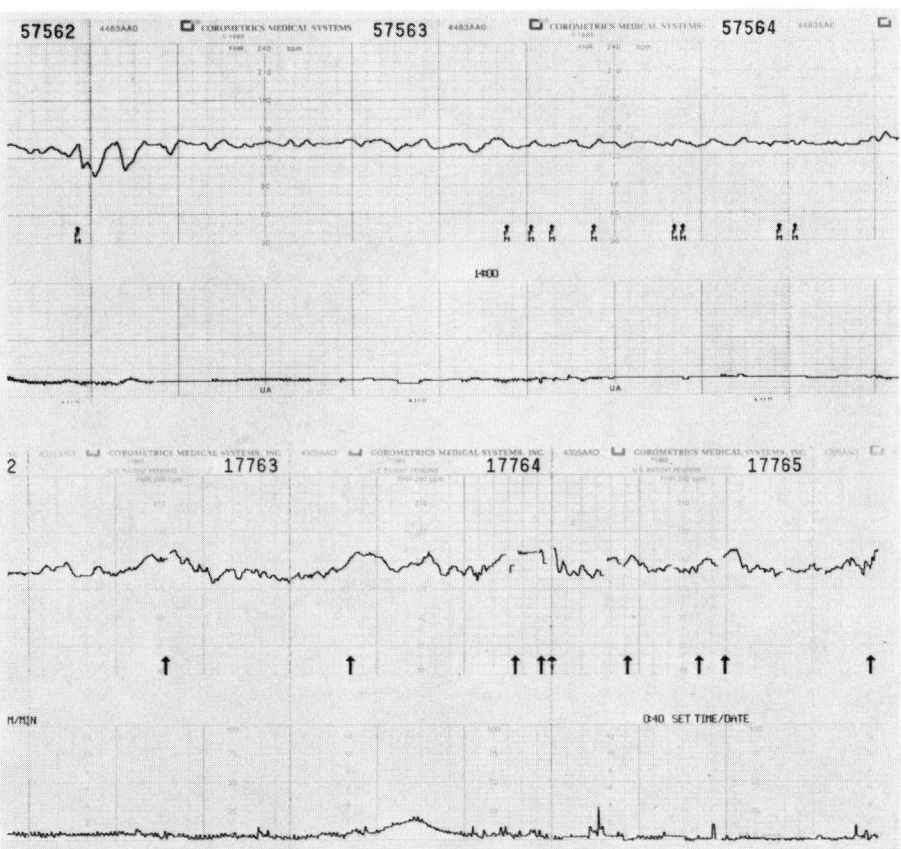

**FIG 3–2.**
Fetal monitoring strips showing a nonreactive nonstress test *(top strip)* and a reactive nonstress test *(bottom strip)*. Fetal heart rate *(FHR)* is represented by the upper tracing and uterine activity *(UA)* by the lower tracing in each strip. Fetal movement marked with *arrows*.

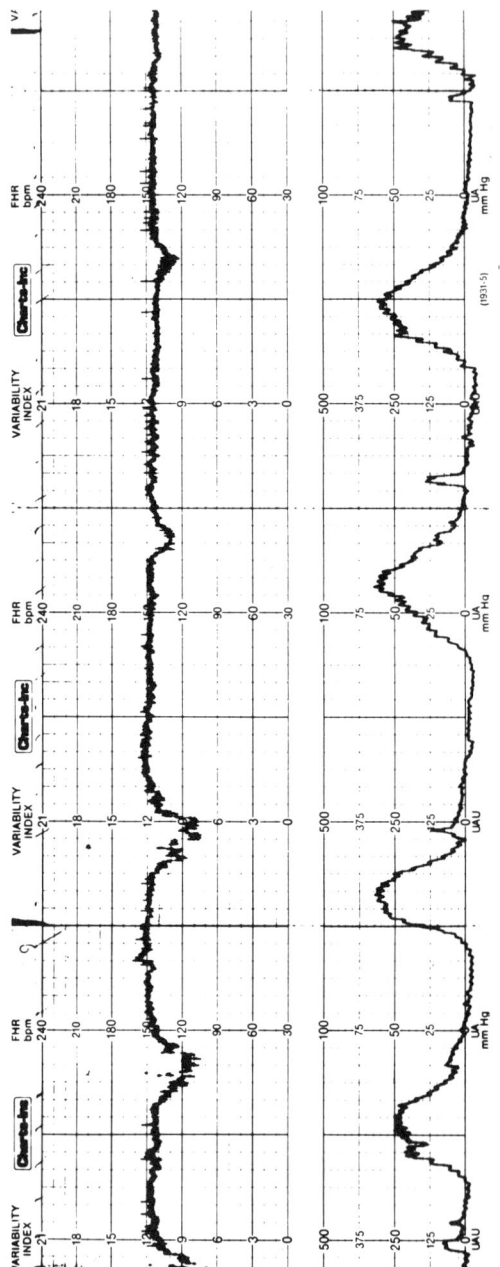

**FIG 3–3.**
Fetal monitoring strip showing a positive CST. Both fetal heart rate *(FHR)* *(upper tracing)* and uterine activity *(UA)* *(lower tracing)* are recorded graphically. The decelerations are persistently late.

2. Positive CST: persistent late decelerations, even with less than three contractions in 10 minutes.
3. Suspicious CST: intermittent late decelerations in 30% of contractions.
4. Unsatisfactory CST: not able to achieve three contractions in 10 minutes. Poor quality recording.

Several schemes are available for antepartum fetal heart rate testing. However, it must be emphasized that patients should be managed with the total clinical situation in mind. A decision to deliver the fetus in the presence of abnormal fetal heart rate testing is strongly influenced by pulmonary maturity. A simplified chain of events would be the following:

| Nonstress Test (NST) | |
| --- | --- |
| Reactive | Nonreactive |
| Repeat once or twice weekly depending on the clinical situation | Continue observation another 30 minutes; if still nonreactive, do CST |
| Contraction Stress Test (CST) | |
| Negative | Positive |
| Go back to NST as the situation demands | Consider delivery |

### Biophysical Profile

A biophysical profile to evaluate fetal condition (Table 3-1) has been proposed and developed by Manning[12] et al. and is rapidly gaining ground in clinical obstetrics. Fetal breathing movements, fetal body movements, fetal tone, qualitative amniotic fluid volume assessment, and the nonstress test are used with a scoring system as described below. Detailed ultrasound assessment is required for the first four variables. This is combined with a nonstress test to give an overall picture of the situation. Combined with clinical data, the biophysical profile appears to be remarkably accurate for evaluation of fetal well-being.

Adding the scores for individual variables produces the final biophysical profile score (BPS). A score of eight or more indicates a satisfactory fetal condition. A score of six is suspect, and the profile should be repeated in 4 to 6 hours. However, if oligohydramnios is present, delivery is indicated. Delivery is indicated with a score of four or less if the fetus is mature enough. It must be emphasized that no tests of fetal well-being are infallible, and therefore they cannot provide com-

**TABLE 3–1.**
Biophysical Profile Scoring

| Biophysical Variable | Normal (BPS = 2) | Abnormal (BPS = 0) |
| --- | --- | --- |
| Fetal Breathing Movements (FBM) | At least 1 episode of FBM lasting ≥30 sec in a 30-min period of observation | Absent FBM or no episode of ≥30 sec in 30 min |
| Gross Body Movement | At least 3 discrete body-limb movements in 30 min (episodes of active continuous movement considered a single movement) | Two or fewer episodes of body-limb movements in 30 min |
| Fetal Tone | At least 1 episode of active extension with return to flexion of fetal limb(s) or trunk (opening and closing of hand considered normal tone) | Either slow extension with return to partial flexion or movement of limb in full extension or absent fetal movement |
| Qualitative Amniotic Fluid Volume (AFV) | At least 1 pocket of amniotic fluid that measures ≥1 cm in two perpendicular planes | Either no amniotic fluid pockets or one ≤1 cm in two perpendicular planes |
| NST: Reactive Fetal Heart | At least two episodes of FHR acceleration of ≥15 beats per minute associated with fetal movement in 30 min | Fewer than two episodes of acceleration of FHR or acceleration ≤15 beats per minute in 30 min |

plete reassurance. Clinical evaluation remains the cornerstone in monitoring the fetus before birth.

## NEONATAL MONITORING

Monitoring of physiologic variables in newborn infants serves the following purposes:

1. Surveillance: Vital functions are monitored continuously, and an alarm sounds as soon as a deviation from the normal range occurs. Surveillance can also be applied to the function of life-supporting equipment used in the nursery.
2. Quality control: Physiologic variables are monitored to give feedback information about the effects of therapies and nursing procedures on these variables. Detrimental effects can be detected and procedures modified.
3. Diagnosis: Continuous monitoring can be used to clarify clinical observations and to identify possible causes of a medical problem. This mostly requires continuous recording of the monitored signal.

4. Research: Monitoring is required to control the environmental and physiologic conditions under which research is performed. To describe physiologic variables and their changes with age, during a disease process, or in response to a specific therapy, continuous monitoring is necessary.

Monitoring can be invasive or noninvasive, continuous, or intermittent. Monitors can be preconfigured or modular. The latter consist of different modules, each capable of monitoring one variable. The monitoring ability is, therefore, flexible and can be tailored to the infant's needs. An oscilloscope and a recorder can also be part of the system. In contrast, preconfigured monitors are less flexible because they are limited to monitoring certain vital functions predetermined by the manufacturer. In most newborn intensive care nurseries, both types of monitors are in use.

During the last 15 years with the advances in electronic circuitry and feedback from the users to the manufacturers, the quality and reliability of monitors has improved. New transducers have been developed that can noninvasively measure physiologic variables that previously could only be measured by invasive techniques. All this has broadened our understanding of neonatal physiology, improving neonatal care.

The least traumatic way of monitoring is noninvasive. The most information is gained by continuous monitoring. In this chapter, the monitoring of heart rate, respiration, blood pressure, temperature, transcutaneous gas tension, and oxygen saturation will be discussed.

## Heart Rate and Respiration

Most *preconfigured* monitors combine the ability to monitor both heart rate and respiration. The electrocardiogram (ECG) is obtained from two electrodes placed on the chest and a third placed on the leg to serve as reference electrode. Visual inspection of the ECG on an oscilloscope is an advantage over digital recording of heart rate alone because artifacts distorting the signal can be appreciated and pathologic conditions such as arrhythmias can be identified. The quality of the ECG obtained is not sufficient to be suitable for more detailed cardiologic evaluations. This is mainly due to improper positioning of the electrodes that also must serve to measure changes in impedance as a reflection of breathing activity.

Heart rate is derived electronically from the QRS complexes by obtaining a moving average of the RR intervals of three to five beats and displayed in digital form. This averaging may mask dramatic beat-to-beat changes in heart rate as may occur with arrhythmias or a sudden vagal stimulus. If beat-to-beat analysis is of interest, a strip chart recorder or a digital storage oscilloscope needs to be used to depict the signal. At present, beat-to-beat heart rate analysis is mainly used as a research tool to reflect vagal and sympathetic responses of newborn infants to various stimuli. Unlike in the fetus, heart rate variability in the newborn does not reflect well-being, stress, or normality of autonomic cardiac function in an easily interpretable way. Computer analysis of the signal for its power spectrum and relation to other physiologic variables may yield more useful information in the future.[13]

Respiration is usually monitored by *impedance pneumography*. Impedance is measured through the two chest leads also used to obtain the ECG and reflects the resistance to flow that a high-frequency current encounters when it flows from one lead to the other. Impedance is determined by the distance and the material between the electrodes. During a respiratory cycle, this distance and tissue composition will change with air entering or leaving the lungs. The resulting changes in impedance are proportional to the size of the tidal volume and are electronically processed to give a respiratory waveform.[14] The waveform can be shown on the oscilloscope and further processed to give respiratory rate.

The limitation of this technique is its extreme sensitivity to motion and position change because this will result in a change in distance of the electrodes and, therefore, in a respiratory signal. This technique cannot reliably detect *obstructive apnea*, a condition where airflow ceases but the infant continues to make respiratory efforts or struggles.[15] Obstructive apnea may be suggested by a sudden decrease in size of the respiratory signal associated with a drop in heart rate.[16]

Newborns are abdominal breathers and show little change in thoracic diameter with each breath. Impedance signals, therefore, require much amplification. This may lead to impedance changes due to cardiac activity being picked up as respiratory signals. Newer cardiorespiratory monitors, therefore, have electronic circuits that compare heart rate with respiratory rate and send an alarm if both should be identical. A better respiratory signal can be detected by placing the electrodes in the midaxillary line in the lower third of the thorax where changes in tissue composition with diaphragmatic activity are more pronounced.

Changes in breathing pattern and the presence of paradoxical breathing may also interfere with the detection of a reliable respiratory signal. The sensitivity of the monitor is therefore frequently increased by the caretaker to avoid false apnea alarms. This will lead to a significant loss of information when the breathing pattern is recorded. Most normal breaths will exceed the limits of the tracing so that their true size cannot be judged and compared to smaller ineffectual or obstructed breaths. All breaths may appear to have the same size, and periods of hypoventilation or hyperventilation cannot be distinguished.

Cardiorespiratory monitors are equipped with alarms for heart rate and respiratory rate. Heart rate alarms can be set for a wide range of heart rates depending on the infant's age and basal heart rate during sleep. Respiratory alarms are usually set to trigger after a period of apnea of 10, 15, or 20 seconds' duration. There are many false alarms because of problems with leads and electrodes or because the signal picked up is too small. Obstructive apnea may not be detected unless bradycardia occurs. Therefore, if only a single variable can be monitored, heart rate should be monitored rather than respiration.

Marking of apneic and bradycardic episodes on the infant's chart in response to the monitor alarms is inaccurate because not all episodes are marked and many episodes are false alarms.[17] The only method to accurately determine frequency, duration, and nature of an infant's apneic and bradycardic episodes is by recording heart rate and respiration over 12 or 24 hours and analyzing the episodes from this hard copy. The recording will also clarify whether a bradycardic episode was triggered by an apnea or whether the bradycardia occurred independently of apnea, the latter suggesting the presence of obstructive apnea. This recording, called a *pneumocardiogram*, has been used widely in preterm infants ready for discharge, in newborns at increased risk for *sudden infant death syndrome* because of family history or other epidemiologic factors, and in older infants with a history of aborted sudden infant death episodes, as an indicator of the risk to suffer a sudden death. Recent prospective studies, however, have shown no correlation between the findings on the pneumocardiogram and outcome.[18]

*Respiratory flow* needs to be monitored to obtain a more detailed analysis of breathing pattern. This can be done noninvasively by taping a *thermistor* or a $CO_2$ sampling capillary to the upper lip below the nostrils. The thermistor is a rapidly responding electronic thermometer that senses temperature differences between inspiratory and expiratory gas. Carbon dioxide in the expiratory gas can be measured by a *capnograph* or a *mass spectrometer* sampling at low flow. Both systems will fail to detect any flow if the infant breathes through the mouth. In older infants, the sensors are difficult to keep in place, and the infants may need to be restrained.

A monitoring unit capable of recording heart rate, respiratory impedance, and nasal airflow will allow the differentiation between central and obstructive apnea and can describe the sequence of events more precisely than a pneumocardiogram alone. This monitoring system can be supplemented by recording *transcutaneous* oxygen tension ($TcPO_2$) and transcutaneous carbon dioxide tension ($TcPCO_2$), and this will indicate whether hypoxia and hypercapnia develop during the episodes or whether blood gas change preceded an episode.[19]

**Blood Pressure**

Blood pressure should be monitored from any arterial catheter placed to obtain blood samples. Umbilical artery catheters are most frequently used in neonates, but accurate blood pressure recordings can also be obtained from peripheral arteries such as the radial or the posterior tibial arteries.[20] The risks and complications associated with indwelling catheters are not increased by connecting the line to a *pressure transducer*. However, much information can be gained about an infant's cardiovascular condition. The tubing connecting the catheter to the transducer should be as short as possible, noncompliant, free of any air bubbles or blood clots, with as few connectors and stopcocks as possible in order not to dampen the pressure signal. The transducer should have a minimal volume displacement with pressure changes and an adequate frequency response.[21] A disposable pressure monitoring kit needs to be used when infusing fluids and electrolytes through the arterial catheter and monitoring blood pressure simultaneously. The whole system consists of a special Y-piece equipped with a valve and the appropriate connectors and must be set up under sterile conditions and kept sterile during its use. Balancing and calibration of the transducer is usually done automatically by the monitor. It is, however, recommended that the calibration be checked with a mercury manometer at regular intervals. The pressure signal can be shown on the oscilloscope and its quality assessed. A signal with a lack of detail suggests dampening, possibly due to blood clots or air bubbles, position of the catheter tip adjacent to the vessel wall, or a problem with the connecting tubing or the transducer itself. The signal is processed electronically, and systolic, diastolic, and mean blood pressures are shown in digital form.

The decision to act therapeutically on an abnormal blood pressure should not be based on one measurement alone. The calibration and proper setup of the entire system should be checked. Blood pressure should be measured by another noninvasive technique before accepting the abnormal value as real. The clinical status, mainly skin perfusion, acid-base balance, and renal output should be taken into consideration.

The *oscillometric* method of measuring arterial blood pressure noninvasively has been perfected and shows good correlation with the directly measured pressure.[21] Only 3.8% of measurements deviate by greater than 10 mm Hg from a simultaneously obtained mean blood pressure through an umbilical artery catheter.[22] However, this difference may be intolerable in infants with very low birth weight whose mean blood pressure may be only 30 mm Hg. Some instruments seem to overestimate pressure in hypotensive infants.[23]

To utilize the oscillometric method for measuring arterial blood pressure, a cuff applied to an extremity is inflated to above systolic pressure. The pressure changes in the cuff due to the pulsation of the arteries beneath are analyzed. Pressure changes are minimal when cuff pressure is above systolic pressure, reach a maximum at approximately mean blood pressure, and then decrease with further decrease in cuff pressure. These changes are analyzed and processed electronically, and mean, systolic, and diastolic blood pressure are displayed digitally and updated every 1 to 5 minutes. The inflation of the cuff and gradual deflation are controlled electronically. The size of the cuff is critical for accurate results. Its width should be half of the circumference of the extremity being used. The error is smaller with a cuff too wide rather than too small. The oscillometric method does not require another sensor (for example, a Doppler sensor to detect flow); it can be used on different extremities and repeated continuously without requiring additional nursing time.

**Temperature**

Thermistors function on the principle of electricity-conducting wires that change their resistance with changes in temperature. These thermistors are very sensitive and 10 times as accurate as the mercury thermometers frequently used to measure the infant's temperature. Thermistors are used to measure core, skin, and environmental temperature. Because of their accuracy and reliability thermistors are used to *servocontrol* the infant's thermal environment in incubators and under radiant warmers. This is done by a feedback loop measuring continuously an infant's skin temperature and adjusting the environmental temperature so that skin temperature is kept at a predetermined level. Metabolic rate is at a minimum when skin is well perfused and warm (36.5°C), and skin temperature is 0 to 0.5°C lower than the core temperature.[24]

A temperature servocontrol system allows small fluctuations in the infant's temperature because the heater is turned on and off, triggered by signals from the skin thermistor. The switch-on is necessarily triggered by a lower temperature than the switch-off. If the thermistor becomes detached from the skin or becomes wet, it will measure a lower temperature than true skin temperature, and the incubator may overheat, leading to hyperthermia and apnea in the infant.[25] The thermistors are sensitive to radiant energy and will measure a higher temperature than true skin temperature if exposed to radiant heat, thus leading to a reduction in heater output and exposure of the infant to cold stress. When radiant warmers are used as sole heat source for the infant or together with an incubator, the thermistor should be shielded with a *heat-reflecting patch*.

When skin temperature is controlled at 36.5°C, the development of hypothermia or hyperthermia may not occur because core temperature will also remain stable. The metabolic equivalents of hypothermia or hyperthermia can be detected, however, by the temperature differences between skin and environmental air. A large difference suggests an increased metabolic rate and reflects a febrile condition. A small difference, or a situation where environmental temperature is warmer than skin temperature, suggests hypothermia, as seen in sepsis, or indicates excessive heat losses by routes other than convection, such as radiation and evaporation.

## Transcutaneous Gas Pressure Monitoring

### Transcutaneous Oxygen Tension

Transcutaneous $PO_2$ ($TcPO_2$) monitors were developed and introduced into the care of the neonate by Huch et al. in 1972.[26] Transcutaneous $PO_2$ monitoring has been widely used since the second half of the seventies, changing neonatal care dramatically. Transcutaneous $PO_2$ is used in the immediate postnatal period to determine inspired oxygen ($FI_{O_2}$) needs and speed up weaning from oxygen in newborns with transient tachypnea and asphyxia who only have a transient pulmonary problem for which no arterial line is placed. Transcutaneous $PO_2$ monitoring has become indispensable in ventilator-dependent infants and provides immediate information and feedback after changes in ventilator settings. The continuous $TcPO_2$ monitoring has improved the understanding and appreciation of the lability of oxygenation in sick newborns and has made caretakers aware of the development of hypoxemia associated with routine nursery procedures such as endotracheal tube suctioning, lumbar puncture, arterial puncture, and position changes.[27, 28] Continuous $TcPO_2$ monitoring has helped to reduce periods of hypoxemia or hyperoxia and has improved the care of sick newborns.[27] Weaning from supplemental oxygen and mechanical ventilation can be faster; fewer arterial blood samples for blood gas analysis need to be drawn; and hospital bills will be lower.[29] The electrode is also helpful in detecting hypoxemia in infants with chronic problems such as *bronchopulmonary dysplasia* or *sleep apnea*.

The function of the oxygen electrode is based on the same principle as the Clark cell. It consists of a gold cathode and a silver anode. The sensing area is covered with a thin membrane and bathed in an electrolyte solution. The output is linear, and calibration can be done by using nitrogen or a reducing solution to determine the zero point, and room air ($PO_2$, 159 mm Hg) to determine the upper part of the calibration curve. The electrode consumes oxygen and depends on a continuous flow of oxygen across the skin. It measures skin $PO_2$, not arterial $PO_2$. Skin $PO_2$ depends on the perfusion of the dermis and on the diffusion of oxygen through the epidermis, which is reduced with increasing skin thickness. Skin $PO_2$ at the surface is normally low because oxygen flow to the skin is sufficient to cover the low metabolic needs of the tissue and not supplied beyond that need. This problem is overcome by heating the skin surface to 43.5° to 44.5°C,[30] which causes vasodilation and maximizes skin perfusion. The increase in temperature also leads to a right shift of the oxygen-hemoglobin dissociation curve thus increasing the capillary $PO_2$. These changes are in part balanced by the skin's oxygen consumption so that the $PO_2$ measured at the skin's surface is close to arterial $PO_2$. Correlations between $TcPO_2$ and arterial $PO_2$ have been published by several investigators, the correlation coefficient varying from 0.85 to 0.93.[29, 30, 31] Correlation is not as close when the arterial $PO_2$ is over 100 mm Hg[32] and is poor or lost completely during hypotension. In older infants with bronchopulmonary dysplasia, correlation may be poor presumably due to increasing skin thickness.[33]

The in vivo lag time from a change in the fraction of oxygen in dry inspired gas ($FI_{O_2}$) to the beginning of a $TcPO_2$ change is 10 to 20 seconds.[30, 34] However, when initiating $TcPO_2$ measurements, 10 to 15 minutes need to elapse until hyperemia and a steady oxygen flow across the skin are established and a stable $TcPO_2$ reading is reached. The electrode functions well for 4 to 6 hours then loses its reliability presumably due to skin changes secondary to the local hyperthermia.[30, 34a] Therefore, the site of the electrode has to be changed every 4 hours. Small red marks reflecting first or mild second-degree burns are left after removal of the electrode but will disappear within a few days.[35] Blistering is usually not observed. In very immature infants with gelatinous skin, skin breakdown may occur mainly due to the tape used to attach the electrode.

Because the electrode does not measure arterial $PO_2$ directly, inaccurate values are possible. Therefore, direct measurements of blood gases from arterial samples may at times be necessary to check the accuracy of the electrode. An arterial blood sample only reflects the arterial $PO_2$ of that very moment when it was drawn and, therefore, has very limited value.[27, 36] When blood samples are drawn by arterial puncture in infants with chronic lung disease or acute respiratory failure, $TcPO_2$ should be measured simultaneously because arterial $PO_2$ may drop during the procedure. Following the $TcPO_2$ readout will prevent this error by documenting the drop and a return of the values into the normal range after the stick. Continuous $TcPO_2$ monitoring can identify the range of $PO_2$ values and their distribution over time in an individual infant. This $TcPO_2$ information can best be handled and made available by a computer prepared *dynamic histogram.*[37]

### Transcutaneous Carbon Dioxide Tension

The $TcPCO_2$ electrode is available as a separate electrode but has also been combined with a $TcPO_2$ electrode into a single sensing device. The basis of the electrode is a pH-sensitive glass electrode. The electrode does not consume $CO_2$ so that skin permeability is not a limiting factor and does not affect the correlation to arterial $PCO_2$. Therefore, blood pressure and gestational age do not influence its function.[38] Nonetheless, $TcPCO_2$ overestimates arterial $PCO_2$ in infants with bronchopulmonary dysplasia.[33] The $TcPCO_2$ electrode works at 37°C, but a more rapid response time is achieved at 42° to 44°C. Even at that temperature, the response is slower than that of the $TcPO_2$ electrode.[39]

Because the $CO_2$ production of the skin increases tissue $PCO_2$ above arterial levels, transcutaneously measured $PCO_2$ values are 1.37 times higher than arterial $PCO_2$.[39] The readout of the monitor may show the uncorrected value of skin $PCO_2$ or an electronically corrected value that approximates arterial $PCO_2$. As with the $TcPO_2$ electrode, the correlation between $TcPCO_2$ and arterial $PCO_2$ is similarly close, and the presence of falsely elevated or falsely low measurements in 18% of the cases also requires the occasional direct determination of arterial $PCO_2$.[40, 41]

The $CO_2$ electrode has been of great help in the management of infants with respiratory problems mainly characterized by hypercapnia. Infants with poor respiratory drive or apnea on mechanical ventilation, infants with bronchopulmonary dysplasia, and infants with upper airway obstruction typically benefit from $TcPCO_2$ monitoring. Monitoring $TcPCO_2$ in infants requiring mechanical ventilation will provide early indication of tolerance to ventilator setting changes. This is especially true for infants with chronic lung disease without arterial lines who frequently show unreliable and misleading blood gas results because of limited pulmonary reserve and breath holding during arterial puncture.

## Oxygen Saturation

Recently a *pulse oximeter* has been developed that measures beat by beat arterial oxygen saturation. The instrument's probe emits light of low intensity with red and infrared spectrum. The probe is attached to a finger or toe in large infants or to the hand or foot in smaller infants. The pulsatile arterial flow through the tissue leads to varying absorption of the emitted light, which is the basis for computation of $O_2$ saturation. No calibration is necessary, response time is rapid, and the results are presented continuously in digital form.

The measurements correlate closely to oxygen saturation determined by co-oximeter and to $TcPO_2$ measurements ($r = 0.96$). The values are not markedly affected by hematocrit, body temperature, acid-base status, percentage of fetal hemoglobin (hemoglobin F), drugs, or anesthetic gases.[42] These are considerable advantages as compared to $TcPO_2$ measurements, which do not reflect changes in affinity of hemoglobin to oxygen and, therefore, may show normal values while $O_2$ saturation is decreased, as may occur during acidosis or hyperthermia. There is no risk of skin burns. However, the instrument is less affected by hypotension than the $TcPO_2$ electrode, although unsuccessful measurements have been reported in infants with low cardiac output. The problem will be apparent from the pulse display of the monitor, whereas a $TcPO_2$ electrode continues to give false readings.[43] The main disadvantage is the sensor's sensitivity to motion and the difficulty in keeping it in place in active, restless infants.

In the steep portion of the oxygen-hemoglobin dissociation curve small changes in arterial $PO_2$ result in large changes in $O_2$ saturation; therefore, the oximeter reflects hypoxemia and oxygen availability to tissues better than $TcPO_2$ measurements. In the flat portion of the oxygen-hemoglobin dissociation curve, large changes in arterial $PO_2$ result in only small changes in $O_2$ saturation. Therefore, hyperoxia cannot be detected reliably when $O_2$ saturation is 95% to 100%. With the $O_2$ saturation reading 80% to 95%, the partial pressure of oxygen in arterial blood ($PaO_2$) was 40–80 mm Hg in 94% of cases.[42]

## PULMONARY FUNCTION TESTING

### Tidal Volume

Tidal volume ($V_T$) is measured easily and accurately with a pneumotachograph,[44] a tube with low resistance through which gas flows in a laminar fashion. The pressure gradient necessary for gas to flow through the pneumotachograph is determined by a differential pressure transducer and is proportional to the flow. Tidal volume is obtained by electronic *integration* of the flow signal.

The size of the pneumotachograph is important because it determines the added deadspace to the respiratory system. If the added deadspace causes hyperventilation and/or hypercapnia, a T-piece with a background flow can be used and the pneumotachograph placed in the outflow part of the system. The signal from the background flow passing through the pneumotachograph is zeroed electronically so that only the flow changes occurring when the infant adds (expiration) or subtracts (inspiration) volume from the system will be measured.[45] The size of the pneumotachograph is also important because it determines the flow range within which the differential pressure is proportional to flow. Exceeding this range will give inaccurate measurements. It is recommended that the pneumotachograph that covers the flows generated by the infant tested be chosen. Using a pneumotachograph with a larger range of flows than produced by the infant will add unnecessary deadspace and will require increased amplification of a faint flow signal, thus introducing artifacts and errors.

*Calibration* of the flow signal needs to be done with known flows using a large spirometer or an electronic or mechanical flowmeter. Calibration of tidal volume can be done with a calibrated glass syringe using the same gas mixture as the infant is breathing during the test, as a difference in viscosity of the gas will lead to a difference in pneumotachograph output. During the measurement, the pneumotachograph needs to be heated to prevent condensation of humidity on the inner walls that could increase the resistance and result in an overestimation of the flow signal.

Before using a pneumotachograph in intubated, mechanically ventilated infants, the pressure ramps generated by a ventilator should be applied to one side of the pneumotachograph while occluding the other side. This should only result in a negligible flow signal if a differential pressure transducer with equal size of its two chambers and stiff pressure tubing of equal length are used to connect the pneumotachograph to the transducer. Tubing should be kept as short as possible.[46] If no significant flow signal occurs when pressure is applied to test the pneumotachograph, any drift in tidal volume (inspired volume larger than expired) observed during mechanical ventilation must be due to a leak around the adaptors or the endotracheal tube. The latter can be corrected by putting mild pressure on the trachea with thumb and index finger. In extubated infants, the pneumotachograph is attached to the airway with nasal prongs or mask using petroleum jelly to avoid leaks. Different size prongs and masks need to be available. Nasal prongs are preferred over a face mask because of the lower deadspace, easier seal, and better tolerance by the infants. Malposition of prongs or face mask can lead to airway obstruction, which can be detected by a sudden increase in esophageal pressure after prongs or mask have been placed. There should only be a minimal increase in esophageal pressure when breathing through the peumotachograph.

## Compliance

*Compliance* ($C_L$) is calculated by dividing the tidal volume ($V_T$) by the pressure change $V_T/\Delta P$ necessary to generate the observed tidal volume. $C_L = V_T/\Delta P$ (ml/cm $H_2O$). In an intubated infant on mechanical ventilation, tidal volume can be measured together with airway pressure (Paw) (Fig 3–4). This can be done from a side port of the endotracheal tube adaptor using a pressure transducer. To obtain quasistatic compliance, inspiration should be prolonged to 0.5 to 1.0 second holding inspiratory pressure at a plateau and allowing tidal volume also to reach plateau (Fig 3–5). Dividing tidal volume by the change in airway pressure, which includes the pressure necessary to distend the lungs as well as the chest wall, gives the *compliance of the respiratory system*. This value is similar to *lung* compliance because in newborn infants *chest wall* compliance is only 1/10 to 1/5 of lung compliance.[48] Therefore, compliance of the respiratory system can well be used to follow pulmonary problems. To determine lung compliance, *transpulmonary pressure* needs to be known. This is the pressure gradient between alveolar and pleural pressure. At periods of no flow, alveolar pressure is equal to airway pressure, and pleural pressure changes are reflected by esophageal pressure changes (Pe). Lung compliance ($C_L$) can then be calculated by dividing $V_T$ by the difference of airway and esophageal pressure changes.

$$C_L = V_T/(\Delta Paw - \Delta Pe)$$

The pressure-volume curve is not necessarily linear and becomes progressively flatter as higher pressures on the ventilator are used, resulting in lower values for compliance. To make daily measurements comparable with previously obtained values, repeat studies should be done at the same pressure or tidal volume.

Reliable measurements cannot be performed in infants whose own breathing is superimposed on mechanically generated breaths. The infants should be paralyzed or their own inspiratory efforts controlled by mild hyperventilation.

In infants breathing spontaneously, compliance of the respiratory system can be determined by occluding the airway at the end of inspiration (Fig 3–6).[49, 50] This is simply done by placing the finger over

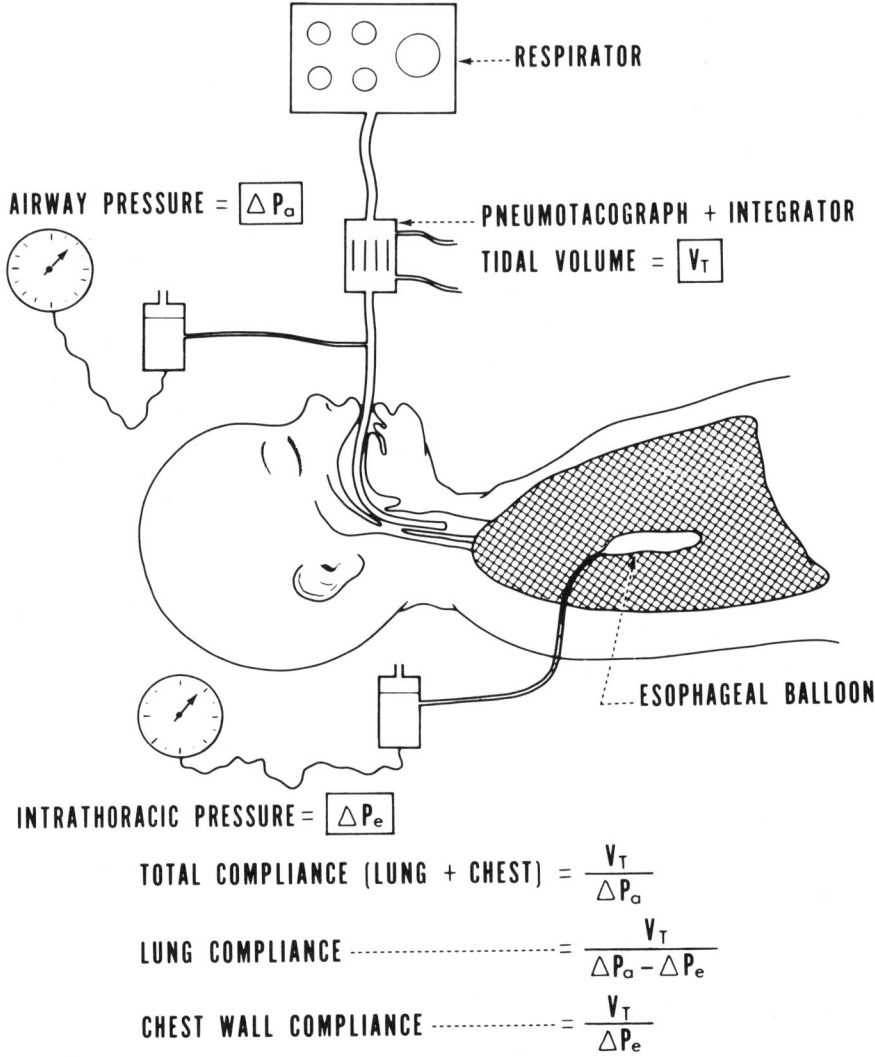

**FIG 3–4.**
System used to determine pulmonary mechanics in intubated and ventilated infants. A water-filled feeding tube to measure intrathoracic pressure is preferred over the esophageal balloon. In spontaneously breathing infants, the pneumotachograph is attached to the airway by mask or nasal prongs. Airway pressure changes are minimal and do not need to be measured. (From Gerhardt T, Bancalari E: Lung compliance in newborns with patent ductus arteriosus before and after surgical ligation. *Biol Neonate* 1980; 38:96. Used by permission.)

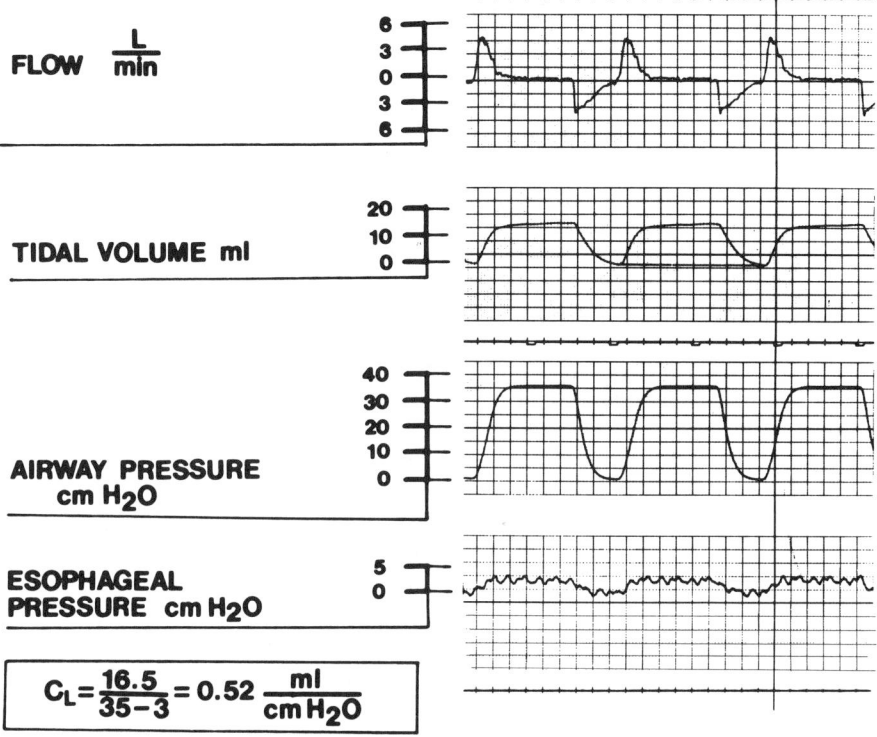

**FIG 3–5.**
Typical tracing of flow, tidal volume, airway pressure, and esophageal pressure in a mechanically ventilated infant. Inspiration is prolonged showing an inspiratory plateau. Speed: 5 divisions ~ 1 second. (From Gerhardt T, Bancalari E: Lung compliance in newborns with patent ductus arteriosus before and after surgical ligation. *Biol Neonate* 1980; 38:96. Used by permission.)

the open part of the pneumotachograph. Due to the *Hering-Breuer reflex*, the infant will relax the respiratory muscles, and airway pressure will rise to a plateau with continuation of the occlusion that will persist for the duration of a normal expiration or longer, depending on the strength of the reflex. If no plateau is reached and the pressure continues to rise, it suggests that the infant is not relaxed and tries to overcome the occlusion by active expiration. Gradual pressure drops after a peak has been reached indicate a leak in the system. Both of these situations are not suitable for analysis. Compliance is again calculated by dividing the tidal volume at which occlusion occurred by the corresponding change in airway pressure. Tidal volume is best derived from the linear part of the flow/volume curve where its extension intersects the volume axis (see Fig 3–6). This value is more accurate than inspired tidal volume because neonates keep their functional residual capacity above

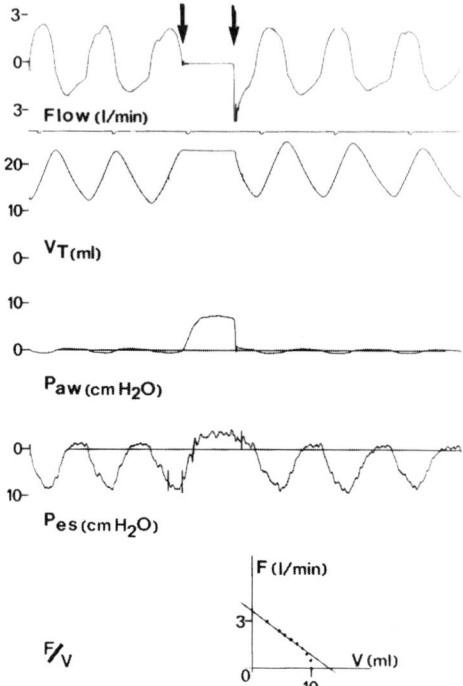

**FIG 3–6.**
Measurement of pulmonary mechanics by the occlusion method. Occlusion starts at the end of inspiration *(first arrow)* resulting in a short period of zero flow, a tidal volume $(V_T)$ plateau, and a rise in airway pressure *(PAW)* to plateau level. Release of the occlusion *(second arrow)* is followed by a relaxed expiration, the flow/volume relation of which is shown in the lowest tracing. Paw is 7.0 cm $H_2O$. The intersection of the straight portion of the flow/volume curve with the volume axis is at 12.5 ml and with the flow axis at 3.6L/minute or 0.06L/second. From these values, compliance of the respiratory system (Crs) can be calculated.

$$Crs = 12.5/7.0 = 1.79 \text{ ml/cm } H_2O$$

and expiratory resistance of the respiratory system (Rrs) is

$$Rrs = 7.0/0.06 = 117 \text{ cm } H_2O/L/second$$

These values compare well with compliance and resistance measurements of the previous unoccluded breath obtained by the classical method of measuring esophageal pressure *(Pes)* changes. Dynamic compliance (Cdyn) is

$$Cdyn = 11.0/6.5 = 1.69 \text{ ml/cm } H_2O$$

and expiratory lung resistance is

$$R_L = 3.75/0.030 = 125 \text{ cm } H_2O/L/second$$

relaxation lung volume by inspiring before expiration is completed. The advantage of this method is that esophageal pressure measurements are not necessary (see Fig 3–6).

If lung compliance is to be measured, an esophageal balloon or a water-filled tube needs to be used to estimate pleural pressure changes. In preterm infants with lung disease, this method has recently been shown to give unreliable results because the negative pressure generated by the diaphragm is not equally distributed through the pleural space and over the mediastinum.[51, 52] This problem can be identified by occluding the airway for a few breaths and observing that simultaneously occurring airway and esophageal pressure changes are of equal magnitude.[53, 54] Esophageal pressure changes can be measured with the same transducer used for blood pressure measurements. Calibration should be done with a water manometer. A fluid-filled catheter gives a more reliable signal and is easier to pass than the balloon system. A size 8 French feeding tube is placed into the lower part of the esophagus by recording pressures while pulling the tube from the stomach into the esophagus. This position reduces cardiac artifacts and produces the most reliable signal. The tube needs to be flushed immediately before each recording to eliminate air bubbles.

Lung compliance is calculated by dividing tidal volume by the esophageal pressure change measured at zero flow between inspiration and expiration. This measurement is called *dynamic compliance*.[55] In infants with airway obstruction (prolonged time constant), dynamic compliance is frequency dependent. With elevated frequencies, compliance measurements are lower than with lower respiratory rates because at the end of inspiration, air flow may continue between areas of the lung that have discrepant time constants although no flow is measured at the airway opening. Swallowing distorts the esophageal signal, and measurements need to be stopped until esophageal pressure has returned to baseline. At least ten quiet, regular breaths should be analyzed. The coefficient of variation should not be more than 10% in a well-done study. Compliance is closely related to body weight or functional residual capacity. The measurements should, therefore, be corrected when comparing infants of different age and weight.

### *Resistance*

The pressure that leads to inflation of the respiratory system does not only have to overcome the elastic forces of the system but also resistance to airflow through the airways and viscous forces of lung and chest wall.

In mechanically ventilated infants, total resistance of the respiratory system can be calculated from the recording of flow, tidal volume, and airway pressure.[47] Resistance is usually measured at half (mid) tidal volume. The points of half inspiration and half expiration are identified on the volume tracing, and the corresponding flows and pressures are marked. The pressure difference measured between the points of half inspiration and half expiration is divided by the sum of inspiratory and expiratory flow measured at the same points in time. To obtain pulmonary resistance in a spontaneously breathing infant, the esophageal pressure tracing is analyzed in the same way as airway pressure in the above example.[55]

Pressure and volume can also be depicted on an x-y recorder or a digital storage oscilloscope to give a pressure-volume loop.[55] The slope of the line connecting zero volume with the peak tidal volume indicates the compliance. The distance between the inspiratory and expiratory lines of the loop measured at any fraction of tidal volume indicates the driving pressure necessary to overcome the resistance of the system at that phase of the respiratory cycle. This pressure divided by the sum of inspiratory and expiratory flow measured at the same time will give the resistance value.

Resistance can also be determined by the occlusion method.[49, 50] After occluding the airway at end of inspiration for a fraction of a second, so that the infant relaxes his respiratory muscles, the airway is opened. A similar situation exists in intubated mechanically ventilated infants: with the opening of the respiratory valve, a passive expiration with the driving force equal to the airway pressure, measured just prior to opening of the airway, occurs. The flow generated by this pressure can be estimated by extrapolation of the linear part of the flow/volume curve of this expiration to its intersection with the y-axis (zero volume). This can be done manually by plotting the flow-volume curve on millimetric paper, by using an x-y recorder, or even faster, by a computerized program (see Fig 3–6). This measurement gives expiratory resistance of the respiratory system. It has the advantage of being noninvasive, not needing placement of an esophageal tube, and giving expiratory resistance, which reflects small airway problems better than total resistance. Again, ten determinations should be made from quiet, regular breaths or well-timed, relaxed expirations after an occlusion. The coefficient of variation should be less than 20%.

### *Forced Expiration*

A forced expiration is a helpful measurement reflecting the state of the small airways. In neonates this can be done by wrapping an inflatable cuff around the chest and abdomen and pressurizing it at the end of inspiration.[56] This will force the air out and empty the lungs below the *functional residual capacity* level. The system pressurizing the cuff must have a short time constant (less than 100 msecond). The pressures applied have to be increased from 40 to 80 mm Hg to make sure that the highest possible flows are reached. The cuff can be inflated by turning a manual valve or by using a solenoid valve triggered by a computer.

The expiratory flow/volume curve in infants with small airway obstruction is concave toward the volume axis, and flow at functional residual capacity is low. This is due to the small airways narrowing toward the end of expiration and thus interfering with unimpeded expiratory flow. A computer program can be used to draw and analyze the flow/volume curves. There is still a lack of normal values for this relatively new method, and results need to be related to functional residual capacity or weight to compare measurements in infants of different size.

Pulmonary function testing as described here used to be a research tool only. However, with equipment specifically made for use in newborns and with increasing understanding and familiarity of neonatologists and respiratory therapists with these techniques, testing has become an important monitoring tool. The effectiveness of drug therapy, such as diuretics for pulmonary edema or bronchodilators in bronchopulmonary dysplasia, can be determined. The recovery from acute respiratory failure, the setbacks with the development of a patent ductus arteriosus, and the early changes in chronic lung disease can be detected and documented when lung function is monitored daily. Clinical monitoring of pulmonary mechanics will allow a more rational use of ventilatory support systems and drug therapy.

## REFERENCES

1. Hon EG: *An Atlas of Fetal Heart Rate Patterns*. New Haven, Conn, Harty Press, 1968.
2. Lowensohn RI: Instrumentation for fetal heart rate monitoring. *J Obstet Gynecol Neonat Nurs* 1976; 75(suppl):7S–10S.
3. Kubli FW, Hon EG, Khazin AF, et al: Observations on heart rate and pH in the human fetus during labor. *Am J Obstet Gynecol* 1969; 104:1190.
4. Myers RE, Mueller-Heubach E, Adamsons K: Predictability of the state of fetal oxygenation for a quantitative analysis of the components of late deceleration. *Am J Obstet Gynecol* 1973; 115:1083.
5. Creasy RK, Resnik R: *Maternal Fetal Medicine: Principles and Practice*. Philadelphia, WB Saunders Co, 1984.
6. Cibils LA: Clinical significance of fetal heart rate patterns during labor: II. Late decelerations. *Am J Obstet Gynecol* 1975; 123:473.

7. Sibai BM, Lipschitz J, Schneider JM, et al: Sinusoidal fetal heart rate pattern. *Obstet Gynecol* 1980; 55:637.
8. Lauersen NH, Hochberg HM: *Clinical Prenatal Biochemical Monitoring.* Baltimore, Williams & Wilkins Co., 1981.
9. Evertson LR, Gauthier RJ, Schifrin BS, et al: Antepartum fetal heart rate testing. *Am J Obstet Gynecol* 1984; 148:18.
10. Phelan JP, Cromartie AD, Smith CV: The nonstress test: The false negative deceleration. *Am J Obstet Gynecol* 1982; 115:1983.
11. Dashow EE, Read JA: Significant fetal bradycardia during antepartum heart rate testing. *Am J Obstet Gynecol* 1984; 148:18.
12. Manning FA, Platt LD, Sipos L: Antepartum fetal evaluation. Development of a fetal biophysical profile. *Am J Obstet Gynecol* 1980; 136:787.
13. Dykes FD, Ahmann PA, Baldzer K, et al: Breath amplitude modulation of heart rate variability in normal full term neonates. *Pediatr Res* 1986; 20:301.
14. Polgar G: Comparison of methods for recording respiration in newborn infants. *Pediatrics* 1965; 36:861.
15. Warburton D, Stark AR, Taeusch HW: Apnea monitor failure in infants with upper airway obstruction. *Pediatrics* 1977; 60:742.
16. Vyas H, Milner AD, Hopkin IE: Relationship between apnea and bradycardia in preterm infants. *Acta Paediatr Scand* 1981; 70:785.
17. Southall DP, Levitt GA, Richards JM, et al: Undetected episodes of prolonged apnea and severe bradycardia in preterm infants. *Pediatrics* 1983; 72:541.
18. Southall DP, Richards JM, Rhoden KJ, et al: Prolonged apnea and cardiac arrhythmias in infants discharged from neonatal intensive care units: Failure to predict an increased risk for sudden death syndrome. *Pediatrics* 1982; 70:844.
19. Hiatt IM, Hegyi T, Indyk L, et al: Continuous monitoring of $PO_2$ during apnea of prematurity. *J Pediatr* 1981; 98:288.
20. Butt WW, Whyte H: Blood pressure monitoring in neonates: Comparison of umbilical and peripheral artery catheter measurements. *J Pediatr* 1984; 105:630.
21. Darnall RA Jr: Noninvasive blood pressure measurement in the neonate. *Clin Perinatol* 1985; 12:31.
22. Briassoulis G: Arterial pressure measurement in preterm infants. *Crit Care Med* 1986; 14:735.
23. Diprose GK, Evans DH, Archer LNJ, et al: Dinamap fails to detect hypotension in very low birth weight infants. *Arch Dis Child* 1986; 61:771.
24. Adamsons K Jr., Gandy GM, James LS: The influence of thermal factors upon oxygen consumption of the newborn human infant. *J Pediatr* 1965; 66:495.
25. Perlstein PH, Edwards NK, Sutherland JM: Apnea in premature infants and incubator-air-temperature changes. *N Engl J Med* 1970; 282:461–466.

26. Huch R, Lubbers W, Huch A: Quantitative continuous measurement of partial oxygen pressure on the skin of adults and newborn babies. *Pflugers Arch* 1972; 337:185.
27. Long LG, Philip AGS, and Lucey JF: Excessive handling as a cause of hypoxemia. *Pediatrics* 1980; 65:203.
28. Peabody JL, Emergy JR: Noninvasive monitoring of blood gases in the newborn. *Clin Perinatol* 1985; 12:147–160.
29. Peevy KJ, Hall MW: Transcutaneous oxygen monitoring: Economic impact on neonatal care. *Pediatrics* 1985; 75:1065–1067.
30. Pollitzer MJ, Whitehead MD, Reynolds EOR, et al: Effect of electrode temperature and in vivo calibration on accuracy of transcutaneous estimation of arterial oxygen tension in infants. *Pediatrics* 1980; 65:515.
31. Okken A, Rubin IL, Martin RJ: Intermittent bag ventilation of preterm infants on continuous positive airway pressure: The effect on transcutaneous $PO_2$. *J Pediatr* 1978; 93:279–282.
32. Martin RJ, Robertson SS, Hopple MM: Relationship between transcutaneous and arterial oxygen tension in sick neonates during mild hyperoxemia. *Crit Care Med* 1982; 10:670–672.
33. Rome ES, Stork EK, Carlo WA, et al: Limitations of transcutaneous $PO_2$ and $PCO_2$ monitoring in infants with bronchopulmonary dysplasia. *Pediatrics* 1984; 74:217.
34. le Souëf PN, Morgan AK, Soutter LP, et al: Comparison of transcutaneous oxygen tension with arterial oxygen tension in newborn infants with severe respiratory illnesses. *Pediatrics* 1978; 62:692.
34a. Abu Osba YK, Thach BT, Brouillette RT: Evaluation of response time of a transcutaneous oxygen tension electrode. *Pediatr Res* 1981; 15:143.
35. Boyle RJ, Oh W: Erythema following transcutaneous $PO_2$ monitoring. *Pediatrics* 1980; 65:333.
36. Lofgren O, Jacobson L: Some characteristics of transcutaneously monitored oxygen partial pressure in normal newborns. *Acta Paediatr Scand* 1979; 68:789.
37. Fallenstein F, Bucher HU, Huch R, et al: The dynamic transcutaneous $PO_2$ histogram or how to deal with immense quantities of monitoring data. *Pediatrics* 1985; 75:608.
38. Hansen TN and Tooley WH: Skin surface carbon dioxide tension in sick infants. *Pediatrics* 1979; 64:942.
39. Herrell N, Martin RJ, Pultusker M, et al: Optimal temperature for the measurement of transcutaneous carbon dioxide tension in the neonate. *J Pediatr* 1980; 97:114.
40. Epstein MF, Cohen AR, Feldman HA, et al: Estimation of $PaCO_2$ by two noninvasive methods in the critically ill newborn infant. *J Pediatr* 1985; 106:282.
41. Wimberely PD, Frederiksen PA, Witt-Hansen J, et al: Evaluation of a transcutaneous oxygen and carbon dioxide monitor in a neonatal intensive care department. *Acta Pediatr Scand* 1985; 74:352.

42. Deckardt R, Steward D: Noninvasive arterial hemoglobin oxygen saturation versus transcutaneous oxygen tension monitoring in the preterm infant. *Crit Care Med* 1984; 12:935.
43. Fanconi S, Doherty P, Edmonds JR, et al: Pulse oximetry in pediatric intensive care: Comparison with measured saturations and transcutaneous oxygen tension. *J Pediatr* 1985; 107:362.
44. Grenvik A, Hedstrand U, Sjogren H: Problems in pneumotachography. *Acta Anaesthesiol Scand* 1966; 10:147.
45. Rigatto H, Brady JP: Periodic breathing and apnea in preterm infants: I. Evidence for hypoventilation possibly due to central respiratory depression. *Pediatrics* 1972; 50:202.
46. Abrahams N, Fisk GC, Churches AE, et al: Errors in pneumotachography in intermittent positive pressure ventilation. *Anaesth Intensive Care* 1975; 3:284.
47. Churches AE, Loughman GC, Fisk N, et al: Measurement errors in pneumotachography due to pressure transducer design. *Anaesth Intensive Care* 1977; 5:19.
48. Gerhardt T, Bancalari E: Chestwall compliance in full-term and premature infants. *Acta Paediatr Scand* 1980; 69:359.
49. Mortola JP, Fisher JT, Smith B, et al: Dynamics of breathing in infants. *J Appl Physiol* 1982; 52:1209.
50. le Souëf PN, England SJ, and Bryan AC: Passive respiratory mechanics in newborns and children. *Am Rev Respir Dis* 1984; 129:552.
51. le Souëf PN, Lopes JM, England SJ, et al: Influence of chest wall distortion on esophageal pressure. *J Appl Physiol* 1983; 55:353.
52. Heaf DP, Turner H, Stocks J, et al: The accuracy of esophageal pressure measurements in convalescent and sick intubated infants. *Pediatr Pulmonol* 1986; 2:5.
53. Beardsmore CS, Helms P, Stocks J, et al: Improved esophageal balloon technique for use in infants. *J Appl Physiol* 1980; 49:735.
54. Baydur A, Behrakis PK, Zin WA, et al: A simple method for assessing the validity of the esophageal balloon technique. *Am Rev Respir Dis* 1982; 126:788.
55. Krieger I: Studies on mechanics of respiration in infancy. *Am J Dis Child* 1963; 105:51.
56. Taussig LM, Landau LI, Godfrey S, et al: Determinants of forced expiratory flows in newborn infants. *J Appl Physiol* 1982; 53:1220.

# 4

# The Airways

Robert E. Wood, Ph.D., M.D.
James M. Sherman, Jr., M.D.

## ANATOMY OF THE AIRWAYS

### The Larynx

The infantile *larynx* is situated higher in the neck than it is in the adult, with the inferior border of the *cricoid cartilage* (the "cricoid ring") at the level of the fourth cervical vertebra. With growth, the larynx gradually moves caudally to eventually assume its adult position with the cricoid ring near C-7.[1] The *epiglottis* in infants is more omega-shaped than in adults but normally maintains a rigid shape. Part of the support for the epiglottis is muscular; with sleep or relaxation, it may become flaccid, with resulting stridor. The epiglottis helps deflect swallowed material into the esophagus and away from the *glottis*, but it is not necessary to prevent aspiration (as is closure of the vocal cords).

The *arytenoid cartilages* are often more prominent in infants than in adults, but the *accessory cartilages*, the *corniculate* and *cuneiform*, are usually much less prominent. In the infant, the *vocal cords* are 4 to 4.5 mm long. Cord movement is effected via the *recurrent laryngeal nerves*, so that lesions in the mediastinum as well as in the neck or brain can result in cord paralysis. The *ventricular folds*, or false cords, lie just above and lateral to the true cords from which they are separated by a lateral slit, the *laryngeal ventricle*.

The subglottic space is bounded by the plane of the glottis (between the true cords), the *thyroid cartilage*, and the *cricoid cartilage*. The inferior margin of the cricoid is a complete ring (in effect, the first tracheal ring) and in infants has the smallest diameter of any part of the upper airway. Therefore, this area is especially vulnerable to damage from endotracheal tubes or instruments passed through the larynx. In premature infants, the diameter of the cricoid ring may be estimated from the following formula[2]:

Cricoid diameter (mm) = (gestational age in weeks/10) + 0.5

## The Trachea

The wall of the *trachea* is composed of U-shaped cartilages joined at their open ends by a muscular membrane. This structure (in contrast to that of the cricoid ring) allows some change in tracheal caliber with changes in intrathoracic pressure or with mechanical stress. The tracheal diameter in a term newborn infant is approximately 5.5 mm.

## The Bronchi

The structure of the larger *bronchi* is similar to that of the trachea. More peripherally, cartilage is gradually lost so that the airways become more compliant and more dependent on tissue elastic forces (and perhaps surface tension) to maintain their patency.

The trachea bifurcates at the *carina* to form the right and left main bronchi. The left main bronchus takes a much sharper angle from the axis of the trachea. Thus, endotracheal tubes and/or suction catheters passed beyond the carina preferentially enter the *right main bronchus*. The right upper-lobe bronchus takes off laterally, just below the carina, and is very short. The right middle-lobe bronchus arises anteriorly, while the lower-lobe bronchus branches directly off the main-stem bronchus. The right lower-lobe and right main bronchi are particularly vulnerable to damage from endotracheal tubes and suction catheters.

The *left main bronchus* is long and straight and is surrounded by vascular structures (the aortic arch, the pulmonary artery, and the left atrium). It branches into the upper and lower lobes. The *lingula* is the left-sided analog of the right middle lobe but is a part of the upper lobe.

# CARE OF THE AIRWAYS

## General Aspects

Under most circumstances, the natural airways function better than any artificial airway (which in any case serves only as a conduit to the natural airways). Therefore, care should be taken to preserve and protect the integrity and function of the natural airways. Adequate humidification of inspired gases should be ensured, and cough should be promoted. Chest physiotherapy may help to mobilize secretions and stimulate cough. Suctioning of the lower airways should be avoided if possible.

**Intubation**

When an artificial airway is necessary, *endotracheal intubation* (see also Chapter 5) is most often preferable to *tracheostomy*, unless a prolonged intubation is planned or there is upper airway pathology that makes intubation undesirable or more difficult. Polyvinyl chloride tubes of uniform outside diameter are used; it must be noted that the outside diameter of such tubes is 1.0 to 1.5 mm greater than the nominal diameter (which is the *inside* diameter).

An endotracheal tube may be passed through the mouth or the nose; there is no general agreement on which route is best. *Orotracheal tubes* are probably more easily passed, while *nasotracheal tubes* are more easily stabilized. Problems with orotracheal tubes include palatal grooving,[3] defective dentition,[4] interference with non-nutritive sucking, and difficulty in achieving stabilization. Problems with nasotracheal tubes include late choanal stenosis, perforation of the nasal septum, and deformity of the nares.[5,6] There is no difference in the incidence of pulmonary or tracheal complications with either route.[7]

Endotracheal tube size should be chosen carefully. The object of intubation is to provide a secure route for air exchange while promoting clearance of respiratory secretions without damaging the natural airway. Based on a prospective study of intubated infants,[8] we recommend that the ratio of nominal tube size to gestational age in infants be less than 0.1. Thus, infants of up to 30 weeks' gestation should receive 2.5-mm tubes; those 31 to 35 weeks, a 3.0-mm tube; and infants greater than 36 weeks, a 3.5-mm tube. An endotracheal tube that is too small will result in significant air leakage and high airway resistance with consequent problems in maintaining ventilation. A tube that is too large will likely damage the subglottic space, resulting in subglottic stenosis. In any patient, the above guidelines must be modified by observation of the patient during and following intubation: the tube should have a small air leak at a pressure of 25 cm $H_2O$. If it is too small or too large, then an appropriate change should be made.

Endotracheal intubation is usually accomplished easily by experienced operators. Because the infantile larynx is small and located anteriorly compared to adults, persons inexperienced with infants may have difficulty in performing intubation. It is rare that intubation is an absolutely emergent procedure; usually ventilation can be maintained with other methods until proper equipment and additional personnel are available. The technique for intubation is described in Chapter 5.

Nasotracheal intubation may be accomplished by passing the tube (well-lubricated with sterile water-soluble lubricant) through one nostril to the posterior pharynx. The laryngoscope is then inserted and the tube advanced under direct vision. The tube may be guided into the larynx by movement of the head and neck (including gentle pressure on the external surface of the neck), or a McGill forceps may be used to grasp the tube near its tip and directly place it into the glottis.

Maintenance of the artificial airway once it is successfully placed requires constant attention to detail. The tube must be kept in proper position, and it must be kept clean. The most common technique for immobilizing endotracheal tubes involves the use of adhesive tape. This must be done carefully in infants, especially premature infants, to avoid damage to the skin. In some centers, a suture or a safety pin is passed through the wall of the tube to provide additional anchoring, although this may interfere with the passage of suction catheters. It is usually easier to secure a nasotracheal tube than an orotracheal tube. Regardless of how the endotracheal tube is attached to the patient, if the tubing connected to the tube is rigidly fixed to the patient's bed, there is danger of accidental extubation if the patient moves around or is moved. The tubing from the ventilator should be positioned and secured so that the patient can be moved without putting significant tension on the endotracheal tube.

The tube must be suctioned at intervals to remove secretions and prevent obstruction. The object of suctioning is to maintain patency of the tube, not to maintain patency of the bronchi. Most infants who require intubation in the nursery do not have copious secretions and may require suctioning as infrequently as once every several hours. Patients with pulmonary infection, however, will have more secretions and will require more frequent suctioning. When the secretions are very thick, instilling up to 1 ml of sterile saline into the tube prior to suctioning may be helpful. Occasionally a patient will have thick secretions that cannot be suctioned through a catheter; these patients usually have atelectasis and will need bronchoscopy to effect bronchial toilet. This may be clinically confusing, since it may seem that there are no secretions (since none are obtained with suctioning). If there is insufficient humidification of the gases supplied to the endotracheal tube, both the tube and the bronchi may become obstructed with inspissated mucus.

Because suctioning removes air from the lungs, patients are often given manual hyperinflations with a bag as part of the suctioning process. This should be done gently so as not to drive secretions toward the periphery of the lung. In addition, a concentration of oxygen no greater than 10% higher than the previous concentration should be used to prevent marked hyperoxia and to reduce the probability of absorption atelectasis produced by inflating a poorly ventilated area of lung with pure oxygen.

There are several potential harmful effects of suctioning. Hypoxemia, transient bacteremia, bradycardia, or even pneumothorax may occur acutely.[9-12] In infants, the diameter of the suction catheter is nearly equal to that of the main-stem bronchi; deep suctioning may collapse the bronchial wall around the catheter and result in substantial mucosal damage, with hypersecretion of mucus, impairment of mucociliary clearance, development of granulation tissue, and eventually bronchial stenosis. Transudation of serum from a denuded epithelial surface may produce a plug of mucus that has the consistency of a stone. Therefore, the suction cathether should be passed no deeper than approximately 1 cm beyond the end of the tube. A 6- or 6.5-F catheter should be used in 2.5-mm tubes, while an 8-F catheter may be used in larger tubes; 5-F catheters are so small that effective suctioning is very difficult.

There are many potential complications of intubation, and neonates should be extubated as promptly as their medical condition allows. Criteria for extubation include an adequately functioning airway and the ability to satisfactorily ventilate spontaneously and handle oral secretions. Before extubation, preparation for reintubation should be made. The patient should be suctioned, bagged, and extubated after a full lung inflation. Often the patient will be stridorous or hoarse following extubation. Laryngeal edema may develop minutes to hours after extubation, so the patient must be closely monitored for some time. An aerosol of epinephrine may help with laryngeal edema and may be repeated as often as twice an hour. The use of high-dose steroids may also help prevent postextubation laryngeal edema. We use dexamethasone, 1.5 mg/kg intravenously (IV), followed by 1 mg/kg IV every 8 hours, beginning 12 hours prior to extubation and continuing for 24 hours after extubation. In some patients, thick secretions may accumulate in the trachea around the endotracheal tube, which may then obstruct the trachea following extubation; immediate tracheal suctioning and/or reintubation may be required.[13]

Other problems that may develop after extubation include atelectasis and respiratory failure. Vigorous chest physical therapy may help prevent or treat atelectasis, but in some patients bronchoscopy may be required.[13]

## Tracheostomy

Under most circumstances endotracheal intubation is the best method for providing an artificial airway, but *tracheostomy* may be required in patients with anatomical problems preventing intubation or in those who have been intubated for prolonged periods. There are no adequate criteria to determine when tracheostomy should be done to prevent the development of subglottic stenosis. In patients with acquired subglottic stenosis, the *cricoid split* procedure may be effective,[14] but subglottic stenosis remains the most common indication for tracheostomy in infants. Other indications may include Pierre Robin anomaly, vocal cord paralysis, severe laryngomalacia or tracheomalacia, tracheal stenosis, tracheoesophageal fistula, laryngeal web, and mass lesions in the airway (including hemangiomas, neurofibromas, and cystic hygromas).

Plastic and metal tracheostomy tubes are available for infants. In general, the plastic tubes are more satisfactory. The most common tube is made by Shiley and comes in two lengths (pediatric and neonatal) and various diameters. The neonatal tube is 1 cm shorter than the pediatric tube but may reach past the carina in premature infants.

The postoperative care of an infant after a tracheostomy is critical. In the days before the stoma heals, accidental decannulation may be fatal and often leads to major complications such as pneumothorax, bleeding, or creation of a false tract. The tube placed at surgery should not be changed during the first week except by someone very skilled in airway management (and only if absolutely necessary). By that time, the stoma usually has healed and a tract formed. If the tube does accidently become dislodged, orotracheal intubation is a satisfactory method for reestablishing an airway if there is any difficulty in recannulation of the stoma (unless there is severe laryngeal stenosis). Recannulation may be facilitated by passing the suction catheter through the tracheostomy tube, and then passing a suction catheter through the stoma into the trachea. The tracheostomy tube may then be passed into the trachea using the suction catheter as a guide.

Tracheostomy tubes usually remain in place much longer than endotracheal tubes. It is essential to provide for humidification of inspired gases and for suctioning. Suction routines should be similar to those outlined for endotracheal intubation; however, simple bulb suctioning will often be sufficient. The tube must be changed at regular intervals: once a week at a minimum and more frequently if secretions are very thick.

Because of the danger of occlusion or dislodgement of the tracheostomy tube, infants with tracheostomies should be kept on a monitor, whether at home or in the hospital. A plugged or displaced tube is an all-too-common cause of death in these patients. A clean tracheostomy tube and scissors (to cut the ties and remove an occluded tube quickly) must be kept at the patient's bedside at all times.

It is quite possible to send infants home with tracheostomies, but the caretakers must be carefully trained. Parents, grandparents, babysitters, and others caring for the child must know suction technique, how to change the tube, and how to do cardiopulmonary resuscitation (CPR). Equipment for humidification and suctioning, a monitor, a self-inflating bag for manual ventilation as well as all consumable supplies must be provided. Home visits to ensure adequate care are necessary in many cases.

Complications of tracheostomy are numerous[15] and may be classified as early (operative) and late. Operative complications include pneumothorax, pneumomediastinum, subcutaneous emphysema, bleeding, and paratracheal insertion of the tube. Late complications include accidental decannulation, plugging of the airway with secretions, traumatic tracheoesophageal fistula, massive hemorrhage (due to erosion of the innominate artery), tracheal stenosis, tracheal granulations, tracheomalacia, bronchial stenosis, bronchial granulations, and infection. Most of these potential complications can be prevented by close attention to details of care.

There are two schools of thought about the most appropriate method for decannulation. If the patient meets the criteria for decannulation (the original indication has resolved; the patient is breathing, coughing, and handling oral secretions well), then the airway must be examined to determine its anatomical and functional patency. At this point, some physicians would replace the tube with successively smaller tubes, hoping to get the patient to breathe around the tube. However, we feel that in most cases it is better to assess the patency of the airway with a small flexible bronchoscope and to remove the tube with the bronchoscope in the airway (and with the patient comfortably sedated). If the airway is functionally patent and the patient breathes satisfactorily, then the patient is carefully observed for at least 48 hours in the hospital. On rare occasions (most often in patients with cerebral dysfunction), a patient will find it difficult to coordinate the function of the upper airway after the tube is removed, even though the airway is anatomically normal (or at least adequate). In this situation, the use of progressively smaller tubes may be helpful, but it must be recognized that placing a smaller tube may significantly increase airway resistance and make it difficult for the patient to ventilate adequately. This is especially true with the plastic tracheostomy tubes (which have thicker walls than the metal tubes).

**TABLE 4-1.**
Congenital Abnormalities of the Airways

| Nasopharynx | Larynx | Lower Airways |
|---|---|---|
| Choanal atresia or stenosis | Laryngomalacia | Tracheomalacia |
| Cystic hygroma | Hemangiomas | Extrinsic compression |
| Hemangiomas | Laryngeal web | Tracheoesophageal fistula |
| Thyroglossal duct cysts | Extrinsic compression | Congenital tracheal stenosis |
| Teratomas and other tumors | Vocal cord paralysis | Abnormal branching |
|  | Congenital subglottic stenosis |  |

## CONGENITAL ABNORMALITIES OF THE AIRWAYS

The congenital abnormalities discussed below are listed in Table 4-1.

### The Nasopharyngeal Airway

Newborn infants are largely obligate nose breathers, and *stenosis or atresia of the choanae* will result in serious respiratory distress. In any infant with respiratory distress, the patency of both nostrils should be assessed by passage of a catheter or detection of airflow. Airway obstruction may be relieved by an oral airway, and the patient should be investigated radiographically or by endoscopy. It may be difficult to pass a catheter through the nose of a normal newborn infant, and patients referred for evaluation of suspected choanal atresia more often than not are normal. Choanal atresia is a rare lesion. Even more rarely, a newborn infant will present with upper airway obstruction due to an *encephalocele* in the nasopharynx.

There are a number of lesions that may obstruct the nasopharyngeal airway.[16,17] They may be evident at birth (or may even be detected on fetal ultrasonography) or may develop in the days or weeks after birth. These include cystic hygroma, hemangioma, thyroglossal duct cyst, teratoma, and other lesions.

*Cystic hygromas* are developmental anomalies of the lymphatic system that tend to expand and involve adjacent tissues. Their management is very difficult, and patients often require a tracheostomy because of airway obstruction at or above the larynx.

*Hemangiomas* may occur in the pharynx or supraglottic area and cause variable degrees of airway obstruction. A mass lesion in the aryepiglottic fold or the lateral aspect of the epiglottis may produce airway obstruction that varies markedly as the patient moves to different positions.

*Thyroglossal duct cysts* result from a persistence of the thyroglossal duct and can produce airway obstruction. These mass lesions, which can be anywhere from the base of the tongue to the infrahyoid area, are treated by excision.

Newborn infants may present with tumors in the oropharynx that produce substantial airway obstruction. Although malignant tumors are rare, teratomas and other lesions may have fatal consequences if airway obstruction occurs.

Micrognathia, cleft palate, Pierre Robin anomaly, and the Treacher Collins syndrome may also result in clinically significant airway obstruction.

**The Larynx**

The most common symptom of laryngeal disorders in infants is stridor,[18] for which there is a very long differential diagnosis. Most stridor in infants is benign and self-limited, but that which persists or causes significant respiratory embarrassment should be investigated (see the later section on laryngoscopy and bronchoscopy).

*Laryngomalacia* is the most common cause of stridor in infants and is due to one of several abnormalities. The epiglottis may be very floppy and may fold along its long and/or short axis to vibrate or even to prolapse into the glottis during inspiration. The symptoms usually improve substantially during the first 6 to 9 months of life, but occasionally a tracheostomy is required for relief of obstruction. Other infants have very large arytenoid cartilages that fall into the glottis during inspiration. This is the most common finding in those infants who require endoscopic examination and may be mistaken on casual laryngoscopy for laryngeal edema, since often the vocal cords are hidden from view. The major importance of definitive diagnosis is the exclusion of other possibilities. In our experience, however, about 15% of patients who had laryngomalacia as a plausible cause of their stridor also had significant abnormalities in the lower airways.[13] Conventional wisdom about laryngomalacia states that the stridor will always decrease in the prone position. In fact, this is often not the case. Laryngomalacia is frequently confused with tracheomalacia. Although both conditions may coexist, they are totally different entities.

*Laryngeal hemangiomas* may produce airway obstruction, although this is unusual at birth.[19] More commonly, symptoms appear during the first several weeks to months of life and are often accompanied by cutaneous hemangiomas. The typical subglottic hemangioma appears as a cystic lesion looking not at all like the common cutaneous strawberry hemangioma, and often biopsy is needed for definitive diagnosis. Any infant with stridor and cutaneous hemangiomas (even if they do not look like the typical strawberry hemangioma) should be suspect for a hemangioma in the airway. Treatment consists of tracheostomy and "tincture of time," although recently laser excision of the tumors as a primary therapy has shown promise. In some patients, high-dose steroid therapy has appeared to be of some benefit.

*Laryngeal webs* probably occur more commonly than they are diagnosed since a thin web may be lysed effectively by intubation in the delivery room and never be diagnosed. Most webs lie between the vocal cords in the anterior part of the glottis, but some are located lower, near the cricoid cartilage. The majority of patients with laryngeal webs that are diagnosed require tracheostomy.

Cystic lesions of the larynx may be present at birth or shortly thereafter and cause extrinsic compression and obstruction. A *laryngocele* is an air-filled cystic lesion that usually arises from the laryngeal ventricle. It is rare and difficult to diagnose. *Saccular cysts* filled with mucus or serous fluid are more common and require surgical intervention for drainage. We have seen one child with a congenital malignant *tumor* occupying the aryepiglottic fold, presenting with stridor on the day of birth.[20]

Newborns may have airway obstruction because of *vocal cord paralysis* either as a congenital defect or as a result of birth trauma. Bilateral abductor paralysis may be an emergency that requires intubation and even tracheostomy. Fortunately, most infants recover spontaneously after several weeks to months. The diagnosis may be difficult, especially if the larynx is examined under general anesthesia. Infants with bilateral vocal cord paralysis must have a thorough neurologic evaluation, including computed tomography of the head, as hydrocephalus and the Arnold-Chiari malformation are not uncommon etiologies.[21] *Congenital subglottic stenosis* is a poorly understood lesion, often presenting several weeks to months after birth as stridor. Many newborns with this defect require *tracheostomy*. Other lesions of the upper airway are reviewed elsewhere.[22,23]

**The Lower Airways**

The most common congenital abnormality of the trachea is *tracheomalacia*. In most patients, this consists of a deformity of the tracheal cartilages such that the membranous portion of the tracheal wall occupies a much greater percentage of the circumference than normally. During forced expiration or cough, the posterior and anterior walls of the trachea touch, producing the characteristic harsh, barky cough. In some infants, the instability of the trachea is such that stenting (with an endotracheal or tracheostomy tube) is necessary. Many patients have these changes limited to the lower half or third of the trachea, and patients with esophageal atresia and tracheoesophageal fistula almost uniformly have tracheomalacia.[24] The respiratory symptoms of tracheomalacia usually consist of wheeze and harsh cough but can be biphasic if the abnormal dynamics extend into the cervical trachea. Here, the relatively negative intratracheal pressure during inspiration produces inspiratory collapse with stridor.

The diagnosis of tracheomalacia can be made radiographically in many infants. Lateral chest films will show a markedly narrowed tracheal diameter (this will not be evident on posteroanterior (PA) or anteroposterior (AP) films) that varies from film to film. Fluoroscopy may be helpful. Definitive diagnosis requires bronchoscopy. The natural history of tracheomalacia is that of gradual improvement with growth. Most patients will become asymptomatic by 2 to 3 years of age, but some will have persistent symptoms into adulthood.

The second most common congenital abnormality of the trachea and major bronchi is *extrinsic compression,* usually due to *vascular anomalies.*[23] The innominate artery normally arises from the proximal part of the aortic arch and passes in front of the trachea. If it arises more distally on the arch, it will compress the trachea anteriorly (usually in the region of the thoracic inlet), producing stridor and/or wheezing. Vascular rings surrounding the esophagus and trachea may produce severe airway compromise, which may not be relieved by intubation (in which case vascular contrast studies and surgical correction are required on an emergency basis). Tracheal compression may produce localized softening and deformity of the cartilage rings, with tracheomalacia persisting for some time after relief of the compression. Extrinsic compression may also be caused by cystic or solid tumors.

*Tracheoesophageal fistula*[24] may occur alone or, more commonly, in association with esophageal atresia. The fistula is usually located near the carina and may be manifest by reflux of gastric contents into the airways (or aspiration from the mouth in patients with esophageal atresia). The H-type fistula may or may not be associated with esophageal abnormalities and is much less common. It is rarely diagnosed in the newborn unless it is part of the complex of esophageal atresia and distal fistula. Mechanical ventilation may be complicated by insufflation of the stomach and intestine by air from the fistula, producing abdominal distention and elevation of the diaphragm.

*Congenital tracheal stenosis* due to complete tracheal rings is rare and may not become symptomatic in the immediate newborn period.

In a small number of patients, there is *abnormal branching of the airways.* A bronchus may arise from the trachea above the carina, almost always on the right. It may serve a small, dysplastic lobe or the normal, right upper lobe. Occasionally it may cause problems with endotracheal tube positioning or suctioning. Abnormal branching of the lobar or segmental airways may also occur, with or without associated pathologic changes.

## ACQUIRED ABNORMALITIES OF THE AIRWAYS

Acquired abnormalities of the airways discussed below are listed in Table 4–2.

### The Larynx

The most common acquired laryngeal abnormality is *laryngeal edema*, which may be infectious (i.e., croup) or iatrogenic. Croup in an infant less than 6 months old should raise the question of congenital subglottic stenosis or a laryngeal mass lesion such as a subglottic hemangioma, especially if the clinical symptoms are severe, prolonged, or recurrent. Because of the small size of the infant larynx, relatively minor degrees of mucosal edema may produce significant airway obstruction. Treatment with topical vasoconstrictors (epinephrine aerosol) may relieve the symptoms but does not alter the natural history of the condition. Since it may obviate the need for intubation, however, it should be tried and, if successful, repeated as often as every 20 to 30 minutes.

*Laryngeal stenosis* is an all-too-common complication of intubation and mechanical ventilation for neonatal respiratory disorders.[8] Pressure of the translaryngeal tube against the mucosa of the subglottic space will produce mucosal ischemia if the pressure exceeds capillary filling pressure (which is about 35 cm $H_2O$). Thus a tube that is too large may, within a few hours, produce mucosal ischemia with subsequent mucosal necrosis. If the ischemia continues, or if infection ensues, the perichondrium of the cricoid cartilage may become involved, and deformity and scarring may develop. In some patients, movement of the endotracheal tube can excoriate the mucosa and produce similar effects.

*Subglottic stenosis* may result from collapse and deformity of the cartilage from scarring, from formation of granulation tissue, or from

**TABLE 4–2.**
Acquired Abnormalities of the Airways

| Larynx | Lower Airways |
|---|---|
| Laryngeal edema | Granulation tissue |
| Laryngeal stenosis | Tracheal deformities |
| Subglottic stenosis | Mucus plug |

the development of submucosal mucous cysts. If the cross-sectional area of the glottis or subglottis is reduced below about 50% of normal, tracheostomy is usually necessary. Treatment of subglottic stenosis is a dismal affair, and every effort should be made to prevent it rather than to attempt treatment after the fact.

**The Lower Airways**

Most acquired lesions of the lower airways of importance in the neonatal period are iatrogenic and associated with trauma to the lower airways from endotracheal or tracheostomy tubes and suction catheters. Repeated mucosal trauma can result in the formation of *granulation tissue*, which then may mature into dense fibrous scar tissue. Such lesions may be seen in the lower trachea, but are more common in the right main bronchus. We have seen infants whose main-stem bronchi were almost totally occluded by granulation tissue within 2 weeks of birth, while others remain intubated for several months without apparent damage. It is not clear why some infants are more susceptible, but precautions should be taken in all infants to prevent these complications. The avoidance of deep suctioning would appear to be of primary importance in this regard.

Infants who have a tracheostomy often develop *tracheal deformities* at the site of the stoma. The tube pushes the cartilage rings posteriorly, and after some time, the deformity may become semipermanent. Granulation tissue usually develops at the superior margin of the stoma. This may act as a ball valve when the tracheostomy tube is not in place, with fatal consequences.

Another complication of endotracheal intubation and suctioning is the development of *mucous plugs* in the airways. Loss of normal mucociliary activity due to mucosal trauma allows the accumulation of mucus. In general, the smaller the infant and the more massive the atelectasis, the more likely it is to be due to a central mucous plug that can be removed by appropriate endobronchial suctioning. In many cases, however, suction catheters will not provide adequate suctioning, and bronchoscopy may be necessary.[13]

# LARYNGOSCOPY AND BRONCHOSCOPY IN NEONATES

The definitive evaluation of airway structure and patency often depends on direct visual inspection. Several instruments are available for endoscopy of the airway in infants; those used depend on the individual patient problem and the physician involved.

Pediatricians often use a *laryngoscope* at the bedside for a "quick and dirty" look at the larynx, but usually the quality of the resulting exam is quick, dirty, not very informative, and often misleading. For maximally effective evaluation, the patient must be relaxed and comfortable, although general anesthesia is not always needed and sometimes can interfere with the examination (it may seriously impair the ability to evaluate vocal cord function, for example). *Rigid laryngoscopy and bronchoscopy* are clearly indicated for study of the fine details of structure, operative procedures requiring dilation or excision of tissue, bronchoscopy in patients who cannot ventilate on their own, and for evaluation of patients with suspected bilateral vocal cord paralysis or H-type tracheoesophageal fistula.

*Flexible fiberoptic instruments*, small enough to be used in even the smallest infants, are now available and give very satisfactory diagnostic results in most cases.[13] However, flexible instruments differ in a very major way from rigid ones: they are solid, and the patient must breathe around them. Most full-term newborns can ventilate around the standard pediatric flexible bronchoscope (3.5-mm diameter), but smaller infants will not. Therefore, procedures must be done very carefully by skilled endoscopists. *Ultrathin bronchoscopes* can be passed through endotracheal or tracheostomy tubes to examine the lower airways without the need for extubation.[25] In most cases, the instruments need to be in the airways for 30 seconds or less so the risk of hypoxia can be significantly minimized, even though the instruments may obstruct the airway.

Flexible laryngoscopy has some advantages over rigid laryngoscopy in the evaluation of the child with stridor. The flexible instrument is passed through the nose instead of the mouth. This means that not only does the operator visualize the nasopharynx (where the pathology sometimes is found), but the larynx is examined with the head and neck in a natural position and with no external forces being applied to it. Rigid laryngoscopy, on the other hand, may distort the larynx because the mandible and tongue must be lifted to allow viewing of the larynx. A second major advantage is that general anesthesia is virtually never required for flexible examinations, which are performed with topical anesthesia and mild sedation (no sedation in infants who are very small or in distress). The complication rate with flexible endoscopy is very low.

There is one general indication for diagnostic laryngoscopy or bronchoscopy in a child: when definitive information necessary for treatment of the patient's condition can be more easily and safely obtained by bronchoscopy than by another technique. If the same information can be obtained by simpler, less invasive methods, then bronchoscopy should not be done. There is one contraindication to bronchoscopy in an infant: when the procedure is unnecessary. Relative contraindications include severe bleeding, cardiovascular instability, airway stenosis, and severe bronchospasm. None of these are absolute contraindications if bronchoscopy really needs to be done.

In the first several months of life, the most common indications for diagnostic bronchoscopy or laryngoscopy include stridor, atelectasis, and evaluation for suspected anomalies. The most common indication for therapeutic bronchoscopy is massive atelectasis not responding to conventional therapy. As noted above, bronchoscopy is much more effective than suction catheters in removing central mucus plugs, and it is our feeling that bronchoscopy done by an expert is less traumatic to the infant than reintubation for deep suctioning. An additional advantage is that the airways can be visually inspected; unsuspected abnormalities are often found.

## REFERENCES

1. Tucker JA, Tucker, GF: A clinical perspective on the development and anatomical aspects of the infant larynx and trachea, in Healy GB, McGill TJI (eds): *Laryngo-Tracheal Problems in the Pediatric Patient.* Springfield, Charles C Thomas, Publishers, 1979, p 3.
2. Fishman RA, Pashley NRT: A study of the preterm neonatal airway. *Otolaryngol Head Neck Surg* 1981; 89:604.
3. Molteni RA, Bumstead DH: Development and severity of palatal grooves in orally intubated newborns: Effect of "soft" endotracheal tubes. *Am J Dis Child* 1986; 140:357.
4. Moylan FMB, Seldin EB, Shannon DC, et al: Defective primary dentition in survivors of neonatal mechanical ventilation. *J Pediatr* 1980; 96:106.
5. Baxter RJ, Johnson JD, Goetzman BN, et al: Cosmetic nasal deformities complicating prolonged nasotracheal intubation in critically ill infants. *Pediatrics* 1975; 55:884.
6. Sherry KM: Ulceration of the inferior turbinate: A complication of prolonged nasotracheal intubation. *Anesthesiology* 1983; 59:148.
7. McMillan DD, Rademaker AW, Buchan KA, et al: Benefits of orotracheal and nasotracheal intubation in neonates requiring ventilatory assistance. *Pediatrics* 1986; 77:39.
8. Sherman JM, Lowitt S, Stephenson C, et al: Factors influencing acquired subglottic stenosis in infants. *J Pediatr* 1986; 109:322.
9. Simbruner G, Coradello H, Fodor M, et al: Effect of tracheal suction on oxygenation, circulation, and lung mechanics in newborn infants. *Arch Dis Child* 1981; 56:326.
10. Storm W: Transient bacteremia following endotracheal suctioning in ventilated newborns. *Pediatrics* 1980; 65:487.

11. Cabal L, Devaskar S, Siassi B, et al: New endotracheal tube adapter reducing cardiopulmonary effects of suctioning. Crit Care Med 1979; 7:552.
12. Vaughan RS, Menke JA, Giacoia GP: Pneumothorax: A complication of endotracheal tube suction. J Pediatr 1978; 92:633.
13. Wood RE: Spelunking in the pediatric airways: Explorations with the flexible bronchoscope. Pediatr Clin North Am 1984; 31:785.
14. Cotton RT, Seid AB: Management of the extubation problem in the premature child: Anterior cricoid split as an alternative to tracheostomy. Ann Otol Rhinol Laryngol 1980; 89:508.
15. Stool SE, Eavey R: Tracheostomy, in Bluestone CD, Stool SE (eds): Pediatric Otolaryngology. Philadelphia, WB Saunders Co, 1983, p 1330.
16. Parkin JL: Congenital malformations of the mouth and pharynx, in Bluestone CD, Stool SE (eds): Pediatric Otolaryngology. Philadelphia, WB Saunders Co, 1983, p 912.
17. Karmody CS: Developmental anomalies of the neck, in Bluestone CD, Stool SE (eds): Pediatric Otolaryngology. Philadelphia, WB Saunders Co, 1983, p 1386.
18. Holinger LD: Etiology of stridor in the neonate, infant, and child. Ann Otol Rhinol Laryngol 1980; 89:397.
19. Liekensohn GV, Benton C, Cotton R: Subglottic hemangioma. J Otolaryngol 1976; 5:487.
20. Abramowsky CR, Witt WJ: Sarcoma of the larynx in a newborn. Cancer 1983; 51:1726.
21. Bluestone CD, Delerme AN, Samuelson GH: Airway obstruction due to vocal cord paralysis in infants with hydrocephalus and meningomyelocele. Ann Otol 1972; 81:778.
22. Bluestone CD, Stool SE (eds). Pediatric Otolaryngology. Philadelphia, WB Saunders Co, 1983.
23. Ferguson CF, Kendig EL (eds): Pediatric Otolaryngology: Disorders of the Respiratory Tract in Children. Philadelphia, WB Saunders Co, vol 2, 1972.
24. Benjamin B: Endoscopy in esophageal atresia and tracheoesophageal fistula. Ann Otol Rhinol Laryngol 1981; 90:376.
25. Wood RE: Clinical applications of ultrathin flexible bronchoscopes. Pediatr Pulmonol 1984; 1:244.

# 5

# Clinical Care Techniques

Marvin D. Lough, R.R.T.
Waldemar A. Carlo, M.D.

One must concede that infants are not just little adults. Therefore, many respiratory care procedures are unique to the infant. Also, the equipment necessary to perform these procedures is either specifically designed or modified. This chapter will discuss some of these procedures as they pertain to respiratory care of the sick newborn infant.

## TRANSPORT

The *regionalization* of perinatal care has placed increased importance on methods of transporting high-risk pregnant women and sick newborn infants to tertiary care centers. If a high-risk situation is identified before delivery, the mother should be transferred to a tertiary care center since the uterus is the ideal "transport incubator." However, pregnancy and labor usually start as low-risk, and insufficient time is available to perform a maternal transport once the high-risk factors are identified.

The timing of the transport is particularly important for the premature infant. Approximately one third of all infant deaths occur within the first 24 hours following birth, and early treatment of many conditions improves outcome. Therefore, for whatever reason the physician considers referring an infant, be it an illness that cannot be handled properly at a particular hospital or inadequate equipment, we recommend early transportation.

To perform safe infant transports, the tertiary (receiving) center should have a specially trained staff that includes physicians, nurses, respiratory therapists, and medical transporters. A medical director

**TABLE 5–1.**
Checklist of Items to be Organized by the Referring Hospital

1. Maternal history
2. Copy of patient's chart
3. Laboratory results
4. All available x-rays
5. List of drugs and treatment given
6. Maternal and cord blood specimens
7. Patient identification
8. Parental agreement concerning transport
9. Telephone number of referring physician

with particular interest in infant transfer should oversee the transport system. A 24-hour hotline should be appropriately staffed by a trained physician who can receive information on the infant's condition as well as provide stabilization and management instructions necessary before the transport team arrives.

Basic principles of care important for most unstable infants should be reviewed with the referring hospital. These include maintenance of airway patency, oxygenation, normovolemia, temperature, and acid-base balance. Instructions related to the infant's specific condition should also be given.

Once the transfer has been requested, all coordination should be performed by the receiving hospital and its transport team. For critically ill infants, the transport team may consist of a physician, a nurse, a respiratory therapist, and a medical transporter. For less ill infants, a smaller transport team is usually sufficient. The transport team will travel to the referring hospital and become acquainted with the infant's condition by performing a clinical history, physical examination, and review of all prior treatment and laboratory results. The transport will be expedited if the referring facility has the items listed in Table 5–1 ready at the time of arrival of the transport team. Stabilization should be completed, and frequently intensive care should be initiated before the infant leaves the referring facility. For the transportation to be accomplished without further insult to the infant, conditions such as pneumothorax, endotracheal tube dislodgment, hypoxemia, hypovolemia, hypoglycemia, hypothermia, acidosis, and seizures should be recognized and treated before transport.

A reasonable time should be alloted for the parents to see the infant. This is a good opportunity to briefly review with the parents the infant's condition, expected clinical course, and long-term prognosis. Though it is obviously impossible to allay all parental fears, a short discussion about the transportation and the nature of the care the infant will receive in the intensive care unit is helpful. Many parents of infants to be transported believe that their baby probably will not survive, and reassurance to the contrary may be appropriate. Parents appreciate a picture of their baby, especially when the infant is transported to another hospital. In our unit, the parents can call directly into the intensive care unit and visit 24 hours a day. It is helpful to work closely with the father, particularly when the mother remains at the referring hospital.

## Equipment and Supplies

A transport system should have the equipment and supplies necessary to handle any neonatal emergency (Table 5–2). A tackle box containing all expendable supplies should be replenished after each trip. Problems of transportation are often related to equipment failure that should be prevented by careful maintenance.

## Transport Vehicles

Vehicles used for infant transport range from simple ground ambulance to jet aircraft especially suited for medical transports. The simplest form of *ground transport* includes a standard ambulance, a transport incubator, and a tackle box with supplies and medications. This system is adequate only for the transport of stable infants. A more sophisticated ground transport consists of a fully equipped ambulance that is essentially a mini-intensive care nursery on wheels. This vehicle should contain the equipment included in Table 5–2 and be large enough for the transport team to work. This ground system is designed for short- and medium-range trips, regardless of the severity of the infant's condition.

Helicopters and fixed-wing *aircraft transport* are particularly useful when distance or time make ground transportation impractical. Aircraft transportation is usually valuable when transport distance is over 100 miles or in selected cases of extreme urgency. A serious complication associated with fixed-wing aircraft transport is the decrease in partial pressure of oxygen at higher altitudes, leading to hypoxia, pneumothorax, and abdominal distention. An altimeter and a barometer should be kept in the cabin to adjust the inspired oxygen concentrations to compensate for the change in atmospheric pressure (Table 5–3). Weather conditions and costs should be taken into consideration when selecting the transport vehicle. Fixed-wing aircraft are usually less noisy than helicopters. Excessive vibrations and noise in a helicopter may make it difficult to adequately evaluate the patient's condition. Guidelines for air and ground transportation have been developed by the American Academy of Pediatrics.[1]

**TABLE 5-2.**
Supplies for Transport

| | |
|---|---|
| Transport incubator with battery | Drugs |
| | Diluted sodium bicarbonate (0.5 mEq/cc) |
| Monitoring | 1:10,000 aqueous epinephrine |
|   Blood pressure monitor | Naloxone |
|   Cardiorespiratory monitor, leads, and electrodes | Atropine sulfate |
| | Calcium gluconate |
|   Transcutaneous oxygen and carbon dioxide monitor | Prostaglandin E |
| | Tolazoline |
|   Saturation monitor | Dopamine |
| | Phenobarbital |
| Respiratory | Antibiotics |
|   Transport ventilator | |
|   Laryngoscope handle with premature (Miller 0) and term infant (Miller 1) blades | Charting |
| |   Intensive care record sheet and progress notes |
|   Precut endotracheal tubes (2.5, 3.0, 3.5, and 4.0 mm ID) |   Transport information and permission forms |
|   Adapters for endotracheal tubes | |
|   Bag and masks of various sizes | Suction pump and suction catheters (6, 8, and 10 F) |
|   Oxygen tank | |
|   Infant airways | |
|   Oxygen hood | Miscellaneous |
| |   Stethoscope |
| Vascular access/fluid administration |   Preparation tray with povidone-iodine (Betadine) |
|   Syringes (1 cc, 3 cc, 5 cc, and 10 cc) | |
|   Needles (20-, 22-, and 25-gauge) |   Thoracotomy tube set |
|   Umbilical vein catheterization set and extra catheters |   Feeding tubes (5 and 8 F) |
| |   Thermometer |
|   Butterfly needles (23 and 25 gauge) |   Hematocrit tubes |
|   Intravenous catheters (22 and 24 gauge) |   Lancets |
|   T-connectors |   Suture material |
|   Intravenous tubing |   Scissors |
|   Three-way stopcocks, sterile |   Adhesive tape |
|   Stopcock plugs (needle caps) |   Dextrostix |
|   Buretrols |   Tape measure |
|   IV solutions (10% and 5% dextrose in water) |   Disposable sterile gloves |
| |   Specimen tubes |
|   Sterile distilled water |   Blood culture tubes |
|   Sterile saline |   Alcohol sponges |
|   Heparinized saline |   Benzoin |
|   Rubber bands |   Suture material |
| |   Instant camera |

**TABLE 5-3.**
Effects of Altitude on Ambient and Alveolar Oxygen

| Altitude | Atmospheric Pressure, mm Hg | Partial Pressure of Oxygen, mm Hg | | |
|---|---|---|---|---|
| | | Ambient | Alveoli | Blood |
| Sea level | 760 | 159 | 105 | 100 |
| 2,000 | 707 | 148 | 97 | 92 |
| 6,000 | 609 | 127 | 84 | 79 |
| 10,000 | 523 | 109 | 74 | 69 |
| 20,000 | 349 | 73 | 40 | 35 |
| 30,000 | 226 | 47 | 21 | 19 |

## THERMOREGULATION

As suggested by the studies of Budin, a pioneer neonatologist, temperature regulation is one of the most important infant care procedures and largely determines ultimate outcome.[2] He demonstrated that keeping small infants warm increased survival by about sevenfold. Even though careful thermoregulation of the newborn is now widely practiced, it should not be taken for granted. Infants should be nursed in their *neutral thermal environment temperature*, i.e., the environmental temperature at which metabolic rate (as well as oxygen consumption and carbon dioxide production) is the lowest (Table 5-4). In addition to the following discussion, Chapter 7 also includes a section on thermoregulation.

### Incubators

The most commonly used device for temperature control of the infant is the *single-walled incubator*. The incubator air is heated to the

**TABLE 5-4.**
Approximate Neutral Thermal Environment Temperatures (°C)

| Age | Weight (gm)* | | | |
|---|---|---|---|---|
| | <1,200 | 1,201-1,500 | 1,501-2,500 | >2,500 (>36 weeks) |
| 0-6 hr | 34.0-35.4 | 33.9-34.4 | 32.8-33.8 | 32.0-33.8 |
| 6-12 hr | 34.0-35.4 | 33.5-34.4 | 32.2-33.8 | 31.4-33.8 |
| 12-24 hr | 34.0-35.4 | 33.3-34.3 | 31.8-33.8 | 31.0-33.7 |
| 24-96 hr | 34.0-35.0 | 33.0-34.2 | 31.1-33.2 | 29.8-32.8 |
| 4-14 days | | 32.6-34.0 | 31.0-33.2 | 29.0-32.6 |
| 2-3 wk | | 32.2-34.0 | 30.5-33.0 | 30.0 |
| 3-4 wk | | 31.6-33.6 | 30.0-32.7 | |
| 4-5 wk | | 31.2-33.0 | 29.5-32.2 | |
| 5-6 wk | | 30.6-32.3 | 29.0-31.8 | |

*Adapted from Klaus MH, Fanaroff AA (ed.): *Care of the High-Risk Neonate,* ed 3. Philadelphia, WB Saunders Co, 1986, p 103.

proper temperature as it passes through a heating coil. High relative humidity (75% to 90%) is achieved as the warm air passes over the water in the humidity reservoir. Due to the slight positive pressure maintained inside the incubator by the air-circulating system, there is always a tendency for air to flow to the outside, thus ensuring a high degree of isolation. The incubator temperature may be manually or servocontrolled.

The single-walled incubator is an efficient method of keeping the infant warm by convection, but because the temperature of the plastic walls cannot be controlled, radiant heat loss from the infant will occur. If the nursery is cool or if the incubator is placed near a cold window or wall, the infant will radiate heat to the cold incubator walls, and it will be virtually impossible to maintain a *thermoneutral environment*. When a small clear plastic *heat shield* is placed over the infant inside the single-walled incubator, the warm incubator air will heat the plastic shield to the same temperature as the air within the incubator. The infant then will radiate only to the warm plastic heat shield, as radiant waves from the infant will not penetrate this shield. *Double-walled incubators* that serve the above combined effect of heat shield and incubator are commercially available.

### Radiant-Warmers

Radiant warmers provide another method for temperature control. Radiant warmers allow easy access to the infant and have become widespread particularly for the critically ill patient. Overheating or underheating may occur but can be easily prevented by using the servocontrol mode and correct placement of the skin probe. The skin temperature over the right upper abdomen should be kept around 36.5°C. An increase in insensible water loss occurs in infants nursed under radiant warmers.

## OXYGEN THERAPY

Oxygen can be delivered to the infant in several ways: (1) hood; (2) nasal cannula; (3) bag and mask; (4) continuous positive airway pressure; and (5) mechanical ventilation. This section will not deal with oxygen delivery by continuous positive airway pressure and mechanical ventilation, which are discussed in detail in Chapter 12.

The simplest and most efficient way to deliver an oxygen-enriched atmosphere to a spontaneously breathing infant is with a clear plastic

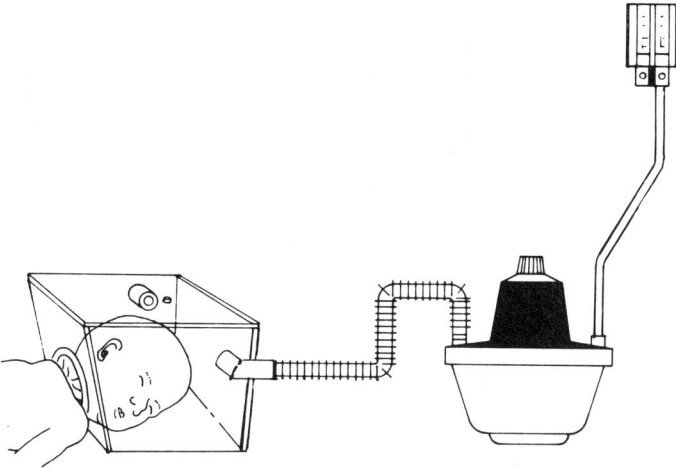

**FIG 5–1.**
An oxygen hood with controlled temperature, humidity, and oxygen.

hood placed over the infant's head. Air and oxygen blenders allow for the delivery of a wide range of oxygen concentrations (21% to 100%) through a cascade humidifier to the oxygen hood (Fig 5–1). The air-oxygen mixture must be humidified and warmed to the same temperature as that of the incubator air, which should be in the range of the thermoneutral environment. The concentration of environmental oxygen should be monitored closely.

A *nasal cannula* is most suitable for older infants who are more active and who may tolerate inadvertent changes in the inspired oxygen concentration. A blender should be used to deliver the appropriate oxygen concentration, although infants may breathe through the mouth or at flows higher than those being supplied by the cannula. Thus, inspired oxygen concentrations may need to be higher than that used with an oxygen hood. Transcutaneous oxygen tension and saturation monitors can be used to determine the inspired oxygen concentration and the rate of flow required for each infant.

Two types of *bag-and-mask systems* are commonly used for newborn infants: flow-inflating and self-inflating. The *flow-inflating* system utilizes a 0.5 to 1 L thin-wall rubber anesthesia bag and a face mask with a soft rubber or air-filled rim. Proper pressure and inflation of the bag can be obtained by varying either the flow of gas or pressure relief valve. A manometer must be placed in line to accurately measure delivered pressures. When applied to the face, the mask should avoid the eyes and allow a small leak around the mask to prevent rebreathing of carbon dioxide and to act as a pressure "pop-off." Unlike the flow-inflating bag, the *self-inflating* bag does not require a source gas. The recoil characteristics of this bag allow for spontaneous reinflation following a manual deflation. This type of bag is necessary when an adequate source of compressed gas is not available. Some of the problems associated with the self-inflating bag-and-mask system are (1) varying and unknown concentration of oxygen; (2) the "feel" for bagging is lost due to the recoil characteristics of the bag; and (3) the safety release valve often is limited to less than 40 cm $H_2O$.

## ENDOTRACHEAL INTUBATION

When upper airway patency cannot be established by mild hyperextension of the neck, an artificial oropharyngeal airway piece may be used. However, at times only endotracheal intubation will assure proper patency. Bag-and-mask ventilation usually is sufficient for resuscitation, but if assisted ventilation is to be initiated, endotracheal intubation will be necessary. Usually bag-and-mask ventilation should be initiated while steps are taken to ensure that all equipment for endotracheal intubation is ready. Bag-and-mask ventilation should not precede endotracheal intubation of infants born meconium stained, as the meconium will be pushed into the distal airways. These infants are often intubated just long enough to aspirate the trachea.

### Orotracheal Intubation

Prior to intubation, all equipment must be at hand (laryngoscope with proper size blade and functioning light; suction catheters; appropriate endotracheal tubes; oxygen line; appropriate mask and bag with adapter for the endotracheal tube; and tape and/or other material for securing the tube to the patient's face). Provide the infant with oxygen continuously before and during the intubation by at least directing a flow of oxygen to the face. If the infant is apneic, then do not interrupt bag-and-mask ventilation longer than 30 to 45 seconds during intubation attempts. Empty the stomach to prevent emesis and aspiration.

Hold the infant so that the head is slightly extended and the shoulders are flat to prevent arching of the back. Grasp the laryngoscope handle between the thumb and the first two fingers of the left hand. Insert the blade (Miller size 0 for premature and Miller size 1 for term infants) into the right side of the mouth, and move it to the midline, gently deflecting the tongue to the left side of the mouth. Stabilize the infant's head by grasping the chin with the third and fourth fingers of the left hand (Fig 5–2). Gently advance the blade into the vallecula,

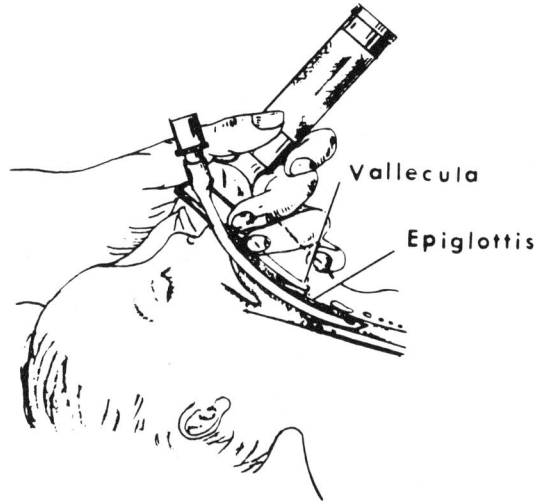

**FIG 5-2.**
Position of bronchoscope and endotracheal tube during endotracheal intubation.

anterior to the epiglottis (a pink flaplike structure at the base of the tongue). Do not pick up the epiglottis with the laryngoscope blade. Gently lift the tip of the blade upward while using the small finger of the left hand to apply pressure over the hyoid bone to move the larynx posteriorly and expose the glottis. Exercise care to prevent the blade from traumatizing the upper gums by lifting, but not rotating, the laryngoscope when trying to expose the larynx. Suctioning of secretions in the oropharynx may be necessary. Insert the endotracheal tube alongside the laryngoscope, not down the barrel of the blade. Insert the tube between the vocal cords, and advance the tip approximately 2 cm beyond them. Then carefully withdraw the laryngoscope blade while the position of the tube is maintained by the right hand. The maximal allowable time for any one attempt is 30 to 45 seconds or until bradycardia occurs. If intubation has not been accomplished within this time, ventilate the infant with bag and mask for at least 2 minutes before a second attempt is made.

Verify correct placement of the tube by (1) the presence of symmetric breath sounds and chest movement bilaterally and (2) the absence of loud inspiratory sounds over the stomach area. Of course, the best verification of endotracheal tube tip position is by x-ray.

Once the endotracheal tube has been inserted to the predetermined distance, securing the tube is of major importance. After drying the mouth and upper lip, paint the cheekbones, upper lip, and endotracheal tube with benzoin. After the benzoin has become tacky, place a piece of half-inch adhesive tape on the right cheek, draw it across the upper lip, and press it firmly to the skin. Continuing, wrap the tape firmly around the tube (2 revolutions) in a counterclockwise direction. Take the excess tape and secure it to the left cheek. Using a second strip of tape, begin on the left cheek, and reverse the procedure, wrapping the tape in a clockwise fashion. Common adhesive tape, as opposed to waterproof adhesive tape, adheres better to polyvinyl chloride endotracheal tubes when moistened with saliva or nasal secretions. A holder that facilitates tube fixation is commercially available.

**Practical Hints**

The following hints will facilitate intubation:

1. Endotracheal tubes should be made of nontoxic polyvinyl chloride that will conform to the trachea when warmed to body temperature. A radiopaque line on the endotracheal tube facilitates radiographic visualization.

2. The following guidelines for length of orotracheal insertion approximated from Figure 5–3 facilitate correct tube tip positioning:

| Infant Weight, gm | Length of Endotracheal Tube Insertion, cm |
|---|---|
| 1,000 | 7 |
| 2,000 | 8 |
| 3,000 | 9 |

At these lengths, the distal end of the endotracheal tube should be at the midtrachea. An extra centimeter should be allowed for securing the endotracheal tube. Endotracheal tubes should be cut to the appropriate length (measured from the lip). The 15-mm endotracheal tube adapter should be in place before intubation.

3. The following guidelines for size (internal diameter) of the endotracheal tube are recommended (see Chapter 4):

| Gestational Age, wk | Size of Endotracheal Tube, mm |
|---|---|
| <30 | 2.5 |
| 30–35 | 3.0 |
| >35 | 3.5 |

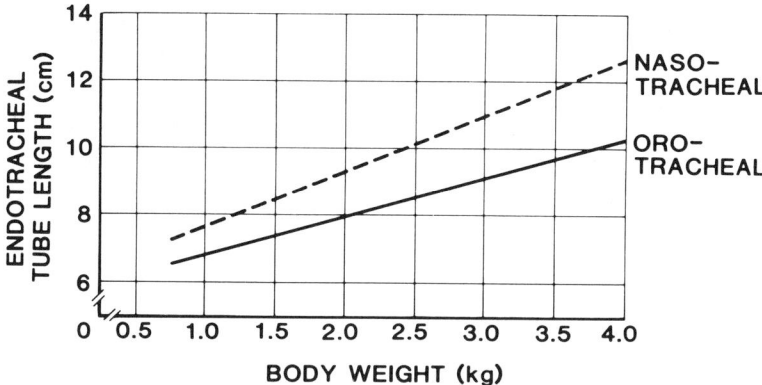

**FIG 5–3.**
Graph for determination of length of insertion of endotracheal tubes. The tip of the endotracheal tube is aimed at the midtrachea. (Adapted from Tochen ML: Orotracheal intubation in the newborn infant: A method for determining depth of tube insertion. *J Pediatr* 1979; 9:1050, and Coldiron JS: Estimation of nasotracheal tube length in neonates. *Pediatrics* 1968; 41:823.)

4. Iced tubes will be stiffer, facilitating intubation without the need of a stylet.

5. If a stylet is used, it should not protrude beyond the distal tip of the endotracheal tube.

6. Extreme hyperextension of the neck elevates the glottis (which is already anteriorly situated in neonates), making visualization and intubation of the trachea more difficult.

7. Oropharyngeal suction will facilitate visualization if excessive secretions are present.

8. Greater air entry in the right than left hemithorax suggests that the endotracheal tube has passed into the right main-stem bronchus, and it must be slowly withdrawn until bilateral air entry is present.

9. A nasogastric tube with its proximal tip placed under water will demonstrate inspiratory gas bubbles during assisted ventilation if the endotracheal tube is in the esophagus.

10. Radiographic confirmation of the tip position is mandatory.

## Nasotracheal Intubation

Fixation of the tube may be easier when introduced via the nasal route. However, nasotracheal intubation requires slightly more time than orotracheal intubation and should be reserved for elective procedures. Trauma and necrosis to the nasal septum suggest that nasal intubation should be used sparingly. However, palatal groove formation that follows prolonged orotracheal intubation will not occur. With a few exceptions, nasotracheal intubation is performed essentially with the same technique as oral intubation. A lubricated tube is inserted through one nostril into the pharyngeal space before the vocal cords are visualized. After the cords are visualized, in the same manner as with oral intubation, a McGill forceps may be necessary to advance the tube into the larynx. Nasotracheal tubes should be cut approximately 20% longer than the length required for orotracheal tubes (see Fig 5–3). A stylet should not be used for nasotracheal intubations.

**Teaching Model for Intubation**

Four-week-old kittens serve as excellent teaching models for endotracheal intubation of the neonate.[3] The kitten should be anesthetized with about 40 mg of ketamine injected into the triceps muscle. Ketamine will take effect in about 5 minutes and leaves the laryngeal reflex intact. The anatomy of the kitten is very similar to that of the infant, with the exception of a slightly larger, broader epiglottis. The kitten can be intubated using a 3.0-mm tube and a Miller size 0 laryngoscope blade and will usually be awake and well in less than 1 hour.

# CHEST PHYSIOTHERAPY

A program of pulmonary physiotherapy facilitates mobilization of pulmonary secretions.[4] Percussion, or "clapping," over the chest and vibration may be combined with postural drainage to facilitate removal of secretions. Position changes of the infant should be made every 2 to 4 hours with percussion and vibration before suctioning of the endotracheal tube. In the acutely ill infant with minimal mucus production, physiotherapy and tube suctioning should be performed less frequently.

Removal of secretions from the bronchi is facilitated by the force of gravity in various positions and by percussion. The lung congestion and the infant's tolerance will dictate the need for postural drainage with percussion and vibration. Figures 5–4 and 5–5 illustrate the various positions for proper drainage of the upper, middle, and lower lobes of the infant. The infant should be placed in a position such that the segment being drained is uppermost and the major airway leading out of the segment is pointed downward.

Percussion or clapping over the thorax in the area of the segment being drained will facilitate the movement of secretions from smaller airways into larger ones. Since the adult hand usually is larger than the infant's thorax, a small plastic medicine cup attached to the clinician's finger will provide effective percussion with a cupping action. Vibration is applied to the chest wall, over the affected area, during the expiratory phase. Vibration is a fine shaking motion, which is

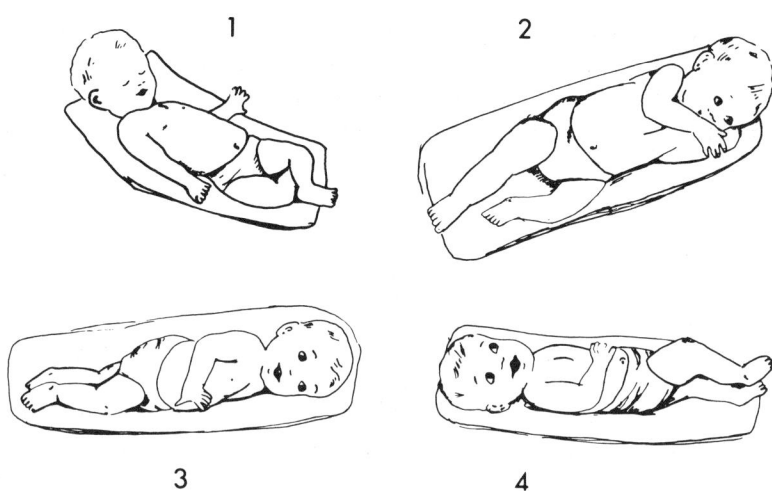

**FIG 5-4.**
Positions for chest physiotherapy: *1*, the anterior segment of the upper lobes is drained in a supine position at a 30° upright angle. *2*, the apical segment of the right lung is drained while the infant lies on his left side at a 30° upright angle. *3*, the posterior segment of the right upper lobe is drained in a prone position with the right side elevated 45°. *4*, the anterior segment of the upper lobe is drained in a supine position.

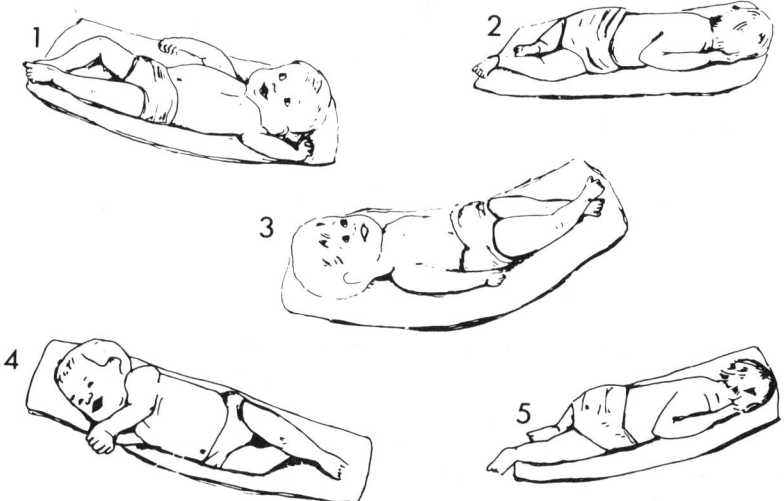

**FIG 5-5.**
*1*, the right middle lobe is drained at a 15° head-down angle with a 45° rotation to the left. The lingula is drained by rotating to the right. *2*, the superior segment of the lower lobes drains in a prone position. *3*, the anterior basal segments of the lower lobes are drained at a 30° head-down position. *4*, the basal segments of the lower lobe are drained at a 30° head-down position while the infant is lying on the side. *5*, the posterior basal segments of the lower lobes are drained at a 30° head-down prone position.

achieved by tightening all the muscles of the arm and shoulders. It may also be applied with a battery-powered vibrator or toothbrush fitted with a soft rubber cup, such as a nipple. All secretions loosened after percussion or vibration must be removed via suctioning following each treatment.

## SUCTIONING

Periodic suctioning of the endotracheal tube is necessary to remove secretions. Suctioning is potentially dangerous because it may result in pneumothoraces, infection, hypoxic episodes, and traumatic lesions in the trachea (if suction is applied beyond the endotracheal tube tip). When necessary, the infant should be suctioned briefly, using strict sterile technique with disposable gloves and suction tubes, and must be allowed to recover between episodes of suctioning. Frequent routine suctioning is not necessary, but suctioning must be performed whenever it is suspected that secretions are present in the endotracheal tube. Instillation of saline facilitates removal of thick, inspissated secretions; however, if adequate humidification is used, this problem is reduced. An endotracheal tube change is indicated if partial or complete blockage cannot be resolved by suctioning. Routine tube changes are not indicated. For further discussions on suctioning, see Chapters 4 and 7.

## TRACHEOSTOMY

See Chapter 4 for a discussion of tracheostomy.

## EXTERNAL CARDIAC MASSAGE

Whenever cardiac massage is indicated, it should be started promptly and maintained without interruption at a constant rhythm of at least 100 compressions per minute. The techniques for infant and pediatric cardiac massage and cardiopulmonary resuscitation (CPR) have been reviewed recently.[5] The sternum should be compressed 1.5 to 2 cm with each stroke. Two techniques of massage currently are acceptable. The first technique (Fig 5–6) is to use the tips of the index and middle finger. These two fingertips are positioned one fingerwidth below an intermammary line where it intersects the sternum. For maximal effectiveness, the infant should be lying supine on a firm surface.

The alternative method is the two-thumb technique. The thumbs

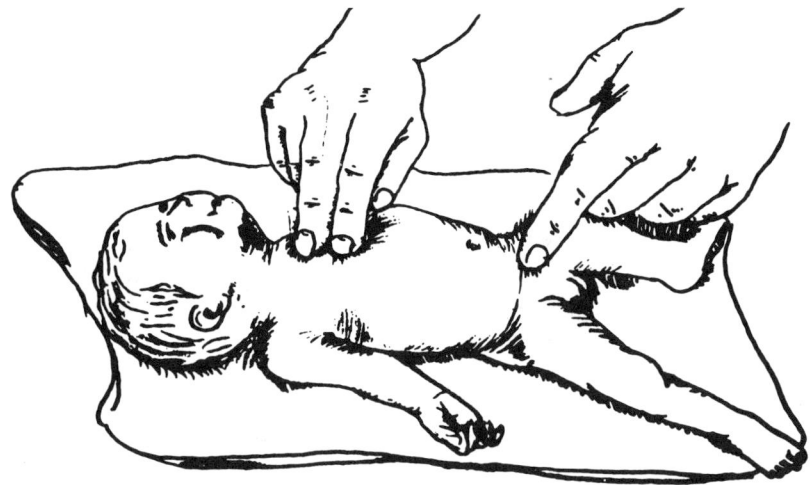

**FIG 5–6.**
Two-finger technique of external cardiac massage.

should be placed on the middle third of the sternum. Both hands then should encircle the infant's chest. Care must be taken to compress with the thumbs and not push upward on the infant's back with the fingers.

With both techniques, chest pressure should be released at the end of each compression (without removing the fingers) to allow the sternum to come to its normal position. The effectiveness of cardiac massage is monitored by the presence of a carotid or femoral pulse. Chest compressions should always be accompanied by assisted ventilation which should be performed at a compression to ventilation ratio of 5 to 1.

## ARTERIAL CATHETERIZATION

Arterial catheterization is indicated in patients requiring frequent arterial blood gas analysis or continuous direct blood pressure monitoring. When intermittent blood sampling is sufficient, peripheral arterial punctures should alternatively be used. New noninvasive blood pressure monitors have reduced the need of arterial catheterization for the sole purpose of measuring systemic pressures.

### Umbilical Artery Catheterization

*Umbilical artery* catheterization should be attempted in critically ill neonates requiring frequent arterial blood gas analysis. The length

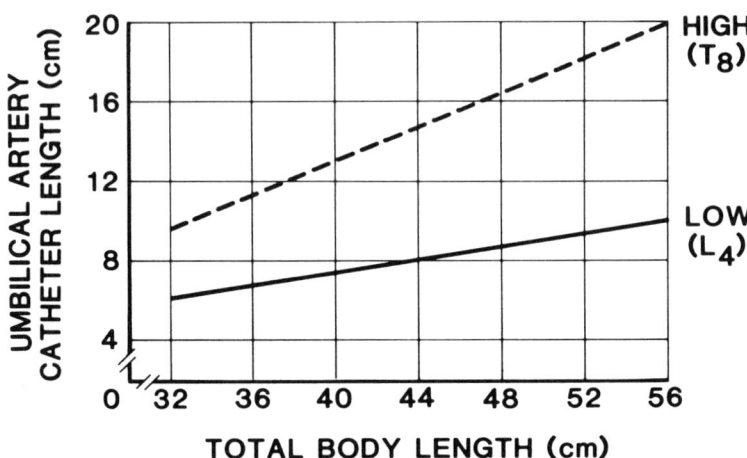

**FIG 5–7.**
Graph for determining the length of insertion of umbilical artery catheter for placement of its tip at high (eighth thoracic [T = 8]) or low (fourth lumbar [L = 4]) levels. The length of the umbilical stump should be added to the obtained values. (Adapted from Rosenfeld W, et al: *J Pediatr* 1980; 96:735 and Rosenfeld W, et al: *J Pediatr* 1981; 98:627.

of insertion of an umbilical arterial catheter necessary for correct tip placement can be predetermined from the body length using the graph in Figure 5–7. The tip of the umbilical artery catheter should be placed in the descending aorta either at the thoracic aorta (vertebral level T-6 to T-10) or at the lumbar aorta (L-3 to L-4). Major arteries such as celiac axis (T-11 to T-12), superior mesenteric (L-1), renal (L-1), and inferior mesenteric (L-2 to L-3) emerge from the aorta at the levels between T-11 and L-3, and avoidance of these regions is warranted.

Low (vertebral level L-3 to L-4) tip placement has been associated with an increased incidence of blanching or cyanosis of the lower extremities. Warming of the contralateral extremity may improve perfusion to the leg, but frequently the catheter has to be removed. We prefer to initially insert a high (T-6 to T-10) line to prevent problems of perfusion to the legs and because the region of correct placement is longer for a high than for a low line. Furthermore, if the catheter is not inserted far enough, or is subsequently partially pulled out accidentally, it can be retracted to a lower position. After initial placement, umbilical catheters should not be advanced further as this would markedly increase the risk of infection. Regardless of tip position, umbilical artery catheterization may be complicated by thromboembolism. This may manifest as decreased perfusion to a leg or toe, hypertension, or impaired renal function.

Catheters that measure intra-arterial oxygen tension or saturation are now available for continuous oxygenation assessment. These catheters are particularly useful in critically ill infants who require continuous blood gas monitoring.

*Procedure*

An umbilical artery catheter (3.5 F for infants less than 1500 gm or a 5.0 F for infants more than 1500 gm) should be marked according to desired length of insertion. The catheter should be soft and transparent and have a rounded tip with a single end hole and a radiopaque line. The catheter is connected to a three-way stopcock and filled with sterile heparinized normal saline solution (1 unit of heparin to 1 ml of sterile saline). The umbilical cord is cut, leaving a stump of 1 to 1.5 cm. The stump and surrounding area are cleansed with an antiseptic solution and a drape placed over the stump. The arteries are small, constricted, thick-walled vessels located at about 4 and 8 o'clock (Fig 5–8). The artery to be used is teased open with a forceps or small obturator. The catheter is inserted into the lumen and gently advanced. It is common

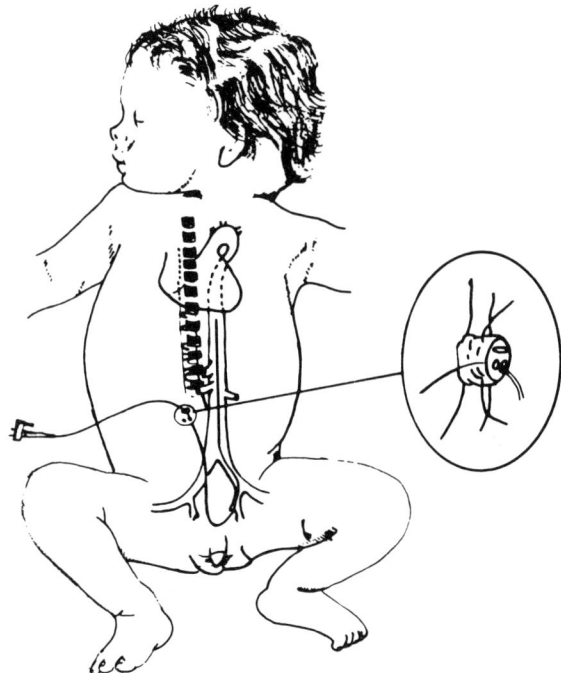

**FIG 5–8.**
Position of umbilical artery catheter and an exploded view of umbilical cord showing position of umbilical arteries.

to meet resistance slightly below the abdominal wall, where the vessel turns caudally, and at the junction of the hypogastric artery (5 to 6 cm). Gentle sustained pressure on the catheter usually will relax the artery and allow the catheter to advance. If gentle pressure is not successful, 0.1 to 0.2 ml of 1% or 2% lidocaine (without epinephrine) can be injected in an attempt to relieve vasospasm. However, the catheter should never be forced past a site of obstruction. If resistance persists, catheterization of the other artery should be attempted. Once the catheter is inserted, it can be held in place by a pursestring suture around the cord stump. The position should be radiographically confirmed. It is extremely important to prevent air embolism through an arterial line. When no longer needed, the last 6 to 8 cm of the catheter should be slowly withdrawn to allow the artery to constrict.

**Peripheral Artery Catheterization**

A *peripheral artery* catheter can be placed if umbilical artery catheterization has been unsuccessful or complicated by side effects. Catheterization of a peripheral artery can only be performed at sites where collateral circulation is present such as the radial, dorsalis pedis, and posterior tibialis arteries. These arteries can be safely catheterized in infants using a 22- or 24-gauge catheter with a needle stylet and a percutaneous technique. Before attempting a peripheral artery catheterization, the *Allen Test* should show evidence of collateral circulation. For this test, blanch the extremity distal to the site to be punctured by first squeezing it and then gently applying pressure to the involved arteries. Next remove pressure from one artery, and look for the extremities to flush as it fills with blood. Repeat the procedure with the other artery. Return of color (disappearance of blanching) indicates the presence of collateral circulation. Local anesthesia can be provided by infiltration of 1 ml of 1% to 2% lidocaine. Thromboembolism is a potential complication, and the circulation of the fingertips should be frequently evaluated.

Transillumination of the extremities for the purpose of arterial catheterization or blood sampling is an easily performed technique with a high degree of success.[6] With the room lights dimmed, the probe is placed against the extremity directly opposite the arterial site to be sampled. Anatomical landmarks and the artery to be sampled are easily visualized. The artery appears as a pulsating linear structure with indistinct edges due to pulsation.

## VENOUS CATHETERIZATION

When urgent vascular access is necessary in a newborn infant, *umbilical vein* catheterization is the easiest and fastest procedure that assures an adequate infusion and sampling site. Other indications for umbilical vein catheterization include exchange transfusion and central venous pressure monitoring. In the first few hours after birth, the ductus venosus is patent, and the umbilical vein catheter may be advanced to the inferior vena cava or right atrium. These sites are reliable for central venous pressure monitoring. Resistance encountered beyond 4 to 7 cm (depending on infant size) indicates inability to pass through the ductus venosus and possible inadvertent catheterization of the portal or other major veins. The catheter should be retracted to 4 to 7 cm until good blood return is obtained. Hypertonic solutions should only be infused if the catheter tip is beyond the ductus venosus. The position of the catheter should be verified radiographically. A lateral view will readily distinguish between an arterial (initially caudal and then posterior) and a venous catheterization (initially cephalic and anterior). Liver necrosis, portal vein thrombosis, and infection are common complications of umbilical vein catheterization. Catheterization of a peripheral vein should replace umbilical vein catheterization as soon as central venous pressure monitoring is no longer necessary.

## INTERMITTENT ARTERIAL BLOOD SAMPLING

When frequent or continuous blood gas monitoring is not essential, intermittent arterial blood sampling may be performed. A technique similar to the percutaneous catheterization of a peripheral artery may be employed by using a scalp vein set or small needle (23 to 27 gauge). Arterial puncture should only be performed using arteries that have adequate collaterals as described for peripheral artery catheterization.

## CAPILLARY BLOOD SAMPLING

Arterial punctures can sometimes be avoided by the use of capillary blood samples. If peripheral perfusion is adequate, capillary blood taken from the extremities will reflect arterial values of pH and carbon dioxide tension ($P_{CO_2}$). Oxygen tension ($P_{O_2}$) values for capillary blood are not reliable indicators of arterial oxygenation. To obtain a capillary blood sample for blood gas analysis, the foot should first be warmed for several minutes to a temperature of 38° to 40°C to stimulate circulation and "arterialize" the capillary blood. After cleaning the site with alcohol, the heel is punctured with a blood lancet, and free-flowing blood is collected in a glass capillary tube. The tube ends are sealed with wax or Critoseal making sure air bubbles are not present in the sample tube. Poor circulation or failure to warm the foot properly may result in slow blood flow from the puncture site and unreliable results. One should resist the temptation to squeeze the heel as this often results in contamination of the sample with interstitial fluid or venous blood and prolongs exposure of the blood to air (which will reduce the $Pco_2$).

## CONTINUOUS BLOOD GAS MONITORING

Techniques recently developed allow for continuous estimation of arterial blood gases and oxygen saturation in neonates. These techniques have improved patient evaluation and reduced the need of other invasive procedures. Continuous monitoring of blood gases is particularly useful to follow critically ill infants and to evaluate the effect of procedures.

### Transcutaneous Blood Gas Monitoring

*Oxygen*

Clark electrodes applied over the skin and heated appropriately (usually 42° to 44°C) may be used to estimate arterial oxygen tension.[7] Transcutaneous oxygen monitoring should be employed in patients receiving oxygen supplementation who do not have indwelling arterial lines. It is also helpful to continuously monitor critically ill patients, accelerate weaning, and reduce the frequency of blood gas analysis in patients who have an indwelling arterial line.

The correlation between the transcutaneous and arterial oxygen tension is usually very good and has a slope that approximates 1.0 with a 0 intercept.[7] Reasons for overestimation of arterial oxygen tension include (1) air bubble or leak between the electrode and skin and (2) improper calibration. Transcutaneous oxygen monitoring may also underestimate arterial oxygen tension. This may be due to (1) decreased tissue perfusion; (2) increasing postnatal age; (3) insufficient heating of the electrode; and (4) improper calibration.

Burns may occur when the heated electrode is applied to the skin, especially in premature infants and when perfusion is compromised. Changing the electrode site every 3 to 4 hours, or more frequently in the most immature infants, will reduce the incidence and severity of skin burns. If right-to-left ductal blood shunting occurs (as in infants with persistent fetal circulation), preductal monitoring sites (right upper chest, right arm, and head) will yield higher transcutaneous $P_{O_2}$ values than postductal sites (rest of body). Simultaneous monitoring of preductal and postductal sites and the resultant oxygen tension gradient provides an index of the degree of shunting and the effect of therapies such as hyperventilation and vasodilators.

### Carbon Dioxide

A heated transcutaneous (Severinghaus) electrode can be used to estimate arterial carbon dioxide tension.[8] Transcutaneous $P_{CO_2}$ monitoring is particularly useful for mechanically ventilated infants who are predisposed to marked changes in arterial $P_{CO_2}$ such as those undergoing assisted ventilation. A combined oxygen and carbon dioxide electrode is also available.[9]

Transcutaneous $P_{CO_2}$ accurately predicts arterial $P_{CO_2}$, but unlike transcutaneous $P_{O_2}$, a correction factor is necessary.[8, 9] Despite this correction, overestimation of arterial $P_{CO_2}$ may occur (1) during hypercapnia, (2) due to poor perfusion, (3) with advancing postnatal age, and (4) with improper calibration. Underestimation may be due to (1) presence of air or leak between the skin and the electrode, (2) insufficient heating of the electrode, and (3) improper calibration.

## Oximetry

Another noninvasive method of oxygen monitoring that has become available during the last few years is photometric measurement of *oxygen saturation*. This measurement is accomplished by evaluation of transmission of red light through the monitoring site. Oxygenated blood reflects more red light than desaturated blood. Although the relation between arterial oxygen tension and saturation is altered by factors such as pH, $P_{CO_2}$, temperature, and 2,3-diphosphoglycerate (2,3-DPG), saturation by itself is of extreme importance as the arterial oxygen content is largely determined by hemoglobin saturation and not by dissolved oxygen (Chapters 2 and 10). In neonates, we usually maintain arterial oxygen saturation between 88% to 92%.

Oximetry offers several advantages over transcutaneous oxygen monitoring that include (1) avoidance of heating the skin and the risk of burns; (2) elimination of a delay period for transducer equilibration; and (3) maintenance of an accurate measurement regardless of patient age, skin characteristics, or chronic lung disease. However, oximetry is insensitive to hyperoxia because hemoglobin approaches 100% saturation for all arterial oxygen tensions above approximately 100 mm Hg.

Several manufacturers have developed photometric oxygen saturation devices for infant and child use with an easily applied wraparound adhesive-bandage–like transducer that can be placed on a hand, foot, finger, or toe.

**Intra-arterial Oxygen Tension or Saturation Monitoring**

Catheters with an embedded oxygen-tension electrode or an infrared light emitter and detector have been developed for continuous monitoring of oxygen tension or saturation, respectively, for use as an indwelling line.[10,11] Major advantages over transcutaneous monitoring include (1) a faster response time (as the sensors are in direct contact with the blood) and (2) independence from peripheral perfusion states. However, these techniques are associated with the hazards of regular invasive indwelling catheters.

# TRANSILLUMINATION OF THE THORAX

Transillumination via fiberoptic probe may be used for the diagnosis of a pneumothorax in infants.[12] This procedure is performed with the overhead nursery lights turned off, but total darkness is not necessary. With the infant in a supine position, the probe is placed superior and then inferior to the nipple on both sides of the chest. If either side of the chest transilluminates more than the other, several spots at varying distances from the sternum should be transilluminated. If abnormal air collections are present (e.g., severe pulmonary interstitial emphysema and subcutaneous air), transillumination will be greater in those affected areas. Unless an urgent intervention is necessary and there is a clear asymmetry between the transillumination of the infant's chest, a confirmatory chest radiograph should be obtained before needle aspiration or chest tube placement is performed.

# THORACOSTOMY TUBE PLACEMENT

Evacuation of air or fluid collected in the pleural space is frequently necessary to restore the negative thoracic pressure and improve lung function. After aseptic and anesthetic (1% lidocaine) preparation, the skin should be cut at the level of one rib inferior to the intercostal spine through which the tube will be inserted. This subcutaneous tunnel will reduce air leakage into the chest. Care should be exercised to cut the skin at a distance from the nipple. Blunt dissection should be performed with a curved mosquito hemostat. A tracer or trocar should not be used in infants because the usually stiff lungs are predisposed to perforation. Because air collects anteriorly, the thoracostomy tube will be more effective if its hole lies in the anterior aspect of the chest.[13] Proper securing of the external portion of the tube will keep the tip in the desired position. Continuous bubbling after connection of the tube to a vacuum source ($-15$ to $-20$ cm $H_2O$) suggests a persistent large intrathoracic air leak (bronchopleural fistula) or a skin leak. Intermittent bubbling occurs with persistent small air leaks, while fluctuations with the respiratory cycle indicate pleural positioning without persistent air leaks. Radiographic confirmation of tube positioning and resolution of the pneumothorax is necessary. The tube can usually be removed 24 to 48 hours after air drainage has stopped.

## REFERENCES

1. American Academy of Pediatrics: Guidelines for air and ground transportation of pediatric patients. *Pediatrics* 1986; 78:943.
2. Budin D: *The Nursing*. Caxton Publishing Co, London, 1907.
3. Kisling J: The kitten as a teaching model for intubation of the human neonate. *Respir Care* 1976; 21:1243.
4. Finer NN, Boyd J: Chest physiotherapy in the neonate: A controlled study. *Pediatrics* 1978; 61:282.
5. American Heart Association: Standards and Guidelines for Cardiopulmonary Resuscitation and Everyday Cardiac Care: IV. *Pediatr Basic Life Support* 1986; 255:2954.
6. Wall PM, Kuhns LR: Percutaneous arterial sampling using transillumination. *Pediatrics* 1977; 59(suppl):1032.
7. Huch R, Huch A, Albani M, et al: Transcutaneous $pO_2$ monitoring in routine management of infants and children with cardiorespiratory problems. *Pediatrics* 1976; 57:681.
8. Herrell N, Martin RJ, Pultusker M, et al: Optimal temperature for the measurement of transcutaneous carbon dioxide tension in the neonate. *J Pediatr* 1980; 97:114.
9. Whitehead M, Pollitzer M, Parker D, et al: Transcutaneous estimation of arterial $pO_2$ and $pCO_2$ in newborn infants with a single electrochemical sensor. *Lancet* 1980; 1:1111.
10. Pollitzer MJ, Soutter LP, Reynolds EOR: Continuous monitoring of arterial oxygen tension in infants: Four years of experience with an intravascular electrode. *Pediatrics* 1980; 66:31.
11. Wilkinson AR, Phibbs RH, Gregory GA: Continuous measurement of oxygen saturation in sick newborn infants. *J Pediatr* 1978; 93:1016.
12. Kuhns LR, Bednarek FJ, Wyman ML, et al: Diagnosis of pneumothorax or pneumomediastinum in the neonate by transillumination. *Pediatrics* 1975; 56:355.
13. Allen RW Jr, Jung AL, Lester PD: Effectiveness of chest tube evacuation of pneumothorax in neonates. *J Pediatr* 1981; 99:629.

# 6

# Delivery Room Management and Resuscitation of the Newborn

William E. Truog, III, M.D.

The birth of a human fetus can be a perilous event because of many factors unique to the time of birth. The embryologic patterns of human development result in a perinate born at a time of virtually complete helplessness, especially compared to other primates. Despite his or her functional immaturity, the term newborn demonstrates third-trimester head growth that imposes a need for significant stretching and distortion of the maternal pelvis. Powerful uterine compressive forces are needed to allow expulsion of the fetus successfully. The entire process is both stressful and strenuous for mother and baby.

The most seemingly benign labor may be marked by periods of relative fetal hypoxia. Reflex bradycardia occurs commonly from compression of the fetal skull against the dilating lower uterine segment and cervix. Although this pattern of bradycardia is considered benign (type 1 or early fetal decelerations), its occurrence is unique to the time of delivery. A misshapen, moulded skull and an occasional subarachnoid hemorrhage attest to the dimensions of the forces sometimes generated to expel the fetus. The stresses of labor and delivery, coupled with an ignorance of normal perinatal physiology, have helped to sustain high perinatal mortality rates, estimated to be 100 to 200 deaths per 1,000 live births, throughout most of human history.[1]

This record has improved concomitantly with a greater understanding of the physiology of the fetal to neonatal transition. With the application of this knowledge in the daily practice of obstetrics and pediatrics, it is now possible to devise rational approaches to the management of distressed newborns and perhaps make inroads against the potentially crippling or lethal effects of perinatal hypoxemia and acidosis. Although uncertainty persists regarding the importance of perinatal asphyxia as a contributing or causative agent in the various forms of static encephalopathy,[2] the prevention or reversal of neonatal hypoxemia and acidosis remains the ultimate task for the delivery room resuscitation team, in order that the new or additional injuries do not occur as a part of the birth process.

Perinatal and neonatal mortality rates are influenced by the incidence of low birth weight (birth weight less than 2,500 gm) and especially very low birth weight (birth weight less than 1,500 gm). For multiple, incompletely understood, medical, and social reasons, the United States has a very low birth weight rate two to three times that of other industrialized nations.[3] Although these premature infants have not experienced the same dramatic in utero head growth as a full-term infant, they are ill-equipped to tolerate labor and delivery and routinely require resuscitation in the delivery suite. Very low birth weight rates in the United States vary slightly from state to state but approach 1% of all live births.[3] Therefore, the goal of lowering perinatal and infant mortality rates in the United States will be achieved partly by solving the problem of preventing the birth of the extremely immature fetus, who is often unequipped for the stresses of labor, delivery, and postnatal transition.

## TRANSITIONAL PHYSIOLOGY AND PATHOPHYSIOLOGY

All perinates are at risk for developing *asphyxia* (hereinafter defined as the combination of metabolic and respiratory acidosis and arterial hypoxemia caused by inadequate respiratory gas exchange) before and during labor and delivery. The two "storage" pools of body oxygen, separate from that carried in the arterial blood, are minimal to absent in the fetus. As the lungs are fluid and not gas filled, there is no storage of oxygen in the functional residual gas, as is true in the adult. Additionally, because both arterial and mixed venous oxygen tensions are considerably lower in the fetus, there is also much less oxygen stored in venous blood. Mixed venous oxygen content in the fetus is only about 6 ml/100 ml of blood vs. 15 ml/100 ml of blood in the adult. Oxygen partial pressure in the placental intervillous space, where fetal gas exchange occurs, is 40 to 45 mm Hg, compared to an alveolar $Po_2$ of 100 torr during postnatal life at sea level. Increased intrauterine pressure with contractions, maternal hypotension or hypertension, or anesthetic agents may all diminish maternal placental blood flow, decreasing oxygen stores in the intervillous space, and hence the availability of oxygen for the fetus. Despite the relatively hypoxemic in utero environment, the fetus is capable of extremely rapid growth at minimal oxygen consumption rates during intrauterine life. However, the particular stresses of labor may compromise all sources of oxygen for the fetus.

## Initiation of Breathing

*Intermittent respiratory movements* are detected in utero, depending on maternal activity level and fetal sleep state. However, the fetus does not engage in *continuous breathing movements*. The so far unexplained conversion from intermittent to continuous breathing with the onset of birth remains one of the mysteries of perinatal medicine. The multiple circulatory, respiratory, and endocrine adjustments that occur with birth contribute to sustaining the *respiratory drive*. The loss of the placental uterine circulation causes hypoxemia and hypercapnia, which may stimulate *peripheral* and possibly *central chemoreceptors*, although profound and sustained hypoxemia and acidosis depress breathing. *Sensory* and perhaps *tactile afferents* in the trigeminal area of the face are stimulated by exposure to the relatively cold, dry air of the delivery room. The interaction of these events and probably others serves to initiate regular respirations. Drug-induced depression of the infant's respiratory center or sudden re-exposure of the peripheral sensory receptors to warm saline may depress or abolish the respiratory drive, resulting in apnea.

## Cardiopulmonary Adjustments With Birth

The fetal lung is a fluid-filled and fluid-secreting organ. This *lung fluid* is relatively rich in chloride and deficient in bicarbonate compared to fetal plasma. The mechanisms governing the rate of secretion and quality of the fluid are as yet unclear but at least in fetal lambs, initiation of labor, with concomitant rises in epinephrine, appears to depress secretion of the fluid, presumably as a first step in preparing the lung for conversion to neonatal life.[4] The squeezing of the fetal chest with delivery also helps expel fluid from the airways. Much of the remainder of the lung fluid is removed by the lymphatic system, beginning at the time of birth. Lung fluid removal is depicted schematically in Figure 6–1.

The first breath rapidly elevates distal airway $PO_2$ and lowers the elevated *pulmonary vascular resistance*, presumably by relieving hypoxic pulmonary vasoconstriction. Other virtually simultaneous

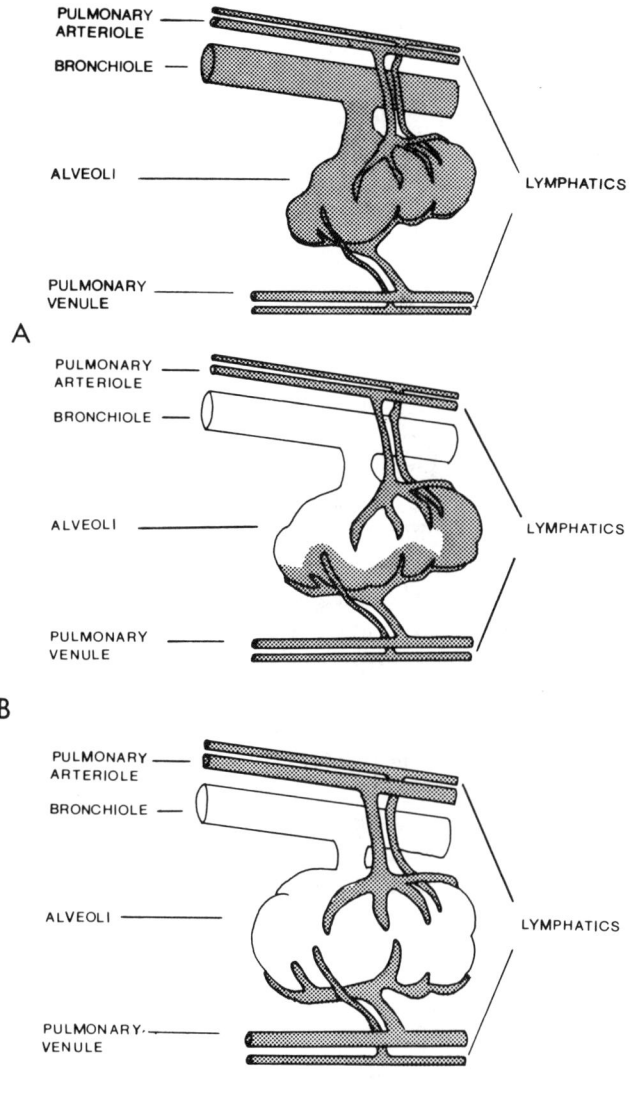

**FIG 6–1.**
Airway fluid is removed from the lungs in several steps before and during birth. **A,** fluid secretion by the lung stops during labor although the air sacs and airways remain fluid filled. **B,** fluid remaining in the airways is squeezed out the mouth and nose and is rapidly reabsorbed into the now-expanded pulmonary capillary bed as well as into the extensive lymphatic drainage system of the lung **(C).**

changes, perhaps also mediated by catecholamines, include elevation of the *systemic vascular resistance*. The change in the ratio of pulmonary to systemic vascular resistance converts the right to left interatrial shunt through the *foramen ovale* into a left to right shunt. Closure of the *ductus arteriosus* presumably occurs more slowly, and functional left to right ductal shunts can be detected for the first 72 hours.[5] Decreased flow via the ductus arteriosus means increased flow into the pulmonary circulation and evenutally to the left atrium, raising left atrial pressure and closing the foramen ovale. The *ductus venosus* also closes, sealing the pathway by which umbilical venous blood avoids the portal circulation and flows directly into the inferior vena caval circulation. Closure of the ductus venosus occurs as flow via the umbilical veins diminishes with cord clamping.

Assuming sustained spontaneous ventilation occurs, there is a rapid rise in arterial $PO_2$ from less than 30 mm Hg to more than 60 mm Hg in the first minutes of life. This dramatic change attests to the efficiency of the lung for oxygen exchange. The increased oxygenation stimulates contraction of the smooth muscle lining the ductus arteriosus, helping close that shunt, and helps constrict the muscular wall of the umbilical arteries. The circulatory transition from fetal to neonatal life is now complete, although ongoing adjustments, such as a continuing decrease in the pulmonary to systemic vascular resistance ratio, continue to occur over the first hours and days of life.

Because of the critical nature and the speed at which these changes must occur, there appears to be redundancy in the controlling systems for these events. The neonate is provided with a variety of vasoactive stimuli to help accomplish these tasks. There is evidence that *prostaglandin metabolites*, especially the vasodilator prostacyclin,[6] as well as polypeptide substances such as bradykinin,[7] participate in this conversion, perhaps by interacting with catecholamines.

## Other Changes With Birth

The conversion from intrauterine to extrauterine life is accompanied by changes in virtually every organ system. Attention has been focused traditionally on the above discussed areas of cardiopulmonary and respiratory changes. However, other changes occur, including an increase in cardiac output and cardiac work,[8] increases in hepatic glucose output, free fatty acid mobilization, and triiodothyronine ($T_3$) production. Umbilical cord cutting itself appears to result in a sudden release of catecholamines,[9] which in turn may be mediators for many of these events. The need for increased heat production is met by nonshivering thermogenesis, by which fat stores are released as glycerol and nonesterified fatty acids.

All of the metabolic phenomena of transition create a unique environment in which resuscitation of the neonate must sometimes be performed. Future research endeavors into the causes and consequences of asphyxia must account for the unique transitional physiology, distinguishing it from other infant and pediatric resuscitation.

## PATHOPHYSIOLOGY OF NEONATAL ASPHYXIA

Figure 6–2 depicts the vicious cycle that may occur following clamping and cutting of the umbilical cord if the fetus fails to initiate and complete the steps in neonatal transition. The major focus of this vicious cycle is the failure to relieve the normally elevated (during fetal life) pulmonary vascular resistance by clearing lung fluid and initiating sustained respirations. Arterial $P_{CO_2}$ rises 7 to 10 torr with each minute of apnea. Arterial $P_{O_2}$ falls at a brisk rate as oxygen consumption continues, but without any replacement for oxygen in the tissues. *Anaerobic metabolism* soon adds lactate to the acid load of the infant. The combination of respiratory and metabolic acidosis produces both constriction of the pulmonary vascular bed and, if allowed to persist, systemic hypotension, bradycardia, and reduced cardiac output. Without prompt intervention, the now cold-stressed and depressed fetus has difficulty reversing this situation on his own. Chemical stimuli may induce breathing efforts, but breathing movement may be ineffectual because of persistently fluid-filled lungs. Agonal gasping efforts may

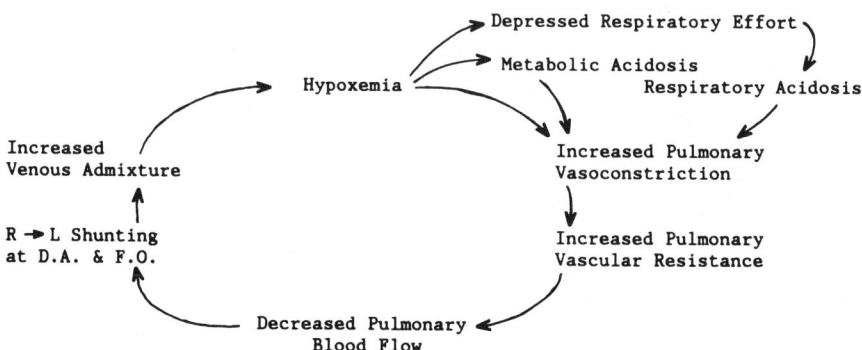

**FIG 6–2.**
The depressed neonate may enter a cycle of increasing hypoxemia producing an increasingly severe combined metabolic and respiratory acidosis. The result is the creation of conditions in which it is increasingly difficult to establish adequate oxygenation and break the cycle. D.A. = ductus arteriosus; F.O. = foramen ovale.

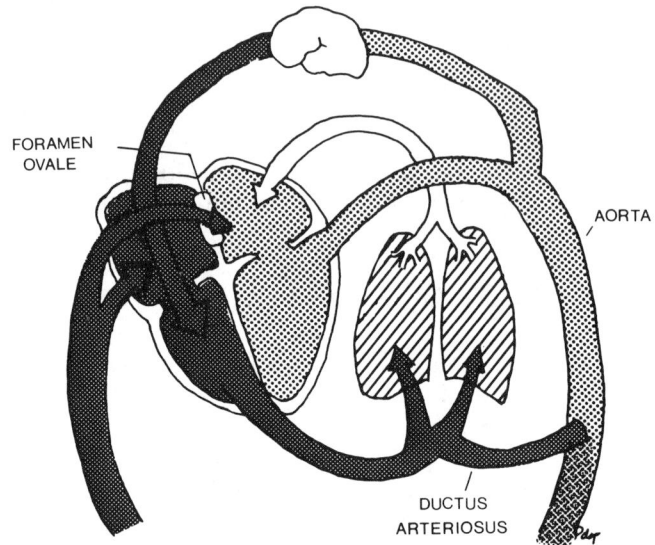

**FIG 6–3.**
A schematic illustration showing that with nonexpanded lungs, persistent right to left shunts at the ductus arteriosus and foramen ovale result in the direct transfer of relatively nonoxygenated venous blood into the systemic circulation. Degree of stippling indicates unoxygenated blood.

produce ineffectual respirations insufficient to inflate the lungs and help to reverse the vicious cycle shown. Figure 6–3 depicts schematically the circulatory patterns that persist in a neonate unable to expand his lungs and decrease pulmonary vascular resistance.

Birth is associated with an increase in metabolic activity and oxygen consumption, a response normally modulated by the immediate postnatal increase in triiodothyronine. The risk of hypothermia with its adverse effects including the development of a coagulopathy is increased with asphyxia. Cold stress alone depresses arterial oxygen tension in term infants, possibly because of persistent right to left shunting.[10] Cold stress may diminish oxygen availability at a time of increased oxygen need for counteracting hypoxemia.

## CAUSES OF NEONATAL DEPRESSION

Because the initial approach to the depressed neonate almost always consists of establishing an airway and providing assisted ventilation, knowing the exact cause of neonatal depression becomes more important only after the first 1 to 2 minutes of resuscitation. Table 6–

**TABLE 6–1.**
Conditions Contributing to Increased Risk of Complications of Labor or Delivery

| Maternal | Fetal |
|---|---|
| Young mother (<17 yr) | Prematurity |
| Older mother (>38 yr), especially if primiparous | Breech or transverse presentation |
| | Meconium staining of amniotic fluid |
| Low socioeconomic status | Twins or multiple gestation |
| Poor nutrition | Large or small for gestational age |
| Diabetes mellitus | Evidence of fetal malformation detected by ultrasound or amniotic fluid examination |
| Drug addiction | |
| Toxemia of pregnancy | Blood group isoimmunization |
| Placental abnormalities (abruptio or placenta previa) | |
| Prolonged labor, first or second stage | |
| Adverse reproductive history | |
| Prolonged rupture of membranes | |
| Chronic renal, cardiac, and pulmonary disease | |

1 indicates both maternal problems and fetal problems that may produce conditions in which resuscitation will be needed.

Particular attention needs to be paid to the extremely premature infant in the delivery room. Shiny pink skin color is not necessarily an accurate reflection of satisfactory arterial oxygen tension. The premature infant's very compliant chest wall produces respiratory efforts that may be ineffectual for establishing gas-filled lungs, as negative intrathoracic pressure insufficient to allow adequate airflow may be generated by his efforts.

## ASSESSMENT OF NEONATAL WELL-BEING

The traditional approach to the assessment of neonatal well-being has depended on the neonatal *Apgar score* (Table 6–2). The limitations of this score are: (1) it does not predict with great accuracy the long-term outcome from perinatal asphyxia; (2) it was not designed with prematures in mind and, hence, the evaluation of tone and even color and reflex irritability become problematic with the smaller infant; (3) as originally designed, the score was calculated at 1 minute and 5 minutes of age, yet one should not wait even the full 1 minute to begin resuscitative efforts in the case of a severely depressed baby. Therefore, an assessment done immediately after birth is useful.

Attempts have been made to find better indicators of long-term outcome than the Apgar score (which was not designed with that purpose in mind). One proposed indicator is the pH obtained by sampling blood from a segment of the clamped umbilical cord. *Umbilical cord*

**TABLE 6-2.**
Apgar Scoring System

| Sign | Score | | |
|---|---|---|---|
| | 0 | 1 | 2 |
| Heart rate | Absent | <100 beats/min | >100 beats/min |
| Respiratory effort | Absent | Slow, irregular | Strong cry |
| Muscle tone | Flaccid | Flexing of extremities | Active |
| Reflex irritability | None | Grimace | Cough or cry |
| Color | Cyanotic, pale | Body pink, extremities blue | Completely pink |

| Cumulative Score After 1 or 5 min | Interpretation |
|---|---|
| 7-10 | No asphyxia; no treatment necessary |
| 4-6 | Moderate asphyxia; continued close observation |
| <4 | Severe asphyxia; immediate intervention with assisted ventilation; further evaluation necessary |

*blood pH* has now become routine for high-risk deliveries in some perinatal centers. The usefulness of this measurement may be greatest in those situations in which Apgar scores are unreliable.[11]

The cornerstone of management of the newborn in the delivery room is serial physical examinations directed toward *heart rate, respiratory rate, and effort,* and to a lesser extent *skin color.* Decisions for intervention can be based on these findings without waiting for any arbitrary period of time following delivery. Table 6-3 outlines these steps.[12] Serial uninterrupted evaluations of the infant by a knowledgeable individual will help provide the best guidelines for the degree of intervention needed.

## APPROACH TO THE ASPHYXIATED INFANT

### Drying and Initial Stabilization

Immediately following delivery, the baby's mouth and nares may be gently suctioned with a bulb syringe to remove any fluid. Suctioning of the mouth should occur first because stimulation of the nares may induce a sudden inspiratory gasp and cause aspiration of any remaining fluid in the mouth. Excessive suctioning produces trauma with mucosal swelling resulting in the potential for partial occlusion of the airways. It also diverts attention from the ongoing tasks of evaluating air entry into the lungs and monitoring heart rate.

**TABLE 6-3.**
Immediate Evaluation of Perinate at Birth

| Assess Heart Rate, Respirations, and Color | Take Appropriate Action |
|---|---|
| If<br>Heart rate ≤60 beats per minute<br>Respirations absent<br>Color cyanotic | Then<br>Resuscitate immediately; dry the infant, suction the upper airway, and immediately apply bag-and-mask–assisted ventilation; if there is no prompt response, perform orotracheal intubation |
| If<br>Heart rate 60–100 beats per minutes<br>Some respiratory efforts<br>Color cyanotic | Then<br>Dry the infant, suction the airway, and apply supplemental oxygen to the face while observing the infant closely; provide tactile stimulation; if there is no improvement, apply bag-and-mask ventilation beginning by 1 min, or sooner if the heart rate becomes progressively slower |
| If<br>Heart rate ≥100 beats per minute | Then<br>Dry the infant; if the infant is cyanotic, apply free-flowing oxygen to the face; if no obvious respirations occur, stimulate the infant by rubbing his or her back or pinching the extremities for 20–30 sec; if the heart rate starts to fall to less than 100 beats per minute, institute bag-and-mask resuscitation |

Adequacy of *respiratory effort* is determined by the presence of air entry sounds by auscultation of the chest, an increase in the anterior to posterior diameter of the chest with inspiratory efforts, audible crying, absence of cyanosis of the lips and mucous membranes in the mouth, absence of marked intercostal retractions after the first several minutes of life, and a pulse rate consistently maintained above 100 beats per minute. Any infant not demonstrating these findings on his or her own within the first minutes after birth demands very detailed evaluation and possible intervention.

Simultaneous with this evaluation, the infant should be dried and moved away from convective currents frequently found in delivery rooms. Infants are born into a wet, cool, drafty environment. Evaporative, radiant and convective heat losses occur immediately, which partly account for the increased oxygen consumption at a time when oxygen supply is marginal. Even the most vigorous infant requires protection from hypothermia by being dried and placed on a prewarmed, nonconductive surface with an overhead radiant warmer. This activity may constitute the entire resuscitative process for most babies. An excellent source of heat for the pink, nondistressed baby may be the mother's own body. Drying of the baby and moving him into a warm place must be accomplished before other measures are instituted for more depressed infants.

*Heart rate* should be measured by chest auscultation or palpation of umbilical cord pulsations. A rate of greater than 100 beats per minute usually indicates the absence of severe asphyxia. Ongoing serial observations without further intervention are indicated. An infant with a heart rate of greater than 100 beats per minute and still cyanotic may benefit from breathing supplemental oxygen flowing over the nose and face but the absolute indications for this minimal intervention are unclear (see Table 6–3). A pulse rate initially less than or falling below 100 beats per minute and especially less than 60 beats per minute signals the need for initiation of assisted ventilation even if the infant is making occasional inspiratory efforts. Persistent bradycardia for the first 1 to 2 minutes following delivery is an indication that assisted ventilation should be instituted.

**Assisted Ventilation**

Assisted ventilation may be delivered by one of two means: (1) a 0.5-L *rubber bag* attached to a molded rubber *mask* or circular plastic mask with rubber edges fitted over the baby's mouth and nares or (2) a rubber bag connected to an *endotracheal tube*. In both cases, the oxygen supply for inflating the bag is connected to the bag by a length of plastic tubing. The choice between bag-and-mask and bag-and-tube ventilation is based on consideration of degree of depression, cause of respiratory distress, size of the infant, and likelihood of need for prolonged resuscitation. The more depressed or premature the baby, the more likely the need for more prolonged resuscitation and assisted ventilation, which can be more easily accomplished by bag-and-tube ventilation. The possibility of a malformation such as congenital diaphragmatic hernia should also prompt the resuscitator to perform intubation and bag-and-tube ventilation. Many authorities, however, believe that bag-and-mask ventilation is sufficient for the majority of mildly to moderately asphyxiated infants. *Meconium-stained infants* benefit from intubation and suctioning of readily removable meconium from the upper airways and trachea before assisted ventilation is initiated.

Initial inspiratory positive pressure may need to exceed 20 cm $H_2O$ and occasionally reach 50 cm $H_2O$ to overcome surface adhesive forces in the airways. Initial assisted inspirations can be delivered slowly, with inspiration sustained for 0.5 to 1.0 seconds.[13]

Failure to mask ventilate effectively may be caused by improper face-mask size precluding a tight seal on the face, airway blockage by the tongue falling against the posterior pharyngeal wall, macroglossia (as in infants with hypothyroidism, Down syndrome, or Beckwith-Wiedemann Syndrome), congenital airway anomalies (such as cleft palate or bilateral choanal atresia), or the presence of micrognathia.

Proper positioning of the infant's head is crucial for either successful bag-and-mask ventilation or for placement of the endotracheal tube (see Fig 5–2). When the infant is correctly positioned, the neck will be neither flexed nor extended. Because the occiput of a full-term infant is large, the neck may become flexed with the infant supine. Placing a small towel under the shoulders, not the neck, helps overcome this problem. This is not, however, a problem in the smallest premature infants. The infant's chin should be extended making him appear to be sniffing the air with his nose. Some physicians insert an oral airway during bag-and-mask ventilation, but its usefulness will be subverted if it becomes pressed against the posterior oropharynx. A feeding tube placed in the stomach with the proximal end open to the atmosphere helps prevent distention of the stomach, as is likely to occur with bag-and-mask ventilation.

The infant who requires prolonged resuscitation with administration of resuscitative medications and external cardiac massage, will have a more stable airway maintained by placement of an endotracheal tube. If inadequate ventilation or bradycardia persists after 1 to 2 minutes of bag-and-mask ventilation, oral tracheal intubation should be undertaken.

The successful intubation is performed with smooth and unhurried movements. The head should be repositioned as described above. Following suctioning of secretions from the oropharynx, the resuscitator passes a straight infant laryngoscope blade (Miller size 0 for the smallest babies; Miller size 1 for full-term babies) between the base of the tongue and anterior surface to the epiglottis, elevating the epiglottis with the tip of the blade, visualizing the glottis and vocal cords. An oral tracheal tube may then be passed with the tip advanced 1 cm beyond the glottis. Appropriate tube size is shown in Table 6–4.

For most asphyxiated babies, establishing an airway and providing assisted ventilation for periods of 2 to 3 minutes should restore nearly normal blood gas tensions and the concomitant onset of spontaneous respirations with normal heart rate, blood pressure, and perfusion. For those infants in whom assisted ventilation for 1 to 2 minutes fails to restore a heart rate of greater than 80 to 100 beats per minute, two

**TABLE 6–4.**
Guidelines for Selection of Endotracheal Tube and Suction Catheters

| Weight, gm | Endotracheal Tube Size, mm inner diameter | Size of Suction Catheter, F |
|---|---|---|
| <1,000 | 2.5 | 5 |
| 1,000–1,500 | 2.5 or 3.0 | 5 or 6 |
| 1,501–2,500 | 3.0 | 6 |
| 2,501–3,000 | 3.0 or 3.5 | 6 or 8 |
| >3,000 | 3.5 | 8 |

additional measures will be necessary. These are external cardiac massage and administration of bicarbonate and epinephrine.

**Establishing Vascular Access**

Each individual involved in resuscitation must determine what route of vascular access he or she can most quickly secure in the depressed neonate. For most babies, placement of a catheter into the *umbilical vein* will be the quickest. The umbilical vein can be cannulated by cutting the umbilicus approximately 1 cm above the abdominal wall through Wharton's jelly. Grasping the edge of the umbilicus, the resuscitator can easily identify the umbilical vein by its large lumen and flaccid wall (Fig 6–4) and insert a catheter directly into it. If the catheter can be advanced approximately 10 cm into the vessel of a full-term infant or approximately 6 to 7 cm in the smallest premature infant, and if blood return occurs readily by gentle aspiration, then one can assume that the catheter has passed through the

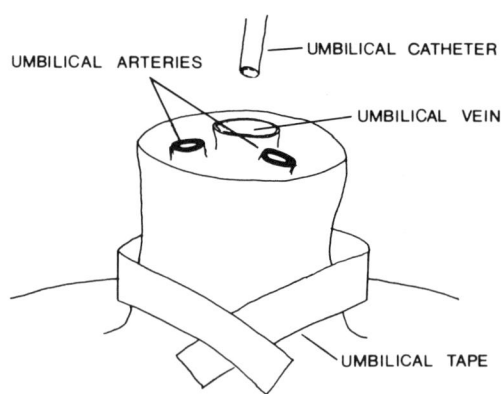

**FIG 6–4.**
The cut surface of the umbilical cord (after constriction with umbilical tape to prevent blood loss) demonstrates two small muscular umbilical arteries and a single umbilical vein.

ductus venosus and inferior vena cava and into the right atrium. If blood cannot be easily aspirated, then the catheter should be withdrawn until the tip is only a distance of 2 to 3 cm into the vessel. In either position, one can administer bicarbonate solution and/or epinephrine.

Alternative routes of administration would include starting an intravenous infusion in a peripheral vein. This procedure is usually more time consuming than umbilical venous catheterization. A catheter can be inserted into the umbilical artery, but this insertion is also more time consuming and requires a less "rapidly moving field" than is likely to exist during neonatal resuscitation.

In the event that no vascular access can be obtained and the infant is continuously bradycardic, *epinephrine* (0.1 ml/kg of 1:10,000 solution increased to a volume of approximately 0.5 to 1 ml with normal saline) can be administered via the endotracheal tube.[14] There is absorption into the circulation by this route, but if the infant is profoundly acidotic, epinephrine may not have as much effect as if the pH had been corrected by adequate ventilation and *bicarbonate* infusion. An appropriate empirical dose of bicarbonate in a severely asphyxiated infant is 2 mEq/kg administered as 0.5 mEq/ml at a rate of infusion of approximately 1 to 2 ml/minute. While bicarbonate is being administerd, it may not be possible to administer epinephrine into the intravascular line because alkalotic solutions will inactivate the epinephrine. Therefore, one could interrupt the infusion, flush the line with normal saline and then administer the epinephrine, or administer the epinephrine into the endotracheal tube while bicarbonate continues to be administered into the intravascular line. A second dose of both may be repeated after 5 to 10 minutes, depending on response to ongoing ventilation and massage.

## External Cardiac Massage

In the event of persistent bradycardia and cyanosis, external cardiac massage should be begun by 3 to 5 minutes of age either concomitant with or immediately after the administration of the medication as described above. Two techniques exist for external cardiac massage. The first involves placing the resuscitator's two thumbs over the middle third of the sternum with the fingers encircling the torso of the infant and supporting the back (Fig 6–5). The thumbs should be positioned on the sternum just below a line drawn between the nipples. The lower portion of the sternum should not be compressed because of the potential damage to the liver or spleen. The second technique applies if the infant is larger or if the resuscitator's hands are too small to encircle the chest completely. Compression of the sternum is accomplished with

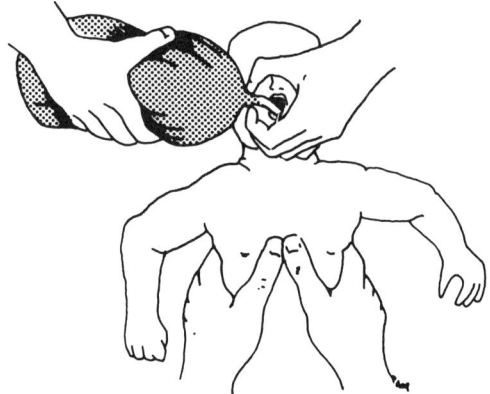

**FIG 6–5.**
External cardiac compression during assisted ventilation of a neonate. This degree of resuscitation requires two trained individuals.

the second and middle fingers just below the nipple line. The other hand may be needed to support the infant's back if the infant is not placed already on a firm surface. The sternum is compressed approximately 1 to 2 cm at a rate of 120 times per minute. Compression should be at approximately a 1:1 ratio between compression and relaxation time. Compression should always be accompanied by positive pressure ventilations continuing at a rate of approximately of 40 to 60 breaths per minute. The stimulus for forward blood flow in these circumstances may be the elevation in pleural pressure rather than forceful expulsion of the blood from the cardiac ventricles, although firm evidence for this in neonates is not available.[15] If adequate ventilation is not being achieved during external massage, then massage should stop briefly to allow 2 to 3 inhaled breaths and then quickly resume. Periodically (approximately every 60 seconds) one should determine the spontaneous pulse rate and its effectiveness by both listening for heart sounds and palpating a peripheral pulse.

**Other Medications**

If ongoing resuscitation is needed beyond the first 5 to 10 minutes, then a bedside reagent stick should be used to check a drop of blood for glucose concentration. Infants have rapid depletion of glucose stores, and a depressed infant has difficulty mobilizing new glucose through glycogenolysis or gluconeogenesis. An infusion of *glucose* (1 to 2 ml/kg of a 10% solution) may be needed, as resuscitation is unlikely to be successful in a profoundly hypoglycemic infant. Although controversy

**TABLE 6-5.**
Potentially Useful Drugs in Resuscitation of the Neonate

| Drug | Indication | Route and Dosage |
|---|---|---|
| Sodium bicarbonate | Metabolic acidosis | 2 mEq/kg I.V. as 0.5 mEq/ml of fluid given at 1–2 ml/min |
| Dextrose | Low blood sugar | 2 ml/kg of 10% dextrose in $H_2O$ IV (200 mg/kg) |
| Epinephrine | Prolonged bradycardia | 0.1 ml/kg of 1:10,000 solution IV or via endotracheal tube |
| Naloxone | Respiratory depression secondary to maternal narcotic administration | 0.01 mg/kg IV or IM |
| Plasma-like substance (normal saline, plasma, or 5% albumin in normal saline) | Low intravascular volume | 10–15 ml/kg |

surrounds the appropriate role of glucose infusions in ameliorating hypoxic-ischemic encephalopathy, well-controlled data in neonatal animals suggest that hypoglycemia is detrimental during such stress.[16]

The *opiate antagonist* naloxone (Narcan neonatal, 0.01 mg/kg) may be a useful adjunct to resuscitation if the primary problem appears to be respiratory depression without other signs of severe asphyxia, and if there is a history of maternal administration of medications likely to induce neonatal depression (i.e., morphine or its synthetic congeners).

There appears to be little role for infusion of *calcium salts* in delivery room resuscitation. Total serum calcium levels in the perinate are actually elevated above maternal levels. It is highly unlikely that ionized calcium is low in neonates because acidosis will lead to an increase in ionized calcium concentration.

*Atropine*, a vagolytic agent, has an unclear role in delivery room resuscitation. An empirical trial of a single dose (0.01 to 0.02 mg/kg/dose) may be useful in persistent bradycardia, but the far more likely reason for bradycardia than increased vagal tone is depression unresponsive to epinephrine. Table 6–5 provides a summary of potentially useful drugs in delivery room resuscitation.

## SPECIAL DELIVERY ROOM SITUATIONS REQUIRING ADDITIONAL INTERVENTIONS

The possibility of *hypovolemia* contributing to asphyxia should be considered in cases of suspected placental abruption, ruptured umbilical placental vessels, or in rare cases, ruptured liver or spleen during the delivery. Pallor (difficult to appreciate with coexistent cyanosis), distant precordial heart sounds, poor peripheral capillary filling, diminished peripheral pulses, and hypotension are signs suggestive of decreased intravascular volume. An initially normal hematocrit does not exclude hypovolemia. Treatment consists of an infusion of fresh whole blood, either cross-matched to the mother or type O negative if available, or isotonic saline or lactated Ringers solution at a dosage of at least 10 ml/kg initially. Blood obtained from the placenta could be used as a last resort. It should be noted, however, that hypotension in asphyxiated infants does not necessarily correlate with hypovolemia, and on the basis of present evidence, automatic intravascular volume expansion should be discouraged in depressed neonates, as overhydration may simply induce pulmonary and soft tissue edema, compounding later problems. In situations in which there may be difficulty interpreting intravascular volume status because of previous losses or preexisting edema, it may be helpful to place an umbilical venous catheter into the right atrium for *central venous pressure* measurements. Umbilical venous catheters are most easily placed in the first 12 hours after birth before closure of the ductus venosus. Central venous pressure measurements are useful when one assesses relative change in pressure following volume expansion or contraction, rather than attempting to interpret a single absolute value.

A particularly severe problem is the infant with clinical features of *hydrops fetalis* (i.e., total body edema) with extremely low hematocrit (slow fetal to maternal transfusion, maternal infant blood group incompatibility). *Abdominal paracentesis* through the flank to partially remove ascitic fluid may help allow better lung expansion. *Thoracentesis* for possible pleural fluid should probably be withheld until after a chest radiograph has been obtained and examined. An isovolemic *partial exchange transfusion* with packed red cells designed to raise the hematocrit from the teens to at least 30% to 35% may be necessary shortly after birth in order to provide adequate oxygen delivery.

*Meconium* expelled from the fetal intestinal tract in utero becomes diluted with amniotic fluid and may be aspirated occasionally in utero or with the first breath. Aspiration produces postnatal hypoxemia and hypercapnia because of obstruction in both large and small airways. Ultimately, an inflammatory response ensues. Rapid suctioning of the oropharynx at delivery and direct laryngoscopy with suctioning of any meconium easily removable from the larynx appears to minimize the occurrence and severity of the aspiration. In this situation, the physician must balance the need to remove meconium with the need to correct concomitant cyanosis and bradycardia.

## EVALUATION OF TREATMENT DURING THE PERIOD IMMEDIATELY FOLLOWING RESUSCITATION

In the first half hour following neonatal resuscitation, the following questions need to be considered by the physician in charge:

1. *Is the infant hypoglycemic?* A continuous infusion of glucose should be started before the infant becomes hypoglycemic. A dose of glucose of about 5 to 6 mg/kg/minute (or 3 to 4 ml/kg/hour of 10% glucose in water) will be necessary. In an effort to protect against severe cerebral edema, fluid restriction may be helpful, which means that infants requiring additional glucose may need more concentrated forms of glucose, which require infusion into a larger vessel, not a peripheral site.

2. *Is the infant still profoundly acidotic, and is his own ventilation satisfactory?* This question can be answered by obtaining a blood sample for blood gas determination. Although arterial blood provides the most accurate assessment of arterial oxygen tension, valuable information can be learned from blood obtained from an umbilical venous catheter, or even by capillary heel sampling, although poor peripheral perfusion may make the latter results unreliable. Infants without severe respiratory distress may have secondary hyperventilation driven by a primary metabolic acidosis. The blood pH may approach normal (>7.20) in this situation, but concomitantly measured $P_{CO_2}$ may be quite low, indicating persisting metabolic acidosis. Serial blood gas determinations will help establish optimal treatment. A baby with an arterial pH greater than 7.20 probably does not need further bicarbonate treatment. Respiratory acidosis (pH <7.25, with $P_{CO_2}$ >60 torr) may indicate central nervous system injury, or pulmonary disease perhaps secondary to resuscitative efforts (i.e., pneumothorax).

3. *Is the infant's cardiovascular system responding appropriately?* Noninvasive blood pressure monitoring via a doppler ultrasound device (Dinamap) is accurate and reliable in infants. This measurement can be correlated with clinical examination of capillary refill (less than 3 seconds), easily palpable pulses, and pink peripheral skin color with a normal blood pressure. Direct blood pressure measurement through an umbilical or peripheral arterial cannula will be necessary in extremely depressed infants.

4. *Is the infant developing seizure activity?* Perinatal asphyxia can result in neonatal seizures beginning shortly after birth. The role of prophylactic phenobarbital in limiting the frequency of the seizures or the severity of encephalopathy following asphyxia is unestablished. However, if the infant appears to be having seizure or seizure-like ac-

tivity, such as posturing, initial treatment with 20 mg/kg of phenobarbital is indicated, given as two 10-mg/kg doses. In the premature infant, prophylactic treatment with phenobarbital does not prevent the development of intracranial hemorrhage.[17]

5. *Is the infant septic?* Unexpected depression at birth can be a sign of bacterial sepsis, as infected infants tolerate the stress of labor poorly. Unexplained depression of a newborn, especially with a history of maternal fever, prolonged ruptured membranes, or foul-smelling amniotic fluid (or infant) is an indication to begin antibiotics.

6. *Does the infant have any unsuspected congenital malformations?* Immediate or severe respiratory distress in a term neonate indicates airway anomalies. These anomalies include tracheoesophageal fistula and congenital diaphragmatic hernia. In both cases immediate respiratory distress is noted. In the case of tracheoesophageal (TE) fistula, there may be frothing of oral secretions in the mouth and immediate choking with any feeding attempt. Management of a TE fistula consists of placing a catheter in the proximal esophageal pouch, with the catheter maintained on continuous suction. The infant is placed in an upright and prone position. Management of congenital diaphragmatic hernia includes basic resuscitation, intubation for severe distress, evacuation of stomach contents, obtaining a chest radiograph to confirm the diagnosis, and arrangements made for surgery as soon as possible. Early paralysis (pancuronium, 0.1 mg/kg) may help control the extreme respiratory embarrassment and minimize the risk of pneumothorax prior to surgery.

## BIRTH INJURIES TO THE NEWBORN NERVOUS SYSTEM

Birth injuries most frequently occur in full-term or large-for-gestational-age infants. They are divided here into injuries to the peripheral nervous system and those to the central nervous system.

### Peripheral Nervous System

Peripheral nervous system injuries occur because of lateral flexion and traction of the neck to allow shoulder delivery.

1. Duchenne-Erb paralysis or brachial plexus injury (injury to the fifth and sixth cervical spinal nerves). The affected arm is adducted; the forearm is pronated; the wrist is flexed; reflexes are absent locally; the grasp reflex is intact. Treatment consists of prevention of further

injury by immobilization; then passive range of motion exercises may be attempted after several days.

2. Klumpke's paralysis (injury to the seventh and eighth cervical and first thoracic spinal nerves). Muscles of the hand are affected, and grasp is absent. In some cases, the entire brachial plexus is injured. Management is similar to that of brachial plexus injury. Recovery is not always complete. Children in whom little or no recovery can be detected by 2 weeks have a much more guarded prognosis for complete recovery.

3. Phrenic nerve injury is usually associated with Duchenne-Erb paralysis. Diaphragmatic paresis or paralysis presents with tachypnea and occasionally results in respiratory failure, necessitating mechanical ventilation. Diagnosis can be confirmed by fluoroscopy. A major hazard is development of aspiration pneumonia. Plication of the diaphragm may be necessary if signs of recovery are not apparent by 1 to 2 weeks after birth.

4. Facial nerve paresis is usually caused by misapplication of forceps. The infant has an asymmetrical face while crying. This injury may produce an unblinking eyelid. The eye will then need protection with methylcellulose eyedrops until lid function returns.

**Central Nervous System**

1. Subdural hematoma usually, but not always, occurs in the fullterm infant. There may be marked discrepancy between the clinical appearance of the infant and the degree of hemorrhage. Treatment of symptoms of localized pressure on the brain, if indicated, is by subdural aspiration of the blood. This may be done via the open fontanel and repeated frequently.

2. Subarachnoid hemorrhage can occur with difficult delivery and may cause seizures or ill-defined neurologic symptoms in infants who otherwise appear well. Computerized tomography (CT) (but not necessarily cranial ultrasound) scanning will demonstrate the lesion.

3. The common finding of cephalohematoma is associated with a 5% incidence of underlying linear skull fracture. No radiograph or special treatment is necessary unless palpation suggests a depressed skull fracture. Occasionally leptomeningeal cysts develop following incomplete resolution of the fracture.

## COMMON ERRORS TO AVOID IN RESUSCITATION

1. Error: Hyperextension of the neck, frequently recommended in adult procedure manuals, to provide a patent airway.
    Result: The infant's airway is occluded.
    Appropriate action: Place the infant's head in a "sniffing" position, using a small shoulder roll that will most effectively provide a patent airway.
2. Error: Failure to vent the stomach during bag-and-mask ventilation.
    Result: Restriction of lung expansion is caused by the air-filled stomach placing pressure on the diaphragm. Gastric rupture may occur, especially in the small premature infant. Reflux of gastric contents, resulting in aspiration, may also occur.
    Appropriate action: Insert an orogastric tube after the first few ventilations for the duration of bagging.
3. Error: Anxiety on behalf of the resuscitator, resulting in a ventilation rate of 80 breaths per minute or greater.
    Result: Hyperventilation alkalosis develops, with a low $P_{CO_2}$, diminishing the infant's stimulus to breathe.
    Appropriate action: Administer assisted ventilation at rates that approximate the normal infant respiratory rate of 40 breaths per minute, checking that adequate lung expansion occurs.
4. Error: Cardiac compression is initiated because of failure of the infant to respond to bagging with spontaneous respirations.
    Result: Presents unnecessary risks from chest compressions.
    Appropriate action: Initiate cardiac compression when the heart rate falls or remains below 80 beats per minute after 3 to 5 minutes of effective ventilatory assistance.
5. Error: Institution of assisted cardiac and respiratory efforts are set at adult levels.
    Result: Ineffective cardiopulmonary resuscitation (CPR).
    Appropriate action: Attempt to achieve newborn normal vital signs: Compress the sternum approximately 120 times per minute; ventilate every third compression.
6. Error: Use of wall suction for the routine management of normal newborn airway secretions.
    Result: High potential for trauma to delicate mucous membranes.
    Appropriate action: Use bulb syringe or deLee mucous trap as these are sufficient for routine management of secretions. Wall or

machine suction set to a "low" setting should be reserved for the management of secretions in endotracheal tubes.

7. Error: Temperature regulation is often ignored or given second place during resuscitation.

Result: The infant frequently suffers rapid and severe heat loss during resuscitation. Because the newborn's physiologic response to cooling or overheating is to demand additional oxygen, maintenance of a neutral thermal environment must be an integral part of the resuscitation effort.

Appropriate action: Dry rapidly, and keep the infant warm during resuscitation (radiant warmer, warm blankets underneath the infant).

## CONCLUDING COMMENTS

Articles describing techniques of neonatal resuscitation routinely focus on the "hows and whys" but often avoid discussion about when to start or stop resuscitation. The 1980s are a time of transition in the development of medical and societal agreement about providing intensive support for even the smallest and sickest infants. Against this background of lack of consensus, immediate decisions about whom to resuscitate must be made. The delivery room is a poor place to make judgments about starting or stopping treatment. At the present time, babies of birth weight less than or equal to 600 gm only rarely survive to discharge, whereas babies of birth weight above 750 to 800 gm are much more frequent survivors with a reasonable likelihood of normal long-term neurologic and intellectual development. It is difficult to distinguish 100- to 150-gram weight differences in the delivery room when one's focus should be attempting to establish an airway and ventilate the baby. Additionally, extremely immature babies are born with a variable level of depression and a variable ability to respond to resuscitative efforts. One approach is to offer initial resuscitative efforts to live-born infants, with ongoing evaluation based on the infant's response, and to expand the available database to include weight, gestational age, and condition of the mother at the time of delivery. No simple rules can be written to govern behavior in this situation.

The second difficult situation is how long to continue attempting to revive an extremely depressed baby. If a spontaneous heart rate is present and persists, resuscitative efforts should continue for at least 20 minutes. In the absence of any spontaneous cardiac activity or any other sign of life following 2 to 3 doses of epinephrine and 10 to 15 minutes of effective resuscitation, further resuscitative efforts are unlikely to result in a baby who can be discharged alive.

Artful inactivity, so useful elsewhere in medical practice has little place in the delivery room when one is confronted with a depressed neonate. A rapidly implemented logical approach to resuscitation will often produce gratifying and potentially life-long benefits for the patients.

## REFERENCES

1. Swyer PR: Organization of perinatal care with particular reference to the newborn, in Avery GB (ed): *Neonatology: Pathophysiology and Management of the Newborn.* Philadelphia, JB Lippincott Co, 1975, Chapter 3, pp 15–34.
2. Nelson K, Ellenberg J: Antecedents of cerebral palsy. N Engl J Med 1986; 315:81.
3. Institute of Medicine: *Preventing low birth weight.* Washington DC. National Academy Press, 1983.
4. Brown M, Olver R, Ramsden C, et al: Effects of adrenaline infusion and of spontaneous labor on lung liquid secretion and absorption in the fetal lamb. J Physiol (Lond) 1981; 313:13.
5. Gentile R, Stevenson G, Dooley T, et al: Pulsed Doppler echocardiographic determination of time of ductal closure in normal newborn infants. J Pediatr 1981; 98:443.
6. Leffler C, Hosler J, Terregno W: Ventilation induced release of prostaglandin like material from fetal lungs. Am J Physiol 1980; 238:282.
7. Melmon K, Cline J, Hughes T, et al: Kinine: Possible mediators of neonatal circulatory changes in man. J Clin Invest 1968; 47:1295.
8. Rudolph AM: Changes in the circulation after birth. Circulation 1970; 41:343.
9. Padbury J, Diakomanolis E, Hobel C, et al: Neonatal adaption: Sympathoadrenal response to umbilical cord clamping. Pediatr Res 1981; 15:1483.
10. Stephenson J, Du J, Oliver T: The effect of cooling on blood gas tensions in newborn infants. J Pediatr 1970; 76:848.
11. Goldenburg R, Huddelston J, Nelson K: Apgar scores and umbilical arterial pH in preterm newborn infants. Am J Obstet Gynecol 1984; 149:651.
12. Hodson WA, Truog WE: *Critical Care of the Newborn.* WB Saunders Co, Philadelphia, 1983.
13. Vyas H, Milner A, Hopkins I, et al: Physiologic responses to prolonged and slow rise inflation in the resuscitation of the complicated newborn infant. J Pediatr 1981; 99:635.
14. Chernow R, Holbrook P, D'Angona D, et al: Epinephrine absorption after intratracheal administration. Anesth Analg 1984; 63:829.
15. Rogers M: New developments in cardiopulmonary resuscitation. Pediatrics 1983; 71:655.

16. Dwyer B, Wasterlain C: Neonatal seizures in monkeys and rabbits: Brain glucose depletion in the face of normoglycemia, prevention by glucose loads. *Pediatr Res* 1985; 19:992.
17. Kuban K, Leviton A, Krishnamoorthy K, et al: Neonatal intracranial hemorrhage and phenobarbital. *Pediatrics* 1986; 77:443.

## SUGGESTED READINGS

Anon: Neonatal advanced life support. *JAMA* 1986; 255:2969.
Truog WE: Care of the newborn in the delivery room, in Kelley VC (ed): *Practice of Pediatrics*. Harper & Row, Philadelphia, 1985.

# 7

# Nursing Care of the Infant With Respiratory Disease

Mary Fran Hazinski, R.N., M.S.N.
Annette Simpson Pacetti, R.N., B.S.N., M.S.N.

Care of the seriously ill neonate requires a team of skilled personnel, including physicians, nurses, respiratory therapists, physical therapists, social workers, laboratory technicians, and x-ray technicians. Each member of the team should be aware of the neonate's condition, plan of care, and risk of particular complications. As part of daily rounds, care givers should communicate changes in plan of care and discuss planned responses to anticipated complications. An excellent patient-care team will be capable of responding in an organized and skilled fashion to sudden changes in the patient's condition. Since a bedside nurse is with the neonate 24 hours a day, the nurse is often the health team member most likely to detect changes in patient condition and to implement care according to the team plan.

The purpose of this chapter is to present information necessary for the assessment and nursing care of the neonate with respiratory disease. Since most of these neonates are seriously ill, the bedside nurse must be able to perform comprehensive assessment of all body systems and detect complications of prematurity as well as those of the respiratory disease or its therapy.

The first section of this chapter presents an overview of assessment and general care of any seriously ill neonate. Following the section entitled "Nursing Assessment and General Care of the Neonate," more specific details about thermoregulation, fluid and electrolyte balance, and nutrition will be addressed. Then detailed information about the care of the neonate receiving oxygen therapy and mechanical ventilatory support is presented. The final sections of the chapter address skin care and psychosocial aspects of neonatal intensive care. Throughout these sections, practical approaches to bedside nursing assessment and care will be included. The chapter concludes with a discussion of infant stimulation and sleep deprivation in the neonatal intensive care unit (NICU), and support of the parents.

## NURSING ASSESSMENT AND GENERAL CARE OF THE NEONATE

### Assessment of General Appearance

Anyone approaching the neonate's bedside must be able to rapidly determine the degree of distress that the infant demonstrates. The nurse will conclude that the neonate either *"looks good"* or *"looks bad."* This is probably the single most important assessment that is made during the infant's hospitalization.[1] In making this assessment, the nurse will note the infant's color, level of activity, position, response to the environment, and (if applicable), feeding behavior (Table 7–1). In addition, the nurse must monitor the neonate's vital signs, noting significant changes since the previous assessment.

### *Assessment of Color*

The infant's color should be uniform (not mottled), and mucous membranes, nailbeds, palms, and soles should be pink. While the very immature neonate may normally have reddened skin with a plethoric appearance, such plethora in the more mature neonate may indicate polycythemia. Poor systemic perfusion or hypoxemia will result in a *mottled* appearance, or a gray *pallor*, and extreme compromise in systemic perfusion or severe hypoxemia will result in *cyanosis* (unless severe anemia is present).[1]

The neonate may develop hyperbilirubinemia and *jaundice* during the first days of life. Hyperbilirubinemia is likely to peak at approxi-

**TABLE 7–1.**
Assessment of General Appearance in the Neonate

General appearance
  "Looks good" vs. "looks bad"
Color
Level of activity
  Spontaneous movement
  Irritability/jitteriness/lethargy
Position
Responsiveness
Feeding Behavior
Vital signs

mately 3 days of age in the term infant and at approximately 5 days of age in the preterm infant.

### Level of Activity

Even the very low birth weight infant will demonstrate spontaneous movements. Every awake neonate beyond 35 weeks' gestation should demonstrate a complete startle (Moro) *reflex* in response to sudden stimulation, and most neonates will demonstrate some movement in response to any sudden stimulation.[2]

A critically ill neonate may initially become irritable or jittery; this may occur spontaneously or following a mild stimulus and may be the result of electrolyte imbalance, sepsis, or neurologic disease. As further deterioration occurs, the neonate will become lethargic and unresponsive. Intraventricular hemorrhage, hypoxemia, hemorrhage, or sepsis may cause a sudden decrease in movement with a deterioration in vital signs.[2] These changes should be brought immediately to the attention of a physician.

### Position

The term or more mature neonate will demonstrate a dominance of flexor *tone,* and the neonate beyond 35 weeks' gestational age will normally assume a position with elbows, hips, and knees flexed. A very immature infant (younger than 28 weeks' gestation) will have less tone, so extremities may remain extended and relatively flaccid.[2] It is important that the nurse be familiar with the neonate's normal position and muscle tone so that changes will be detected immediately. Decreased tone may occur as the result of electrolyte imbalance (including hypoglycemia), hypoxemia, intraventricular hemorrhage, sepsis, or seizure activity.

### Responsiveness

The neonate's responsiveness can easily be determined during routine care. Response to a change in body position may include a change in *facial expression* or *movement* (extension or flexion) of extremities. The neonate will normally attempt to withdraw from a painful stimulus, such as a heel-stick, and should move extremities or cough during suctioning.

If the infant is receiving anticonvulsant drugs, sedatives, or pharmacologic paralyzing agents, these agents will, of course, blunt the infant's response. Electrolyte imbalance, hypoxemia, sepsis, or neurologic problems may also produce lethargy and unresponsiveness.

While it is important to avoid excessive stimulation of the extremely immature infant, it will be necessary to document the neonate's responses to normal care activities at least once during each nursing care shift. Any change in responsiveness should be brought to the attention of a physician.

### Feeding Behavior

If the neonate is able to take normal feedings by nipple or tolerate gavage or tube feedings, the infant's activity during and following such feedings should be assessed. Early signs of cardiorespiratory distress include inability to suck, prolongation of feeding times, significant increase in respiratory rate and effort after feedings, vomiting, and abdominal distention. While these signs may simply indicate that the neonate has been overfed, they may also signify the presence of increased respiratory distress, sepsis, intraventricular hemorrhage, necrotizing enterocolitis (NEC), gastrointestinal obstruction, extreme immaturity, or congestive heart failure.

### Assessment of Vital Signs

The neonate's *respiratory rate and effort* (or rate and degree of chest expansion if the neonate is receiving positive-pressure ventilation), *heart rate*, and *blood pressure* (as displayed by cardiac monitor) should be observed before the neonate is disturbed.[3] The clinician should then perform auscultation to determine the infant's heart rate, respiratory rate, and breath sounds.

The neonate's heart rate will normally be approximately 120 to 160 beats per minute, and the respiratory rate will vary between 40 and 60 breaths per minute. Small changes in heart rate or respiratory rate may occur from hour to hour, but the development of a trend may indicate increasing distress or deterioration. The blood pressure should be recorded at least every 2 to 4 hours, and hourly in the seriously ill infant. Systolic, diastolic, and mean blood pressure should be documented, and these pressures should be evaluated in light of the neonate's age, maturity, and birth weight (see Appendix, Table A-12 for normal blood pressures in neonates). A fall in diastolic pressure with a widened pulse pressure may indicate the presence of a large shunt through a patent ductus arteriosus.[4] Since small quantitative changes in blood pressure may be qualitatively significant,[3] any consistent changes in blood pressure should be reported to a physician.

The clinician should be familiar with normal vital signs for age, as well as trends in the individual patient's vital signs. *Normal vital signs may not be appropriate vital signs for the critically ill neonate.*[3] For example, tachycardia and tachypnea are expected in the sick newborn; bradycardia or slowing of the respiratory rate to "normal" levels in the compromised infant may indicate impending cardiopulmonary arrest.

## Systems Assessment and Care—The Eight-Point Check

Recall of important assessment and nursing care information is usually increased by use of a standardized approach. The assessment and general care information presented below has been organized using the first eight letters of the alphabet to promote ease in recall (Table 7–2). The nurse will monitor the following characteristics: Aeration, Brain function (neurologic status), Circulation, Drips and Drug therapy, Electrolytes, Fluid balance and therapy, Gastrointestinal and Genitourinary function, and Heat (thermoregulation).[1] This approach may be useful during the orientation of new nursing staff or as a method of recalling essential information during nursing report or charting.

### *Aeration*
**Developmental Changes in Pulmonary Function.**—The neonate is at risk for the development of respiratory distress and failure for several reasons. In these patients, an immature control of breathing, small airway size, compliant chest wall, immature respiratory muscles, and immature or injured lung tissue can all contribute to the development of respiratory failure.

The *central nervous system*, which controls breathing, is immature; as a result, the neonate is prone to apneic episodes. The neonate's *airways* are small, and minimal bronchoconstriction, mucus accumulation, or edema can tremendously reduce airway radius and increase resistance to air flow; this will contribute to increased work of breathing and serious airway obstruction.

The *chest wall* is very compliant and will easily retract inward when the neonate attempts to inspire; as a result, retractions will be evident during periods of respiratory distress. Severe retractions may

**TABLE 7–2.**
Assessment and General Care of the Critically Ill Neonate: The Eight-Point Check*

1. Aeration
2. Brain (central nervous system) function
3. Circulation
4. Drips and drug therapy
5. Electrolytes
6. Fluid balance and therapy
7. Gastrointestinal and genitourinary function
8. Heat (thermoregulation)

*Modified from Hazinski MF: Nursing care of the critically ill child: The seven-point check, *Pediatr Nurs* 1985; 11:453.

limit the infant's ability to generate an adequate tidal volume and may reduce efficiency of ventilation.[5]

*Respiratory muscles* include the chest wall muscles (specifically the diaphragm and intercostal muscles) and muscles of the upper airway (which help to maintain airway patency). These muscles are immature during the neonatal period; they have reduced tone, strength, and coordination. The diaphragm is the chief muscle of respiration, and if it is paralyzed or immobilized, the neonate will be incapable of generating an adequate tidal volume.[5] Decreased upper airway muscle activity may lead to obstructive apnea.

*Lung tissue* is incompletely developed in the premature neonate. Terminal airways begin to develop during the 24th week of gestation, and surfactant production starts during gestational weeks 22 to 35. When surfactant production is insufficient, a condition known as respiratory distress syndrome (RDS) or hyaline membrane disease can occur. While maternal corticosteroid administration can hasten the production of surfactant, and surfactant administration can supplement the neonate's supply, respiratory failure may still develop.[6] In these infants, atelectasis with a subsequent shunt of blood away from the collapsed lung units is likely to develop.

The neonate may also be more susceptible to the development of pulmonary edema than the older infant; such edema will be likely to develop during episodes of respiratory distress or excessive fluid administration. All of these conditions can produce hypoxemia, which may, in turn, cause significant pulmonary arterial and venous constriction. These changes may ultimately result in decreased pulmonary blood flow or increased risk of pulmonary edema.

**Assessment of Respiratory Function.**—The neonate with respiratory distress will demonstrate tachypnea (respiratory rate persistently > 60/minute), apnea, nasal flaring, and retractions. If severe distress is present, grunting will be noted. The color, respiratory rate and effort, and quality of breath sounds of any seriously ill neonate should be recorded at least hourly. Since respiratory distress and resultant hypoxemia may contribute to cardiovascular dysfunction, the infant's heart rate, and evidence of systemic perfusion should also be noted hourly, or whenever there is a change in patient condition or therapy.

Effectiveness of ventilation should be assessed by observation of chest movement and auscultation of breath sounds. During both spontaneous and positive-pressure ventilation inspiration, chest movement should be symmetrical, and some chest expansion should be noted. During positive-pressure ventilation, the chest should rise symmetrically during inspiration. Breath sounds should be equal and adequate bilaterally. Documentation of intensity and quality of breath sounds should be made at least every 1 to 2 hours during the acute phase of respiratory failure, or when any deterioration in patient condition occurs.

If the infant is receiving oxygen therapy, the inspired oxygen concentration should be determined and recorded hourly. If mechanical ventilatory support is required, the ventilator variables (including rate, peak inspiratory pressure, inspired oxygen concentration, ratio of inspiratory time to expiratory time, etc.) should also be monitored and recorded at the same time. If noninvasive blood gas monitoring is utilized (including pulse oximetry, transcutaneous oxygen, and transcutaneous carbon dioxide monitoring), results should be monitored and recorded every 15 minutes during the acute phase of respiratory care, and particularly during intervention or deterioration in patient condition. Alarm limits for high and low inspired oxygen concentration, hemoglobin saturation, transcutaneous oxygen, and carbon dioxide levels, and mechanical ventilator settings should be set and checked periodically according to unit protocol.

**Support of Ventilatory Function and Maintenance of a Patent Airway.**—Unless mechanical ventilatory support is provided, the infant with respiratory distress should be placed prone, with the head of the bed elevated 30 degrees; this will reduce the tendency of the diaphragm to draw the lower ribs inward, and it will drop abdominal contents away from the diaphragm.[5] If the neonate must be placed supine, a soft roll should be placed under the infant's shoulders to slightly extend (but not hyperextend) the airway.

The nurse should ensure that emergency equipment is readily available at all times. This equipment includes a manual resuscitator bag (with positive end-expiratory pressure—or PEEP—valve) and mask of appropriate size, oxygen source, and intubation equipment. This equipment must be available at each bedside and checked each nursing shift to ensure that it is in working order. The nurse should always be prepared to provide hand ventilation whenever there is any question of effectiveness of either spontaneous respiratory effort or mechanical ventilation.

If apnea develops as the result of central nervous system depression and hypoventilation, the infant may initially respond to tactile stimulation alone. Aminophylline may also be prescribed to prevent neonatal apnea. Naloxone (0.01 mg/kg) may be administered for neonatal respiratory depression due to narcotic administration to mother or infant. Favorable response to either of these agents will include an increase in respiratory rate (with appropriate improvement in arterial or noninvasive blood gas monitoring results), and a decrease in apneic episodes. Intubation and mechanical ventilation will be required if the neonate demonstrates ineffective airway clearance or fails to improve ventilation following physical or pharmacologic stimulation.

If respiratory failure develops as the result of upper airway obstruction, the infant's condition may improve following positioning. The neck should be extended (but not hyperextended), and the infant's head should be positioned in the "sniff" position to increase airway patency. Suctioning should be performed as needed to remove mucus that may be compromising airway radius. Inhalation treatments (with nebulized racemic epinephrine or β-agonist drugs) or parenteral bronchodilators may be prescribed to reduce upper airway edema or relieve bronchospasm. During bronchodilator therapy, the clinician should monitor patient response to therapy, and heart rate and systemic perfusion. Favorable response will include improvement in air exchange with a reduction of respiratory effort and wheezing. Excessive tachycardia is a potential side effect of these drugs, which may limit their use in the critically ill neonate.

Intubation may be necessary to maintain an adequate airway or to provide mechanical ventilatory support. Selection of the appropriate endotracheal tube will be based on the neonate's size and gestational age (see Chapter 5). A Miller size 0 straight laryngoscope blade will be utilized during the intubation (although a Miller size 1 straight blade may be necessary for larger neonates). Preparation for intubation and assessment of tube position and patency is discussed later in this chapter (see "Care of the Neonate Requiring Mechanical Ventilatory Support," and Chapter 5).

If respiratory failure occurs as the result of parenchymal disease, diaphragm paralysis, or respiratory muscle fatigue, mechanical ventilatory support will be required. Signs of failure will include the development of respiratory acidosis with signs that the neonate is "tiring" (with the development of decreased chest excursion or slowing of the respiratory rate, accompanied by a deterioration in blood gases).

**Maximization of Arterial Oxygen Delivery.**—If respiratory failure develops as a result of intrapulmonary shunting, ventilation-perfusion mismatch, or pulmonary edema, it will be necessary to improve the neonate's oxygen delivery. This may be accomplished in several ways.

If the neonate is hypoxemic but not hypercapnic, administration of supplemental oxygen alone, or oxygen therapy with continuous positive airway pressure (CPAP) may be sufficient to improve oxygenation. Continuous positive airway pressure may be delivered via an endotracheal tube or via nasal cannulas (refer to section entitled "Care of the Neonate Requiring Oxygen Therapy" in this chapter). Favorable response will include an improvement in arterial oxygen content, with a decrease in respiratory effort and rate. Mechanical ventilation will be required if the neonate develops respiratory acidosis, or increased respiratory effort accompanied by evidence of fatigue.

Methods of improving oxygenation can be considered by using the equation of oxygen delivery (see Chapter 2):

$$O_2 \text{ delivery} = \text{arterial } O_2 \text{ content} \times \text{cardiac output}$$

where arterial $O_2$ content is determined by hemoglobin and oxygen saturation (see Chapter 2, equation 4). Thus an increase in hemoglobin (blood transfusion) and oxygen saturation (increase in fraction of oxygen in dry inspired gas ($F_{I_{O_2}}$), CPAP, or mean airway pressure) will increase oxygen delivery. The product of heart rate and stroke volume will determine cardiac output. Inotropic drugs, volume therapy, and vasodilators will increase stroke volume and improve oxygen delivery.

### *Brain (Central Nervous System) Function*
**Developmental Changes in Neurologic Function.**—At birth, the term infant's neurologic system functions largely at a subcortical level; this means that brain stem functions (such as respiration and heart rate) and spinal cord reflexes (such as some postural reflexes) are normally present, but cortical functions (such as fine motor coordination and specific neurologic responses to specific stimuli) are incompletely developed. In addition, the autonomic nervous system is intact, but immature, so thermoregulation and heart rate are less precisely regulated than in the older infant. Most cranial nerves are present and myelinated in the term infant, so specific examination of cranial nerve function may be performed.[2]

At approximately 28 weeks' gestational age, the infant should startle in response to sound or sudden touch, although a complete Moro response will not be observed. At this age, the neonate will usually blink, and pupils will constrict in response to light.[2] The premature infant may cry in response to painful stimuli by 26 to 28 weeks' gestational age, and spontaneous cry may be observed by 30 to 32 weeks' gestation. Facial expression resembling smiling can be observed during sleep when the neonate is approximately 29 weeks' gestational age, and periods of wakefulness will be observed by approximately week 30.[2] The muscles necessary to suck and swallow may function as early as 28 weeks' gestation, but coordination of sucking and swallowing is usually not effective until the neonate is 32 to 34 weeks' gestational age.

The infant's skull is not rigid since the cranial bones do not fuse until approximately 16 to 18 months of age. If the neonate develops a gradual increase in intracranial volume (such as may occur with the development of hydrocephalus), head circumference may increase, and the anterior fontanelle may feel tense to palpation and may "bulge" outward.

**Assessment of Neurologic Function.**—Evaluation of the neonate's neurologic function is based largely on observation of the level of consciousness (including alertness and responsiveness), spontaneous movements, reflexes, and muscle tone and strength. If there is deterioration in neurologic function, the neonate will be less alert and responsive and will move infrequently; reflexes may be diminished or absent; muscle tone will diminish; and strength of movements will be decreased.[7] While such deterioration can be associated with generalized cardiorespiratory distress, it may also indicate specific neurologic problems, including sepsis with meningitis.

The neonate's head circumference should be measured on admission to the newborn unit and daily thereafter. More frequent measurement and documentation of head circumference will be necessary if neurologic complications develop. The fontanelle should be palpated at least once per shift and a description written in the nursing notes or on the infant's chart.

Signs of an acute increase in intracranial pressure include a deterioration in level of activity, decreased responsiveness, bulging anterior fontanelle, bradycardia, and poor systemic perfusion with a metabolic acidosis. Pupil dilation with decreased response to light, seizure activity, or posturing (including decorticate or decerebrate posturing) may be noted.

Intraventricular hemorrhage may complicate the care of the premature or immature neonate with respiratory disease. Characteristics that have been associated with increased risk of intraventricular hemorrhage (IVH) include immaturity (<32 weeks' gestation); low birth weight (<1,500 gm); low Apgar scores; perinatal asphyxia; hypoxia; intrauterine growth retardation; respiratory distress; pneumothoraces; stress; severe head trauma at birth; symptomatic patent ductus arteriosus; sepsis; necrotizing enterocolitis; and vigorous fluid resuscitation.[7] Clearly, many of these risk factors are present in the neonate with respiratory disease.

Signs of intraventricular hemorrhage include decrease in responsiveness; jitteriness (which will progress to lethargy as the infant's condition deteriorates); fullness of anterior fontanelle; temperature instability; hyperglycemia; and a fall in hematocrit (unresponsive to transfusion). Seizures may be noted in a small number of patients, and significant IVH may produce cardiovascular instability, shock, and death.

Ultrasonography is used to confirm or rule out an IVH and to follow its progression or resolution.

Seizures in the neonate may be difficult to recognize. Rhythmic sucking, lip smacking, or tongue thrusting may indicate seizure activity. Seizure activity may also be manifested as "bicycling" of the legs or unilateral/bilateral jerking of the extremities. Jitteriness in the sick newborn is common; seizures are not. A gross method for differentiating jitteriness from seizures requires restraint of the affected extremity. Jitteriness will cease when the limb is held; seizures will be unaffected.[8,9] If seizures develop, the neonate's heel-stick glucose concentration and electrolyte balance should be assessed, and the duration, distribution, and characteristics of the seizure activity should be recorded and reported to a physician.

Single seizures require investigation, and frequent seizures unrelated to metabolic problems usually are treated. Continuous seizures, or seizures that result in cardiorespiratory compromise require immediate treatment with anticonvulsants. Phenobarbital, 10 mg/kg intravenously, is usually the anticonvulsant of choice. Whenever these drugs are administered, the nurse should closely monitor the infant's respiratory function and be prepared to provide hand ventilation and assist with intubation, should respiratory depression develop.

If the neonate with respiratory failure is receiving pharmacologic agents that cause paralysis to ensure effective ventilatory support, it will be virtually impossible to detect seizure activity through clinical examination alone. In these paralyzed patients, seizure activity should be suspected whenever sudden deterioration occurs, particularly if such deterioration is associated with pupil dilation, or tachycardia with beat-to-beat fluctuations in blood pressure. An electroencephalogram (EEG) will be required to diagnose seizure activity in the pharmacologically paralyzed neonate.

**Care of the Neonate With Increased Intracranial Pressure.**—If the neonate develops increased intracranial pressure (ICP), the head of the bed should be elevated, and the head should be maintained in midline (to facilitate cerebral venous return). A mild respiratory alkalosis will be maintained, if possible, since this will reduce cerebral blood volume. Hypercapnia and hypoxemia are to be avoided since these may contribute to cerebral vasodilation and an increase in cerebral blood volume and increased intracranial pressure. Suctioning should be performed only when absolutely necessary (as needed to maintain airway patency), and stimulation should be kept to a minimum. Extreme elevations in central venous pressure are to be avoided. Fluid restriction and diuretic therapy may be prescribed in an effort to minimize cerebral edema.

Administration of hypotonic fluids and any sudden reduction in serum sodium are to be avoided since these will produce a fall in serum osmolality and may contribute to increased cerebral edema.

### Circulation (Cardiovascular Function/Systemic Perfusion)

**Perinatal Circulatory Development.**—Neonatal cardiovascular function is different from that of the older infant or adult in several important ways. Normal cardiac output in the neonate is approximately 200 ml/kg/minute; this is nearly twice the normal cardiac output (per kilogram body weight) of the adult.[10] This high *cardiac output* is a product of heart rate and stroke volume (the volume of blood ejected by the left ventricle with each contraction); if either of these components decreases without a commensurate and compensatory increase in the other component, cardiac output will fall.

The neonate's *heart rate* is normally very rapid, and the ventricular *stroke volume* is normally very small (only approximately 5 ml). Neonatal myocardium has less contractile elements than adult myocardium; therefore, it is stiffer and less able to increase strength of contraction than adult myocardium. As a result, the neonate may be incapable of increasing stroke volume during periods of stress or following volume administration.[11,12] For these reasons, the neonate's cardiac output is extremely dependent on a high heart rate. While periodic episodes of bradycardia may be normal during sleep, a persistent or profound fall in heart rate is likely to produce a fall in cardiac output.

Sympathetic nervous system innervation to the newborn myocardium is incomplete; during periods of stress, the heart rate and strength of ventricular contraction may not increase significantly.[11] Parasympathetic nervous system innervation to the newborn myocardium is complete, however. As a result, the neonate will readily develop bradycardia in response to vagal stimulation such as suctioning but may be incapable of increasing heart rate during episodes of stress.

Neonatal myocardium seems to be more sensitive to increased afterload (increased resistance to ejection) than adult myocardium. Heart failure or low cardiac output is likely to develop if the right or left ventricle is forced to eject into a high resistance circulatory pathway.[11,12]

Increased pulmonary vascular resistance (pulmonary vasoconstriction) will produce an increase in right ventricular afterload. Specific conditions that may contribute to pulmonary vasoconstriction in the neonate are listed in Table 7–3; these conditions are to be avoided in the neonate with pulmonary hypertension (such as occurs with persistent fetal circulation or some congenital heart defects). Increased left ventricular afterload will be present if systemic vascular resistance is high (such as occurs when the neonate develops very poor systemic

**TABLE 7–3.**
Conditions Contributing to Pulmonary Vasoconstriction

Alveolar hypoxia
Hypoxemia
Hypercapnia
Acidosis
Hypothermia
Pain/agitation

perfusion), or if a congenital heart lesion producing left heart or aortic obstruction is present (such as coarctation of the aorta or critical aortic valvular stenosis).

**Assessment of Systemic Perfusion and Cardiovascular Function.—** An important part of the hourly assessment of any critically ill neonate is the assessment of systemic perfusion. If the neonate is well perfused, extremities will be warm; skin color will be uniform; and mucous membranes, palms, and soles should be pink. Peripheral pulses (including brachial, radial, femoral, dorsalis pedis, and posterior tibial) should all be strong and equal. Decreased intensity of peripheral pulses may occur when systemic perfusion is poor, or if aortic obstruction is present, and bounding pulses may be noted when the neonate has a large shunt through a patent ductus arteriosus. Capillary refill should be brisk (1 to 2 seconds); prolonged capillary refill may be associated with poor systemic perfusion or aortic obstruction.

The warmth of the neonate's extremities, strength of peripheral pulses, and briskness of capillary refill should be charted at least hourly while the neonate is acutely ill. It is especially important to assess systemic perfusion in the neonate with cardiovascular compromise. Lower extremity perfusion should be assessed closely while an umbilical artery line is in place and immediately following its removal, since aortic thrombus formation has been reported in association with these catheters.

Urine output will average 2 to 4 ml/kg/hour in the well-hydrated neonate. If the infant's fluid intake is restricted, or if dehydration or increased insensible water losses are present, urine output of 1 to 2 ml/kg/hour may be acceptable. Decreased urine output may occur as a result of decreased renal perfusion associated with congestive heart failure, poor systemic perfusion, or hypovolemia. In addition, a decrease in glomerular filtration rate and urine volume will usually be observed following indomethacin administration to promote constriction of the ductus arteriosus. Decreased urine volume in the presence of adequate fluid intake and good systemic perfusion often indicates the presence of decreased renal function.

Signs of poor systemic perfusion in the neonate include tachycardia; cool extremities with prolonged capillary refill; decreased urine output; decreased intensity of peripheral pulses; and a metabolic acidosis. The seriously ill neonate with poor systemic perfusion will often develop hypoglycemia, hypocalcemia, and temperature instability. Arterial blood pressure will often remain stable despite initial compromise in systemic perfusion; hypotension, and bradycardia often develop only as very late signs of poor perfusion in the neonate.

Signs of congestive heart failure in the neonate include: tachycardia, decreased urine output, periorbital edema, hepatomegaly, peripheral edema, excessive weight gain, and an active precordium. If the neonate is breathing spontaneously, tachypnea with increased respiratory effort, or apnea may be noted. If mechanical ventilation is provided, the neonate will often require increased levels of support, including an increase in inspired oxygen concentration, increased peak inspiratory pressure, or increased positive end-expiratory pressure. If the infant is receiving feedings by nipple, prolonged feeding times and increased respiratory effort during feedings may be noted.

**Assessment of Cardiac Rate and Rhythm.**—The neonate's cardiac rate and rhythm should be documented whenever vital signs are taken. Most *arrhythmias* observed in the newborn intensive care unit are benign and do not compromise systemic perfusion. The neonate with underlying cardiovascular disease, however, is more likely to become symptomatic as the result of an arrhythmia. Whenever an arrhythmia is present, it is imperative that the neonate's systemic perfusion be assessed and supported as needed. If the arrhythmia results in a loss of all pulses, cardiac compression, ventilation, and resuscitation will be required.

The most common clinically significant arrhythmias seen in the newborn intensive care unit are bradycardia and supraventricular tachycardia (SVT). *Bradycardia* is a heart rate that is too slow for the infant's clinical condition; it will result in signs of poor systemic perfusion. Two common causes of bradycardia in the newborn intensive care unit are hypoxemia and vagal stimulation (such as occurs during suctioning).

*Supraventricular tachycardia* will produce an atrial and ventricular rate that is too fast; once the ventricular rate exceeds approximately 210 to 220 beats per minute, ventricular diastolic filling time and coronary artery perfusion time will be inadequate, and stroke volume and cardiac output will fall dramatically within minutes or hours. Neonates with supraventricular tachycardia often have aberrant intracardiac conduction pathways that must be treated pharmacologically.

**Support of Heart Rate.**—Good systemic perfusion requires a heart rate that is appropriate for clinical condition and a stroke volume that is not compromised. Since bradycardia in the neonate can result from hypoxemia or vagal stimulation, the care giver should ensure that the infant's respiratory rate and effort are adequate. If the bradycardic neonate is intubated and mechanically ventilated, hand ventilation should be provided to ensure that the neonate is effectively ventilated. Endotracheal tube placement and patency should be verified. If bradycardia does not respond to hand ventilation, and if systemic perfusion and peripheral pulses are inadequate, cardiac compression may be necessary. Cardiac compression should also be performed if the heart rate is persistently below 60 beats per minute, despite the presence of effective ventilation with supplemental oxygen. The neonate's electrolyte balance should also be assessed, and attempts should be made to determine the cause of the bradycardia. Administration of sympathomimetic agents (including epinephrine) or parasympatholytic agents (such as atropine) will usually be required.

Atrial pacing through use of an esophageal pacing catheter may be performed if bradycardia *without* heart block is present despite correction of any reversible metabolic conditions. If the neonate develops bradycardia *with* atrioventricular block, administration of sympathomimetic drugs and transvenous, epicardial, or transdermal pacemaker therapy will usually be necessary.

If the neonate develops SVT, vagal stimulation or pharmacologic therapy may be prescribed. If the SVT produces profound reduction in systemic perfusion, however, synchronized cardioversion should be performed on an urgent basis.

**Support of Cardiac Function and Systemic Perfusion.**—The neonate's stroke volume may be increased slightly through manipulation of ventricular preload, contractility, and afterload. Manipulation of ventricular preload is accomplished through judicious titration of fluid to optimize the ventricular filling pressures. Contractility will be improved through correction of any existing acid-base imbalances and administration of sympathomimetic drugs, such as dopamine, dobutamine, or epinephrine by continuous infusion (see "Drips and Drugs," below). Manipulation of ventricular afterload is accomplished through vasodilator therapy. Reduction in right ventricular afterload may be accomplished through relief of pulmonary vasoconstriction (such as may be accomplished through maintenance of mild alkalosis and avoidance of conditions such as alveolar hypoxia, which may promote pulmonary vasoconstriction).[13]

Treatment of congestive heart failure requires elimination of excess intravascular fluid and improvement in cardiac contractility. Reduction of the neonate's fluid intake often results in improvement in clinical condition. If diuretic therapy is required, furosemide (1 to 2 mg/kg/dose) is often the drug of choice. However, since it may produce hypokalemia, hypochloremia, and metabolic alkalosis, the infant's electrolyte balance should be monitored closely during therapy.

Administration of a digitalis derivative in the treatment of congestive heart failure has been associated with a high incidence of clinical toxicity.[14] As a result, many centers have abandoned the use of this drug in the treatment of neonatal congestive heart failure. Improvement in cardiac function is usually achieved through administration of sympathomimetic drugs or through vasodilator therapy (see "Drips and Drugs," below).

### Drips and Drug Therapy

Before any drug is administered to a neonate, it is important to verify the dosage, physician order, compatibility of the drug with other medications that the infant is receiving, and the metabolism or excretion of the drug. Finally, the nurse should monitor the effectiveness of the drug and note in the nursing care plan any potential side or toxic effects of the drug.

If any vasoactive drugs are administered, the drugs should be titrated carefully at the bedside, with careful evaluation of patient response. Administration tubing should be labeled to prevent inadvertent "bolus" administration of the drug by tubing "flushes."

Vasoactive medications may be administered through a peripheral or central intravenous line; each route has some advantages and disadvantages. If the vasoactive drug is administerd through a peripheral catheter, a separate infusion site may be utilized for each medication; thus, the nurse will not have to worry about compatibility of the drug or variation in administration rate, since no other drugs will be added to the line. However, infiltration of a vasoactive drug into tissue may produce severe burns and would result in inadequate drug delivery to the infant.

Central line infusion will provide a reliable route of administration of vasoactive drugs, unless the line must also be used for infusion of other substances, such as parenteral alimentation, antibiotics, or emergency drugs. If a vasoactive drug is administered through a central venous line, it is imperative to ensure uninterrupted delivery of the medication.

Intravenous antibiotics should be administered at precise time intervals to maintain constant serum levels. These drugs must be carefully diluted and administered over specific minimal times to prevent harmful toxic effects. Standard antibiotic dilutions should be prepared by pharmacy personnel, or the dilutions should be posted prominently in the nursing care unit (Table 7–4).

Whenever intravenous medications are administered, the nurse must include the fluid used to dilute the medication in calculating the infant's total fluid intake. Often, a great deal of ingenuity is required to provide needed medications within required fluid restrictions. The nurse must also know the "dead space" within each fluid administration set (that is, the amount of fluid required to "flush" the tubing from the syringe or infusion pump to the patient), so that this volume can be considered when planning to administer drugs within a prescribed time. Microbore tubing is now commercially available for use with syringe or other infusion devices; this tiny tubing may have a dead space volume of as little as 0.1 cc for a 12–in. length of tubing.

Whenever drugs are administered by intravenous infusion, the nurse should check the infusion system at least every 15 minutes to ensure that all connections are tight and that the medication is infusing as expected. Loose connections or improperly set infusion pumps may result in inadequate or excessive drug administration.

All intravenous infusion sites should be checked hourly and their appearance described in the nursing notes or on the nursing chart. Severe burns can result from tissue infiltration of parenteral alimentation fluids, calcium, glucose (greater than 10% glucose solutions), antibiotics, or vasoactive drugs. If infiltration occurs, hyaluronidase may be prescribed to enhance drug absorption.[15] The infiltrated site should be kept elevated, if possible, and a physician should be consulted if a burn develops.

In addition to this section on drips and drug therapy, see also Chapter 9 on pharmacology.

### *Electrolytes*

The most common electrolyte imbalances encountered in the NICU include glucose, calcium, sodium, and potassium imbalances. Close observation and careful fluid and electrolyte administration should prevent most of these imbalances.

The neonate has high *glucose* needs and low glycogen stores. As a result, when the neonate becomes critically ill, hypoglycemia may develop; since such hypoglycemia can contribute to the development of seizures and poor systemic perfusion, it must be prevented or rapidly detected and treated. Unexplained hypoglycemia or hyperglycemia may be a sign of infection in the neonate. Infants of diabetic mothers may also demonstrate glucose instability, particularly 2 to 3 hours after birth.

Hypoglycemia may be prevented if heel-stick glucose concentration is monitored closely and if a constant source of glucose is provided. Heel-stick glucose concentration should be checked hourly when the neonate is unstable and should be checked 30 minutes following any change in electrolyte infusion. Once the neonate is stable, heel-stick glucose concentration should be checked every 4 hours.

The neonate less than 1,500 gm should receive 7.5% dextrose solution with water as a maintenance fluid, and the neonate weighing more than 1,500 gm should receive 10% dextrose and water. These fluids should be administered without interruption; if the intravenous line becomes infiltrated, resulting in extravasation of the glucose solution, the neonate may become hypoglycemic. Treatment of hypoglycemia requires administration of glucose solution. However, attempts should be made to provide a constant source of glucose and maintenance of a steady serum glucose concentration. Frequent bolus administration of glucose in response to hypoglycemia will result in undesirable fluctuations in serum glucose concentration.

Regulation of serum ionized *calcium* concentration may be imprecise in the premature neonate because of transient hypoparathyroidism. As a result, the serum calcium concentration should be monitored closely in the critically ill premature neonate. Hypocalcemia is prevented through daily addition of calcium gluconate in maintenance fluids (approximately 10 mEq/L), and bolus administration of calcium should be avoided (since much of the calcium administered in this manner is excreted in the urine). Occasional supplementation of calcium gluconate may be necessary in the asphyxiated neonate or the neonate with persistent fetal circulation; such supplements should total approximately 20 mg/kg and should be administered over several hours.

*Sodium* is the major intravascular ion, and acute changes in serum sodium concentration may be associated with changes in serum osmolality. In the NICU, the most common cause of changes in serum sodium concentration is a change in the neonate's level of hydration. A fall in serum sodium concentration, particularly if associated with weight gain, usually indicates excessive fluid administration. A rise in serum sodium concentration, particularly if associated with a weight loss (or lack of weight gain), usually indicates dehydration and the need for more liberal fluid administration (refer also to following section entitled "Fluid Balance and Therapy"). Acute hyponatremia is to be avoided, since it will be associated with a fall in serum osmolality and may be associated with a fluid shift from the intravascular to the interstitial and cellular spaces. Such a fluid shift may produce pulmonary or cerebral edema.

*Potassium* is the major intracellular ion, and it plays an important role in the excitability of nerve and muscle cells. Potassium imbalances

**TABLE 7-4.**
Recommended Medication Dilutions*†

| Drug (Trade name) | Method of Administration | Nursing Implications |
|---|---|---|
| Amikacin (Amikin) | Dilute to concentration of 25 mg/10ml. Administer by continuous infusion over 30–120 min. | Administer slowly as noted. |
| Aminophylline | IV administration or orally. | Toxicity includes tachycardia, jitteriness, and signs of gastrointestinal dysfunction. |
| Ampicillin | Dilute with sterile water to concentration of 100 mg/ml. Do not mix with other medications. | Give by slow IV push at maximum rate of 1 ml/min. Store diluted medication in refrigerator when mixed. Flush tubing with saline after dose administered. |
| Caffeine | Administer orally or IV. | See aminophylline. |
| Carbenicillin | IV administration preferable, although IM route may be used if volume is small. Dilute to 1 gm/10 ml. | Observe for bleeding. Contains large amount of sodium and may produce high potassium losses so monitor sodium and potassium closely. |
| Cefazolin | Dilute in normal saline or 5% dextrose and water. May be administered by IV or IM route. | Preferred infusion over 30–60 min. May also be administered by slow IV push. May be nephrotoxic, so monitor urine output closely. Manufacturer does not recommend for use in infants less than 1 mo. of age. |
| Ceftriaxone | Dilute in normal saline or sterile water according to manufacturer's instructions. Intravenous route. | Administer over 15–30 min. |
| Cephalothin (Keflin) | Dilute in normal saline or 5% dextrose and water. May be administered IV or IM. | Administer slowly over 3–5 min. IM injection may be very painful. |
| Chloral hydrate (Noctec) | May be administered orally. | Irritating to stomach; therefore, dilute or administer with a feeding. May cause laryngospasm if aspirated. |
| Dexamethasone sodium phosphate (Decadron) | Dilute to minimum of half strength (with at least equal volume of diluent). Do not mix with other drugs. | Administer slow IV push over 10 minutes. May be used to treat laryngeal edema. Probably not effective in treatment of cerebral edema. Monitor serum glucose, weight, BP, and serum electrolytes. Must wean dose gradually before drug is discontinued. May increase risk of GI ulceration or infection. |

| Drug | Nursing considerations | Comments |
|---|---|---|
| Diazepam (Valium) | May produce vascular irritation—do not administer through umbilical artery catheter. Do not mix with any drugs. | Administer slow IV push over 3–5 min. Give with caution to infants not receiving mechanical ventilatory support, and monitor respiratory status closely for evidence of respiratory depression (keep resuscitation equipment at the bedside). May potentiate hypotension when administered in conjunction with thiazide diuretics, so monitor BP. Flush IV line well before and after administration. |
| Digoxin (Lanoxin) | Double-check dose, and verify proper loading and maintenance doses and route of administration (dose for IV administration will be $2/3$ of that recommended for oral administration). If dose totals volume of less than 0.1 ml, dilute medication to ensure delivery of entire dose. | Administer IV dose slowly over 1 min. Prior to administration, check heart rate, and notify physician and hold dose if less than 120. Digoxin toxicity may produce virtually any arrhythmia, and toxicity is more likely if hypokalemia present, so monitor serum potassium closely. This drug is a gastric irritant, so infant may vomit following administration of oral dose on an empty stomach. Vomiting may also be sign of digitalis toxicity. Monitor digitalis levels closely—particularly if renal failure present. |
| Furosemide (Lasix) | May be administered orally (elixir form), or IV or IM. May be administered undiluted. Do not mix with other drugs. | Monitor infant's diuretic response (diuresis should follow IV dose within 15 min and oral dose within 90 min). Failure to respond to previously successful dose may indicate worsening congestive heart failure or poor systemic perfusion. Will result in increased potassium and chloride excretion in urine, so monitor serum concentration of these electrolytes. Hypokalemia or hypochloremia may produce metabolic alkalosis and decreased diuretic response. May be ototoxic, and nephrotoxic if given in conjunction with aminoglycosides. May compete for albumin binding sites with bilirubin, so administer with caution to the neonate with hyperbilirubinemia. Oral dose may be higher than effective IV dose. |
| Gentamicin (Garamycin) | Mix in fluids as needed so concentration no higher than 1 mg/ml, and so dose is administered over 30–120 min. May be given IM, but is very irritating to muscle. Do not mix with other drugs. | May be ototoxic or nephrotoxic. Administer IV slowly, and monitor urine output closely. Also check *peak* and *trough* serum levels to monitor for toxicity. May potentiate neuromuscular blocking agents. |

(*Continued.*)

**TABLE 7-4 (cont.).**

| Drug (Trade name) | Method of Administration | Nursing Implications |
| --- | --- | --- |
| Indomethacin (Indocin) | 0.2 mg IV, NG, or rectally. IV administration of IV form of drug provides much more consistent drug absorption, levels, and effects. May repeat dose times 2. | Will produce a decrease in renal perfusion and glomerular filtration rate, so monitor urine output closely. Will also compete for albumin binding sites with bilirubin, so give with caution to neonates with hyperbilirubinemia (may be contraindicated). May produce coagulopathies, so monitor for evidence of blood in stool, and for GI drainage. |
| Meperidine hydrochloride (Demerol) | Dilute in 2–3 ml of normal saline for IV administration. May be given IM (do not dilute). | Administer IV over 5 min. Monitor respiratory rate and effort—may produce respiratory depression (keep resuscitation equipment at bedside, and naloxone in unit). |
| Methicillin | IV dose preferable. Dilute to 1 gm/50 ml. May administer IM if volume small. | May be nephrotoxic. Monitor urine output closely. |
| Morphine sulfate | IV route: dilute in 2–3 ml of normal saline. May also administer subcutaneously. | May produce respiratory depression so monitor respiratory rate and effort (keep resuscitation equipment at bedside). May contribute to an increase in intracranial pressure, so administer with caution to neonates with IVH or asphyxia. Monitor for evidence of urinary retention, decreased gastrointestinal motility. Reverse with naloxone. |
| Nafcillin | IM route preferred. Dilute 1 gm to at least 30 ml if administered IV. | Manufacturer recommends IM route of administration. Give IV over a 5- to 10-min period. |
| Naloxone (Narcan) | May give undiluted IV or IM. May administer by sublingual route in emergency (when no line available). Adult dilution may be used to decrease volume for IM injection. | May induce narcotic withdrawal in neonate of addicted mother. |
| Pancuronium bromide (Pavulon) | Administer IV undiluted. Do not mix with other drugs. | May be given quickly. Will produce total muscle paralysis, so administer only if infant is receiving total respiratory support. This drug has no analgesic properties, so should be given in conjunction with analgesic. May produce tachycardia, increased salivation. Monitor for urinary retention. Peripheral edema may result from total muscle paralysis. Must provide artificial tears. |

| Drug | Administration | Comments |
|---|---|---|
| Phenobarbital | Give slowly IV. Do not administer through umbilical artery catheter; do not mix with other drugs. Elixir may be administered orally or via OG tube. | Administer over 5 to 15 min. Monitor respiratory rate and effort—may produce respiratory depression. Solution must be administered within 30 min of reconstitution. Extravasation of IV solution may produce tissue sloughing. Elixir may act as gastric irritant. |
| Phenytoin (Dilantin) | Do not dilute for IV administration, and do not administer through umbilical artery catheter. Administer loading dose very slowly, and maintenance doses slowly, and flush IV line before and after administration. Do not mix with other drugs. | Adverse effects include hypotension, respiratory depression, bradycardia, heart block, ventricular arrhythmias. Monitor serum levels. Administer loading dose over minimum of 15 min, maintenance dose over minimum of 5 min. |
| Prostaglandin E$_1$ (Alprostadil; Prostin VR) | Dilute to concentration of 0.15 mg/50 ml (equivalent of 3 μg/ml; then administer 1 ml/kg/hr of this solution by *continuous IV infusion*, for dose of 0.05 μg/kg/min. | If used to promote ductal patency in neonate with cyanotic heart disease, effective response will include an increase in arterial oxygen saturation and PaO$_2$. If administered to promote ductal patency in the neonate with ductal-dependent systemic perfusion, effective response should include improvement in urine output and lower extremity perfusion. May produce apnea, so monitor respiratory rate and effort closely (keep resuscitation equipment at bedside). May also produce seizure-like activity that disappears once alprostadil is discontinued. Increased pulmonary blood flow may be associated with development or worsening of congestive heart failure. May produce false positive sweat-chloride test for cystic fibrosis. Fever, erythema may also be observed. |
| Ticarcillin | See carbenicillin. | See carbenicillin. |
| Tolazoline (Priscoline) | May mix in 10 mg/kg of plasma expander. Central line infusion preferred; if central infusion impossible, administer in vein above heart (scalp or upper extremity). | May produce severe hypotension, especially if patient hypovolemic (have volume expanders at bedside). May produce bleeding. |

*Material taken from the following sources:
Cloherty JP, Stark AR: *Manual of Neonatal Care*, Boston, Little, Brown & Co, 1980.
McCracken GH, Jr, Nelson JD: *Antimicrobial Therapy for the Newborn*, New York, Grune & Stratton, 1977.
Nelson JD: *Pocketbook of Pediatric Antimicrobial Therapy*, ed 5, Dallas, Jodone Publishing Co, 1983.
Noerr B: Commonly used drugs in the neonatal intensive care setting: Policies and Procedures Section (unnumbered). *Neonatal Network* 1984; 2.
See also Chapter 9 for further details.
†IV = intravenously; IM = intramuscularly; BP = blood pressure; GI = gastrointestinal; NG = nasogastric; OG = orogastric.

are uncommon in the NICU, and those that occur are usually associated with changes in acid-base balance or diuretic therapy. Intravascular potassium concentration will fall as the serum pH rises as a result of a shift of potassium from the intravascular to the intracellular compartment. The intravascular potassium concentration will rise and the serum pH will fall as the result of a shift of potassium ions from the intracellular to the intravascular space. Therefore, changes in serum potassium concentration should be evaluated with consideration of the neonate's acid-base balance.

Furosemide therapy may be prescribed for the older neonate (beyond approximately 3 weeks of age) with chronic lung disease. While this drug may improve lung mechanics, the diuretic effect will enhance potassium and chloride excretion in the urine and may be associated with the development of a hypokalemic or hypochloremic metabolic alkalosis.[16] Therefore, if furosemide is administered, the infant's electrolyte and acid-base balance should be monitored closely. A normal or elevated pH in the hypercapneic infant receiving furosemide therapy most probably indicates the presence of potassium and chloride depletion, and he or she requires increased supplementation of these ions if diuretic therapy is to continue.

### *Fluid Balance and Therapy*

The neonate's fluid balance can only be maintained with careful evaluation of the clinical appearance, daily (or up to three times daily) weight, and electrolyte balance. The nurse must continuously evaluate total fluid intake and total fluid output and discuss excessive fluid administration or loss with a physician.

At birth, excessive extracellular fluid is present; this fluid is normally excreted in the urine during the first days of life.[17] As a result, the premature neonate will normally lose a small amount of weight (5% to 10% of birth weight) during these first days of life and should demonstrate a urine output of 2 to 4 ml/kg/hour. Weight gain in the neonate during the first 72 hours of life usually only occurs if fluid administration is excessive and fluid retention occurs.

An average fluid administration rate for the neonate should total approximately 60 to 80 ml/kg/day. This fluid administration rate should be reduced if the neonate has severe respiratory disease and may be liberalized if the neonate is healthy. Any unit protocol regarding fluid administration rates should serve only as an initial guide to fluid therapy, and the neonate's fluid balance and fluid requirements must be evaluated several times each day.

Excessive fluid administration is undesirable in the neonate since it may worsen respiratory distress and pulmonary edema. In addition, excessive fluid administration to the premature neonate has been linked to the development of symptomatic patent ductus arteriosus. Signs of fluid retention in the critically ill neonate include a fall in serum sodium concentration and a rise in weight (or failure to lose weight) during the first days of life. This fluid retention may be associated with clinical or radiographic evidence of pulmonary edema or increased ventilatory support requirements.

Signs of inadequate fluid administration include a rise in the serum sodium concentration and a weight loss exceeding 5% to 10% of body weight during the first 3 days of life. In addition, urine output may total less than 2 ml/kg/hour.

When the neonate's fluid balance is calculated, all sources of fluid intake must be considered, including those used to flush monitoring lines and dilute medications. All intravenous fluids should be administered through use of infusion pumps, and syringe pumps with microbore tubing may be helpful in reducing tubing dead space. Each fluid administration system should be checked hourly to ensure proper function and to assess for signs of subcutaneous fluid infiltration. The nurse should literally touch each part of the infusion system to verify that all connections and stopcocks are secure and that the fluid is infusing at the proper rate.[1] Each infusion system should be equipped with alarms to indicate occlusion, air in line, and completion of infusion.

All sources of fluid loss must be totaled, weighed, or estimated. Urine output can be measured directly through collection of urine, but it is more commonly estimated by weighing diapers (or bed linens) before and after use; a 1-gm increase in weight indicates approximately 1 ml of fluid output.

Additional sources of fluid loss in the neonate may include fluid lost in stool, vomitus, and insensible losses. Insensible water losses may be increased by 50% to 100% when the neonate receives phototherapy or is under a radiant warmer.[18] Such insensible losses may be as high as 1 to 3 ml/kg/hour.

To accurately evaluate the neonate's fluid balance, it is imperative that accurate weights be obtained. Daily weights are required throughout the neonate's hospitalization, and twice-daily or more frequent weights should be obtained while the neonate is critically ill. The use of in-bed scales should be considered whenever the neonate requires careful fluid titration, particularly if the neonate has demonstrated intolerance of stimulation during nursing care activities.

### *Gastrointestinal and Genitourinary Function*

Intravenous alimentation will generally be provided for the premature neonate and the critically ill neonate. As noted above, the muscles necessary to suck and swallow may be present in the neonate as early as 28 weeks, but coordination of sucking and swallowing will usually not be effective until the neonate is approximately 32 to 34 weeks' gestational age.[2] In addition, the critically ill neonate may have decreased perfusion of the gut, so early feeding may increase the risk of necrotizing enterocolitis.

Regardless of the type of feeding provided, the nurse is responsible for provision of the prescribed volume and content of feeding and for monitoring the neonate's tolerance of the feeding. Further details about nutritional support are provided in the section entitled "Fluid Requirements and Fluid Therapy" in this chapter.

Assessment of gastrointestinal function requires regular observation of the appearance of the abdomen and measurement of abdominal girth at least every 4 hours. An increase in abdominal girth with rigidity, tenderness, or visible bowel loops may indicate the development of necrotizing enterocolitis (NEC). Other signs of NEC include thermolability, lethargy, signs of poor systemic perfusion, and guaiac-positive stools.[19]

Once oral or nasogastric feedings are begun, the neonate's total caloric intake and tolerance of the feedings must be monitored. Signs of feeding intolerance will include abdominal distention, vomiting, increased volume of residual formula in stomach between feedings, or diarrhea.

Every neonate should pass stools within the first 24 hours after birth. Stools should be tested for the presence of blood, and any positive results reported to a physician.

A decrease in urine output may occur as the result of inadequate fluid intake or decreased renal function. Some oliguria is anticipated following indomethacin administration, but a sharp decline in urine volume should be discussed with a physician.

### *Heat (Thermoregulation)*

The neonate is unable to shiver to generate heat, so if the neonate is subjected to a cold environmental temperature, brown fat will be broken down to generate heat and maintain body temperature. This breakdown of brown fat, however, is an energy- requiring process called "nonshivering thermogenesis" and will increase the infant's oxygen consumption.[20]

An important part of the hourly assessment of the critically ill neonate should include an evaluation of the neonate's body temperature. In addition, the environmental temperature should be controlled to provide a neutral thermal environment (the environmental temperature at which the neonate maintains a normal temperature with the lowest oxygen consumption). Maintenance of a neutral thermal environment is discussed further in the following section of the chapter.

If the neonate demonstrates a labile body temperature, infection or sepsis should be ruled out. If the neonate demonstrates cooling of extremities with delayed capillary refill, poor systemic perfusion should be suspected. Such clinical signs should be reported to a physician.

### Summary

The preceding eight-point check should serve as a general review of important aspects of the general assessment and care of the neonate with respiratory disease. More specific information regarding thermoregulation, fluid therapy and nutrition, and care of the neonate requiring oxygen therapy and mechanical ventilation will be discussed in subsequent sections of this chapter.

## THERMOREGULATION DURING THE NEONATAL PERIOD

### Normal Heat Production

Heat production in humans occurs in four major ways: through metabolism, voluntary muscle activity, involuntary muscle activity, and nonshivering thermogenesis. Heat is generated during metabolism; the higher the metabolic rate, the greater the heat generated.

While active older infants and children are able to generate significant heat during voluntary exercise, the critically ill neonate usually demonstrates decreased spontaneous movement. Heat may be produced through involuntary muscle activity, or shivering; however, the young infant is incapable of shivering until reaching several months of age. As stated previously, chemical heat production occurs as the result of breakdown of brown fat in a process called, "nonshivering thermogenesis." The breakdown of brown fat occurs following norepinephrine secretion and results in increased oxygen consumption. This heat generation in response to cold stress may be blunted by sepsis, drugs, hormonal imbalance, shock, or central nervous system damage. In addition, depleted brown fat stores will not be regenerated unless glucose intake is adequate.

### Mechanisms of Heat Loss

Heat loss in the neonate can occur as the result of internal gradients or external gradients. Internal gradients produce a loss of heat from within the body to the surface of the body. This heat loss will increase if the neonate develops vasodilation and can be reduced if peripheral vasoconstriction develops.

The most common cause of heat loss in the neonate is the result of an external gradient—the neonate loses heat from the body surface to the environment as the result of radiation, evaporation, conduction, and convection. Since the neonate has a large surface-area-to-volume ratio, a great deal of heat may be lost through this external gradient. The neonate also lacks significant quantities of subcutaneous fat (which acts as an insulator) and is unable to assume a posture conducive to heat retention.

**Neutral Thermal Environment**

To prevent nonshivering thermogenesis (and consequent increased oxygen requirements) during the neonatal period, the neonate should be nursed in a *neutral thermal environment*. A neutral thermal environment is that environmental temperature at which a neonate maintains a normal temperature with the lowest oxygen consumption.[20] The nurse is responsible for maintaining a neutral thermal environment throughout the neonate's hospital stay. Maintenance of thermoneutrality will be especially important for neonates with respiratory disease, since these neonates will probably not be able to increase oxygen consumption or oxygen delivery if nonshivering thermogenesis becomes necessary.

It is important to note that the presence of a neutral thermal environment cannot be ensured merely by observing the neonate's temperature—the neonate may demonstrate a "normal" skin temperature yet be utilizing nonshivering thermogenesis (and increased oxygen consumption) to do so. It is impractical to measure the infant's oxygen consumption in the clinical setting for direct evidence of thermoneutrality. Indirect evidence of thermoneutrality including the neonate's general appearance, skin temperature, and environmental temperature should be monitored and the relationship between ambient heat (and warming sources) and the neonate's temperature should be determined. Fortunately, the approximate ranges of neutral thermal environments have been experimentally determined (see Chapter 5), based on the neonate's age, maturity, and weight. These suggested ranges should serve to guide the nurse for initial provision of environmental temperature and should be modified according to the neonate's response.

Virtually every seriously ill or immature neonate will require some adjustment in environmental temperature, yet it is impractical to attempt to adjust the unit temperature and airflow patterns to the needs of each infant. Therefore, incubators or overbed warmers are commonly utilized. However, each of these devices has limitations, and the nurse must be aware of the proper operation and signs of malfunction for each device. Finally, the nurse must be aware of mechanisms of heat loss in the young infant and be prepared to institute appropriate therapy to minimize heat loss and cold stress.

## Prevention of Heat Loss in the Neonate

As noted above, the neonate may lose a great deal of heat from the body surface to the environment through radiation, evaporation, conduction, and convection.

### *Radiation*

*Radiation* causes loss of heat from the body due to the transmission of thermal energy by electromagnetic waves. All objects radiate thermal energy and hence tend to lose heat. However, since radiant energy can be reflected and absorbed as well as given off, the use of Plexiglas heat shields and double-walled incubators can reduce the heat loss by containing body heat within a small, isolated space.[21, 22]

Overbed radiant warmers were designed to counteract radiant heat loss by providing a source of radiant energy that the body can absorb, ideally at the same rate that it loses radiant energy so that body temperature remains constant. These heaters utilize a servocontrol mechanism to warm the air surrounding the neonate and maintain a neutral thermal environment as long as drafts are not present. Blankets and other clothing should not cover the neonate's trunk during warming, since heat from the warmer will not penetrate the material, and cooling of the infant may occur.

The overbed warmers should only be used with a servocontrol mechanism. This mechanism utilizes a temperature probe that is placed on the infant's trunk with a cushioned adhesive reflector pad. It is important that the probe be placed over a well-perfused area of the trunk on a nondependent surface of the skin (i.e., the neonate should not be lying on the probe). When the infant's skin temperature falls below the set range, heat output of the warmer will increase until the infant's skin temperature falls within the range desired. All warmers should be equipped with a functioning high/low temperature alarm, probe disconnect alarm, and a high-output heat alarm that signals if the infant requires constant heating.

Radiant heat will warm Plexiglas but will not penetrate the Plexiglas to warm the neonate. Therefore, while the infant is under a radiant warmer, no Plexiglas should be placed between the infant and the radiant warmer. Plexiglas sides may be used to create the frame of a

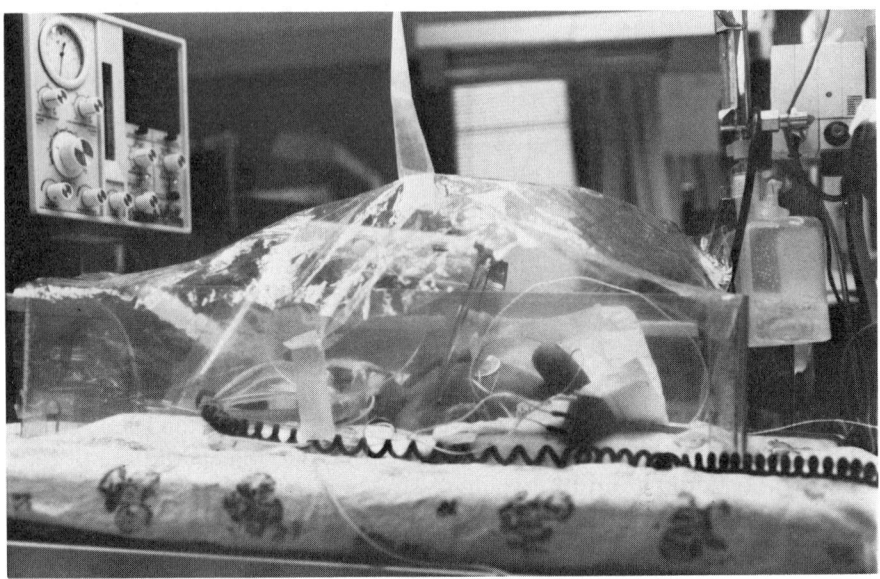

**FIG 7–1.**
This neonate is under a radiant warmer within the Plexiglas frame. The plastic cover can clearly be seen above the plastic frame. Note that a ribbon of tape prevents the plastic from coming into contact with the neonate's skin. This neonate is receiving nasal continuous positive airway pressure (CPAP) (via nasal prongs) and therefore is also under a head hood (to ensure adequate inspired oxygen concentrations). See the Section in this chapter on "Care of the Neonate Requiring Oxygen Therapy" for further information about provision of CPAP by nasal prongs.

shield, and plastic wrap may be used to cover the neonate (Fig 7–1). This set up will prevent drafts, while allowing effective warming of the neonate.

The neonate's head is relatively large and provides a large surface for heat loss. As a result, radiant heat loss can be reduced if the neonate's head is covered with a hat. These hats may be crocheted or knit by family members or volunteers, or purchased commercially. Stockinette tubing (such as the material used under casts) can also be knotted at one end and utilized for a hat. The hats should be warmed to body temperature before they are utilized to prevent conductive heat loss. Then, once the hats are in place, they will be warmed by the same device used to warm the neonate.[21]

### *Evaporation*

*Evaporation* causes loss of heat through the changing of water from a liquid to a gas state on the body surface. While some evaporative heat losses are unavoidable, excessive evaporative heat loss can be prevented by ensuring that the skin of the neonate is kept dry. It is imperative that the neonate be dried thoroughly in the delivery room. In addition, condensed water from oxygen hoods or heat shields should not be allowed to accumulate on the neonate's skin. Bathing is not necessary while the neonate is critically ill, and it may result in significant evaporative heat losses. Infants weighing less than 1,500 gm should only be bathed under an external heat source.

Increased evaporative water losses will occur during use of the overbed warmer or during bilirubin phototherapy; when such equipment is utilized, allowance must be made for this source of fluid loss.[18] Excessive evaporative heat and water losses can also occur if inspired air (especially that delivered during mechanical ventilation) is inadequately humidified. All *inspired gases* delivered to the premature neonate (whether by hood, nasal CPAP, "blow-by" oxygen, or mechanical ventilation) should be warmed to within 1° to 2°C of the neutral thermal environmental temperature for that infant. Such warming will prevent heat loss and will also ensure maximal humidification of the inspired air (since warm air holds more water in vapor form than cool air).

Humidification of *ambient* air will also facilitate maintenance of thermoneutrality and will reduce evaporative heat loss. Such humidification can be maintained in an incubator or under a warmer bed with a heat shield.[21]

### *Conduction*

*Conduction* causes loss of heat by transferring thermal energy from the body to a cooler surface that is in direct contact with the skin. Conductive heat loss in the NICU commonly occurs when the neonate is placed on a cool (room temperature) x-ray plate, scale, or treatment table. Such heat loss can be reduced if warm (body temperature) blankets are placed on any surface that will come into contact with the neonate.

### *Convection*

*Convection* causes loss of heat through the movement of air currents across the body that carry away thermal energy. Convective heat losses most frequently occur in the NICU when the neonate is under an overbed warmer in a drafty room. The nurse should ensure that open beds are placed well away from air vents. Air drafts can easily be detected with a small strip of tissue or crepe paper taped to both ends of the neonate's bed. If air currents are present, the paper strips will blow vigorously. If such air currents are present, the infant bed should be moved to another area of the unit, or nearby air vents should be shielded until drafts are absent.

Incubators allow care of the neonate in controlled environments. However, the temperature and humidity in the incubator will only be maintained if the incubator is entered infrequently through the insulated portholes; thus, this is an impractical method of controlling environmental temperature for a neonate who requires constant intervention. In addition, most commercially available incubators are heated through convection, which may result in creation of air drafts and may allow the infant's environmental temperature to vary by several degrees every hour. If the incubator is not double-walled, the walls may cool to room temperature, and the nude neonate will lose heat to the cooler (room temperature) walls. Such convective heat loss can be prevented if the incubator walls are warmed to 1° to 2°C warmer than the ambient temperature or if a Plexiglas heat shield is utilized to cover the infant in the incubator.

Convective and radiant heat loss may also be reduced through the use of Plexiglas shields or plastic sheeting. Such shields are most frequently used during care of neonates less than 1,500 gm. Plexiglas is an ideal material for construction of the shields, as it will allow the infant to remain visible while shielded from air drafts. The shield should be warmed prior to use and then will be kept warm by the air in the incubator.[22]

## Treatment of Hypothermia

If the infant demonstrates persistent hypothermia, sepsis, shock, or electrolyte imbalance should be ruled out. If the neonate is inadvertently subjected to a cold ambient temperature (such as during transport), careful, gradual warming should be provided while the infant is closely observed.

During rewarming, the ambient temperature should be kept approximately 1° to $1^1/_2$°C above the infant's core temperature, or a maximum of 35° to 36°C. The infant's skin temperature should be checked at least every 15 minutes and the ambient temperature adjusted to prevent rapid temperature rise or fall. The neonate will probably maintain temperature better if the humidity of the ambient air is maintained at approximately 60% to 70%.

The infant should be observed closely during the rewarming, since apnea may occur if warming is too rapid. Contact with the infant should be minimal since stimulation may contribute to a fall in temperature. Direct application of heat (such as through use of a warming mattress) should be avoided, as this form of heat will provide only local warmth and may result in a burn.

## Hyperthermia

Hyperthermia is to be avoided in the neonate with respiratory disease since it will result in an increase in metabolic rate and oxygen requirements. The most common cause of hyperthermia in the NICU is excessive warming from exogenous sources. It is imperative that all warming devices function properly to prevent such problems. If the neonate demonstrates hyperthermia despite appropriate ambient temperature, central nervous system disease should be suspected, and the infant's condition should be discussed with a physician. Occasionally, sepsis may produce fever in the neonate; however, most neonates demonstrate thermolability and hypothermia in response to infection.

## FLUID REQUIREMENTS AND FLUID THERAPY

### Neonatal Maintenance Fluid Requirements

The neonate has high maintenance fluid requirements per kilogram of body weight. A large proportion of the neonate's body weight is body water. In addition, a large proportion of this body water is extracellular. During the first days of life, the neonate normally demonstrates a natural diuresis and eliminates part of the extracellular water. As a result, the normal premature neonate can be expected to demonstrate weight loss of approximately 5% to 10% of body weight during the first 72 hours of life. In fact, consistent weight gain during the first days of life, or failure to lose weight, usually indicates that excessive fluid administration has occurred.

The neonatal kidney is incapable of excreting a concentrated urine. For this reason, if high solute loads are administered to the neonate, these solute loads must be excreted in relatively high urine volumes. Therefore, fluid and nutritional therapy should be calculated to provide renal solute loads that do not require maximal renal concentration or dilution.[23]

Maintenance fluid requirements for a low birth weight neonate during the first 72 hours of life total approximately 60 to 80 ml/kg/day. Maintenance fluid requirements beyond the first days of life may be liberalized if needed to total 100 to 150 ml/kg/day. The very low birth weight infant may require higher fluid administration rates as the result of greater insensible water losses through evaporation.

The infant nursed under a phototherapy light or radiant warmer will demonstrate greater evaporative losses than the infant nursed in a humidified incubator or under a shield. The neonate receiving mechanical ventilation with adequate humidification of the inspired air may have reduced insensible water losses through the respiratory tract, but these neonates may also develop pulmonary interstitial edema with even modest fluid intake. For all of these reasons, it is clear that any fluid administration rate must be individualized according to the infant's condition and must be constantly evaluated and modified according to the patient's response.

It is clear that the incidence of symptomatic patent ductus arteriosus will increase among neonates receiving high (> 100 ml/kg/day) fluid volume during the first days of life.[24,25] As a result, these levels of fluid administration will usually be avoided until the neonate is older.

## Assessment of Fluid Balance and Hydration

Assessment of level of hydration requires careful clinical examination and evaluation of daily weight and fluid balance. The clinical examination includes observation of the neonate's systemic perfusion and urine volume. The mucous membranes should be moist (observation should be made of the moistness inside the mouth), and the skin should not remain "tented" after it is pinched (although some tenting may be due to reduced amounts of subcutaneous fat in the premature neonate). Urine volume should average 2 to 4 ml/kg/hour, and urine osmolality should range from 150 to 400 mOsm/L, with a specific gravity of 1.002 to 1.012.

Fluid retention will result in periorbital and sacral edema, and edema may be noted in the hands and feet. In addition, overhydration will produce a fall in serum sodium concentration. Significant dehydration will result in compromise of systemic perfusion. Moderate dehydration will be associated with drying of the mucous membranes, poor skin turgor, and significant elevation in serum sodium concentration.[23]

Accurate body weight should be measured and recorded daily or more often when the neonate is critically ill. Use of in-bed scales will reduce the need for movement of the neonate for weighing. The same scale should be used throughout the neonate's care. The neonate should be weighed at the same time(s) of day to avoid variations in weight resulting from diuretic therapy or feedings.

All sources of fluid intake and output must be meticulously documented using flow sheets (see Appendix, Fig A-3). Fluid intake will include feedings, fluids used to dilute medications, and those needed to flush monitoring lines and blood sampling lines.

Fluid lost in urine, stool, nasogastric drainage, ostomy drainage, vomitus, and chest tube drainage should be totaled hourly. Documentation of accurate urine output can be difficult unless the neonate has an indwelling urinary catheter. Since such catheters are only available for the larger neonate, and since they will increase the risk of infection and urethral stenosis, catheters are generally used only when the neonate is extremely unstable.

Other methods of urine collection may require a great deal of creativity. Disposable diapers may be weighed before and after use, and any gram of weight increase in the diaper is assumed to be caused by 1 ml of fluid output. However, if the infant is under a radiant warmer or phototherapy light, the urine on the diaper may evaporate before it is measured; therefore, the nurse must be sure to remove and weigh the diapers as soon as the infant voids or has a stool. If it is necessary to obtain a urine sample from the surface of the diaper, a syringe (without needle) may be used to aspirate urine from the surface of the diaper; however, this method of urine collection will not necessarily obtain a representative sample of urine (since solutes may remain in the diaper and relatively free water may be drawn into the syringe). Plastic sheets or pants may be used to collect urine samples. However, plastic may irritate the neonate's skin so should not be left in place for extended periods. Urine bags (with adhesive surfaces) are usually avoided since they usually produce skin breakdown.

### Blood Sampling from Indwelling Lines

Scrupulous technique must be utilized when sampling blood from indwelling lines, or infection or vascular injury can result. The amount of blood that is lost or drawn for laboratory sampling should be recorded and totaled on the neonate's chart, and blood administration should be planned if the blood loss totals 5% to 7% of the neonate's circulating blood volume (calculated at 85 ml/kg), or if the hematocrit falls below 30% to 40%. Strict asepsis must be employed during sampling, and excessive blood loss or fluid administration must be avoided. The technique used for blood sampling from indwelling lines should be consistent throughout the unit. (See Chapter 5.)

### Feeding the Neonate

#### Nutritional Requirements

The seriously ill neonate requires good nutrition to ensure adequate growth and development and to hasten recovery from disease. Nutritional support should be planned to provide maintenance fluids as well as necessary calories, electrolytes, proteins, minerals, and vitamins.

Nutritional support of the premature neonate with respiratory disease offers several challenges. The muscles required for sucking and swallowing are not coordinated until the neonate reaches 32 to 34 weeks' gestational age. Therefore, orogastric or transpyloric feedings or parenteral alimentation will often be required. In addition, the gastrointestinal tract is immature, and the premature neonate may be intolerant of long-chain triglycerides and may absorb vitamins and minerals poorly.[23, 25]

The normal neonate is thought to require approximately 100 to 120 kcal/kg/day, and the low birth weight neonate is thought to require at least 75 to 95 kcal/kg/day during the first week of life. If the neonate with respiratory disease is breathing spontaneously, an enormous percentage of daily calories may be utilized to perform the increased work of breathing. Under these conditions, very high caloric intake (perhaps exceeding 150 kcal/kg/day) may be required to ensure appropriate weight gain. When the neonate with respiratory disease is admitted to the unit, good intravenous access must be established, and a plan must be made to nourish the infant and provide appropriate fluid and electrolyte therapy.

### *Oral Feedings*

Oral feedings are the preferred route of feedings for the relatively stable neonate greater than 34 weeks' gestational age and weighing more than 1,500 gm. Prior to initiation of oral feedings, the nurse must document the presence of a strong suck and a gag reflex. Bowel sounds should also be present.[26, 27]

Oral feedings should not be initiated if the infant demonstrates tachypnea (with respiratory rate greater than 60 breaths per minute), or tachycardia, as these clinical signs often indicate distress.[26, 27] In addition, the tachypneic neonate will usually tire during feedings and may swallow large quantities of air; as a result, feedings will not be tolerated, and the risk of vomiting and aspiration will be increased.

The infant should be fed by bottle (or Volufeeder) initially to assess exact fluid and caloric intake and strength of suck. Once the infant has demonstrated tolerance of feedings, breast feedings may be provided. The neonate should be weighed before and after each breast feeding to estimate the volume of feedings consumed.

During the feeding, the head of the neonate should be held so the infant is semi-upright, and the nurse or parent should maintain control of the infant's head (then, if the infant vomits or develops distress during feedings, the head can be turned or positioned to prevent aspiration). Feedings should be planned to follow a quiet period of rest and should not immediately follow tiresome treatments or suctioning. All feedings should be provided in a quiet environment.

The initial feeding may consist of sterile water.[26, 27] If this is tolerated, the next feeding can be advanced to half-strength or full-strength formula. Once the neonate has demonstrated the ability to suck and retain feedings, the volume and concentration of the feeding may be increased in an orderly fashion. It is important, however, that only the volume or the concentration of the feeding be advanced at any one time, and feedings, in general, should be advanced slowly.

Oral feedings should be offered for a maximum of 20 minutes—longer feeding times will probably exhaust the neonate. After each feeding, the infant should be burped and then placed in the prone position or on the side; these positions facilitate gastric emptying and reduce the risk of aspiration if vomiting occurs. The head of the bed should be slightly elevated.

If the neonate tires excessively during oral feedings, the feeding schedule should be varied to provide smaller, more frequent feedings. If such feedings still result in excessive fatigue, the nurse should allow the infant to take every other feeding by mouth and provide the other feedings by the orogastric route. Alternatively, the nurse may place an orogastric tube prior to the feeding and then allow the infant to suck as tolerated and provide any remaining formula through the orogastric tube.

When the infant has limited strength to take oral feedings, attempts should be made to maximize the caloric content of the feedings. Supplementation of formula with additional carbohydrates may increase caloric content but will also increase the osmolality of the feeding and may result in diarrhea. Medium-chain triglyceride oil may also be added to the formula, but this may also produce diarrhea. Breast milk supplements may be added to breast milk to increase caloric concentration as high as 30 kcal/oz. Whenever supplementation of feedings is provided, the caloric content of the feeding should be increased gradually and the infant's tolerance of the change assessed carefully. Vomiting, diarrhea, or abdominal distention will indicate intolerance of the feeding.

### *Orogastric (or Nasogastric) Feedings*

Orogastric feedings will be provided for the neonate with tachypnea and tachycardia, who demonstrates a weak suck, weak or absent gag reflex, or other neurologic impairment that may lead to loss of airway protective reflexes.[27] Nasogastric tubes may obstruct the neonate's nares. Since the neonate is thought to be predominantly a nose breather, it is thought that use of such tubes may contribute to increased respiratory distress. If nasogastric feedings are provided, the nurse must ensure that the presence of the tube itself does not result in an increase in the neonate's respiratory rate or effort.

Eight-F feeding tubes are utilized for infants weighing greater than 1,000 gm, and 5- or 6-F feeding tubes are utilized for infants less than

1,000 gms. The nurse should measure the appropriate length of tube insertion by placing the distal tip of the tube at the level of the infant's stomach (just below the sternum). While anchoring the distal tip at the stomach, the remainder of the tubing is held to the infant's ear and angled to the level of the infant's lip; this mimics the course of the orogastric tube. An indelible mark or piece of tape should be placed on the portion of the tube that corresponds to the level of the patient's lip to indicate the appropriate depth of tube insertion. The tube should be moistened with water-soluble lubricant and passed gently from the infant's mouth into the esophagus and stomach. Once the appropriate depth of insertion (as indicated by the mark or tape) is reached, the tube is taped in place.

The nurse should verify that the tube is in the stomach by injecting a small amount (0.5 to 1.0 ml) of air through the tube while listening with a stethoscope over the stomach. If the orogastric tube is in the stomach, a clear "whoosh" of air will be heard as the air is injected through the tube; the air should then be aspirated from the stomach. If there is any question of proper placement, the nurse can submerge the proximal end of the tube in water or saline. If the tube is in the lungs, air will bubble from the tube during spontaneous exhalation; if the tube is in the stomach, no respiratory bubbling should be observed. The nurse should also aspirate fluid from the tube and check the pH of the aspirate, stomach contents will have an acidic pH.

If there is any question of proper tube placement, the tube should be withdrawn and another orogastric tube inserted prior to feeding. Once proper tube placement is achieved, the tube should be taped securely. The nurse should always wait several minutes after tube insertion before beginning feedings to see if the infant develops reflex bradycardia or other complications of vagal stimulation. If no such complications develop, the feeding can continue.

Gastric contents should be gently aspirated prior to any tube feeding to determine the volume of residual feeding in the stomach. If formula totaling one third or more of the previous feeding remains in the stomach, the infant will probably not tolerate any increase in volume or concentration of formula for the subsequent feeding. If the residual formula totals half or more of the previous feeding, the subsequent feeding should be held, and a physician should be notified.[27] Any residual formula aspirated at the beginning of a feeding should be returned to the infant and the volume subtracted from the subsequent feeding.

Orogastric feedings should be provided through the barrel of a syringe attached to the distal portion of the tube. The feedings should be provided using gravity drainage only, and the syringe barrel should be elevated so the feeding will be completed over 10 to 15 minutes. Throughout the feeding, a pacifier should be placed in the infant's mouth to encourage sucking; this will help the infant associate sucking with the sensation of satiety. At the end of the feeding, the infant should be burped and placed prone or on the side with the head of the bed slightly elevated.

### *Transpyloric Feedings*

Transpyloric (orojejunal) feedings are indicated if the infant is intolerant of bolus or continuous gastric feedings. Such intolerance may be due to respiratory distress or gastroesophageal reflux. Transpyloric feedings are often provided if the infant is intubated or receiving CPAP.[27]

Orojejunal tubes are inserted using a method similar to that described above (see orogastric feedings). However, when the nurse determines the appropriate depth of tube insertion, the distal tube tip should be placed 2 to 3 cm below the xiphoid process to mimic the placement of the tube tip in the jejunum.

Polyvinyl tubes should be changed every 1 to 3 days since these tubes tend to become stiff within a few hours or days after placement. Silastic feeding tubes are manufactured with a weighted tip to facilitate transpyloric placement and prevent tube migration. These tubes are equipped with an introducer that should be removed before the tube is inserted (the stiff introducer is not necessary for placement, and it may contribute to perforation). Silastic tubes may remain in place for 1 to 3 months.

Verification of proper placement of the orojejunal tube is accomplished through aspiration of bile through the tube; the pH of the bile will be greater than 7 if the tube has passed the pyloric sphincter (from the stomach into the jejunum). An abdominal radiograph may also be obtained to verify that the tube has passed beyond the stomach.[27]

Transpyloric feedings are provided continuously using a volume pump. The formula in the pump reservoir should be changed every 4 hours, and the pump tubing should be changed every 8 hours to reduce the risk of contamination or separation of the formula. During feedings, an orogastric tube should be inserted at regular intervals (every 4 to 6 hours) to check for evidence of reflux of formula into the stomach or evidence that the tube has migrated into the stomach (providing orogastric feedings). If a significant amount of formula is present in the stomach (approximating the volume in one hour's feeding), the feedings should be stopped and a physician notified.

### Assessment of Tolerance of Feedings

The best method of determining patient tolerance of feedings is careful observation by the nurse. The nurse should continuously monitor the neonate's heart rate, respiratory rate and effort, and color, and these variables should be charted on the infant's flow sheet prior to and following any feeding. In addition, the abdominal girth should be recorded at least every 4 hours, and any consistent increase in girth should be reported to a physician. The observation of dilated loops of bowel on the surface of the abdomen may indicate the presence of intestinal distention or obstruction. Vomiting, diarrhea, or the presence of large residual feeding in the stomach may also indicate feeding intolerance.[26, 27]

The development of respiratory distress, poor color, or bradycardia during oral or orogastric feedings may indicate intolerance of the feeding or aspiration; if these signs develop, the feeding should be discontinued immediately, and a physician should be notified. Oral feedings should also be discontinued if the infant shows signs of fatigue; if such exhaustion occurs frequently, consideration should be given to providing orogastric feedings until the infant is stronger.

Following any feeding, the nurse should record the volume, concentration, and substance of the feeding. In addition, the duration of the feeding and the infant's tolerance of the feeding should be charted.

The infant's heel-stick glucose concentration should be monitored whenever feedings are initiated or if the method of feeding changes. Urine volume should be assessed, and urine specific gravity and presence (and quantity) or absence of glucosuria should be documented. Glucosuria should be reported to a physician since it may indicate excessive glucose intake or infection.

The frequency, color, and consistency of all stools should be reported, and any increase or decrease in stool output should be discussed with a physician. All stools should be tested for the presence of blood since the presence of blood in the stool may be an early sign of necrotizing enterocolitis. The presence of blood in the stool should be reported to a physician.

If at all possible, the infant should be held during feedings. This may require careful covering of the infant to prevent thermal loss. In addition, oxygen therapy or other respiratory support must continue uninterrupted. The parents should be involved in the feeding process so they are able to participate in nurturing the child. The mother or father may wish to hold the infant or provide the pacifier during the feeding, and this should be encouraged.

Vitamin supplements may be ordered once the neonate is tolerating feedings. Such supplements may include multivitamins, iron, and vitamins E and A.[28]

## Parenteral Alimentation

Parenteral alimentation may be necessary if the neonate demonstrates inability to absorb appropriate quantities of nutrients through the gastrointestinal tract. Such infants include those with major gastrointestinal anomalies or intractable diarrhea. While there is no question that parenteral alimentation can provide adequate nutrition for these neonates, this form of feeding will not provide hyperalimentation.

Parenteral alimentation is begun gradually, and the neonate's tolerance of the continuous infusion is assessed carefully. Glucose concentrations of up to 12.5% may be administered peripherally, and higher concentrations will be administered through a central line. Calories will be provided in the form of glucose, fat emulsion, and protein. In addition, electrolytes and minerals will be included.

The nurse is responsible for checking the alimentation label against the alimentation formula ordered by the physician. In addition, the nurse should total the fluid volume and caloric content of the parenteral alimentation to ensure that the infant is receiving appropriate quantities of each. Glucose provides 4 kcal/gm (so 5% glucose solution contains 5 gm of glucose per 100 ml or 20 kcal/100 ml). Protein also contains 4 kcal/gm, and fat contains 9 kcal/gm. Intravenous 10% fat emulsion solutions usually contain approximately 1.1 kcal/ml. If the total fluid and caloric content of the parenteral alimentation solution is inappropriate, the nurse should discuss this with a physician.

Once parenteral alimentation is begun, the infusion should be administered in an uninterrupted fashion. The rate should not be increased or decreased since such changes may produce wide fluctuations in serum glucose concentration. If the alimentation is administered through a peripheral line, it may be helpful if an additional working intravenous catheter is in place. Then, if the alimentation catheter ceases to function, the alternative line may be used immediately. If the peripheral alimentation must be interrupted while a new catheter is inserted, the neonate may rapidly become hypoglycemic.

The neonate's heel-stick and serum glucose concentrations should be monitored closely when the alimentation is begun and whenever changes in the solution are made. Initially, the infant's electrolyte balance, blood urea nitrogen (BUN), calcium, phosphorus, magnesium, protein, albumin, and liver enzymes will be monitored closely, but these studies may be reduced to weekly intervals once the infant is receiving a stable fluid volume and glucose concentration.

The most common complications of intravenous alimentation include infection and catheter-related complications. Infection may occur since the alimentation solution provides an excellent medium for bacterial growth. For this reason, most hospitals require that the intravenous tubing be changed every 12 hours using strict aseptic technique. If at all possible, the alimentation line should be utilized only for alimentation and should not be entered to administer other drugs or fluids, since this will increase the risk of contamination and infection.

Catheter-related complications include catheter migration, thrombosis, and infiltration of the solution into subcutaneous tissue. Concentrated glucose solutions may cause serious burns and may require treatment with hyaluronidase.[15] Additional complications of parenteral alimentation include electrolyte imbalances (especially hyperglycemia) and hepatic dysfunction.

## CARE OF THE NEONATE REQUIRING OXYGEN THERAPY

### General Nursing Observations

Whenever the neonate has respiratory distress, the clinician should monitor the infant's condition closely. Continuous monitoring of heart rate and rhythm should be provided with alarms set to signal bradycardia or tachycardia. Heart rate and respiratory rate and effort should be charted hourly, and presence and severity of grunting, nasal flaring, and retractions should be noted. A physician should be contacted immediately if the neonate demonstrates increased distress.

The neonate's color and adequacy of systemic perfusion should be monitored continuously, including specific documentation of warmth of extremities, intensity of peripheral pulses, briskness of capillary refill, and urine volume. Blood pressure should be recorded hourly if the neonate is unstable, and at least every 4 hours if respiratory distress is present.

Breath sounds should be auscultated hourly when the neonate is unstable, and chest expansion should be noted. Particular attention should be given to a decrease in intensity of breath sounds or unilateral change in pitch of breath sounds since these signs may indicate the presence of atelectasis, pneumothorax, or pleural fluid.

During periods of acute distress, the neonate should be positioned with the head of the bed elevated. Many neonates will demonstrate improvement in oxygenation when placed in the prone or side-lying position; determination of optimal patient position is made through assessment of arterial blood gases (and noninvasive blood gas monitoring) and clinical examination. Any patient with respiratory distress should be positioned to maximize oxygenation and minimize respiratory effort. If the supine position is utilized, a soft roll should be placed under the infant's shoulders to extend (but not hyperextend) the airway. Stimulation should be minimized, and a neutral thermal environment must be provided to reduce oxygen consumption.

Most infants with respiratory distress will swallow air; this can produce gastric distention and compromise diaphragm excursion. As a result, an orogastric tube should be placed whenever respiratory distress is present. Such tubes should always be inserted when the infant is receiving nasal CPAP. A 5–F feeding tube will be utilized for neonates less than 1,000 gm, and an 8–F feeding tube will be utilized for neonates greater than 1,000 gm. These tubes should be placed to gravity drainage, to allow evacuation of gastric air.[29]

Oral or orogastric feedings should be withheld when respiratory distress is present. If intubation is required and the neonate has a full stomach, vomiting and aspiration of stomach contents may occur.

The nares should be free of obstruction by tubes or tape since the neonate is predominantly a nose breather. Feeding tubes, endotracheal tube tape, and phototherapy eye pads should be positioned so that they are not restricting air exchange. The mouth should be swabbed every 2 to 4 hours with sterile water. Lemon and glycerin swabs should not be used since they often dry the oral mucous membranes.[29]

**Chest Physiotherapy**

The need for chest physiotherapy should be assessed at least every shift. Suctioning should be performed as needed to maintain airway patency, and preoxygenation and hyperventilation should be provided whenever suctioning is required.

Chest percussion and postural drainage may be ordered if the infant develops atelectasis or pneumonia. The Trendelenberg (head-down) position is *not* recommended during the care of the premature neonate since it may contribute to increased intracranial pressure and intraventricular hemorrhage.

Patient tolerance of any physiotherapy must be carefully assessed and adequate rest periods provided during the therapy. Physiotherapy should be interrupted immediately if the neonate's color or clinical condition deteriorates. Chest physiotherapy is also discussed in Chapter 5.

**Noninvasive Blood Gas Monitoring**

Whenever the infant receives oxygen therapy, the inspired oxygen concentration should be verified at least hourly. In addition, the infant's oxygenation should be monitored closely using arterial blood gas analysis, transcutaneous blood gas monitoring, or pulse oximetry.

If transcutaneous blood gas monitoring is utilized, the clinician must ensure that the monitoring equipment is properly calibrated and that the heated electrode is placed on a well-perfused area of the neonate's trunk. Since the heated electrode may cause a dermal burn (similar to a sunburn), the electrode should never be placed on the infant's head or face. The appearance of the burn should be discussed with the parents. Correlation between the transcutaneous oxygen and carbon dioxide tensions and arterial oxygen and carbon dioxide tensions should be established (see Chapter 5).

Pulse oximetry is now widely used to monitor the neonate's hemoglobin saturation. Since hemoglobin saturation directly determines arterial oxygen content, this method of noninvasive monitoring can be extremely useful for determining effectiveness of oxygenation in the neonate with respiratory disease. However, pulse oximetry will provide no information about effectiveness of ventilation (and carbon dioxide removal); thus it will be less useful when carbon dioxide retention is present.[30] In addition, since pulse oximetry indicates hemoglobin saturation and not arterial oxygen tension, the oximeter will not generate an alarm when the neonate develops dangerously high arterial oxygen tension levels (> 100 torr). Therefore, once the neonate's hemoglobin saturation approaches 90% to 95%, the arterial oxygen tension should be checked, as reduction of supplemental oxygen therapy may be indicated.

Noninvasive blood gas monitoring is an extremely useful adjunct to nursing care of the seriously ill neonate. Continuous monitoring will permit immediate recognition of deterioration in gas exchange and facilitate prompt intervention. Such feedback also enables the staff to perfect suctioning and hand ventilation technique so that oxygenation is maintained. In addition, the clinician will be easily able to determine patient positions associated with optimal blood gases. Finally, responses to medications (including vasoactive drug therapy and analgesics) and therapy may be instantly assessed.

**Oxygen Therapy**

Whenever the neonate requires delivery of increased inspired oxygen concentrations, the clinician is responsible for ensuring uninterrupted delivery of the appropriate oxygen concentration (dose) and for monitoring the infant's response to therapy. The method of oxygen delivery will be determined by the level of inspired oxygen required and by the neonate's general condition. If the neonate requires small amounts of supplemental oxygen therapy, this oxygen may be delivered into the infant's incubator. If the neonate requires an inspired oxygen concentration greater than 0.4, this oxygen must usually be administered through a head hood.

### Oxygen Therapy Via Incubator

Inspired oxygen concentrations of up to 0.4 may be provided by the flow of humidified oxygen directly into an incubator. If the neonate weighs less than 1,500 gm, the oxygen should be provided in a mist heated to 31° to 34°C to minimize the infant's heat and water loss.[29] This form of oxygen therapy may be ideal for the neonate who requires minimal nursing care but will not be desirable if the incubator must be entered frequently, since the inspired oxygen concentration will fall significantly every time a porthole is opened.

### Oxygen Therapy Through Head Hood

Inspired oxygen concentrations of up to 0.9 to 1.00 L may be provided through use of a head hood. If this form of oxygen therapy is provided, flow rates of at least 4 to 5 L/minute should be provided to maintain oxygen concentration and prevent carbon dioxide accumulation.

## Continuous Positive Airway Pressure

### Therapeutic Effects of Continuous Positive Airway Pressure

Oxygen therapy with continuous positive airway pressure is the ideal form of ventilatory support for the neonate with hypoxemia and acceptable respiratory effort. Continuous positive airway pressure will not, however, improve carbon dioxide elimination in the neonate with hypoventilation or inadequate respiratory effort; in these neonates, mechanical ventilation will probably be required. For further discussion of the effects of CPAP, see Chapter 5.

The optimal level of CPAP will be the lowest continuous airway pressure consistent with maximal oxygen delivery (arterial oxygen content × cardiac output). In general, determination of the optimal level is made through analysis of arterial oxygen tension and indirect evidence of systemic perfusion. The CPAP should be increased only as needed to improve systemic arterial oxygenation and should not be increased to levels that result in a decrease in urine volume or prolongation of capillary refill (signs of decreased systemic perfusion).

Whenever the infant receives CPAP therapy, the inspired oxygen concentration as well as the level of positive airway pressure provided must be checked at least hourly. These levels should be documented on the nursing chart and the respiratory therapy sheet.

### Delivery of Continuous Positive Airway Pressure by Nasal Cannulas

While CPAP may be provided in a variety of ways, nasal CPAP delivered through nasal prongs is the most widely used form of CPAP in the NICU. To ensure effective therapy, the prongs must fit properly. Small neonatal prongs should be used for neonates less than 1,500 gm.

The nasal prongs must be securely held in place at all times; this is probably the most challenging aspect of this therapy. If the prongs are held too loosely in the nares, effective airway pressures will not be achieved. If the prongs are held too tightly in the nares, erosion of the nasal septum may occur.

Head slings or tape may be used to anchor the nasal prongs. However, these materials may produce skin irritation or breakdown. A stockinette or crocheted cap and twill tape will effectively anchor the nasal prongs without the need for tape or tight headpieces (Fig 7—2,A and B).[29]

Every infant receiving nasal CPAP therapy should have two sets of nasal prongs. The prongs are changed and cleaned every shift—when one set is cleaned, the second set may be inserted to avoid interruption in CPAP therapy. Sterile water and cotton-tipped applicators should be used to clean the prongs, and the spare set of prongs should be stored in a sterile container at the bedside.

Nares care should be provided every 4 hours during nasal CPAP therapy. The nurse should suction the nasopharynx and oropharynx using a bulb syringe. In addition, the nasal prongs should be briefly removed from the nares and inspected. Any secretions or crusts forming on the prongs should be removed with sterile water and a cotton-tipped applicator. Obstructed prongs should be replaced immediately. During nares care, the nares should be gently massaged.[29] Hydrocortisone cream should not be used during nares care since it may cause breakdown of the skin or nasal septum.

Many infants swallow large amounts of air during nasal CPAP therapy. As a result, many physicians request that orogastric tubes be placed prior to CPAP therapy to allow evacuation of gastric air (and prevention of gastric distention). For this reason, transpyloric feedings may be preferred over orogastric feedings during CPAP therapy. The nurse should monitor for signs of abdominal distention or vomiting during therapy.

In our institution, neonates receiving nasal CPAP also receive humidified oxygen therapy by head hood.[29] This ensures adequate inspired oxygen concentrations even if the neonate breathes by mouth. If the neonate weighs less than 1,500 gm, all sources of inspired air should be heated to approximately 31° to 34°C. Infants receiving CPAP should be encouraged to suck on a pacifier. During sucking, the neonate's mouth will be closed, and mouth breathing will be prevented; as a result, most ventilation will occur through the nose, with effective CPAP.

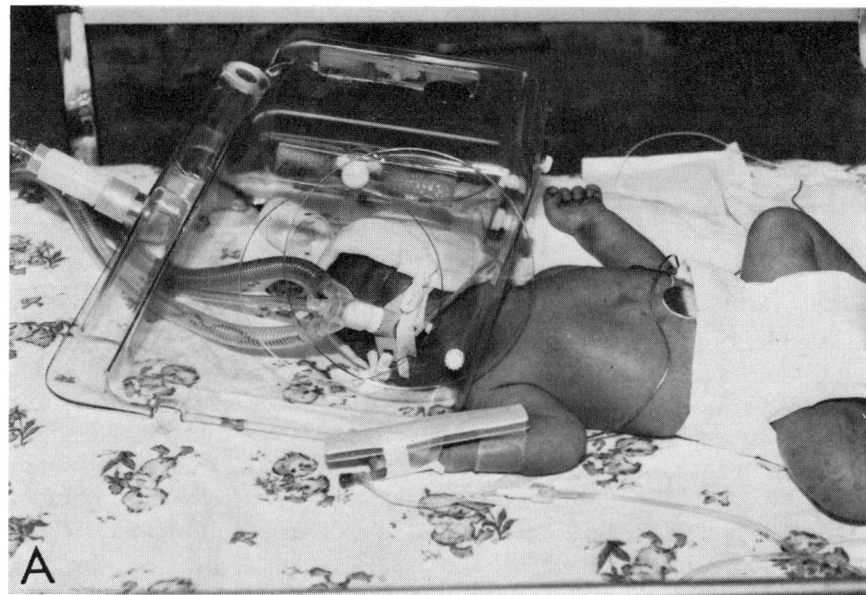

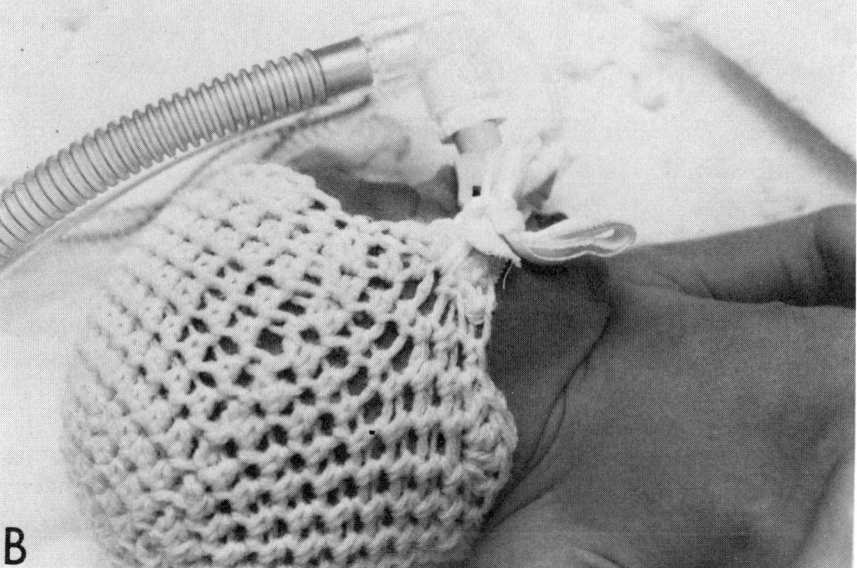

**FIG 7–2.**
Neonate receiving nasal continuous positive airway pressure (CPAP). **A,** neonate under radiant warmer. CPAP nasal prongs are held in place using a crocheted cap and twill tape ties. Note that the neonate is also receiving increased inspired oxygen via head hood, since some mouth breathing may occur. **B,** crocheted cap with twill-tape ties effectively anchors the CPAP nasal prongs. Note presence of orogastric tube (to eliminate swallowed air).

Some neonates receiving CPAP therapy will require occasional provision of manual "sighs" to improve oxygenation and control carbon dioxide levels. If such manual breaths are required, they are provided with a bag equipped with a PEEP valve to maintain the CPAP during hand ventilation.

### Potential Complications of Continuous Positive Airway Pressure Therapy

Throughout therapy, the nurse should monitor the neonate's color, heart rate, respiratory rate and effort, and systemic perfusion. Noninvasive blood gas monitoring will enable evaluation of oxygenation.

Potential complications of CPAP include reduction in cardiac output and barotrauma. These complications are less likely to develop if positive airway pressures of 8 cm $H_2O$ or less are utilized (see Chapter 5). Signs of intolerance of CPAP therapy include an increase in respiratory rate and effort or apnea, bradycardia, and deterioration in blood gases. These signs should be reported to a physician immediately, and mechanical ventilation may be required.

## NURSING CARE OF THE NEONATE REQUIRING MECHANICAL VENTILATION

### Intubation and Initiation of Mechanical Ventilatory Support

Intubation will be required whenever the infant has difficulty maintaining a patent airway, when severe upper airway obstruction is present, or if mechanical ventilation will be required. If at all possible, this intubation should be accomplished on an elective basis, and the most skilled personnel should always be at the bedside. All necessary equipment, including the laryngoscope handle, Miller size 0 and 1 straight blades with working bulbs, hand resuscitator, mask, oxygen source, large suction catheter (to suction the pharynx and vocal cords), and suction catheter that will easily pass into the selected endotracheal tube, should be available. To avoid the need for a stylette (which may perforate the trachea or a bronchus), the endotracheal tubes may be frozen or placed on ice prior to use; this will ensure that they are stiff enough to pass through the vocal cords. Tape and tincture of benzoin should also be prepared.

Selection of the endotracheal tube will be based on unit protocol and on the neonate's gestational age and weight (see Chapter 5). Two types of endotracheal tubes are commonly used in the NICU. Oral tubes are shorter in length and stiffer than standard endotracheal tubes and may be preferred for orotracheal intubation since they are less likely to kink. Softer blue endotracheal tubes may be desirable since they may be less traumatic. If the soft tube is utilized, the external portion of the tube (that portion of the tube between the neonate's lips and the connector and mechanical ventilator tubing) can be reinforced to prevent kinking through use of clear connection tubing. This connection tubing is readily available and is commonly used between suction catheters and the suction cannister. If a short piece of this tubing is cut longitudinally, it may be wrapped around the external portion of the soft endotracheal tube to provide reinforcement. Endotracheal tubes should have a radiopaque line to enable radiographic verification of tube placement.

The appropriate suction catheter size that will easily pass into the endotracheal tube may be estimated by multiplying the endotracheal tube size (in millimeters) by two. The next size suction catheter above this calculated catheter size should also easily pass into the tube.

Before intubation is attempted, the infant should be hand-ventilated with bag and mask to ensure effective oxygenation and carbon dioxide removal. The QRS tone on the cardiac monitor should be audible so that everyone at the bedside will hear the infant's heart rate and be aware if the heart rate falls during intubation. The infant should be positioned with the neck slightly extended. For further discussion of the actual intubation procedure, the reader is referred to Chapter 5.

Once the tube is passed, assessment of tube position is necessary. Chest expansion should be observed during manual ventilation; it is most helpful if a skilled clinician observes chest expansion from the foot of the bed to ensure that chest expansion is equal and adequate bilaterally. Since the infant's chest is compliant, it should rise during positive-pressure ventilation—if the chest does not rise during positive-pressure ventilation, the infant is not effectively ventilated. The clinician should listen to breath sounds bilaterally, and over the stomach area to verify appropriate tube position. If the tube is in the esophagus, breath sounds will be heard more loudly over the stomach than over the lung fields.

Since the neonate's trachea is relatively short, inadvertent right main-stem bronchus intubation can easily occur. This will result in relatively loud breath sounds heard over the right lung fields and diminished breath sounds heard over the left lung fields. In addition, the left chest will probably not expand effectively during positive-pressure ventilation. The neonate's chest wall is thin, so breath sounds from one area of the lung can easily be referred to other areas of the lung; as a result, endotracheal tube migration or unilateral pulmonary pathology may produce a change in pitch as well as a change in intensity of breath sounds. A chest radiograph should also be performed to verify proper tube placement.

Several excellent methods of securing the endotracheal tube have been reported in the literature.[31,32] The reader is referred to these reports. It is important that a consistent method of endotracheal tube taping be adopted by the nursing and medical staff and the respiratory therapists, to enable anyone to assess the security of the tube and assist with retaping of the tube. The tape should not pull on the lips and should prevent tube movement into and out of the mouth (or nares). If spontaneous extubation occurs frequently in the NICU, the incidence of extubation should be documented, other methods of tube taping explored, and the most desirable method of securing the tube adopted. Finally, the effectiveness of the change in technique can be shown through documentation of a decrease in the rate of spontaneous extubation.

Stoma adhesive or a bio-occlusive dressing should be applied to the extremely immature neonate's cheeks before applying tape to secure the endotracheal tube. This should reduce the incidence of skin breakdown under the tape. Taping or retaping of the endotracheal tube always requires participation by two experienced staff—one person stabilizes the tube, and the second person tapes the tube in place.

When the endotracheal tube is inserted, the number or letter printed on the part of the endotracheal tube that lies at the infant's lip (or external nares, if nasotracheal intubation is performed) should be noted. This information should be written on the nursing care card. In addition, the distance between the infant's lip (or nares) and the connector on the endotracheal tube should be measured and recorded. This information will allow immediate detection of tube migration or displacement.

Movement of the neonate's head will result in movement of the orotracheal tube. Extension of the neonate's neck (and upward movement of the chin) will move the tip of the orotracheal tube out of the trachea. Flexion (and movement of the chin toward the chest) will move the tip of the orotracheal tube into the trachea (this may result in right main-stem bronchus intubation). Rotation of the head will also move the tip of the orotracheal tube out of the trachea.[33] As a result, when an endotracheal tube is in place, the neonate's head must be kept in a neutral position.

## Suctioning

Suctioning should be performed as often as necessary to maintain airway and endotracheal tube patency. Although suctioning is a routine part of the care of the intubated patient, it is a technique that is often performed carelessly, with potential complications.[34] Skilled suctioning should result in removal of secretions with minimal tracheal mucosal trauma, without development of hypoxemia or bradycardia.

If suctioning produces hypoxemia, the neonate may deteriorate rapidly. Hypoxemia may contribute to pulmonary vasoconstriction. This can increase right ventricular afterload and result in worsening heart failure or reduced pulmonary blood flow. In addition, improper suctioning (and resultant hypoxemia and hypercapnia) can contribute to a rise in intracranial pressure.[34] For these reasons, two skilled people should participate in the suctioning of an unstable infant (particularly one with severe respiratory disease or pulmonary hypertension, or increased intracranial pressure).

Before suctioning, the neonate should be ventilated with inspired oxygen concentrations slightly (10% to 20%) above baseline levels.[35] Ventilation may be delivered using a bag equipped with appropriate CPAP valve (to maintain the baseline CPAP) and pressure manometer. Peak inspiratory pressure delivered during hand ventilation should be approximately equal to the proximal airway pressure provided during conventional mechanical ventilation. During hand ventilation, the clinician should assess the infant's breath sounds, chest expansion, and lung compliance.

The infant should be positioned so the face is visible during suctioning. In addition, the QRS audible tone on the cardiac monitor should be increased, so the heart rate may be heard. Finally, the noninvasive blood gas monitors should be easily visible so values can be monitored during suctioning. The infant's heart rate, color, and systemic perfusion should also be closely monitored.

Suctioning time should be only a few seconds in duration. If the tube appears to be patent and minimal secretions are present, a single pass with the suction catheter may be sufficient to ensure effective secretion removal. If tube obstruction is suspected, however, several passes with the suction catheter may be necessary to remove the obstruction.

The neonate should be allowed to rest between any suction attempts, and suctioning should be interrupted if bradycardia develops or if the infant demonstrates deterioration in color or blood gases (as assessed with noninvasive monitors). Suction should be applied only as the catheter is withdrawn.

Care must be taken to insert the catheter only as deep as needed to suction the tube. The suction catheter should not be inserted until resistance is felt. Deep suction technique is thought to contribute to irritation and ulceration of tracheobronchial mucosa and may stimulate granulation tissue formation.

Suction catheters are commercially available that are marked with centimeter markings. The clinician can then note the endotracheal tube centimeter marking at the neonate's lip and insert the marked suction catheter to the same centimeter depth (allowing an additional 1 to 3 cm for the connector). Since the marked catheters are more costly than the unmarked catheters, the nurse may wish to simply mark a sample catheter to the appropriate suction depth (by measuring the centimeter length on the catheter that corresponds to the endotracheal tube at the infant's lip and then allowing for connection length). If this marked catheter is mounted on a sign at the head of the infant's bed, every clinician will be reminded of the approximate appropriate suction depth.

Strict aseptic technique must be maintained during suctioning. Contamination of the suction catheter will increase the infant's risk of pneumonia.

Following suctioning, the neonate should be manually ventilated with inspired oxygen concentrations 10% to 20% above baseline (as prior to suctioning) and inspiratory pressure approximately equal to those delivered by the ventilator.[35] It is important to assess the neonate's color, heart rate, chest expansion, breath sounds, and lung compliance and continue to provide manual ventilation until the neonate is stable. Potential complications of suctioning include hypoxemia, pulmonary vasoconstriction, pneumothorax, atelectasis, and tube displacement.

**Assessment of Adequacy of Positive-Pressure Ventilation**

Any mechanical ventilator used in the NICU must be capable of providing small tidal volumes at rapid rates and low inspiratory pressure. The ventilator should be equipped with high- and low-pressure and disconnect alarms, as well as alarms to indicate low gas/oxygen flow, power failure, and high or low inspired air temperature. The alarms must remain activated at all times since they may provide the only signal that tubing has become disconnected, or the ventilator has malfunctioned.

The neonate receiving mechanical ventilatory support may not be adequately ventilated. The clinician must constantly assess the neonate's clinical condition and ensure proper function of the ventilator. The best tools for evaluation of effectiveness of ventilatory support include careful clinical examination and analysis of (invasive or noninvasive) blood gases. The infant's vital signs and clinical appearance should be appropriate for the infant's clinical condition. The infant's chest should rise symmetrically with positive-pressure ventilation, and breath sounds should be equal in pitch and intensity bilaterally.

If there is any question about effectiveness of mechanical ventilatory support, the neonate should be removed from the ventilator and hand ventilation should be performed. The clinician should assess ventilation and tube patency immediately. The reader is referred to Chapters 12 and 13 for a detailed review of techniques of mechanical ventilatory support and its complications.

## SKIN CARE

Premature neonates have extremely fragile skin. As a result, particular care must be taken when the skin is cleaned or when tape is applied to the skin. The purpose of this section is to summarize some helpful hints about skin care.

The skin should be cleansed carefully. Excessive use of iodine solutions should be avoided since they may burn the skin. Diluted povidone-iodine (Betadine) solutions have been found to be effective in reducing skin trauma without reduction in infection control. Presaturated iodine swabs will effectively cleanse the skin without trapping excess iodine solution that will remain on the infant's skin. Immediately following any procedure, all iodine solutions should be removed from the skin.[36]

Application of tape over the abdomen should be avoided. Umbilical artery catheters may be taped in place if a bio-occlusive skin barrier (such as Comfeel or Hollihesive) is placed on the skin; then the catheter may be taped to the skin barrier. When temperature probes are placed, the same skin barriers should be used. However, a small hole should be placed in the skin barrier (slightly larger than the size of the temperature probe). Then, the probe can be allowed to touch the infant's abdominal skin directly, but it can be secured with tape placed over the probe and the skin barrier.

Skin barriers should also be placed on the neonate's cheeks before the endotracheal tube is taped in place. These barriers will allow the tube to be taped securely without concern that the tape will injure the infant's cheeks. Barriers should also be used to secure intravenous catheters and chest tubes.

Any adhesive will injure the skin unless it is removed properly with care and patience. A soft gauze pad moistened with water should be used to gently break the bond between the tape and the skin.

Electrodes may be attached to the infant's limbs without use of the electrode adhesive. All adhesive can be trimmed from the electrode, leaving the central electrode itself and the cushion of conductive gel. Soft gauze can be wrapped around the infant's extremity, holding the electrode firmly in place without restricting circulation. A slit made in the gauze will allow the electrode "snap" to be attached to a cardiac monitor cable.

Burn sheets and water mattresses also provide ways to reduce damage to fragile skin. If skin breakdown or irritation continues to be a problem, the nurse should search to find alternative methods of securing tubes and catheters.

## PSYCHOSOCIAL SUPPORT OF THE NEONATE AND FAMILY

### Minimizing Stimulation

In recent years, several studies have explored the effects of stress on the critically ill neonate. This research has demonstrated that stress is associated with assessment and care procedures commonly performed in the NICU. The infant demonstrates stress through physiologic mechanisms, including development of apnea, bradycardia, or lethargy, or the development of arterial oxygen desaturation or poor perfusion.[37]

Many standard NICU procedures, including repositioning, heelsticks, suctioning, and measurement of vital signs, have now been associated with the development of hypoxemia in the neonate. The development of hypoxemia may be prevented or the magnitude of the hypoxemia decreased if such procedures are grouped together, with adequate rest periods allowed between periods of stimulation.

Whenever practical, noninvasive methods of assessing the infant's oxygenation should be employed. Noninvasive monitoring will enable the clinicians to evaluate the neonate's tolerance of procedures such as suctioning and chest physiotherapy. Following any stressful procedure, the infant should be left undisturbed (barring emergencies) until monitoring indicates that arterial oxygenation has returned to and been maintained at baseline levels for 30 to 60 minutes.

Whenever possible, the neonate's vital signs should be obtained from the cardiac monitor. The neonate's respiratory rate can be counted without disturbing the infant. When auscultation of heart and breath sounds is necessary, the stethoscope head should be warmed before use.

The neonate who demonstrates signs of overstimulation or failure to gain weight should be moved to a quiet part of the unit. This quiet area should be free of traffic, and lights should be dimmed (at least at night). Staff conversation should be minimal, and loud noises prevented. If it is not possible to control all of the lighting in the unit, the nurses may construct curtains around the bed, to be used during sleep or nap times. Such barriers should never, however, interfere with observation of the neonate.

## Support of the Parents

The parents of the seriously ill newborn deserve very special care. They are often thrust from the middle of a seemingly normal pregnancy into the newborn intensive care unit. Parents anticipating the birth of a child have dreams and hopes for that child that must suddenly be revised when the newborn is ill or imperfect.[38,39]

The neonate's parents are often extremely tired, frustrated, angry, and frightened. They must have the opportunity to mourn over the loss of their fantasized, desired child. Characteristic grief responses may include shock and disbelief; a stunned, numb state; and remorse. Unfortunately, the parents of the premature neonate with respiratory disease must often immediately make decisions about their infant's care; consequently they are often not allowed time to deal with the reality of their loss.[37]

Many parents will experience guilt and attempt to identify specific behaviors or events that may have caused their infant's premature birth or disease. The parents may also be angry that something is wrong—they may attempt to assign guilt to a member of the health care team for causing their child's illness or treating it inadequately. This anger is a normal response since it is easier to focus anger on a person than to feel guilty or angry or frustrated at themselves or "fate." The parents may also be frightened—frightened that their baby will die—and intimidated by all of the knowledgeable professionals and sophisticated equipment in the intensive care unit.[38,39]

Parents of the critically ill neonate need rest, the opportunity to review their thoughts and feelings about the child they dreamed of, realistic and consistent information about their new infant, and an active role in planning for the care of their neonate. The parents require accurate information about their child's condition, delivered in a manner that they can understand. The specific information and prognosis provided to the parents should be noted on the nursing care card so all members of the health care team can use consistent words and phrases when discussing the child's care and condition.

The parents report that early visits to the nursery are helpful in coping with their child's illness. Even parents of the sickest infants report that they imagined the infant to look much worse than the infant actually did. Tours of the NICU should be given to high-risk antepartum mothers and their spouses, so the parents will see the unit and its equipment before their infant is born. These tours seem to help the parents prepare for the possible premature birth of their infant and give the parents confidence and faith in the unit. For further information about support of the parents, the reader is referred to Chapter 8.

## Support of the Nursing Staff

There is no question that intensive care nursing is extremely stressful. In fact, surveys of critical care nurses reveal that ICU nurses like the constant challenges, opportunities, and unpredictability of the critical care environment. The most stressful aspects of the newborn intensive care unit include the acuity of the patients, the sophistication of the equipment, shortage of nursing staff (as the result of the nursing shortage or hospital budgetary cutbacks), competition among nurses (for promotion, or for parents' trust), conflicts with physicians or hospital or nursing administrators, and parent teaching and support responsibilities.[40]

Nurses often attempt to be "all things to all people," and tend to take more time for emotional support of parents, patients, and other members of the health care team than they take for themselves or for their fellow nurses. To minimize nursing staff turnover and maximize nursing job satisfaction, it is essential to create a supportive, teaching environment in the NICU. Each member of the health care team must be committed to the care of the patients and families and to the support of one another. Everyone must feel responsible for teaching and learning on a daily basis.

A supportive nursing environment may begin with the unit orientation program. Each new nurse should be assigned to a preceptor or supportive colleague. Primary nursing will allow the nurse to plan care for a neonate and family, and care for that family over time. However, occasionally, the nurse will need a break from the care of an extremely ill neonate.

Frequent opportunities for continuing education should be provided in the unit and at the bedside, in the form of nursing and team rounds, and in the form of minilectures. The nurses should be involved in decisions about nursing care techniques and protocols and should also participate in the health care team rounds conducted by physicians.

The NICU can be a wonderfully nurturing environment if the health care team strives to make it so. Nurses should know that they practice both an art and a science. While every patient may not survive to be discharged from the hospital, the nurse may gain satisfaction from providing the best nursing care possible for the infant and valuable support for the family during their time of crisis.

# REFERENCES

1. Hazinski MF: Nursing care of the critically ill child: The seven-point check. *Pediatr Nurs* 1985; 11:453.
2. Hack M: The sensorimotor development of the preterm infant, in Fanaroff AA, Martin RJ (eds): *Behrman's Neonatal-Perinatal Medicine*, ed 3. St Louis, CV Mosby Co, 1984, chap 21.
3. Hazinski MF: Children are different, in Hazinski MF (ed.): *Nursing Care of the Critically Ill Child*, St Louis, CV Mosby Co, 1984, chap 1.
4. Cabal LA, Larrazabel C, Siassi B: Hemodynamic variables in infants weighing less than 1,000 gms. *Clin Perinatol* 1986; 13:327.
5. Muller NL, Bryan AC: Chest wall mechanics and respiratory muscles in infants. *Pediatr Clin North Am* 1979; 26:503.
6. Carlo WA, Martin RJ: Principles of neonatal assisted ventilation. *Pediatr Clin North Am* 1986; 33:221.
7. Brann AW Jr, Schwartz JF: Central nervous system disturbances, in Fanaroff AA, Martin RJ (eds): *Behrman's Neonatal-Perinatal Medicine*, ed. 3. St Louis, CV Mosby Co, 1984, chap 22.
8. Painter MJ, Bergman I, Crumorine P: Neonatal seizures. *Pediatr Clin North Am* 1986; 33:91.
9. Levy SR: Neonatal seizures. *Semin Perinatol* 1986; 11:155.
10. Rudolph AM: Changes in the circulation after birth, in Rudolph AM: *Congenital Diseases of the Heart*. Chicago, Year Book Medical Publishers, 1974, chap 2.
11. Friedman WF: The intrinsic physiologic properties of the developing heart, in Friedman WF, et al (eds): *Neonatal Heart Disease*. New York, Grune & Stratton, 1973, chap 3.
12. Riemenschneider TA, Brenner RA, Mason DT: Maturational changes in myocardial contractile state of newborn lambs. *Pediatr Res* 1981; 15:349.
13. Schreiber MD, Heymann MA, Soifer SJ: Increased arterial pH, not decreased $PaCO_2$ attenuates hypoxia-induced pulmonary vasoconstriction in newborn lambs. *Pediatr Res* 1986; 20:113.
14. Berman W Jr: The relationship of age to the effects and toxicity of digoxin in sheep, in Heymann MA, Rudolph AM (eds): *The Ductus Arteriosus*, Report of the 75th Ross Conference in Pediatric Research. Columbus, Ohio, Ross Laboratories, 1978.
15. Howell L: Effect of hyaluronidase in the treatment of medication burns. University of California at San Francisco Medical Center, unpublished data, 1987.
16. Hazinski TA: Furosemide decreases ventilation in young rabbits. *J Pediatr* 1985; 106:81.
17. Winters RW: Maintenance requirements, in Winters RW (ed): *Principles of Pediatric Fluid Therapy*. New York, Abbott Laboratories, 1975, p 46.
18. Hammerlund K, Sedin G: Transepidermal water loss in newborn infants: VI. Heat exchange with the environment in relation to gestational age. *Acta Paediatrica Scandinavia* 1982; 71:191.

19. Sunshine P, Sinatra FR, Mitchell CH, et al: Necrotizing enterocolitis, in Fanaroff AA, Martin RJ (eds): *Behrman's Neonatal-Perinatal Medicine,* ed. 3, St Louis, CV Mosby Co, 1984, p 512.
20. Hey EN, Katz G: The optimum thermal environment for naked babies. *Arch Dis Child* 1978; 45:328.
21. Glover A: Protocol for thermoregulation of the infant in the NICU. Vanderbilt University Medical Center Neonatal Intensive Care Unit, Nashville, Tenn, unpublished protocol, 1986.
22. Fitch CW, Korones SB: Heat shield reduces water loss. *Arch Dis Child* 1984; 59:886.
23. Nash MA: Provision of water and electrolytes, in Fanaroff AA, Martin RJ (eds): *Behrman's Neonatal-Perinatal Medicine,* ed 3. St Louis, CV Mosby Co, 1984, p 314.
24. Bell EF, et al: Effect of fluid administration on the development of symptomatic patent ductus arteriosus in the premature infant. *N Engl J Med* 1980; 302:598.
25. Cotton RB, Lindstrom DP, Stahlman MT: Early prediction of symptomatic patent ductus arteriosus from perinatal risk factors: A discriminant analysis. *Acta Paediatr Scand* 1981; 70:723.
26. Bragdon DB: A basis for the nursing management of feeding the premature infant. *J Obstet Gynecol Nurs* 1983; (suppl) 83:51.
27. Kraus K: Protocol for the care of the infant receiving enteral feedings in the NICU. Vanderbilt University Medical Center Neonatal Intensive Care Unit, Nashville, Tenn, unpublished protocol, 1986.
28. Shenai JP, Kennedy KA, Chytil F, et al: Clinical trial of vitamin A supplementation in infants susceptible to bronchopulmonary dysplasia. *J Pediatr* 1987; 111:269.
29. Vaughn S: Protocol for the care of the infant with respiratory distress in the NICU. Vanderbilt University Medical Center Neonatal Intensive Care Unit, Nashville, Tenn, unpublished protocol, 1986.
30. Romanathan R, Duirand M, Larrazabal C: Pulse oximetry in very low birth weight infants with acute and chronic lung disease. *Pediatrics* 1987; 79:612.
31. Seaver P: Endotracheal tube stabilization. *Neonatal Network* 1984; 2:52.
32. Nieves JA: Avoiding spontaneous extubation of nasotracheal or oral tracheal tubes. *Pediatr Nurs* 1986; 12:215.
33. Donn SM, Kuhns LR: Mechanisms of endotracheal tube movement with change of head position in the neonate. *Pediatr Radiol* 1980; 9:39.
34. Perlman JM, Volpe JJ: Suctioning in the preterm infant: Effects on cerebral blood velocity, intracranial pressure, and arterial blood pressure. *Pediatrics* 1983; 72:329.
35. Cassami VL: Hypoxemia secondary to suctioning in the neonate. *Neonatal Network* 1984; 2:8.
36. Unfer S: Effective dilution of iodine antiseptic against colonization bacteria of the neonate that reduce the occurrence of chemical burns. Presented at the Mead Johnson Symposium in Perinatal and Developmental Medicine at Marco Island, Fla, Dec 7, 1982.

37. Gorski PA: Behavioral and environmental care: New frontiers in neonatal nursing. *Neonatal Network,* 1985; 5:21.
38. Lemons PM, Weaver DD: Beyond the birth of a defective child. *Neonatal Network* 1986; 5:13.
39. Fraley AM: Chronic sorrow in parents of premature children. *Children's Health Care* 1986; 15:114.
40. Simone JA: The intensity of newborn intensive care: Caring for the caregivers. *Neonatal Network* 1984; 2:27.

# 8

## Care of the Parents

John H. Kennell, M.D.
Marshall H. Klaus, M.D.

In our work managing nurseries for normal and sick newborn infants, we both became aware how difficult it was for some mothers to become attached to their premature or sick infants. For example, we encountered one mother who had successfully managed two full-term infants well but who was uncertain and anxious as she started to care for a newborn premature infant. She required extra support and instruction to feed the baby and change his diapers and had endless questions during the first 3 months after he went home. From this and a number of similar observations, we were stimulated to take a closer look at how parents become attached to their infants. The importance of understanding this was emphasized by a study in our own nursery and reports from other large neonatal intensive care units (NICUs) showing that a disproportionate percentage of babies who were discharged from the nursery in good condition returned days or weeks later battered and abused, or failing to thrive without any organic cause.

From our efforts to understand the bonding process and to unravel the mystery of these problems of attachment, we have developed our present understanding and recommendations.

To begin, it is important to state that attachment is crucial to the survival and development of the infant. The parents' bond to their child may be the strongest of all human ties. The power of this attachment is so great that it enables the mother and father to make the unusual sacrifices necessary for the care of their infant day after day, night after night; attending to his crying, protecting him from danger, changing his diapers, giving feedings in the middle of the night. Over the last decade the term *bond* has come to refer to a tie from parent to infant. A bond can be defined as a unique relationship between two people that is specific and endures through time. Bonding is not a simple or a rapid process.

The difficulties that parents of premature infants experienced in learning to cope with their infants provided the stimulus to explore how normal parents develop a close attachment to their infants. In this chapter we will attempt to integrate studies from a large number of sources into a general framework from which we will develop some clinical recommendations. By observing and studying the human mother during the period prior to pregnancy, during pregnancy, and after the birth, we can begin to fit together the interlocking pieces that lay the foundations of attachment.

## PRIOR TO PREGNANCY

Long before a woman becomes a mother, she has obtained a repertoire of mothering behaviors through observation, play, and practice. She has already learned whether infants are picked up when they cry, how much they are carried, and whether they should be chubby or thin. It is an interesting phenomenon that these modes of conduct, absorbed when children are very young, become unquestioned imperatives for them throughout later life.

## PREGNANCY

### Acceptance of Pregnancy

During the first stage of pregnancy a woman must come to terms with the knowledge that she will be a mother. When she first realizes that she is pregnant, a mother will often have mixed feelings. A large number of considerations, ranging from a change in her familiar patterns to more serious matters such as economic and housing hardships or interpersonal difficulties, all influence her acceptance of the pregnancy.

### Perception of the Fetus as a Separate Individual

The second stage involves a growing awareness of the baby in the uterus as a separate individual. It usually starts with the remarkably powerful event of quickening, the sensation of fetal movement. It appears to occur earlier for mothers who see their baby and its movements on the screen during ultrasonography. After quickening, a woman will usually begin to have fantasies about what the baby will be like, attributing some personality characteristics and developing feelings of attachment. At this time she may go a step further in accepting her pregnancy and show significant changes in attitude toward the fetus. Objectively, there will usually be some outward evidence of the mother's preparation. She may purchase clothes or a crib, select a name, and rearrange her home to accommodate a baby.

The production of a normal child is a major goal of most women. Yet most pregnant women have hidden fears that the infant may be abnormal or reveal some of their own secret inner weaknesses. The caregiver's ability to help parents during the emotional turmoil that occurs during pregnancy probably has a strong influence in determining whether the pregnancy will be a positive or negative experience in the woman's life. Cohen,[1] however, emphasizes that any stress, such as moving to a new geographic area, marital infidelity, death of a close friend or relative, previous abortions, or loss of previous children, that leaves the mother feeling unloved or unsupported, or that precipitates concern for the health and survival of either her infant or herself, may delay preparation for the infant and retard bond formation.

It is difficult to define all the factors that determine the interactional and parenting behavior of an adult human who has lived for 20 to 30 years. A mother's and father's behavior toward their infant is derived from a complex combination of their own genetic endowments, the infant's responses to them, a long history of interpersonal relationships with their own families and with each other, experiences with this or previous pregnancies, the absorption of the practices and values of their cultures, and, probably most important, the way in which each was raised by his or her own parents. The mothering and fathering behavior of each woman and man, the ability of each to tolerate stresses, and the needs each has for special attention differ greatly and depend on a mixture of these factors.

Figure 8–1 is a schematic diagram of the major influences on parental behavior and the resulting disturbances that we hypothesize may arise from them. At the time the infant is conceived, some of these determinants, such as the mothering that the father and mother received when they were infants, the practices of their culture, their endowments, and their relationships with their own families, are contributed by the parents. We originally believed these determinants fixed and unchangeable. However, Harmon and Emde (personal communication) have argued that the influence of some of these may be changed during the crisis of birth. Other determinants relate to the hospital culture. For example, the attitudes, statements, and practices of the nurses and physicians in the hospital; whether there is separation from the infant in the first days of life; the infant's temperament; and whether he is

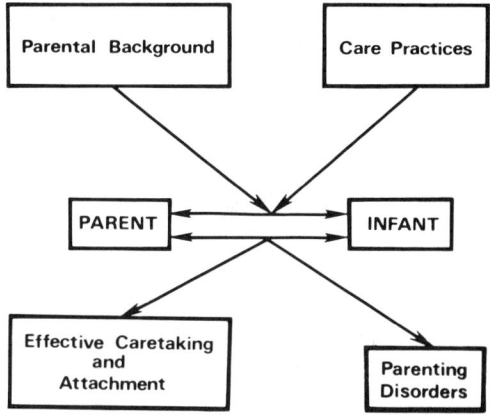

**FIG 8-1.**
Major influences on parent-infant attachment and the resulting outcomes. (From Klaus MH, Kennell JH: *Parent-Infant Bonding.* St Louis, CV Mosby Co, 1982. Used by permission.)

healthy, sick, or malformed obviously also affect the relationship. The vast majority of mothers and fathers develop warm and close attachments with their infants. However, a series of *mothering disorders* ranging from mild anxiety, such as persistent concerns about a baby after a minor problem that has been completely resolved in the nursery, to the most severe manifestation—the *battered child syndrome*—occur in a small number of parents. It is our hypothesis that some problems result in part from separation and other unusual circumstances that occur in the early newborn period as a consequence of present hospital care policies. Experiences during labor, parent-infant separation, and hospital practices during the first hours and days of life are the most easily manipulated variables in this scheme. Recent studies have partly clarified some of the steps in mother-infant attachment during this early period.

## LABOR

Before childbirth moved from the home to the hospital, it was the practice in industrialized nations for family members to support the mother in labor, often with the assistance of a trained or untrained midwife. Although more fathers, relatives, and friends have been allowed into labor and delivery rooms in the past 20 years, a significant number of mothers still labor and deliver in some hospitals without the presence of family members or close friends. Even though fathers are allowed in many hospitals they frequently are unsure, ill at ease, often in the way, and not able to provide active support. Two recent

**TABLE 8–1.**
Effect of Supportive Companion (Doula) on Perinatal Problems*

| Characteristic | Control Group, % (No.) (N=95) | Experimental Group, % (No.) (N=32) |
| --- | --- | --- |
| No problems | 21 (20) | 63 (20) |
| Problems or intervention | 79 (75) | 37 (12) |
| Meconium staining | 25 (24) | 9 (3) |
| Depressed newborn | 3 (3) | 0 (0) |
| Stillbirth | 2 (2) | 0 (0) |
| Cesarean section | 27 (26) | 19 (6) |
| Oxytocin augmentation | 17 (16) | 6 (2) |
| Forceps | 5 (4) | 3 (1) |

*From Sosa R, Kennell JH, Klaus MH, et al: The effect of a supportive companion on perinatal problems, length of labor, and mother-infant interaction. *N Engl J Med* 1980; 303:597. Used by permission.

studies in Guatemala were designed to investigate the effects of a supportive companion (Raphael termed such a person a *doula*) on perinatal complications and mother-infant interaction after delivery, in an obstetric setting in which mothers routinely labor alone.[2,3]

Initial assignment of mothers to the experimental (doula) or control group was random, but controls showed a higher rate ($P<.001$) of subsequent perinatal problems (e.g., cesarean section, meconium staining) (Table 8–1). In both studies the length of time from admission to delivery was much shorter in the experimental group, 9 vs. 19 hours in the first study and 8 in contrast to 14 hours in the second ($P<.001$).

Significantly more mothers who had a *doula* present during labor remained awake after delivery and were more interactive with their infants during the time they were awake. These observations suggest there are major perinatal benefits of constant human support during labor.

## AFTER BIRTH

Immediately after the birth, there is a unique period for the parents that lasts a short time and during which the parents' attachment to their infant sometimes begins to blossom. We have called this the *maternal sensitive period*.

The first feelings of love for the infant are not necessarily instantaneous with the initial contact. The relation between the time when a mother falls in love with her baby and the sensitive period is not clear at present. Several mothers have shared with us their distress and disappointment when they did not experience feelings of love for their baby in the first minutes or hours after birth. It should be reassuring for them and mothers like them to learn about a study of normal, healthy mothers in England. MacFarlane and associates[4] asked 97 Oxford mothers, "When did you first feel love for your baby?" The replies were as follows: during pregnancy, 41%; at birth, 24%; first week, 27%; and after the first week, 8%.

Donald Winnicott[5] who started as a pediatrician and became a distinguished psychoanalyst, has made remarkably perceptive observations that suggest he was describing the sensitive period. From these observations Winnicott proposed that a healthy mother goes through a period of *primary maternal preoccupation*. He observed that "the mother who developed this state . . . provided a setting for the infant's constitution to begin to make itself evident." It was his belief that only if a mother was able to reach this state of heightened sensitivity could "she feel herself into her infant's place, and so meet the infant's needs."

It is interesting that the timing and course of primary maternal preoccupation are similar to those described for the maternal sensitive period (Figure 8–2). Interestingly, the heightened sensitivity of primary maternal preoccupation is sometimes misinterpreted by physicians and nurses as excessive anxiety. Studies of other cultures are important in this regard because in most societies the mother and baby are placed together with support, protection, and isolation for at least seven days

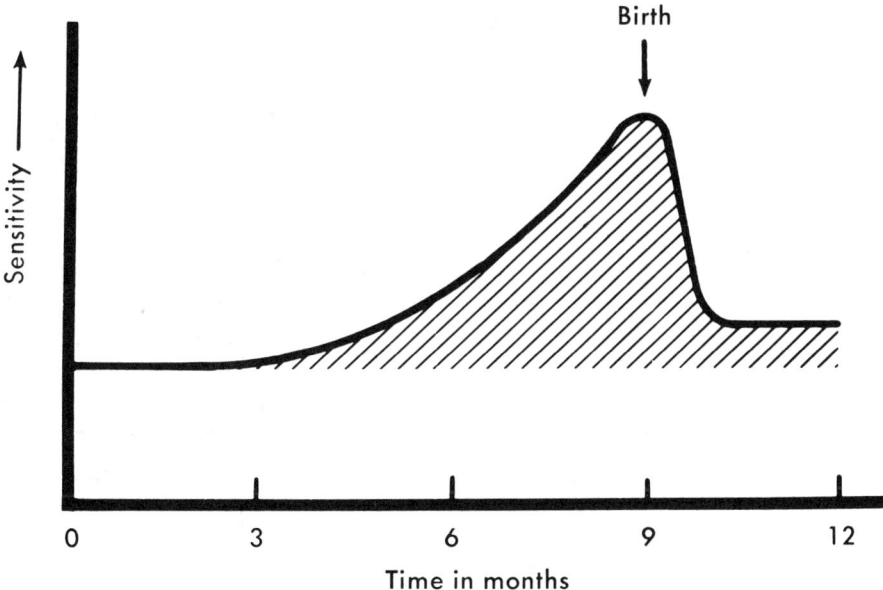

**FIG 8–2.**
Hypothesized change in maternal sensitivity during pregnancy and in the postnatal period. (From Klaus MH, Kennell JH: *Parent-Infant Bonding.* St Louis, CV Mosby Co, 1982. Used by permission.)

after birth. The provision of food and water and a private time for the mother and infant to get to know each other, are common in most cultures.

Anxieties a mother has about her baby in the first few days after birth, even about a problem that is easily resolved, may affect her relationship with the child long afterward. Relatively mild illness in the newborn, such as slight elevations of bilirubin levels, slow feeding, additional oxygen for 1 to 2 hours, and the need for incubator care in the first 24 hours for mild respiratory distress, appear to affect the relationship between mother and infant. The mother's behavior is often disturbed during the first year or more of the infant's life, even though the infant's problems are completely resolved prior to discharge and often within a few hours. That early events have long-lasting effects is one of our principles of attachment.

In the past 15 years, 17 separate studies have focused on whether additional time for close contact of the mother and infant in the first minutes, hours, and days of life alters the quality of the attachment.

Figure 8–3 illustrates the timing of the contact in the 17 human studies. In three studies, the extra time was added not only during the first 3 hours but also during the next 3 days of life.[6] At 1 month the mothers in the group who had extra contact showed significantly more affectionate behavior toward their infants. They stood closer and watched

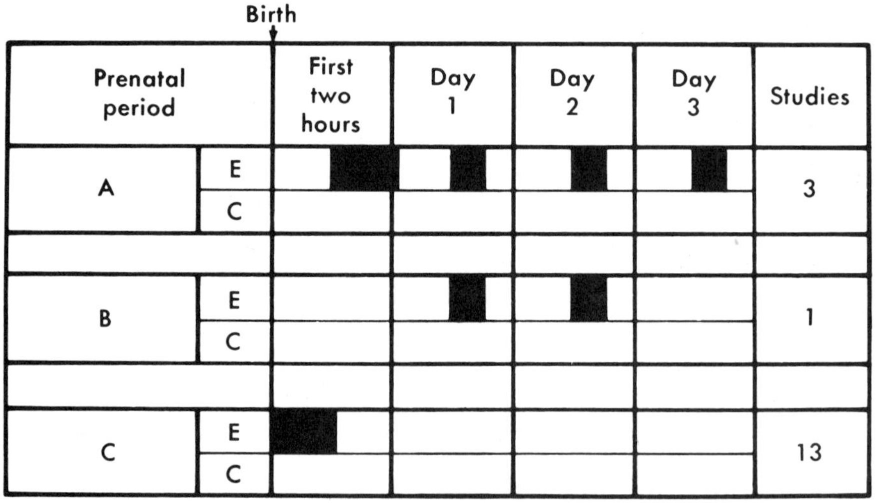

| Prenatal period | | First two hours | Day 1 | Day 2 | Day 3 | Studies |
|---|---|---|---|---|---|---|
| A | E | ■ | ■ | ■ | ■ | 3 |
|   | C |   |   |   |   |   |
|   |   |   |   |   |   |   |
| B | E |   | ■ | ■ |   | 1 |
|   | C |   |   |   |   |   |
|   |   |   |   |   |   |   |
| C | E | ■ |   |   |   | 13 |
|   | C |   |   |   |   |   |

**FIG 8–3.**
Time patterns and number of three types of controlled studies (A, B, and C) in which one group of mothers has additional contact (E) with their infants compared to another group with routine contact (C). (From Klaus MH, Kennell JH: Parent-Infant Bonding. St Louis, CV Mosby Co, 1982. Used by permission.)

over them more during the physical examination, soothed them more when they cried, engaged in more eye-to-eye contact and fondling during feeding, and were more reluctant to leave them with someone else. At 1 year, the two groups of mothers were again significantly different, with extra-contact mothers spending more time assisting and soothing their infants during stressful office visits. In 13 studies, the additional mother-infant contact occurred only during the first hour of life. In 10 of these studies significant differences in the behavior of the mothers were noted. In 7 of 9 studies, breast-feeding was significantly increased by permitting the mother additional time with her infant in the first hour.

When additional time is given for close mother-infant contact following the first 8 hours post partum (see Fig 8–3, type B and Table 8–2), there are also differences in later mothering behavior. In a study of 301 primiparous patients, O'Connor[7] noted that increasing the time by 12 hours (6 hours on days 1 and 2) significantly decreased the number of mothering disorders with 10 such occurrences in the control group but only 2 in the group of mothers who received extra time with their infants (see Table 8–2). Siegel and associates,[8] in a group composed of primiparous and multiparous mothers, did find differences in parenting at 4 and 12 months but no difference in mothering disorders. A woman was defined as having a mothering disorder if her infant was battered, had nonorganic failure to thrive, was abandoned, or was given up for an unplanned adoption.

In the first hour after birth, the newborn infant is in a heightened state of alertness and responsivity. Interestingly, no matter when increased amounts of contact between mother and infant are added in the first 3 postpartum days, there appears to be improved mothering behavior. At present it is not known why such striking alterations in caretaking have been noted when mother-infant contact is increased for such a short time in the first hours of life.

**TABLE 8–2.**
Child Abuse or Neglect in the First Year of Life*

| Study | Total | Abuse or Neglect |
|---|---|---|
| O'Connor et al. (1980)[7] | | |
|     Extended contact | 134 | 2 |
|     Control | 143 | 10† |
| Siegel et al. (1980)[8] | | |
|     Extended contact | 97 | 7 |
|     Control | 105 | 10 |

*From Klaus MH, Kennell JH: *Parent-Infant Bonding*. St Louis, CV Mosby Co, 1982. Used by permission.
†$P<.05$.

## Talents of the Infant

Recent information in a closely related field has greatly augmented our understanding of parent-to-infant attachment. Detailed studies of the amazing behavioral capacities of the normal neonate have shown that the infant sees, hears, imitates facial gestures, and moves in rhythm to his mother's voice in the first minute and hours of life, resulting in a beautiful linking of the reactions of the two and a synchronized "dance" between the mother and infant. The infant's appearance, coupled with his broad array of sensory and motor abilities, evokes responses from the mother and father and provides several channels of communication that are helpful in the process of attachment and the initiation of a series of reciprocal interactions.

MacFarlane[9] has shown that 6 days after birth the infant will have the ability to distinguish reliably by scent his own mother's breast pad from the breast pads of other women. The mother has an intense interest in looking at her newborn baby's open eyes. In the first 45 minutes of life the infant is awake and alert and will follow his mother for 180 degrees with his own eyes. The licking of the nipple will induce a marked increase in prolactin secretion in the mother, and at the same time an increase in oxytocin, to contract the uterus and decrease bleeding. With the mother's strong desire to touch and see her child, evolution has provided for the immediate and essential union of the two. The alert newborn rewards his mother for her efforts by following her with his eyes, thus maintaining their interaction and kindling the tired mother's fascination with her baby. These intricate interactions have focused our attention on the cascade of interlocking sensory patterns that quickly develop between mother and infant in the first hours of life (Fig 8–4).

There is suggestive evidence that many of these early interactions also take place between the father and his newborn child. Parke[12] in particular has demonstrated that when fathers are given the opportunity to be alone with their newborns, they spend almost exactly the same amount of time as mothers, holding, touching, and looking at them. In an interesting observation of fathers, Rödholm and Larsson[10] noted that paternal caregiving was markedly increased when the father was allowed to interact with his infant and establish eye-to-eye contact with him for 1 hour during the first hours of life. Keller et al.[11] have recently reported that the group of fathers who received extended postpartum hospital contact with their infants, compared to a traditional contact group, engaged in greater amounts of en face behavior and vocalization with their infants and were more involved in infant caretaking responsibilities 6 weeks after the baby's birth. They also had higher self-esteem scores than the other group of fathers. Parke[12] believes that the father

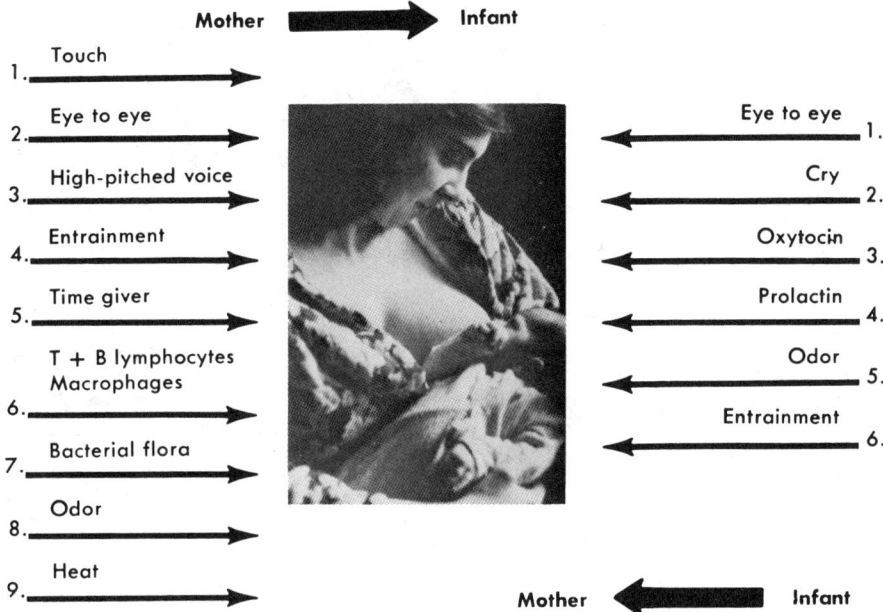

**FIG 8–4.**
Mother-to-infant and infant-to-mother interactions that can occur simultaneously in the first days of life. (From Klaus MH, Kennell JH: *Parent-Infant Bonding.* St Louis, CV Mosby Co, 1982. Used by permission.)

must have an extensive early exposure to the infant in the hospital where the parent-infant bond is initially formed. Parke interpreted his findings as indicating that the father is much more interested in and responsive toward his infant than United States culture has acknowledged.

On the basis of our observations and the reports of parents, we believe that every mother has a task to perform during the postpartum period. She must look and "take in" her real live baby and reconcile the fantasized image of the infant she anticipated with the one she actually delivered (Fig 8–5). Many cultures recognize this need by providing the mother with a *doula*, or "aunt," who mothers her and relieves her of other responsibilities so that she can devote herself completely to this task.

Despite a lack of early contact experience by mothers in hospital births in the past 20 to 30 years, almost all these parents became bonded to their babies. Some misinterpretations of studies of early and extended mother-infant contact may have resulted from a too literal acceptance of the word bonding. The human is highly adaptable, and there are many fail-safe routes to attachment. Sadly, some parents who miss the

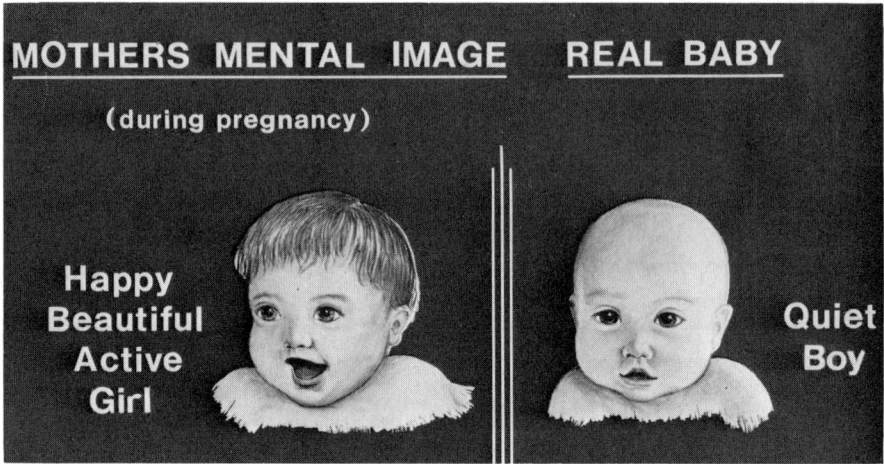

**FIG 8–5.**
The mental image of the baby his mother planned to have is completely different from the baby she has. (From Klaus MH, Kennell JH: *Parent-Infant Bonding.* St Louis, CV Mosby Co, 1982. Used by permission.)

bonding experience have felt that all was lost for their future relationship. This was (and is) completely incorrect. There are still large hospitals that have never provided for early and extended contact, and the mothers who miss out are often those at the limits of adaptability and who may benefit the most—the poor, the single, the unsupported, the teenaged mothers. It is precisely in this group of mothers that studies by Anisfeld and Lipper[13] show that early contact has its greatest effect.

We believe that there is strong evidence that at least 30 to 60 minutes of early contact in privacy should be provided for every parent and infant to enhance the bonding experience and that they should remain together as much as possible throughout the hospital period. It would appear that additional contact in both the first hours and the first days will help mothers become attached to their babies. For some mothers, one period may be more important than the other. If the health of the mother or infant makes this early contact impossible, then discussion, support, and reassurance should help the parents appreciate that they can become as completely attached to their infant as if they had the usual bonding experience, although it may require more time and effort. Obviously the infant should only be alone with the mother and father if the infant is known to be physically normal and appropriate temperature control is utilized. We believe that in the near future, placement in the large central nursery will be phased out for most babies. Allowing the infant to be with the mother will permit both mother and father to have longer periods to learn about their baby and to develop a strong tie in the first week of life.

Each parent does not react in a standard or predictable fashion to the multiple environmental influences that occur during the early postnatal period. Not every mother and father develops a close tie to their infant within a few minutes of the first contact. This is not evidence against a sensitive period but more likely represents multiple individual differences of mothers and fathers. When we make it possible for parents to be together with their baby, in privacy, for the first hour and throughout the hospital stay, we establish the most beneficial and supportive environment for the beginning of the bonding process.

It is our belief that other principles also govern the attachment process. Although solid evidence is scanty, the following additional rules appear to be important:

1. The process of attachment is structured so that the father and mother will become attached optimally to only one infant at a time.
2. During the early process of the mother's attachment to her infant, it is necessary that the infant respond to the mother by some signal such as body or eye movements.
3. People who witness the birth process become strongly attached to the infant.
4. It is difficult and possibly mutually incompatible for some people to both become attached and detached at the same time, as in simultaneously attempting to go through the processes of attachment to one person while mourning the loss or threatened loss of the same or another person.
5. Early events have long-lasting effects. Anxieties in the first day about the well-being of a baby with a temporary disorder may result in long-lasting concerns that may adversely shape the development of the child.

## PRACTICAL CONSIDERATIONS

Most of the traditional customs to provide support for the woman passing through the perinatal period have been lost so a number of support systems have developed. The wide assortment of *childbirth classes*, which attempt to continue previous customs, are good examples. These groups help the mother through the delivery period as well as aiding her in later infant and child care. They also lessen the tensions, fears, and fantasies that occur during normal pregnancies. By joining a group of mothers with whom she can chat and share her feelings, a woman can alleviate many of the emotional upsets that occur during normal pregnancies. We therefore believe that these courses, particularly those in which mothers participate actively with the father, have a valuable supportive role during pregnancy.

To minimize the number of unknowns for a mother while she is in the hospital, she and the father (or other supportive companion who will stay with her throughout labor and delivery) should visit the maternity unit to see where labor and delivery will take place. She should also learn about the type of anesthesia (if she is to receive it), delivery routines, and all the procedures and medication she will receive before, during, and after delivery. By reducing the possibility of surprise, such *advance preparation* will increase confidence during labor and delivery. For an adult, just as for a child entering the hospital for surgery, the more meticulously every step and event is detailed in advance, the less the subsequent anxiety. The less anxiety the mother experiences while delivering and becoming attached to her baby, the better will be her immediate relationship with the infant.

The mother must have *continuing support and reassurance* during her labor and delivery, whether from her husband, the father, her mother, or other female family member or friend, a midwife, or a nurse. She also must be satisfied with the arrangements that have been made to maintain her home during her hospitalization. To reduce the amount of tension on the mother, she should labor and deliver in the same room, preventing the necessity of rushing to a delivery room in the last minutes of labor. Once the delivery is completed and the mother has had a quick glance at the infant, it is important for her to have a few seconds to regain her composure and, in a sense, catch her breath before she proceeds to the next task—taking on the infant. This breath catching usually occurs during the period when the placenta is being delivered, while the mother is being cleansed and is having any necessary suturing. It has been our experience that it is best not to give a mother her baby until she indicates that she is ready. It should be her decision.

After delivery it is extremely valuable for the father, mother, and baby to have an *early contact period* alone in either the labor and delivery room or an adjacent room (e.g., a recovery room). Obviously this is only possible if the infant is normal and the mother is well. The mother should have the infant with her on the bed so that she can hold him. The infant should not be off in a bassinet where the face cannot be seen. The parents should be given the baby undressed so that they can perform a complete inspection. A heat panel easily maintains or, if need be, increases the body temperature of the infant (Fig 8–6). Several mothers have told us of the unforgettable experience of holding their naked baby against their own bare chest, so we recommend skin-

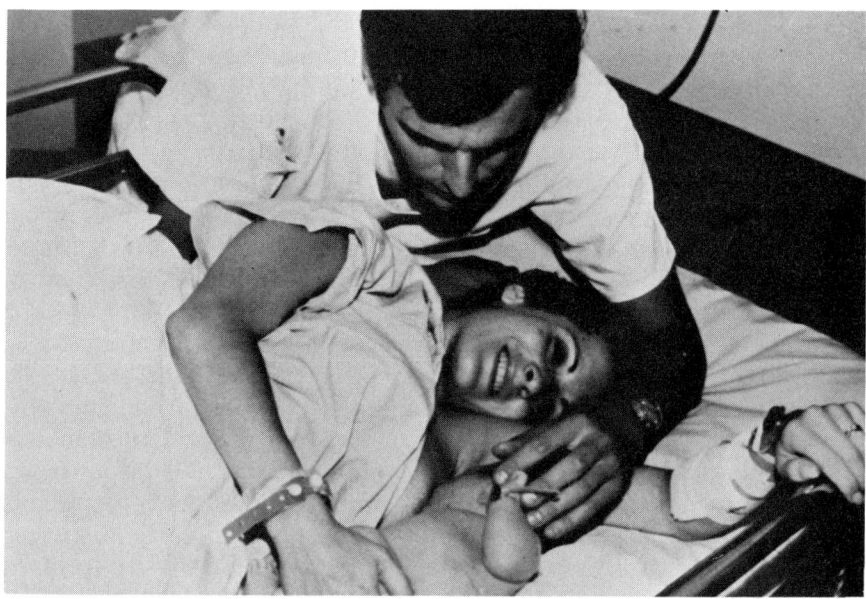

**FIG 8-6.**
A mother nursing her infant a few minutes after birth as the father looks on. (From Klaus MH, Kennell JH: *Parent-Infant Bonding*. St Louis, CV Mosby Co, 1982, photograph by Ken Condo. Used by permission.)

to-skin contact. The father sits or stands at the side of the bed by the infant. This allows the parents and infant to become acquainted. Because the eyes are so important for both the parents and baby, we withhold the application of silver nitrate ($AgNO_3$) or erythromycin ophthalmic ointment to the eyes until after this meeting. We have found it valuable for the mother, father, and infant to be together for at least 30 to 60 minutes. We must emphasize that up to 40% of normal mothers take a week or longer before they feel the baby is really theirs. Obviously close contact with the husband is also important.

## PREMATURE OR SICK NEONATES

In recent years a number of investigators have looked closely at the complex and confusing ecology parents encounter when the birth of a premature, sick or malformed infant brings them into an intensive care nursery.[14] Research in these blinking and buzzing intensive care units is not easy or straightforward but, rather, is frequently confounded by harassed, overworked nurses and physicians, overwhelmed parents, and critically sick infants. Recent observations based on the completed studies suggest a number of interventions that appear to have merit and deserve further investigation in the traditional hospital environment. A few brave investigators have been refreshingly innovative and have broken down the walls of the intensive care unit to create a new and more positive environment for parents of sick infants.

In the years since *parental visiting* has been permitted in the intensive care nursery, a number of studies have revealed that most parents continue to suffer severe emotional stress. Harper et al.[15] noted that this occurred even when parents had close contact with their infants. However, despite their anxiety, they believed the opportunity to have this contact was helpful, and over 90% of parents questioned were opposed to restricting their contact with their infant. Most parents felt that holding their infant made the infant feel more loved. Benfield[16] and associates also noted that most parents of transported infants experienced grief reactions. Interestingly, the level of their response was unrelated to the severity of the baby's problems. Green[17] graphically described the parents' plight when he noted "geographically displaced, their work and lives disrupted, their biologic rhythms in disarray, bewildered, anxious and terribly tired parents in the delirium of crisis are simply unable to comprehend what is happening."

From interviews and observations Mason,[18] Newman,[19] and Minde et al.[20] suggested that *early parental reactions* predicted how the mother would manage with her infant in the early weeks at home. From interviews, Mason found that if the mother expressed a fairly high level of anxiety, actively sought information about the condition of her baby, showed strong maternal feelings for the baby, and had strong support from the father there was usually a favorable outcome. If the mother showed a low level of anxiety and activity, chances were that her relationship with her child would be poor. Minde noted that the most important variable was the mother's own relationship to her mother, her relationship to her father, and whether or not the mother had a previous abortion. Highly interacting mothers in the nursery visited and telephoned the nursery more frequently while the infants were hospitalized and later stimulated their infants more at home. However, Minde noted perceptively that mothers who touched and fondled their infants more in the nursery had infants with increased eye openings. Minde noted the contingency between the infant's eyes being open and the mother's touching and also between gross motor stretches and the mother's smiling. He and his colleagues could not determine to what extent the sequence of touching and eye opening reflected the primary contribution to the mother or the infant. Thus, Mason, Newman, and Minde noted that mothers who become involved, interested, and anxious about their infants will have an easier time when the infant is taken home.

Additional *infant stimulation* may improve the clinical course in some premature infants. In the last 15 years numerous studies have revealed that if a small, premature infant is either touched, rocked, fondled, or cuddled daily during the stay in the nursery, he may have significantly fewer apneic periods, increased weight gain, fewer stools, and, in some studies, even an advance in certain areas of higher central nervous system functioning that persists for a short time after discharge from the hospital. As a result, parents and caretakers have often begun additional stimulation of the preterm infant. As a result of studies by several perceptive researchers, our conceptual framework about stimulation after discharge to home, and possibly before discharge, may be drastically altered.

In a series of creative experimental manipulations of *infant-mother face-to-face interactions*, Field[21] noted that the mother and the normal full-term infant were each interacting about 70% of the time in their spontaneous play. However, when the mother was asked to increase her attention-getting behavior (stimulation), her activity increased to 80% of the time, and strikingly, the infant's gaze decreased to 50%. When the mother was told to imitate the movements of the infant, which greatly reduced her activity, the infant's gaze time greatly increased. Field noted that in the spontaneous situation, the mothers of high-risk preterm infants were interacting up to 90% of the time, whereas the infant was looking only 30% of the time. If the mother was told to use attention-getting gestures, her activity increased even above 90% of the time and the infant's gaze decreased further. If her interactions were decreased by asking her to imitate the baby's movements, there was then a striking increase in the infant's gaze. Although generally the parents' activity was aimed at encouraging more activity or responsiveness from the premature infant, the approach appeared to be counterproductive, leading to less instead of more infant responsiveness.

There is much to be studied and defined about the mother's efforts to increase interaction with her premature infant. How should stimulation be provided? By whom? When? Should it be stimulation or imitation?

**Interventions**

A number of interventions have been introduced to help parents deal with the stressful situation of having a sick or small infant. In some cases they have involved the parents and infant together, whereas others have focused on either the parent or the infant. It should be noted that the ecology of the intensive care nursery is a difficult environment in which to make detailed and definitive assessments. Nurseries not only differ in their physical environment but also in patient population and physician interests, background, training, and sensitivity. Despite this, there are sufficient data and measurements from several nurseries to enable us to begin to make recommendations. However, in assessing the potential value of any intervention, it may be inappropriate to generalize to a much wider population from a study carried out in one premature unit. The following interventions have been adopted:

1. Opening the intensive care nursery to parents
2. Transporting the mother to be near her infant
3. Transporting the healthy premature infant to the mother
4. Programmed contact and reciprocal interaction
5. Rooming-in for the parent of a premature infant
6. Maternal day care for premature infants
7. Listening to parents (interviewing) during the infant's hospitalization
8. Parent groups
9. Nesting
10. Home-based intervention for young parents
11. Discussions with the parents after discharge

## Practical Suggestions for Caregivers of Parents of Premature or Sick Neonates

We recommend the following procedures to caregivers of parents of premature or sick neonates:

1. We have found it useful and safe for the mother to have the baby placed in her bed in the first hour of life with a heat panel above them when a premature baby weighing 1.5 to 2.5 kg is delivered and appears to be doing well without grunting and retractions. We do not recommend this approach unless the physician feels relaxed about the health of the infant.

2. We have found it helpful, if the baby does have to be moved to an intensive care unit or to another hospital, to give the mother a chance to see and touch her infant, even if he is very small, has respiratory distress, and is in an oxygen hood. The house officer or the attending physician stops in the mother's room with the transport incubator and encourages her to touch and look at her baby at close hand. A comment about the baby's strength and healthy features may be long remembered and appreciated.

3. A mother and her infant should be kept near each other in the same hospital, ideally on the same floor. When the long-term significance of early mother-infant contact is kept in mind, a modification of restrictions and territorial traditions can usually be arranged.

4. We encourage the father to follow the transport team to our hospital so he can see what is happening with his baby. He uses his own transportation so that he can stay in the premature unit for 3 to 4 hours. This extra time allows him to get to know the nurses and physicians in the unit, to find out how the infant is being treated, and to talk with the physician in a relaxed fashion about what he or she expects will happen to the baby in the succeeding days. We allow him to come into the nursery and explain in detail everything that is going on with the infant, often offering him a cup of coffee. We ask him to help act as a link between us and his family by carrying information back to his wife, and we request that he come to our unit before he visits his wife so that he can let her know how the baby is doing. We suggest that he take a Polaroid photograph, even if the infant is on a respirator, so that he can describe the baby's care to his wife in detail.

5. Transportation of the mother from the community hospital before delivery to the maternity division of the medical center, so she will be together with her baby after birth, is occurring in many communities, as is transportation of the mother with the baby after delivery.

6. A mother should be permitted to enter the premature nursery as soon as she is able to maneuver easily. When she makes her first visit, it is important to anticipate that she may become faint or dizzy when she looks at her infant. We always have a stool nearby so that she can sit down. A nurse stays at her side during most of the visit describing in detail the procedures being carried out, such as the monitoring of respiration and heart rate, the umbilical catheter, nasal CPAP, endotracheal tube, feeding through the various infusion lines, and the functioning of the incubator and ventilator.

7. We also encourage grandparents, brothers, sisters, and other relatives to view the infant through the glass window of the nursery so they will begin to know and to feel attached to the infant. We believe it is important to arrange for the grandparents and special close friends or relatives to enter the nursery and visit the baby, particularly when the baby is very ill or expected to die, so that they can provide firsthand support and understanding to the parents. We have increasingly allowed siblings to enter the nursery with careful preparation and support. When arranged in this manner, we believe it relieves a child's confusion and anxiety.

8. It is necessary to find out what the mother believes is going to happen or what she has read about the problem. We try to move at her pace during any discussion to ensure that she understands.

9. In discussing the infant's condition by telephone with the mother, who is still in the referring hospital, we ask the father to stand nearby so that we can talk to them both at the same time and they can hear the same message. This group communication reduces misunderstandings and usually is helpful in assuring the mother that we are telling her the whole story.

10. If there is any chance that the infant will survive, we are optimistic with the parents from the beginning. There is no evidence that, if a favorable prediction proves to be incorrect and the baby expires, the parents will be harmed by early optimism. There is almost always time to prepare them before the baby actually dies. If the physician has been pessimistic and the infant lives, it is more difficult for parents to become closely attached after they have figuratively dug a few shovelsful of earth. We recognize that this recommendation is contrary to many old customs and places a heavy burden on the physician. It is our belief that, if the infant does expire, we must continue to work with the mother and father and help them with their mourning reactions.

11. Once the possibility that a baby has brain damage has been mentioned, the parents will not forget it. However, with the present frequent use of brain ultrasound and CT scans, many babies will have hemorrhages identified. This information must be shared with the parents, but it is wise to temper this with appropriate degrees of optimism plus follow-up discussions based on subsequent studies and the baby's progress. In other situations such as jaundiced, large babies, we do not mention the possibility of any brain damage or retardation to the parents unless we are convinced that the baby is damaged or the parents inquire.

12. It is important to emphasize that if there is a clear objective finding such as a cardiac abnormality, an intraventricular hemorrhage, or a specific congenital malformation, we see no reason to hide it from the parents.

13. As soon as possible, we describe to both the father and the mother the value of touching the infant in helping them to get to know him or her, in reducing the number of apneic episodes (if this is a problem), and possibly increasing weight gain, thus hastening discharge from the unit.

14. It is important to remember that feelings of love for the baby are often elicited through eye-to-eye contact. Therefore, if an infant is under bilirubin lights, we turn them off and remove the eye patches so the mother and her infant can really see each other.

15. From our previous observations, we have found that keeping a book in which to record parental phone calls and visits is useful in determining which mothers are likely to require additional help from a social worker or extra discussions about the health of their infant. If

a mother visited our nursery less than three times in 2 weeks, the chances of her developing some sort of mothering disorder were increased. Therefore, if the visiting pattern of the mother is less than that of most other mothers, she is given extra help in adapting to the hospitalization.

16. Parent groups have been shown by Minde et al.[22] to be especially effective in helping parents.

## CONGENITAL MALFORMATIONS

The birth of an infant with a congenital malformation presents complex challenges to the physician who will care for the affected child and his family. Despite the relatively large number of infants with congenital anomalies, our understanding of how parents develop an attachment to a malformed child remains incomplete. Although previous investigators agree that the birth of a child with a congenital malformation often precipitates major family stress, relatively few have described the process of family adaptation during the infant's first year of life. A major advance was Solnit and Stark's[23] conceptualization of parental reactions. They emphasized that a significant aspect of adaptation is the necessity for parents to mourn the loss of the normal child they had expected. Other observers have noted the pathologic aspects of family reactions, including the chronic sorrow that envelops the family of a defective child. Less attention has been given to the more adaptive aspects of parental attachment to children with malformations.

Parental reactions to the birth of a child with a congenital malformation appear to follow a predictable course. For most parents, initial *shock, denial,* and a period of *intense emotional upset* (including *sadness, anger, guilt, and anxiety*) are followed by a period of gradual *equilibrium and adaptation* that is marked by a lessening of intense anxiety and emotional reaction and ultimate *reorganization* (Fig 8–7). This adaptation is characterized by an increased satisfaction with and ability to care for the baby. These stages in parental reactions are similar to those reported in other crisis situations, such as terminally ill children. The shock and denial reported by many parents seem to be an understandable attempt to escape the traumatic news of the baby's malformation, so different than their expectations for a normal healthy newborn.

Solnit and Stark[23] have likened the crisis of the birth of a child with a malformation to the emotional crisis following the death of a child in that the mother must mourn the loss of her expected, normal

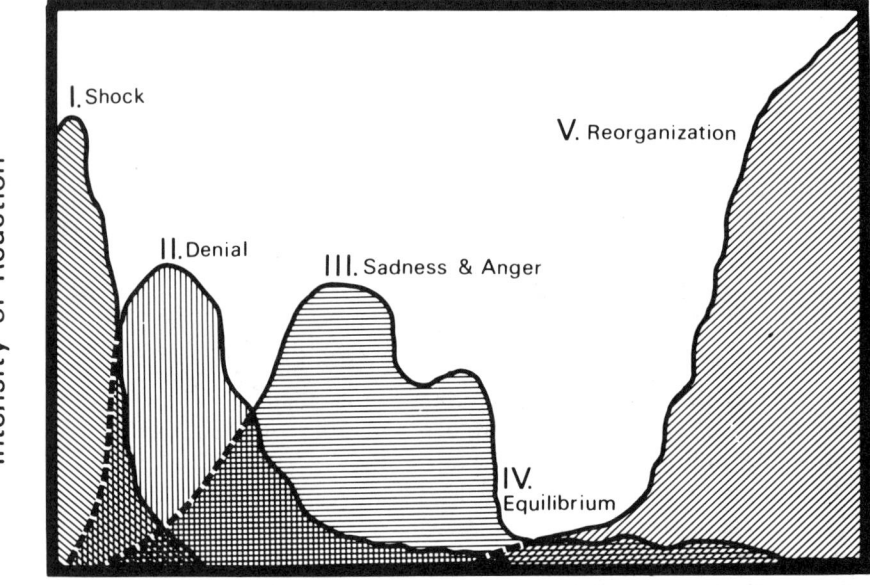

**FIG 8-7.**
Hypothetical model of a normal sequence of parental reactions to the birth of a malformed infant. (From Drotar D, Baskiewicz, A, Irvin N, et al: The adaptation of parents to the birth of an infant with a congenital malformation: A hypothetical model. *Pediatrics* 1975; 56:710. Used by permission.)

infant. In addition, she must become attached to her actual living, damaged child. However, the sequence of parental reactions to the birth of a baby with a malformation differs from that following the death of a child in yet another respect. The mourning or grief work appears not to take place in the usual manner because of the complex issues raised by continuation of the child's life and the demands of his physical care. The parents' sadness, which is important initially in their relationship with their child, diminishes in most instances once the parents take over the physical care. Most parents reach a point at which they are able to care adequately for their children and cope effectively with disrupting feelings of sadness and anger. The mother's initiation of the relationship with her child is a major step in the reduction of anxiety and emotional upset associated with the trauma of the birth. As with normal children, the parents' initial experience with their infant seems to release positive feelings that aid the mother-child relationship following the stresses associated with the news of the child's anomaly and, in many instances, the separation of mother and child in the hospital.

## Practical Suggestions for Caregivers of Parents of Malformed Infants

We suggest the following to caregivers of parents of malformed infants:

1. We believe it is better to leave the infant with the mother for the first 2 or 3 days, if medically feasible. If the child is rushed to the hospital where special surgery will eventually be done, the mother will not have enough opportunity to become attached to him. Even if the surgery is required immediately, as for bowel obstruction, it is best to bring the baby to the mother first, allowing her to touch and handle him and point out to her how normal the infant is in all other respects.

2. It is our impression that the parents' mental picture of the anomaly is often far more alarming than the actual problem. Any delay in bringing the infant and parents together, during which the parents suspect that there may be a problem, greatly heightens their anxiety and causes their imaginations to run wild. Therefore, we suggest that it is helpful to bring the baby to both parents, when they are together, as soon after delivery as possible.

3. We have arranged for the father to stay with the mother and sleep in her room on the maternity division on several occasions. We believe that this opportunity to support each other, to cry and curse and talk together, is highly beneficial. We use the process of early crisis intervention, meeting several times with the parents, whether the father lives in with the mother or not. During these discussions, we ask the mother how she is doing, how she feels her husband is doing, and how he feels about the infant. We then reverse the questions and ask the father how he is doing and how he thinks his wife is progressing. The hope is that they will think not only about their own reactions but will begin to consider each other's as well.

4. We believe that parents should not be given tranquilizers. These tend to blunt their responses and slow their adaptation to the problem. A small dose of secobarbital (Seconal) at night, however, is often helpful.

5. It has been our clinical experience that parents who are initially adapting reasonably well often ask many questions and at times appear to be almost overinvolved in clinical care. In our unit, we are pleased by this and more concerned about parents who ask few questions and who appear stunned and overwhelmed by the problem.

6. Many anomalies are very frustrating, not only to the parents but also to the physicians and nurses as well. There is a temptation for the physician to withdraw from the parents and their infant. The many questions asked by the parent who is trying to understand the problem are often very frustrating for the physician. The parent often appears to forget and asks the same questions over and over again.

7. Each parent may move through the process of shock, denial,

sadness and anger, adaptation and reorganization at a different pace, so the two parents may not be synchronized with one another. If they are unable to talk with each other about the baby, there may be a marked disruption in their relationship. We have found it best to move at the parents' pace. If we move too quickly, we run the risk of losing the parents along the way. It is beneficial to ask the parents how they view their infant: "Maybe you could tell me how you see the infant."

## SUMMARY

Since the newborn baby is utterly dependent on his parents for his survival and optimum development, it is essential to understand the process of bonding as it develops from the first moments after the child is born. Although we have only a beginning understanding of this complex phenomenon, those responsible for the care of mothers and infants would be wise to reevaluate hospital procedures that interfere with early, sustained mother-infant contact, to consider measures that promote a mother's contact with her infant, and to help her appreciate the wide range of sensory and motor responses of her neonate.

## REFERENCES

1. Cohen RL: Some maladaptive syndromes of pregnancy and the puerperium. *Obstet Gynecol* 1966; 25:562.
2. Sosa R, Kennell JH, Klaus MH, et al: The effect of a supportive companion on perinatal problems, length of labor, and mother-infant interaction. *N Engl J Med* 1980; 303:597.
3. Klaus MH, Kennell JH, Robertson SS: Effects of social support during parturition on maternal and infant morbidity. *Br Med J* 1986; 293:585.
4. MacFarlane JA, Smith DM, and Garrow DH: The relationship between mother and neonate, in Kitzinger S, Davis JA, (eds): *The Place of Birth.* New York, Oxford University Press, 1978.
5. Winnicott DW: Collected Papers: Through Paediatrics to Psycho-Analysis. New York, Basic Books, 1958.
6. Klaus MH, Jerauld R, Kreger N, et al: Maternal attachment: Importance of the first post-partum days. *N Engl J Med* 1972; 286:460.
7. O'Connor S, Vietze P, Sherrod K, et al: Reduced incidence of parenting inadequacy following rooming-in. *Pediatrics* 1980; 66:176.
8. Siegel E, Bauman K, Schaefer E, et al: Hospital and home support during infancy: Impact on maternal attachment, child abuse and neglect, and health care utilization. *Pediatrics* 1980; 66:183.
9. MacFarlane JA: Olfaction in the development of social preferences in the human neonate, in Ciba Foundation, Symposium 33, Parent-Infant Interaction. Amsterdam, Elsevier, 1975, pp 103–117.

10. Rödholm M, Larsson K: Father-infant interaction at the first contact after delivery. *Early Hum Dev* 1979; 3:21.
11. Keller WD, Hildebrandt KA, and Richards M: Effects of extended father-infant contact during the newborn period. *Infant Behav Dev* 1985; 8:337.
12. Parke RD, Power TG, Tinsley BR, et al: The father's role in the family system. *Semin Perinatol* 1979; 3:25.
13. Anisfeld E, Lipper E: Early contact, social support and mother-infant bonding. *Pediatrics* 1983; 72:79.
14. Gottfried AW, Gaiter JL (eds): Infant stress under intensive care. *Environmental Neonatology*. Baltimore, University Park Press, 1985.
15. Harper RG, Sia C, Sokal S, et al: Observations on unrestricted parental contact with infants in the neonatal intensive care unit. *J Pediatr* 1976; 89:441.
16. Benfield DG, Leib SA, Reutor J: Grief response of parents following referral of the critically ill newborn. *N Engl J Med* 1976; 194:975.
17. Green M: Parent care in the intensive care unit. *Am J Dis Child* 1979; 133:1119.
18. Mason EA: A method of predicting crisis outcome for mothers of premature babies. *Public Health Rep* 1963; 78:1031.
19. Newman LF: Parents' perceptions of their low birth weight infants. *Paediatrician* 1980; 9:182.
20. Minde K, Trehub S, Corter C, et al: Mother-child relationships in the premature nursery: An observational study. *Pediatrics* 1978; 61:373.
21. Field TM: Effects of early separation, interactive deficits and experimental manipulations on infant-mother face-to-face interaction. *Child Dev* 1977; 48:763.
22. Minde K, Shosenberg B, Marton P, et al: Self-help groups in a premature nursery—a controlled evaluation. *J Pediatr* 1980; 96:933.
23. Solnit AJ, Stark MH: Mourning and the birth of a defective child. *Psychoanal Study Child* 1961; 16:523.
24. Drotar D, Baskiewicz A, Irvin N, et al: The adaptation of parents to the birth of an infant with a congenital malformation: A hypothetical model. *Pediatrics* 1975; 56:710.

## SUGGESTED READING

Klaus MH, Kennell JH: *Parent-Infant Bonding*, ed 2. St Louis, CV Mosby Co, 1982.

# 9

# Neonatal Clinical Pharmacology: Principles and Practice

Michael D. Reed, Pharm.D., F.C.C.P.
James B. Besunder, D.O.
Jeffrey L. Blumer, Ph.D., M.D.

Historically, our understanding of clinical pharmacology in pediatric patients has been limited. This has posed a particular problem for premature and newborn infants. Frequently, we have had to rely on pharmacologic data derived primarily from adults to determine what may seem to be appropriate dosage guidelines for drug use in children. It is only during the past decade that we have begun to gain a greater appreciation of the pharmacokinetic and pharmacodynamic characteristics of many drugs during the newborn period. Despite this fact, the editorial comment by Shirkey in 1968[1] referring to children as "therapeutic orphans" sadly remains relevant today.

The quest for expanding our data base in perinatal pharmacology has been tempered by the unfortunate experiences with the sulfonamides (bilirubin-albumin-binding displacement) and chloramphenicol (the "gray baby syndrome"), as well as a relative lack of sensitive and specific microanalytic methodology. Although these disastrous experiences have often been used as reasons to restrict evaluations in newborn infants, it is important to recall that these misadventures occurred primarily due to our lack of understanding of the clinical pharmacology of drugs in these patients. In this chapter, we will review drug disposition in newborn infants, emphasizing the importance of developmental changes in pharmacokinetic-pharmacodynamic processes and the many interrelationships to disease-induced physiologic alterations.

## PHARMACOKINETIC ASPECTS OF PLACENTAL DRUG TRANSFER

The placenta, once believed to be a relatively impenetrable barrier protecting the fetus from unwanted or "nonphysiologic" substances present in maternal circulation, is a multilayered structure that serves as a temporary organ for fetal absorption and elimination. It is now recognized that the fetus may be exposed to a plethora of xenobiotics in utero. However, our understanding of the placental transfer of pharmacologically active compounds throughout gestation is hampered by obvious ethical and physical considerations. As a result, we have had to depend largely on studies performed in various species of laboratory animals. In this regard, it is important to recognize that diverse anatomical variations are present in placentas and extrapolated data should be interpreted with caution.[2]

The basic mechanisms of placental transfer appear to be similar to those governing the transport of compounds across any biologic membrane and include the *concentration gradient* (between maternal and fetal circulations), the type of *transport process* involved, and the compound's *in vivo physicochemical characteristics*. Simple diffusion appears to be the primary process by which drugs cross the placenta.[2] As a result, the total amount of a drug that crosses the placenta and the rate at which it crosses depends largely on the physicochemical properties of the drug and the ambient physiologic and/or pathophysiologic conditions that prevail.[2,3] In general, lipophilic, unionized, low molecular weight drugs present in their free non-protein-bound state tend to diffuse readily and rapidly across biologic membranes including the placenta.[2,3] The membrane passage of drugs that possess these physicochemical characteristics under physiologic and/or pathophysiologic conditions may be limited only by the blood flow to the particular anatomical region. Examples of such drugs that cross the placenta rapidly with transfer rates dependent primarily on maternal placental blood flow (i.e., "flow-limited drugs") include barbiturates, narcotic analgesics, and local anesthetics.[2,4–6] Alterations in maternal blood flow to the placenta may reduce the placental passage of these agents. Normal uterine contractions during labor,[7,8] oxytocic drugs,[8] exogenously administered sympathomimetics,[9] or β-adrenergic blocking agents[10] all have effects on maternal and fetal hemodynamics that may modify maternal distribution and placental transfer of pharmacologic agents.

As mentioned above, the degree to which a drug is ionized and/or protein bound can influence the total quantity available to cross the placenta. Of the drugs used clinically, most are either weak acids or weak bases with pKa values that fall within the range of physiologic pH.[2] However, many pathophysiologic conditions (e.g., hypoxemia, infection) may modify blood and biologic fluid pH, altering the relative proportion of ionized to unionized drug. Depending on the pH, the placental passage of a drug could be augmented or reduced in either the maternal or fetal circulation. For nonionized lipid-soluble drugs, transfer across the placenta is proportional to the degree of binding to circulating maternal proteins. As stated above, it is the free (unbound) fraction of a drug that is pharmacologically active and capable of diffusing into tissues and traversing cellular membranes.[11] Drugs that possess a high affinity for circulating maternal proteins would be expected to exhibit a relatively reduced total amount in the fetal circulation. Once drug molecules cross the placenta and are present in the fetal circulation, a new equilibrium between free and bound drug will be achieved depending on the compound's affinity for fetal proteins.

Numerous studies in humans have described measurable concentrations of a large number of maternally administered drugs in the fetal circulation and amniotic fluid. Although measurable cord blood and amniotic fluid drug concentrations provide us with some insight into the characteristics of transplacental drug transfer, these data should be interpreted with caution. The available human data are often difficult to interpret due to differences in analytic techniques, duration of maternal drug therapy, method and times of biologic fluid sampling relative to drug administration, single sample determinations, and the random nature of sampling times. In addition, the representation of amniotic fluid or fetal blood drug concentrations as a ratio of maternal blood concentrations may be misleading as this does not account for the probable delay in drug distribution from mother to fetus, or probable differences in fetal drug elimination characteristics. Obviously, ethical and technical constraints limit our ability to obtain optimally timed, consecutive samples from either the mother or fetus. Thus, we must depend on data obtained from animal models.

## In Utero Drug Therapy

Pharmacologic intervention for the treatment of the unborn infant represents a relatively new and challenging therapeutic approach. At present, most research and clinical experience has focused on the in utero treatment of supraventricular tachycardia and in the acceleration of fetal lung maturity.

### *Fetal Supraventricular Tachycardia*

Supraventricular tachycardia (SVT) represents the most common and clinically important fetal cardiac arrhythmia. It appears that the most common reason for the development of fetal SVT is an atrioventricular (AV) nodal reentrant tachycardia. Thus, antiarrhythmic drugs that consistently cross the placenta and block conduction through the AV node prolonging its refractory period should be selected as initial therapy. Digoxin, propranolol, verapamil, procainamide, and quinidine have all been reported to convert in utero SVT to a normal sinus rhythm.[12,13] In the series of Kleinman et al.,[12] 15 of 16 patients were successfully treated in utero—6 with digoxin alone, 1 with digoxin and propranolol, and 8 with the combination of digoxin and verapamil.

From the available experience, it is our opinion that digoxin, at present, is the drug of choice in treatment of in utero SVT. In those cases that do not respond to digoxin, verapamil would appear a viable alternative.[12] However, due to the drug's negative inotropic properties, verapamil should be used with caution in the presence of severe congestive heart failure.

### *Fetal Lung Maturity*

Interest in antenatal therapy to reduce the incidence of neonatal respiratory distress syndrome (RDS) has been long-standing. The first controlled human trial by Liggins and Howie[14] in 1972 demonstrated a significant difference in early neonatal mortality (3.2% vs. 15%) and RDS (9% vs. 26%) between glucocorticosteroid-treated and control patients. These differences, however, were only significant for babies less than 32 weeks' gestation whose mothers received steroid at least 24 hours prior to delivery. Further controlled critical analysis provided by the Collaborative Group on Antenatal Steroid Therapy[15] demonstrated a significant reduction in the incidence of RDS in treated (dexamethasone, 5 mg IM every 12 hours for four doses) vs. control groups with no differences observed in the occurrence of fetal or neonatal deaths. Though some interesting sex and race differences in response rates were observed in this study, newborns between 30 and 34 weeks' gestational age who were delivered between 24 hours and 7 days after initiation of dexamethasone therapy demonstrated the most marked effect.[15] In a follow-up study, the Collaborative Group[16] found no growth, physical, motor, or development deficiencies within the first 3 years of life in the dexamethasone treated vs. control group. From these data, it would appear that antenatal dexamethasone therapy may be effective in accelerating lung maturation in neonates less than 34 weeks' gestation when given at least 24 hours prior to delivery.

# PRINCIPLES OF NEONATAL CLINICAL PHARMACOLOGY

## Basic Concepts

The determination of an optimal drug dose and dosing interval for pharmacotherapeutic intervention is based on an understanding of a drug's overall biodisposition in the body. A drug's biodisposition profile is a composite based on a complex interplay between a variety of host factors and the physicochemical characteristics of the drug. *Pharmacokinetics* is the detailed study and description of the changes in drug distribution through time and can be subdivided into the processes of absorption, distribution, metabolism, and excretion. The clinical utility of understanding a drug's pharmacokinetics is underscored by the fact that drug concentrations determined in biologic fluids, most notably serum or plasma, correlate more directly and predictably with pharmacologic response than do standardized drug doses.

## Drug Absorption

Drugs administered extravascularly, including the sublingual, buccal, oral, intramuscular, subcutaneous, rectal, or topical routes, must cross multiple membranes to reach the systemic circulation and ultimately distribute to sites of action. Absorption into the systemic circulation depends on both the physicochemical properties of a drug and a variety of host factors.[17] These variables, as they relate to the absorption of orally administered agents, are outlined in Table 9–1. Although *active transport* and *facilitated diffusion* mechanisms exist for the gas-

**TABLE 9–1.**
Variables Affecting the Absorption of Drugs Administered Orally

| Physicochemical properties |
|---|
| Molecular weight |
| Formulation characteristics |
|     Disintegration characteristics (solid dosage formulation) |
|     Dissolution rate (solid dosage formulation) |
|     Release characteristics (sustained-release formulations) |
| Degree of lipid solubility |
| pKa of drug |
| Patient factors |
| Gastric and duodenal pH |
| Gastric content and emptying time |
| Size of bile salt pool |
| GI tract bacterial colonization |
| Underlying disease states |

trointestinal absorption of substrates and nutrients, the majority of drugs are absorbed via the process of *passive diffusion*. Important patient factors that regulate the gastrointestinal absorption of drugs include pH-dependent diffusion, the gastric milieu, and gastric emptying time. The integrity and capacity of these latter physiologic processes are highly dependent on age.

### Gastric pH

Gastric pH at birth approaches neutrality but within the first few hours falls rapidly to between 1.5 and 3.0. From the available data, these findings appear quite variable but independent of birth weight or gestational age.[18]

### Gastric Emptying Time

Since most drugs are absorbed in the small intestine, the rate of gastric emptying is an important determinant of the rate and extent of drug absorption. The rate of gastric emptying during the neonatal period is variable and appears to be a result of irregular and unpredictable peristaltic activity. It is directly affected by gestational maturity and postnatal age and is altered by the type of feeding used.[19, 20] The rate of gastric emptying during the newborn period is prolonged when compared to adult values. Gastric emptying rates in preterm infants are longer than those observed in term infants.[20]

### Additional Factors

The ontogeny of additional physiologic and disease processes may influence the gastrointestinal absorption of xenobiotics. The rate of synthesis and pool size of bile salts are reduced in newborn infants as compared to adults.[21] This decreased availability of bile salts may result in a reduced capacity for the oral absorption of certain lipid-soluble drugs that is exemplified by the decreased oral absorption in newborn infants of vitamin D and E.[22] In addition, developmental rates for the colonization of gastrointestinal bacterial flora have also been described and been shown to differ depending on gestational age, type of delivery, and type of feeding.[23] These changes in the bacterial flora during the neonatal period may be of importance in the hydrolysis of drug conjugates secreted in the bile.

### Absorption via Alternative Routes

Other than the oral route, the primary means of extravascular drug administration in infancy is intramuscular (IM) administration. The same physiologic and physicochemical factors that affect the rate and extent of drug absorption from the gastrointestinal tract also influence the absorption of drugs from injection sites and through the skin.[24] For drugs administered IM, the drug must be water soluble at physiologic pH to prevent precipitation and resultant decreased, delayed, and/or erratic absorption at the injection site. The lipid solubility of a drug favors rapid diffusion into the capillaries. Blood flow to and from the site of injection must be competent to assure adequate absorption into systemic circulation.

The skin represents an often overlooked but important organ for the absorption of compounds. This fact has been exemplified by the various toxicities experienced by newborns dermally exposed to hexachlorophene, aniline-containing disinfectant solutions, pentachlorophenol-containing laundry detergents, and hydrocortisone.[25-27] The percutaneous absorption of a compound is directly related to the degree of skin hydration and inversely related to the thickness of the stratum corneum. The skin of full-term newborns appears to be a relatively intact functional barrier.[28] In contrast, the skin of premature infants appears to be immature and a poor barrier.[29] Furthermore, the ratio of the newborn's skin surface area to body weight is approximately three times that of an adult.[28] As a result, the systemic availability (i.e., bioavailability) for an identical percutaneous dose of a drug will be greater in an infant than in an adult.

**Distribution**

The movement of drugs and other compounds from the systemic circulation into various body compartments, tissues, and cells is termed distribution. The apparent volume of distribution, $V_d$, is a pharmacokinetic parameter estimate that describes the relationship between the amount of a drug in the body and its serum concentration. It is assumed that a dynamic equilibrium between a compound's concentrations in tissue and blood is eventually established. Physiologic variables that influence drug distribution include the overall size of water and fat compartments and the composition and quality of circulating plasma proteins (i.e., drug-protein binding), whereas pathophysiologic variables include hemodynamic factors such as cardiac output, regional blood flow, and membrane permeability.

During development, there are continuous changes in body weight and relative body composition that continue throughout infancy and childhood.[30] Dramatic differences exist between premature and newborn infants and adults, particularly with respect to fat and water content. In newborn infants, total body water (TBW) comprises between 70% and 75% (greater for premature infants) of the body weight compared to 55% to 60% in adults. The extracellular water is also increased whereas the quantity of the intracellular water remains relatively constant, fluctuating between 35% and 45%.

**Metabolism and Excretion**

The process of drug removal from the body starts the instant a drug molecule is present within the body. The overall rate of drug removal by the body is described by the pharmacokinetic parameter estimate *clearance*, which can be divided into such types as renal, hepatic, or total body clearance. The body clearance is a summation of all clearance mechanisms involved in removing a drug from the body.

The primary organ for drug *metabolism* is the liver, though the kidney, intestine, and skin are also capable of biotransforming certain compounds.[31] Although biotransformation of most drugs generally results in pharmacologically weaker or inactive compounds, parent compounds may be transformed into active metabolites or intermediates such as theophylline to caffeine. Conversely, pharmacologically inactive parent compounds or pro-drugs may be converted to their active moiety (e.g., chloramphenicol succinate to active chloramphenicol base), and then undergo subsequent biotransformation by processes that promote body elimination.

Drug biotransformation within the hepatocyte involves two primary enzymatic processes; phase I or nonsynthetic, and phase II or synthetic reactions. Phase I reactions include oxidation, reduction, hydrolysis, and hydroxylation reactions, whereas phase II reactions primarily involve conjugation with glycine, glucuronide, or sulfate. Most drug-metabolizing enzymes are located in the smooth endoplastic reticulum of cells that are recovered as the microsomal fraction on homogenation. The phase II enzymatic reactions are primarily responsible for the synthesis of more water-soluble compounds to augment the renal elimination of drugs. Attempts have been made to stimulate or induce the activity of both phase I and phase II enzyme systems by maternal or fetal administration of a known enzyme inducer, such as phenobarbital.[32]

An age-dependent increase in the functional capacity of the kidney is also observed. Most drugs and/or their water-soluble metabolites undergo *excretion* from the body via the kidney. The amount of drug filtered by the glomerulus per unit of time is dependent on the integrity of renal blood flow and the extent of drug-protein binding. With respect to protein binding, the amount of drug filtered is inversely related to the degree of protein binding. For renal blood flow, increases are observed with age primarily due to overall functional maturation, combined with increases in cardiac output and a reduction in peripheral vascular resistance.

Glomerular filtration rate (GFR) approximates 2 to 4 ml/minute in full-term infants and increases to about 8 to 20 ml/minute by 2 to 3 days of life, approaching adult values by about 3 to 5 months of age.[33] The variation observed in the overall maturation of processes that control GFR reflects the dependency of GFR on gestational age (GA) and postconceptional age (PCA). The ontogeny of these processes correlates directly with GA for infants of 34 or more weeks' GA.[33] Tubular secretory function matures at a much slower rate than the processes that control GFR. In contrast, the capacity and ontogeny of tubular reabsorptive mechanisms remain ill-defined, but also appear to mature relative to postconceptional age.[33]

## NEONATAL PHARMACOTHERAPY

Due to the often compromised cardiac output and peripheral perfusion of seriously ill infants, IV drug administration is generally considered the ideal route for drug administration to assure adequate systemic availability.[34] Despite the clinically desirable characteristics and frequent use of IV-administered drugs in these patients, multiple problems are encountered with this method of administration including the dilution and timed administration of small dosage volumes, critical maintenance of fluid balance, and the effect of drug administration technique on resultant serum concentrations. To circumvent these problems and assure accurate and complete drug delivery, uniform guidelines for IV drug administration within an institution or patient unit should be developed and strictly adhered to.

### The Antibiotics

The antibiotics represent the most common class of drugs used in neonates and infants. Bacterial sepsis, pneumonia, necrotizing enterocolitis, and meningitis, either as primary or secondary infectious diseases, are frequent clinical challenges facing the practitioner. The antibiotics effective against common pathogens infecting newborns, including the β-lactams, aminoglycosides, and glycopeptides, are primarily eliminated from the body unchanged via the kidney. Thus, the elimination of these drugs from the body and their resultant doses and dosage intervals are dependent on the ontogeny of renal function. Table 9–2 lists currently recommended dosages and dosage intervals relative to age for selected antimicrobial agents frequently used in pediatric practice.[35, 36]

### TABLE 9–2.
Antimicrobial Agents Commonly Used in Neonates, Infants, and Children

| Drug | Neonates, Days of Postnatal Life | | Children |
|---|---|---|---|
| | 0–7 | 8–30 | |
| *Aminoglycosides*\*† | | | |
| Amikacin | 15–20‡ | 20–30‡§ | 20–30‡§ |
| Gentamicin | 5‡ | 5–7.5§ | 5–7.5§ |
| Kanamycin | 15–20‡ | 20–30‡§ | 20–30‡§ |
| Tobramycin | 5‡ | 5–7.5§ | 5–7.5§ |
| β *Lactams* | | | |
| Ampicillin | 100–300‡ | 100–300§‖ | 100–300‖ |
| Cefotaxime | 100‡ | 100–200§‖ | 100–200§‖ |
| Ceftazidime | 60‡ | 100§ | 100–150§ |
| Ceftriaxone | | | |
| Penicillin G | 100–200K‡ | 100–250K§‖ | 100–300K‖¶ |
| Nafcillin | 100–150‡§ | 100–200§‖ | 100–200‖¶ |
| Ticarcillin | 150–225‡§ | 225–300§‖ | 225–300‖¶ |
| *Others*\*† | | | |
| Chloramphenicol | 25‡ | 50§ | 75–100‖ |
| Vancomycin | 20‡ | 30§ | 40–60‖ |

\*Adapted from McCracken GH Jr, Nelson JD: *Antimicrobial Therapy for Newborns,* ed 2. New York, Grune & Stratton, 1983 and *Pediatrics* 1986; 78(suppl):959.
†Serum drug concentrations should be monitored.
‡Drug doses (mg/kg/day) are equally divided and administered every 12 hours.
§Drug doses (mg/kg/day) are equally divided and administered every 8 hours.
‖Drug doses (mg/kg/day) are equally divided and administered every 6 hours.
¶Drug doses (mg/kg/day) are equally divided and administered every 4 hours.

For specific drugs, routine therapeutic drug monitoring capabilities by means of serum drug-concentration determinations has augmented our ability to tailor drug therapy to specific patient populations and prevent toxicity (Table 9–3).

### TABLE 9–3.
Therapeutic and Toxic Concentrations of Frequently Monitored Antibiotics\*

| | Therapeutic Concentrations | Toxic Concentrations | Potential Toxicity |
|---|---|---|---|
| Aminoglycosides | | Peak ≥10–12 ml/L; trough ≥2 mg/L | Ototoxicity and nephrotoxicity |
| Vancomycin | Peak 25–40 mg/L; trough 5–10 mg/L | Peak ≥60 mg/L | Ototoxicity and nephrotoxicity |
| Chloramphenicol | Peak 20–30 mg/L; trough ≤10 mg/L | ≥50–75 mg/L | Bone marrow suppression: "gray baby" |

\*Serum concentration correlates primarily derived from adult patients.

## Cardiovascular Medications

In contrast to adults and older pediatric patients, neonates most often manifest hemodynamic instability in association with noncardiac illnesses. These include primary pulmonary processes, central nervous system disorders, systemic infections, and severe metabolic derangements. In addition, the responsiveness of the premature and newborn infant heart to the various cardiotonic agents in current clinical use is somewhat different from that observed in the more mature myocardium.[37] The contractile elements in the immature heart tend to be poorly organized, and the response to $\beta_1$-agonist agents appears confined to their chronotropic effects rather than the inotropic effects that are often the therapeutic intent of their administration.[37]

The goal of pharmacologic intervention during cardiopulmonary resuscitation is twofold: to optimize cardiac output and to maintain tissue oxygen delivery. Pharmacologic support of the heart and circulation must commence when, on clinical grounds, patients manifest cardiac output insufficient to support vital organ function and/or marked impairment of tissue oxygen delivery.[38] In newborn resuscitations, *oxygen* remains the most important drug to administer. Hypoxemia due to pulmonary immaturity and/or vascular shunting is the chief cause of cardiovascular compromise in the newborn infant. During resuscitation, 100% oxygen should always be employed, and direct, intratracheal administration is the preferred route of administration. *Sodium bicarbonate* should be employed to correct the metabolic component of the acidemia associated with cardiopulmonary arrest, but its overzealous use can result in an exacerbation of the respiratory acidosis associated with poor ventilation.

Intravenous *fluid* administration is another key therapeutic maneuver during cardiopulmonary resuscitation. The goal of this fluid resuscitation is repletion of the intravascular volume to achieve hemodynamic stability. Agents such as physiologic saline, Ringer's lactate, and 5% albumin should be considered as options for selected infants requiring resuscitation.

*Catecholamines* constitute the mainstay of therapy for cardiopulmonary resuscitation. They are administered both as intravenous boluses during the acute phases of resuscitation and as continuous infusions during the maintenance therapy involved in postresuscitative stabilization. Table 9–4 lists catecholamines currently available for clinical practice and some of their physiologic effects.[37] Inotropic, chronotropic, and dromotropic (affects the conductivity of a nerve fiber; not listed in Table 9–4) effects are mediated through $\beta_1$-receptors in the heart. The pressor effects are mediated via the $\alpha$-receptors and vasodilatory effects through the $\beta_2$-receptors lining the peripheral vascular beds. Because

**TABLE 9–4.**
Catecholamines Used for Cardiopulmonary Resuscitation*

|  | Positive Inotrope | Positive Chronotrope | Direct Pressor | Indirect Pressor | Vasodilator |
|---|---|---|---|---|---|
| Dopamine | + + | + | +/– | + + | +† |
| Dobutamine | + + | +/– | – | – | +/– |
| Epinephrine | + + + | + + + | + + + | – | – |
| Isoproterenol | + + + | + + + | – | – | + + |
| Norepinephrine | + + + | + + + | + + | – | – |

*Activity scale 0 to 3+ : + = present; – = absent.
†Primarily splanchnic and cerebral beds.

of the reported relatively short half-lives of these drugs in circulation, (on the order of 2 to 3 minutes) following the initial resuscitative procedures with potent agents such as epinephrine and/or isoproterenol, further support should consist of continuous infusion therapy.[37] Catecholamine therapy should be directed toward the patient's individual needs and titrated to the desired target response. For example, patients with normal blood pressures who require increased contractility effects may benefit from dobutamine and isoproterenol,[39] whereas patients who require inotropic support, as well as blood pressure support, are more likely to benefit from dopamine or epinephrine.[40] It is recommended that therapy with catecholamines be initiated with the least potent agent available. As the agents increase in potency, for example, going from dopamine to epinephrine, they also increase in their relative toxicity. Thus, epinephrine, isoproterenol, and norepinephrine are more likely to be arrhythmogenic and their administration is more likely to result in subendocardial ischemia than is administration of dopamine and dobutamine. The primary response to catecholamine infusions in the newborn is a chronotropic one in which an increase in heart rate may be the sole basis for an increase in cardiac output. Thus, it is important to ensure that the tachycardia does not preclude adequate ventricular filling.

Atropine is the *anticholinergic agent* of choice during cardiopulmonary resuscitation. Atropine should be reserved for those patients who have true supraventricular or junctional bradyarrhythmia. The idea that cardiac standstill might be related to overstimulation of the parasympathetic nervous system requires further investigation in pediatric patients before atropine can be recommended for cardiac standstill.

Lidocaine remains the *antiarrhythmic agent* of choice for serious sustained ventricular arrhythmias. It is important in using lidocaine that the continuous infusion used for maintenance therapy be started right after the intravenous bolus is administered. This will sustain the serum concentrations achieved by the bolus dose. Once lidocaine therapy is initiated, serum-concentration monitoring is mandatory as its accumulation predisposes to seizures.[41] Finally, sustained antiarrhythmic therapy in pediatric patients should be undertaken with phenytoin as the drug of choice. Phenytoin is used because of its lack of negative inotropic effects and its minimal effects on atrioventricular conduction. Loading and maintenance therapy should be undertaken in a fashion similar to that used for anticonvulsive therapy. However, clinical experience in our center, as well as in others, has suggested that higher serum concentrations may be necessary to achieve adequate control of ventricular arrhythmias.

In stabilizing patients, once blood pressure and heart rate have returned, *vasodilators* are often indicated. Nitroprusside is the vasodilator most frequently use in pediatric patients.[42] It produces both increased venous capacitance and decreased arterial resistance. The dosage may be individualized over a relatively wide range by monitoring of serum thiocyanate concentrations. Since the biodisposition of nitroprusside in the newborn has not been studied, thiocyanate concentrations should be obtained when side effects such as unexplained metabolic acidosis and/or central nervous system excitation, confusion and disorientation associated with increasing venous oxygen tension ($PO_2$) occur. Intravenous nitroglycerin may also be used as a vasodilator.[43] Its effects occur primarily on the capacitance vessels, and it has the added advantage that its administration can be switched to oral, sublingual, or cutaneous therapy once an appropriate dosing regimen has been developed. When considering vasodilator therapy, it should also be recalled that isoproterenol is a potent, effective vasodilator, as well as a positive inotrope.[37] It may be used as a single agent when combination inotropic/vasodilator therapy would be otherwise employed.

The final group of drugs to be discussed are those that are really endogenous substances. Children with malnutrition, severe dehydration, diarrhea, or failure to thrive may, in fact, sustain cardiopulmonary arrest due to hypoglycemia. In patients whose nutritional status is questionable, a *glucose* bolus, as well as continued glucose infusion, may be lifesaving. *Calcium* is another endogenous compound that may be extremely useful during cardiopulmonary resuscitation. Calcium is a naturally occurring inotrope and may improve contractility when administered on a bolus basis. Only the chloride salt of calcium should be used during resuscitation procedures. In this way, the calcium is immediately bioavailable and can act directly. The administration of calcium should be by slow intravenous infusion. Rapid bolus infusions can result in profound hypotension and cardiac standstill.

**TABLE 9-5.**
Drug Doses for Cardiopulmonary Resuscitation*

| | |
|---|---|
| Oxygen | 100% humidified. |
| Bicarbonate | 1 mg/kg bolus; if arrest >2 min, then 0.25 mg/kg bolus every 15 min |
| Fluid | Use colloid or crystalloid tailored to patient's physiologic needs |
| Dopamine | 0.5–2 µg/kg/min splanchnic dilation |
| | 2–7 µg/kg/min inotrope |
| | 7–>30 µg/kg/min inotrope + pressor |
| Dobutamine | 2–>30 µg/kg/min relatively pure inotrope |
| Epinephrine/ Norepinephrine | 0.05–2 µg/kg/min inotrope + pressor. May cause subendocardial ischemia and arrhythmias |
| Isoproterenol | 0.05–5 µg/kg/min inotrope + vasodilator |
| | Chronotropic response may limit dose |
| | May cause subendocardial ischemia and arrhythmias |
| Atropine | 0.01 mg/kg per dose up to 2 mg |
| | Should increase dose if no effect seen |
| Lidocaine | 1 mg/kg bolus followed by 20–50 ug/kg/min by a continuous infusion; serum concentration monitoring essential |
| Bretylium | 5 mg/kg IV bolus; may repeat up to 8 times |
| Phenytoin | 15 mg/kg loading dose; titrate maintenance therapy to serum concentrations of 15–30 µg/ml |
| Nitroprusside | 0.5–>10 µg/kg/min by continuous infusion |
| Nitroglycerin | 0.2–10 µg/kg/min by continuous infusion |
| Glucose | 2 ml/kg 50% dextrose; follow Dextrostix |
| Calcium | 25 mg/kg calcium chloride |

*Drug doses listed are initial starting recommendations. Dosages may require adjustment based on individual patient responses and the changing physiologic status of each patient during the recovery period. See text for details.

Table 9–5 depicts some recommended doses of drugs to be used during cardiopulmonary resuscitation. Dosage adjustments should be made based on individual patient responses and the changing physiologic status of each patient during the recovery period. The doses listed are simply recommended starting points, and suggested ranges and should not be adhered to rigorously.

## Methylxanthines

During the neonatal period, theophylline compounds are used most often in the treatment of apnea of prematurity. However, the efficacy of theophylline in this syndrome may be related to the additive or synergistic action of caffeine, which accumulates in the serum of infants receiving theophylline therapy. The N-methylation of theophylline to caffeine occurs in preterm infants even beyond the newborn period and is clinically important since caffeine has a prolonged half-life that results in its significant accumulation.[44] However, caffeine is rarely detectable in the serum of older infants, children, or adults treated with theophylline. Table 9-6 compares the pharmacokinetic parameter estimates for theophylline and caffeine in preterm infants.

The total body elimination of theophylline in infancy is markedly prolonged due primarily to the immaturity of hepatic metabolism mechanisms.[44] The major metabolic pathways for theophylline involve demethylation and hydroxylation reactions by the cytochrome P450 monooxygenase system. Although neonates methylate theophylline at the N-7 position to caffeine, about 50% of parent theophylline is excreted unchanged in the urine as compared to about 10% in older children and adults.[44,45] These differences in theophylline biodisposition in preterm and full-term infants are reflected in the current theophylline dosage recommendations[46] (see below).

The efficacy of theophylline and/or caffeine in the treatment of neonatal apnea is well established with serum concentrations between 5 and 10 mg/L.[44-47] In contrast, therapeutic serum theophylline concentrations between 10 and 20 mg/L are used in older children and adults with reversible bronchoconstriction. The reason(s) for this discrepancy in "therapeutic" serum concentrations is unknown, though it may reflect different primary actions of the drug for two different pathophysiologic entities. Moreover, the additive or synergistic effects of caffeine combined with the greater amount of free active theophylline available (i.e., decreased plasma protein binding) in newborns must be considered. As a result, for the treatment of apnea of prematurity we recommend an initial theophylline loading dose of 5.5 mg/kg (6.5 mg/kg aminophylline) followed by a maintenance dose of theophylline of 1.1 mg/kg every 8 hours. This dosing regimen usually achieves serum theophylline concentrations between 5 and 10 mg/L; however, due to the tremendous variability in theophylline metabolism in neonates, serum concentrations should be monitored to assure optimal drug dosing.

Theophylline has also been shown to be efficacious in the prevention of postextubation respiratory failure in infants weighing less than 1,250 gm. In one critical evaluation, 5 of 14 theophylline-treated infants vs. 10 of 11 control infants required reintubation within 5 days.[48] Although not clearly understood, theophylline's efficacy in this setting may be due to the drug's enhancement of diaphragmatic contractility.

**TABLE 9-6.**
Pharmacokinetic Parameter Estimates for Theophylline and Caffeine in Premature Infants

| Parameter | Theophylline | Caffeine |
|---|---|---|
| $t_{1/2}$, hr | 19-36 | 65-103 |
| Vd, L/kg | 0.5-1 | 0.76-0.92 |
| Cl, ml/kg/hr | 17-39 | 8.5-8.9 |

Numerous investigators have described the efficacy of caffeine alone in preventing apnea in preterm infants. Turmen and colleagues[49] demonstrated that infant breathing patterns improved markedly as serum concentrations increased toward 10 mg/L. Aranda et al.[50] have reported efficacy of caffeine with serum concentrations between 5 and 20 mg/L with no toxicity observed in infants with serum caffeine concentrations less than 50 mg/L. Available caffeine pharmacokinetic data on infants suggest that an initial loading dose of 10 mg/kg of caffeine results in postdistribution serum concentrations of about 11 to 13 mg/L. A maintenance dose of 2.5 mg/kg administered every 24 hours should maintain therapeutic steady-state caffeine serum concentrations. The variability of theophylline metabolism, combined with the narrow therapeutic index, mandates the routine monitoring of serum theophylline concentrations. If serum theophylline concentrations are between 5 and 10 mg/L and a desirable clinical response has been realized without drug-related toxicity, concurrent measurements of caffeine concentrations are unwarranted. For neonates demonstrating drug-related toxicities, both theophylline and caffeine serum concentrations should be quantitated. It appears that the relative potency of caffeine is about 50% to 75% of theophylline. Thus, when interpreting concurrent serum theophylline and caffeine concentrations in difficult-to-treat neonates, we frequently add two thirds of the caffeine concentration to the measured theophylline concentration to determine "total" plasma methylxanthine.

## Digoxin

Digoxin is an important cardiac glycoside frequently used in the treatment of a variety of myocardial disturbances in neonates, infants, and children.[51] Despite the drug's widespread clinical use and study, much of the available neonatal pharmacology data remains in question. Digoxin-like immunoreactive substance(s) present in the serum of newborn infants cross-react such that current immunoassay techniques give rise to falsely high values.[52] Nevertheless, serum digoxin concentrations should be monitored in infants demonstrating possible digoxin toxicity or in patients receiving drugs known to decrease the body clearance of digoxin (i.e., quinidine).

Pharmacodynamic correlates with the echocardiogram and determinations of systolic time intervals have provided insight into the therapeutic dose of digoxin. Recommendations for digoxin therapy in preterm and full-term infants are shown in Table 9–7.[53, 54]

**TABLE 9-7.**
Initial Digoxin Dosing in Neonates*†

|  | Total Digitalizing Dose, μg/kg | | Maintenance Dose, μg/kg/Day | |
| --- | --- | --- | --- | --- |
|  | IV | PO | IV | PO |
| Premature infant | 20 | 25–27 | 5 | 6–7 |
| Full-term infant | 22–25 | 30 | 5.5–6.5 | 7.5–10 |

*IV = intravenous; PO = oral
†Higher doses may be required for supraventricular tachycardia. Maintenance doses are generally given in two equally divided doses daily.

## Indomethacin

Similar to other nonsteroidal anti-inflammatory agents, indomethacin is a potent inhibitor of prostaglandin synthesis through its inhibition of cyclooxygenase activity. Since its introduction into clinical medicine in the mid-1960s, the drug has been used extensively in adults for a variety of inflammatory disorders including rheumatoid arthritis and osteoarthritis. In pediatric pharmacotherapeutics, indomethacin has found a role in the nonsurgical treatment of patent ductus arteriosus (PDA).

The biodisposition of indomethacin in neonates remains ill defined. The drug demonstrates poor and erratic absorption when administered orally,[55] thus the clinical dependence on IV drug administration. Although the drug is extensively bound to serum albumin (about 98%) and responsible for protein-displacement drug interactions in adults, the low serum concentrations used to promote PDA closure in neonates do not appear to displace bilirubin.[56] In a national collaborative study[57] of 149 infants with a hemodynamically significant PDA who were given indomethacin, 79 demonstrated ductal closure within 48 hours as compared to 28 of 270 infants who received only conventional medical therapy (fluid restriction). Moreover, 65 of the control infants ultimately required surgical ligation of their PDA vs. only 21 of infants receiving indomethacin (13 in whom indomethacin therapy initially failed and 8 in whom the ductus reopened). Although this study failed to detect a significant correlation between ductal closure and birth weight, gestational age, gender, race, or serum indomethacin concentration, closure rates were substantially greater for infants initially treated when they were older than 5 days of age.

The current dosing recommendations for pharmacologic closure of the PDA using indomethacin relative to an infant's postnatal age is shown in Table 9–8. If PDA closure does not result after the first indomethacin dose, up to two additional doses may be administered at 12-hour intervals. For those infants who initially respond to indo-

**TABLE 9–8.**
Indomethacin Dosage Recommendations for Pharmacologic Closure of a Patent Ductus Arteriosus

| | Indomethacin Dose, mg/kg | |
|---|---|---|
| Postnatal Age | Initial Dose | Second and Third Doses* |
| 0–48 hr | 0.2 | 0.1 |
| 2–7 days | 0.2 | 0.2 |
| ≥8 days | 0.25 | 0.25 |

*Second and third doses if needed are administered every 12 hours. See text for details.

methacin but in whom the ductus reopens 48 hours after therapy, most clinicians would attempt a second course of therapy. Surgical ligation of the PDA should be considered for those infants with a significant PDA if the infant fails a second course of indomethacin.

The use of indomethacin in neonates is associated with a number of important and potentially serious drug-induced complications. Depending on the parameter used to define a decrease in renal function, greater than 50% of infants receiving indomethacin experience an acute impairment of renal function. The most common findings are decreases in urine output and GFR, which are usually transient and reversible.[58, 59] These changes in renal dynamics result from suppression of systemic and renal prostaglandin synthesis. Moreover, due to indomethacin effects on renal function and in particular GFR, dosages of other drugs dependent on GFR for body elimination (e.g., digoxin, aminoglycosides) should be closely monitored in infants receiving concurrent indomethacin therapy. In addition, thrombocytopenia and a tendency for increased bleeding may also be associated with the use of indomethacin in newborns. Studies by Maher and colleagues[60] and Ment et al.[61] were unable to ascertain any deleterious effects of indomethacin in preterm infants with intraventricular hemorrhage. Thus, surgical ligation may be indicated in infants with a significant PDA who have renal insufficiency (i.e., blood urea nitrogen greater than or equal to 30 mg/dl and/or serum creatinine greater than 1.8 mg/dl), a platelet count less than or equal to 60,000/cu mm, evidence of significant bleeding, or the presence of necrotizing enterocolitis.

## Diuretics

In perinatal practice, the correction of fluid and electrolyte abnormalities remains a common therapeutic challenge. Pathophysiologic processes including anatomical anomalies, asphyxia, primary pulmonary disease, and renal compromise often lead to fluid and electrolyte imbalance requiring the judicious administration of both electrolyte-containing fluids and diuretic drugs. The clinical importance of these drugs is directly related to their ability to increase renal water and electrolyte excretion. The ability to excrete a sodium or water load is decreased in the neonate due, at least partially, to the decrease in GFR[33] and the elevated concentrations of aldosterone present in both preterm and term infants.[62] In addition, the urinary excretion of prostaglandin $E_2$, calcium, and bicarbonate are increased in neonates. The target organ for diuretic action is the kidney,[63] and thus, the ontogeny of these processes would be expected to markedly influence the pharmacokinetics and pharmacodynamics of diuretic drugs.

The most commonly used diuretics in neonates and infants are the so-called "high efficacy," "high ceiling," or "loop" diuretics, which include furosemide, bumetanide, and ethacrynic acid. These drugs work from within the tubular lumen inhibiting sodium-potassium-chloride co-transport in the thick ascending limb of Henle's loop. At their maximal efficacy, the loop diuretics inhibit reabsorption of greater than 15% of filtered sodium, and their diuretic effects are independent of the patient's acid-base status.[63] Their onset of diuretic action usually occurs within 30 minutes of IV administration with peak effects observed 1 to 2 hours after an IV dose.

In neonates, approximately 97% of furosemide is bound to plasma protein.[64] Although in vitro studies suggested that furosemide, a sulfonamide derivative, was equal to or more potent than sulfisoxazole in displacing bilirubin from albumin binding sites, the concentrations used far exceeded serum furosemide concentrations observed after clinical use of the drug. Aranda and colleagues[64] were unable to demonstrate any significant bilirubin displacement in infants receiving 1 to 1.5 mg/kg furosemide parenterally.

Ethacrynic acid is a phenoxyacetic acid derivative that possesses pharmacokinetic and pharmacodynamic properties very similar to furosemide.[65] Unlike furosemide, ethacrynic acid does not appear to inhibit carbonic anhydrase activity nor alter urinary excretion of bicarbonate.[63] Adverse effects including ototoxicity and gastrointestinal intolerance appear to occur more frequently with ethacrynic acid than with other loop diuretics. As a result, the clinical use of ethacrynic acid is largely reserved for those patients who are allergic to the sulfonamide-derivative loop diuretics.

Current recommendations suggest that furosemide therapy should be initiated with a 1 mg/kg per IV dose or 2 mg/kg per oral dose.[63] At present, individual doses of furosemide should not exceed 6 mg/kg per IV dose or 12mg/kg per oral dose. In term infants, furosemide dose may be repeated every 6 to 8 hours. In contrast, individual furosemide doses should generally not be administered more often than every 12 hours in preterm infants due to their markedly limited capacity to eliminate the drug. The dose of ethacrynic acid is 1 mg/kg per dose either IV or orally. At present, no dosage guidelines have been established for bumetanide in pediatric patients.

The most common adverse effects associated with loop diuretics are fluid and electrolyte abnormalities. Hearing loss, which is usually transient, has been reported with the use of furosemide, often when the drug is concurrently administered with other ototoxic drugs.[63] Nephrolithiasis and secondary hyperparathyroidism and bone disease have been well documented in premature infants receiving chronic furosemide therapy.[66] In addition, Green and colleagues[67] reported an increased incidence of PDA in 33 premature infants who received furosemide as compared to 33 infants given chlorothiazide. As furosemide is a stimulator of renal prostaglandin $E_2$ synthesis, urinary prostaglandin $E_2$ excretion tripled between the first and fifth day of life. Despite these findings, no differences were observed in the number of patients requiring ductal ligation. Yeh and colleagues,[68] in a later study, were unable to document an increased incidence of PDA in a similar group of preterm infants treated with furosemide.

## CONCLUSIONS

Over the past decade, we have witnessed a greater appreciation for understanding and documenting the pharmacokinetic-pharmacodynamic characteristics of drugs used during the perinatal period. It is clear that a myriad of patient-specific variables directly influences an individual's clinical response to drugs and thus our ability to design optimal pharmacotherapeutic regimens. Most important in the care of preterm and full-term infants is our appreciation of the complex interrelationships between the ontogeny of drug-receptor sensitivity and organ function. However, despite our progress to date, an exact description of the clinical pharmacology of drugs in neonates is available for only a few selected compounds. The dynamic ontologic changes characteristic of neonates underscores our need to strive for continued critical evaluation of drugs to be used in perinatal practice.

## REFERENCES

1. Shirkey H: Therapeutic orphans (editorial). *J Pediatr* 1968; 72:119.
2. McKercher HG, Raddi IC: Placental transfer of drugs and fetal pharmacology, in MacLeod SM, Radde IC (eds): *Textbook of Pediatric Clinical Pharmacology*. Littletown, Mass, PSG Publishing Co Inc, 1985, p 293.

3. Mirkin BL, Singh S: Placental transfer of pharmacologically active molecules, in Mirkin BL (ed): *Perinatal Pharmacology and Therapeutics.* New York, Academic Press, 1976.
4. Blechner JN, Makowski EL, Cotter JR, et al: Nitrous oxide transfer from mother to fetus in sheep and goats. *Am J Obstet Gynecol* 1969; 105:368.
5. Finster M, Morishima HO, Mark LC, et al: Tissue thiopental concentrations in the fetus and newborn. *Anesthesiology* 1972; 36:155.
6. Szeto HH, Mann LI, Ghakthavathsalan A, et al: Meperidine pharmacokinetics in the maternal-fetal unit. *J Pharmacol Exp Ther* 1978; 206:448.
7. Borell U, Fernstorm I, Ohlson L, et al: Influence of uterine contractions on the uteroplacental blood flow at term. *Am J Obstet Gynecol* 1965; 93:44.
8. Greiss FC, Jr: Effect of labor on uterine blood flow. *Am J Obstet Gynecol* 1965; 93:917.
9. Adamsons K, Mueller-Heubach E, Myers RE: Production of fetal asphyxia in the rhesus monkey by administration of catecholamines to the mother. *Am J Obstet Gynecol* 1971; 109:248.
10. Lieberman BA, Stirrat GM, Cohen SL, et al: The possible adverse effects of propranolol on the fetus in pregnancies complicated by severe hypertension. *Br J Obstet Gynaecol* 1978; 85:678.
11. Goldstein A: The interaction of drugs and plasma proteins. *Pharmacol Rev* 1949; 1:102.
12. Kleinman CS, Copel JA, Weinstein EM, et al: In utero diagnosis and treatment of fetal supraventricular tachycardia. *Semin Perinatol* 1985; 9:113.
13. Rotmensch HH, Rotmensch S, Elkayam W: Management of cardiac arrhythmia during pregnancy: Current concepts. *Drugs* 1987; 33:623.
14. Liggins GC, Howie RN: A controlled trial of antepartum glucocorticoid treatment for prevention of the respiratory distress syndrome in premature infants. *Pediatrics* 1972; 50:515.
15. Collaborative Group on Antenatal Steroid Therapy: Effect of antenatal dexamethasone administration on the prevention of respiratory distress syndrome. *Am J Obstet Gynecol* 1981; 141:276.
16. Collaborative Group on Antenatal Steroid Therapy: Effect of antenatal dexamethasone administration in the infant: Long-term follow-up. *J Pediatr* 1984; 104:259.
17. Parsons RL: Drug absorption in gastrointestinal disease with particular reference to malabsorption syndromes. *Clin Pharmacokinet* 1977; 2:45.
18. Ames MD: Gastric acidity in the first ten days of life of the prematurely born baby. *Am J Dis Child* 1960; 100:252.
19. Gupta M, Brans YW: Gastric retention in neonates. *Pediatrics* 1978; 62:26.
20. Cavell B: Gastric emptying in preterm infants. *Acta Paediatr Scand* 1979; 68:725.
21. Watkins JB, Ingall D, Szczepanik P, et al: Bile salt metabolism in the newborn. *N Engl J Med* 1973; 288:431.

22. Hillman JS, Martin LA, Haddad JG: Absorption and maintenance dosage of 25-hydroxycholecalciferol (25-HCC) in premature infants. Pediatric Res 1979; 13:400.
23. Long SS, Swenson RM: Development of anaerobic fecal flora in healthy newborn infants. J Pediatr 1977; 91:298.
24. Greenblatt DJ, Koch-Weser J: Intramuscular injection of drugs. N Engl J Med 1976; 295:542.
25. Tyrala EE, Hillman LS, Hillman RE, et al: Clinical pharmacology of hexachlorophene in newborn infants. J Pediatr 1977; 91:481.
26. Fisch RO, Berglund EB, Bridge AG, et al: Methemoglobinemia in a hospital nursery. JAMA 1963; 185:760.
27. Feinblatt BI, Aceto T, Beckhorn G, et al: Percutaneous absorption of hydrocortisone in children. Am J Dis Child 1966; 112:218.
28. Lester RS: Topical formulary for the pediatrician. Pediatr Clin North Am 1983; 30:749.
29. Nachman RL, Esterly NB: Increased skin permeability in preterm infants. J Pediatr 1971; 79:628.
30. Friis-Hansen B: Water distribution in the foetus and newborn infant. Acta Paediatr Scand 1983; 305(suppl):7.
31. Litterst CL, Mimnaugh EG, Reagan RL, et al: Comparison of in vitro drug metabolism by lung, liver and kidney of several common laboratory species. Drug Metab Dispos 1975; 3:165.
32. Talafant E, Hoskova A, Pojerova A: Glucaric acid excretion as an index of hepatic glucuronidation in neonates after phenobarbital treatment. Pediatr Res 1975; 9:480.
33. Arant BS Jr: Developmental patterns of renal functional maturation compared in the human neonate. J Pediatr 1978; 92:705.
34. Roberts RJ: Intravenous administration of medication in pediatric patients: Problems and solutions. Pediatr Clin North Am 1981; 28:23.
35. McCracken GH Jr, Nelson JD: Antimicrobial Therapy for Newborns, ed 2. New York, Grune & Stratton, 1983.
36. Blumer JL, Reed MD: Aminoglycoside antibiotics in pediatric practice. Pediatr Clin North Am 1983; 30:177.
37. Zaritsky A, Chernow B: Use of catecholamines in pediatrics. J Pediatr 1984; 105:341.
38. Blumer JL: Pharmacologic approach to cardiopulmonary resuscitation in children. Pediatric Ann 1985; 14:313.
39. Driscoll DJ, Gillette PC, Lewis RM, et al: Comparative hemodynamic effects of isoproterenol, dopamine and dobutamine in the newborn dog. Pediatr Res 1979; 13:1006.
40. Lang P, Williams RG, Norwood WI, et al.: The hemodynamic effects of dopamine in infants after corrective cardiac surgery. J Pediatr 1980; 96:630.
41. Pentel P, Benowitz N: Pharmacokinetic and pharmacodynamic considerations in drug therapy of cardiac emergencies. Clin Pharmacokinet 1984; 9:273.

42. Gordillo-Paniaqua G, Velasquez-Jones L, Martini R, et al.: Sodium nitroprusside treatment of severe arterial hypertension in children. J Pediatr 1975; 87:799.
43. Benson LN, Bohn D, Edmonds JF, et al: Nitroglycerine therapy in children with low cardiac index after heart surgery. Cardiovasc Med 1979; 4:207.
44. Hendeles L, Weinberger M: Theophylline: A state of the art review. Pharmacotherapy 1983; 3:2.
45. Tserng KY, King KC, Takieddine FN: Theophylline metabolism in premature infants. Clin Pharmacol Ther 1981; 29:594.
46. Aranda JV, Sitar DS, Parsons WD, et al: Pharmacokinetic aspects of theophylline in premature newborns. N Engl J Med 1976; 295:413.
47. Shannon DC, Gotay F, Stein IM, et al: Prevention of apnea and bradycardia in low-birthweight infants. Pediatrics 1975; 55:589.
48. Viscardi RM, Faix RG, Nicks JJ, et al: Efficacy of theophylline for prevention of post-extubation respiratory failure in very low birthweight infants. J Pediatr 1985; 107:469.
49. Turmen T, David J, Aranda JV: Relationship of dose and plasma concentrations of caffeine and ventilation in neonatal apnea. Semin Perinatal 1981; 5:326.
50. Aranda JV, Cook CE, Gorman W, et al: Pharmacokinetic profile of caffeine in the premature newborn infant with apnea. J Pediatr 1979; 94:663.
51 Park MK: Use of digoxin in infants and children, with specific emphasis on dosage. J Pediatr 1986; 108:871.
52. Phelps SJ, Kamper CA, Bottorff MB, et al: Effect of age and serum creatinine on endogenous digoxin-like substances in infants and children. J Pediatr 1987; 110:136.
53. Pinsky WW, Jacobsen JR, Gillette PC, et al: Dosage of digoxin in premature infants. J Pediatr 1979; 96:639.
54. Lang D, Von Bernuth G: Serum concentrations and serum half-life of digoxin in premature and mature newborns. Pediatrics 1977; 59:902.
55. Evans M, Bhat R, Vidyasagar D: A comparison of oral and intravenous indomethacin disposition in the premature infant with patent ductus arteriosus. Pediatr Pharmacol 1981; 1:251.
56. Shankaran S, Pantoja A, Poland RL: Indomethacin and bilirubin-albumin binding. Dev Pharmacol Ther 1982; 4:124.
57. Gersony WM, Peckham GJ, Ellison RC, et al: Effects of indomethacin in premature infants with patent ductus arteriosus: Results of a national collaborative study. J Pediatr 1983; 102:895.
58. Halliday HL, Hirata T, Brady JP: Indomethacin therapy for large patent ductus arteriosus in the very low birth weight infant: Results and complications. Pediatrics 1979; 64:154.
59. Seyberth HW, Rascher W, Hackenthal R, et al: Effect of prolonged indomethacin therapy on renal function and selected vasoactive hormones in very low birth weight infants with symptomatic patent ductus arteriosus. J Pediatr 1983; 103:979.

60. Maher PM, Lane B, Ballard R, et al: Does indomethacin cause extension of intracranial hemorrhages: A preliminary study. Pediatrics 1985; 75:497.
61. Ment LR, Duncan CC, Ehrenkranz RA, et al: Randomized indomethacin trial for prevention of intraventricular hemorrhage in very low birth weight infants. J Pediatr 1985; 107:937.
62. Sulyok E, Nemeth M, Tenyi I, et al: Postnatal development of renin-angiotensin-aldosterone system in relation to electrolyte balance in premature infants. Pediatr Res 1979; 13:817.
63. Witte MK, Stork JE, Blumer JL: Diuretic therapeutics in the pediatric patient. Am J Cardiol 1986; 57(suppl):44A.
64. Aranda JV, Perez J, Sitar DS, et al: Pharmacokinetic disposition and protein binding of furosemide in newborn infants. J Pediatr 1978; 93:507.
65. Scalais E, Papageorgiou A, Aranda JV: Effects of ethacrynic acid in the newborn infant. J Pediatr 1984; 104:947.
66. Hufnagle KG, Khan SH, Penn D, et al: Renal calcifications: A complication of long-term furosemide therapy in preterm infants. Pediatrics 1982; 70:360.
67. Green TP, Thompson TR, Johnson DE, et al: Furosemide promotes patent ductus arteriosus in premature infants with the respiratory distress syndrome. N Engl J Med 1983; 308:743.
68. Yeh TF, Shibli A, Leu ST, et al: Early furosemide therapy in premature infants ($\leq$2000 gm) with respiratory distress syndrome: A randomized, controlled trial. J Pediatr 1984; 105:603.

# 10

# Respiratory Diseases of the Newborn

Michele C. Walsh, M.D.
Waldemar A. Carlo, M.D.
Martha J. Miller, M.D., Ph.D.

Disorders of the respiratory system account for the largest number of admissions to neonatal intensive care nurseries and are the main cause of mortality and morbidity in the newborn period. Respiratory disorders of newborn infants are frequently life threatening and demand prompt diagnostic evaluation and appropriate therapeutic intervention. While many diseases may present with signs of respiratory distress, a brief evaluation is usually sufficient to arrive at a preliminary differential diagnosis. This chapter will review the clinical evaluation of neonates with respiratory distress with emphasis on the differential diagnosis.

## HISTORY

A brief review of the maternal and perinatal history will be essential when evaluating a neonate with respiratory distress (Table 10–1). Preterm gestation may result in lung immaturity and respiratory distress syndrome (RDS). Maternal diabetes mellitus may also predispose to RDS as well as to congenital cyanotic heart disease. Premature or prolonged rupture of membranes (more than 18 hours) and maternal infection may result in neonatal pneumonia. Oligohydramnios is associated with lung hypoplasia while polyhydramnios may occur when gastrointestinal obstruction is present, such as occurs with some types of tracheoesophageal fistula. Infants who experience hypoxia in utero may pass meconium into the amniotic fluid; and bradycardia may be seen on fetal heart rate monitoring.

**TABLE 10–1.**
Brief Evaluation for Neonates With Respiratory Distress

| History | Physical Examination | Laboratory Workup |
|---|---|---|
| Gestational age | Major signs of respiratory distress: cyanosis, tachypnea, grunting, retraction, flaring | Chest roentgenogram |
| Maternal diseases | | Arterial blood gas analysis |
|   Diabetes | | Central hematocrit |
|   Infections | | Blood glucose |
| Fetal distress | Temperature | Consider: blood culture, complete blood cell count, gastric aspirate Gram stain |
| Meconium-stained fluid | Blood pressure | |
| | Skin perfusion | |

## PHYSICAL EXAMINATION

A brief but thorough physical examination should be performed in every neonate with respiratory distress. The major signs of neonatal respiratory distress are discussed below. Temperature and blood pressure are essential parts of this evaluation as both hypothermia and hyperthermia as well as hypotension and hypovolemia may manifest with signs of respiratory distress. Poor perfusion occurs in infants with cardiovascular decompensation such as in septic shock or obstruction to the left outflow tract of the heart (see Table 10–1).

### Major Signs of Respiratory Distress

Five clinical signs are frequently observed in neonates with respiratory distress. These are *cyanosis, tachypnea, retractions, nasal flaring, and grunting*. A frequent misconception in neonatal care is to equate these signs with RDS. These signs are not pathognomonic of RDS and may be observed with many other diseases that cause respiratory compromise.

#### *Cyanosis*

Cyanosis is a slight bluish to purple discoloration of the skin due to the presence of an elevated amount of unsaturated, or reduced, hemoglobin. Cyanosis can be classified as central or peripheral. *Central cyanosis* is due to a low arterial oxygen saturation and manifests as a discoloration of tissues that reflect arterial blood oxygenation such as the tongue and lips. Central cyanosis may be caused by pulmonary disease, cyanotic cardiac lesions, hematologic abnormality (congenital methemoglobinemia), and central nervous system diseases. In contrast, in *peripheral cyanosis* there is normal oxygen saturation of arterial blood but low oxygen saturation of localized areas such as the nailbeds of the hands and feet in newborn infants. Cyanosis of the hands and feet is frequently observed in newborn infants during the first days of life and, when present as the sole finding, is normal.

Detection of cyanosis is dependent on the total amount of unsaturated hemoglobin, which, in turn, depends on both oxygen saturation and hemoglobin level. Central cyanosis is clinically appreciated when a total of 3 to 6 gm/dl of hemoglobin is unsaturated.[1] Thus, for the same oxygen saturation, infants with polycythemia (elevated hemoglobin concentration) will manifest cyanosis earlier than infants with a normal hemoglobin concentration. Central cyanosis may even be noted in polycythemic infants despite a normal $PaO_2$ and oxygen saturation.

### Tachypnea

Respiratory rates up to 60 breaths per minute are normal in the first hours of life, but persistently elevated rates require careful clinical evaluation. The respiratory rate is largely controlled by chemical and mechanoreceptor reflexes. Either hypercapnia or low lung volume may increase respiratory rate. Thus, tachypnea does not have to be accompanied by hypercapnia.

Infants with pulmonary disease attempt to minimize work of breathing by controlling respiratory rate. The total work of breathing consists of elastic and resistive components. The elastic component represents the work required to stretch the lungs, whereas the resistive component is the work required to overcome the resistance to the movement of gases through the airways. In patients with RDS, respirations are shallow and rapid. By breathing shallowly, work of breathing is decreased as less work is done to expand, or stretch, the lungs. In contrast, patients with airway obstruction tend to breathe more deeply and slowly to reduce work due to resistance.

### Retractions

Retraction of the chest wall during inspiration is commonly seen in neonates. The chest wall of neonates, particularly those born prematurely, is highly compliant, and the negative pleural pressures created during inspiration may cause retractions. Depending on the local compliance of portions of the chest wall and the magnitude of the pressure developed, retractions may be present in one or more of the following areas: substernal, subcostal, and intercostal. There is no diagnostic or prognostic value related to the specific area in which retractions occur. In addition, inward movement of the upper chest simultaneous with outward movement of the abdomen during inspiration (asynchronous chest-wall movements) is frequently observed, particularly during active sleep. Retractions or asynchrony of the chest wall may occur in the absence of other signs of respiratory distress and reflect normal maturational stages. This is particularly true in preterm infants in whom asynchronous chest-wall movements occur frequently, particularly in the absence of respiratory disease.[2]

### Nasal Flaring

Nasal flaring, the enlargement of the nostrils produced by activation of the alae nasi muscles, is a sign frequently observed in both normal and sick neonates. Nasal flaring in the absence of respiratory distress is frequently observed in the immediate postnatal period, during active sleep and during feedings. However, when flaring is persistently present beyond the first hours of life or accompanied by other signs of respiratory distress, further evaluation is indicated.

Newborn infants preferentially breathe nasally. However, spontaneous oral breathing has been observed in 30% of infants during sleep. Nasal and pharyngeal resistances contribute up to 50% of the total lung resistance. The enlargement of the nasal passages produced by nasal flaring results in a marked reduction in nasal resistance and work of breathing. Furthermore, it has been shown that nasal flaring, as well as activity of some other upper airway muscles, precedes diaphragm activity by a fraction of a second, and this preactivation is thought to be an important mechanism that reduces resistance and maintains airway patency.[3]

### Grunting

In both healthy neonates and adults, the vocal cords are normally abducted during inspiration and adducted during expiration. However, neonates are unable to passively maintain a normal functional residual capacity largely because their chest wall is highly compliant. Adduction of the vocal cords with delayed expiration (or braking of expiration) is one of the mechanisms used by neonates to maintain their functional residual capacity. This mechanism is frequently not clinically obvious, but careful auscultation may reveal delayed expiratory airflow. In the presence of respiratory disorders, marked adduction of the vocal cords during expiration holds air in the lungs, and during the late phase of expiration, the gas is rapidly propelled, causing a loud, audible grunt. Increased lung volume and airway pressure during the braked expiration results in improved gas exchange, and disruption of this mechanism impairs oxygenation.[4] The grunting mechanism maintains an oxygenation comparable to that during application of a continuous distending pressure of 2 to 3 cm $H_2O$.[5]

## LABORATORY DATA

The clinical evaluation necessary in a neonate with respiratory distress is listed in Table 10–1. An anteroposterior chest radiograph is usually sufficient; however, lateral x-rays may be useful if fluid, masses, or free air are present. Arterial blood is preferred for analysis of oxygenation and ventilation. Noninvasive methods to assess gas exchange such as transcutaneous blood gas measurements or oxygen saturation may also be used. A central hematocrit sample (venous or arterial) is preferred as peripheral samples obtained from the capillary bed may result in an overestimate of hematocrit by up to 10%. Hypoglycemia can be easily ruled out with a quantitative or qualitative blood sugar determination. If the history contains factors known to be associated with a high rate of sepsis, such as rupture of membranes for greater than 18 hours, maternal fever, or signs of chorioamnionitis, then a full evaluation for sepsis is indicated. An evaluation for sepsis should include cultures of the blood and cerebrospinal fluid, and a white blood cell and differential cell count.

## DIFFERENTIAL DIAGNOSIS

A classification of pulmonary and extrapulmonary disorders that cause neonatal respiratory distress is included in Table 10–2.

## RESPIRATORY DISTRESS SYNDROME

Respiratory distress syndrome is the most common single cause of respiratory distress in neonates. Previously, RDS was called hyaline membrane disease, but the latter term has fallen into disuse as hyaline membrane is a nonspecific response of the lungs to various insults, including assisted ventilation. Advances in neonatal care, in particular, in assisted ventilation, have dramatically improved the prognosis in neonates with RDS. However, newer approaches to the care of patients with RDS need to be developed as this disease is the leading cause of neonatal mortality, accounting for approximately 20% of neonatal deaths.[6]

### Etiology and Pathophysiology

For years there has been major controversy relating to the cause of RDS. It is widely accepted that pulmonary immaturity, associated with

**TABLE 10-2.**
Differential Diagnosis of Respiratory Distress During the First Days of Life

| Pulmonary Disorders | | |
|---|---|---|
| Common | Less Common | Uncommon |
| Respiratory distress syndrome | Pulmonary hemorrhage | Congenital lung cysts, tumors |
| Transient tachypnea of the newborn | Pulmonary hypoplasia/agenesis | Congenital lobar emphysema |
| Meconium aspiration | Wilson-Mikity syndrome | Tracheoesophageal fistula |
| Congenital pneumonia | Upper airway obstruction | Pulmonary lymphangiectasia |
| Pneumothorax/air leaks | Tracheomalacia | Tracheal lesions |
| Persistent fetal circulation | Abdominal distention | Rib cage anomalies |
|  | Pleural effusion/chylothorax | Extrinsic masses |
|  | Diaphragmatic hernia |  |
| Extrapulmonary Disorders | | |
| Cardiovascular | Metabolic | Neurologic/Muscular |
| Hypovolemia | Acidosis | Cerebral edema |
| Anemia | Hypoglycemia | Cerebral hemorrhage |
| Polycythemia | Hypothermia | Drugs |
| Persistent fetal circulation | Hyperthermia | Muscle disorders |
| Cyanotic heart disease |  | Spinal cord diseases |
| Congestive heart failure |  | Phrenic nerve damage |

surfactant deficiency, is the principal factor in the pathophysiology of the disease. Surfactant is a complex mixture of phospholipids and proteins that forms a coat over the inner surface of the alveoli, decreasing their natural tendency to collapse. Low surfactant production by alveolar type II pneumocytes results in increased surface tension, alveolar collapse, diffuse atelectasis, and decreased lung compliance. Together these factors increase pulmonary artery pressure. Pulmonary artery hypertension leads to extrapulmonary right-to-left shunting of blood and increased alveolar to arterial oxygen gradient and ventilation perfusion mismatching as evidenced by the high arterial to alveolar carbon dioxide gradient.[7]

Prematurity is the single most important risk factor for development of RDS. In fact, the incidence and severity of RDS markedly decreases with advancing gestational age; nevertheless, preterm infants of 36 to 37 weeks gestation may develop severe RDS. However, RDS is rarely observed in infants of greater than 38 weeks' gestation. Some perinatal complications may increase the incidence or severity of RDS. These include asphyxia, maternal diabetes, and delivery by cesarean section, particularly in the absence of labor. The incidence of RDS is higher in males than in females. Similarly, the second infant of a pair of twins may have more severe RDS than the firstborn twin.

## Clinical Manifestations

Infants with RDS present with multiple signs of respiratory distress soon after birth, usually within the first 4 hours of life. Rare cases that have a late presentation have been described; these cases may represent mildly ill infants who were overlooked during the early phase of disease. Retractions may be particularly prominent in preterm infants as the chest wall is highly compliant whereas the lungs are stiff. Grunting is frequently present, but in mildly ill patients, only an expiratory whine or cry may be heard. In addition to cyanosis, nasal flaring, and tachypnea, infants with RDS also have diminished breath sounds and poor gas entry.

The clinical course of infants with RDS is characterized by gradual worsening during the first 2 to 3 days of life. Sudden deterioration occurs frequently but is usually due to complications of RDS such as pneumothorax, endotracheal tube displacement, obstruction of the endotracheal tube, or development of a patent ductus arteriosus. In some infants, fluctuations in pulmonary artery pressure caused by arterial constriction also may alter blood gases dramatically. Finally, recovery is preceded by a spontaneous diuresis. In very ill and very immature patients who tend to develop bronchopulmonary dysplasia, a protracted recovery is observed frequently.

## Laboratory Data

Surfactant maturity can be assessed by measurement of the lipid ratio of lecithin to sphingomyelin (L:S ratio); these lipids are present in the amniotic fluid due to a net movement of liquid from the fetal lung into the amniotic cavity. An L:S ratio greater than 2:1 indicates surfactant maturity. During the first 6 hours of postnatal life, this test can also be performed on gastric aspirate as swallowed amniotic fluid compromises the majority of gastric fluid. The "shake test" may also indicate surfactant maturation but is not as accurate as the L:S ratio. More recently the presence of the lipid phosphatidylglycerol (PG) has also been found to correlate better with surfactant maturity than the L:S ratio alone.

*Blood gas analysis* usually reveals hypoxia (an increased alveolar to arterial oxygen gradient) and hypercapnia. Blood analysis should be performed on arterial blood, for the venous or arterialized capillary $Po_2$ does not predict arterial oxygenation. However, as oxygenation is in part determined by cardiac output (oxygen transport = cardiac output × [oxygen bound to hemoglobin + dissolved oxygen]), arterial $Po_2$ in itself will not correctly indicate oxygen delivery. Indwelling arterial lines (umbilical or peripheral) should be used in critically ill infants with RDS for evaluation of Pa$o_2$, particularly those requiring more than 30% supplemental oxygen (see Chapter 5). *Transcutaneous oxygen and carbon dioxide* analysis and pulse oximetry are recently introduced and extremely helpful techniques that should be used in addition to frequent arterial blood gas analysis. Infants with RDS typically have *abnormal pulmonary function* characterized by decreased compliance and increased work of breathing. However, airway resistance is normal.

Radiographic findings are characteristic in infants with RDS (see Chapter 11). With air bronchograms, diffuse alveolar collapse surrounding open bronchi produces a typical reticulogranular pattern that has been described as "ground glass." Diffuse atelectasis also results in decreased lung volume. However, the radiographs are not pathognomonic of RDS as similar findings may also be observed in neonatal pneumonia, particularly pneumonia caused by group B *Streptococcus*. The initial radiograph may show mild disease or even be normal. Radiographic findings worsen during the first 12 to 24 hours of life, particularly when the patient is managed without assisted ventilation.

A differential diagnosis of common disorders that cause respiratory distress in neonates is included in Tables 10–3 and 10–4. Bronchopulmonary dysplasia is discussed in Chapter 13.

## Treatment

### Assisted Ventilation

The mainstay of treatment of infants with RDS consists of oxygen supplementation and assisted ventilation with continuous distending pressure, conventional mechanical ventilation, or high-frequency ventilation (see Chapters 12 and 14).

### Surfactant

After the observations that RDS was associated with deficiency or inactivation of lung surfactant, efforts were made to treat neonates with surfactant replacement. Initial studies were unsuccessful, but only the phospholipid components of surfactant, dipalmitoyl-phosphatidylcholine and phosphatidylglycerol, were administered. Recent studies have shown that natural lung surfactant is a mixture of various phospholipids and proteins, but the exact components of lung surfactant that are responsible for the surface-active, adsorptive, and spreadable properties have not yet been determined. Proteins are thought to constitute an essential component, as they may be responsible for modulating surface properties. This lack of understanding has delayed the development and application of effective surfactant replacement preparations. In addition, the optimal mode of delivery (aerosol vs. direct

**TABLE 10–3.**
Differential Diagnosis of the Common Pulmonary Disorders That Cause Respiratory Distress During the First Days of Life

| | Respiratory Distress Syndrome | Transient Tachypnea of the Newborn | Meconium Aspiration | Congenital Pneumonia | Pneumothorax | Persistent Fetal Circulation |
|---|---|---|---|---|---|---|
| Etiology | Surfactant deficiency | Increased lung fluid | Chemical pneumonitis; ball-valve effect | Maternal infection | Air dissection | Pulmonary artery hypertension |
| Predisposing factors | Prematurity | Cesarean section | Passage of meconium with asphyxia | Prolonged rupture of membranes; maternal infection | Resuscitation; renal anomalies | Chronic or acute asphyxia |
| Prominent clinical features | Multiple signs of respiratory distress | Tachypnea | Chest overinflation | Shock; sepsis; metabolic acidosis; neutropenia | Sudden deterioration | Severe hypoxemia with instability |
| Chest radiograph | Reticulogranular appearance; underinflation; air bronchogram | Increased lung fluid and vascular markings | Bilateral infiltrates; overinflation | Diffuse alveolar densities; infiltrates; RDS-like | Free air in pleural space | Hypoperfusion |
| Treatment | CPAP; assisted ventilation with marked $O_2$ supplementation | None or minimal oxygen supplementation | Mild to marked $O_2$ supplementation and assisted ventilation | Mild to marked $O_2$ supplementation and assisted ventilation | Evacuation of air | Hyperventilation and alkalosis |
| Prognosis (mortality) | ~10% | ~0% | ~10% | ~30% | ~0% | ~40%–50% |

**TABLE 10–4.**
Differential Diagnosis of Chronic Respiratory Distress in Neonates

| | Bronchopulmonary Dysplasia | Pneumonia | Wilson-Mikity Syndrome | Chronic Pulmonary Insufficiency | Aspiration Pneumonia |
|---|---|---|---|---|---|
| Etiology | Barotrauma; oxygen toxicity | Bacterial; fungal; viral | Unknown | Diffuse alveolar collapse | Milk aspiration |
| Predisposing factors | Ventilatory therapy | Prematurity | Prematurity; infections? | Prematurity; compliant chest wall? surfactant deficiency? | Recurrent apnea; gastroesophageal reflux |
| Prominent clinical features | Chronic respiratory distress | Sepsis; apnea | Tachypnea | Tachypnea | Apnea |
| Chest radiograph | Cystic lucencies with atelectatic areas | Bilateral infiltrates | BPD-like* | RDS-like | Right upper lobe infiltrates |
| Treatment | Ventilatory support; $O_2$ supplementation; steroids; fluid restriction and diuretics | Antibiotics; antifungal therapy | Nonspecific | Continuous distending pressure | Prevent recurrences; antibiotics? |

*BPD = bronchopulmonary dysplasia

tracheal instillation), time of initial treatment (before the first breath vs. during the course of worsening RDS), and frequency of treatment are unknown at this moment.

In initial clinical trials, administration of natural surfactant to neonates who have clinical signs of RDS, or as prophylactic treatment of asymptomatic premature infants who are at high risk for RDS, usually has produced a milder clinical course.[8-12] Most studies have shown that surfactant treatment improves gas exchange, and treated infants require lower airway pressures and oxygen supplementation than control infants; long-term improvement was not always observed. A recent randomized, controlled trial revealed that in addition to improved gas exchange, there was lower mortality and morbidity due to bronchopulmonary dysplasia, pneumothorax, and interstitial emphysema.[13] One complication of surfactant treatment may be the development of a hemodynamically significant patent ductus arteriosus. However, other potential complications such as infection and immunologic reactions, which were feared, have not been observed. It is likely that surfactant will be a useful adjunct in the care of preterm infants for treatment or even prevention of severe RDS.

### Nonrespiratory Care

Other aspects of neonatal care may be particularly important in patients with RDS (Table 10–5). The ductus arteriosus is normally patent in very premature infants but frequently becomes symptomatic and complicates the course of RDS. In the asymptomatic patient, the presence of a murmur of a patent ductus arteriosus does not require intervention. If the expected recovery of a ventilated patient with RDS does not occur at 3 to 4 days of life, a patent ductus arteriosus should be suspected, particularly when signs of fluid overload such as excessive weight gain, hepatomegaly, or pulmonary edema are present. Fluid restriction, indomethacin therapy (see Chapter 9), or surgical ligation may be necessary to treat patients with a hemodynamically significant

**TABLE 10–5.**
Nonrespiratory Care of Infants With Respiratory Distress Syndrome

Prevention and treatment of patent ductus arteriosus
Temperature regulation
Maintenance of fluid balance
Maintenance of blood pressure
Adequate caloric intake
Prevention of severe anemia
Treatment of metabolic acidosis
Antibiotic therapy
Minimal stimulation

patent ductus arteriosus. Placing the infant in a neutral thermal environment (the thermal conditions at which metabolic demands are the lowest) reduces metabolism, oxygen and caloric consumption, and carbon dioxide production. This is usually accomplished by maintaining the infant's skin temperature at 36.5°C (98°F). However, overheating as well as cooling of the infant will increase metabolism. Adequate fluid intake will prevent dehydration, while fluid overload impairs gas exchange. In addition, it is important to maintain adequate blood pressure, blood volume, and caloric intake. Packed red blood cell transfusions may be required to prevent severe anemia, particularly in the presence of bleeding or frequent blood drawing. Sodium bicarbonate infusions are needed if severe metabolic acidosis ensues. Antibiotics are initially indicated in most infants with RDS because the clinical and radiographic findings may be indistinguishable from bacterial pneumonia, particularly group B streptococcal pneumonia. Finally, minimal stimulation and handling may be appropriate, as such minor interventions as changing a diaper or stroking the infant may be followed by blood gas deterioration.[14]

The prognosis of infants with RDS is as variable as the severity of the original disease. Mildly ill infants who do not require assisted ventilation have an early resolution without sequelae. However, air leaks and bronchopulmonary dysplasia frequently complicate the clinical course in critically ill and very immature infants (see Chapter 13). Despite the improved survival of infants with RDS, this condition remains the leading cause of neonatal mortality and morbidity. Survivors of severe RDS require frequent hospitalizations for upper respiratory tract infections and have persistently abnormal pulmonary function primarily related to increased airway resistance, and an increased incidence of neurodevelopmental sequelae.

## TRANSIENT TACHYPNEA OF THE NEWBORN

Transient tachypnea of the newborn (TTN) occurs most commonly in infants born by cesarean section. It is manifested by tachypnea, frequently without other signs of respiratory distress. Cyanosis and hypercapnia are not prominent features, although a few infants may require up to 35% to 40% oxygen. Assisted ventilation is usually not necessary. The chest radiograph may show increased lung fluid, including fluid in the fissures. Vascular markings may be prominent. The pathogenesis is unclear, but it appears to be secondary to increased lung fluid. Tachypnea usually resolves by the first to third day of life without any sequelae.

## MECONIUM ASPIRATION

Meconium-stained amniotic fluid is present in about 10% to 15% of all deliveries, particularly at term or post-term. Intrauterine passage of meconium may be a sign of fetal distress, especially when it is accompanied by pathologic fetal heart rate decelerations or fetal acidosis (see Chapter 3). Therefore, if meconium is noticed during labor, preparations must be made so that, if needed, prompt resuscitation can be performed at birth. Nasopharyngeal and oropharyngeal suctioning using a DeLee catheter before delivery of the thorax and the first cry is important to reduce the risk of postnatal aspiration.[15] Immediately after the infant is born, direct laryngoscopy with endotracheal intubation should be performed and meconium aspirated from the trachea.[16, 17] This procedure should be rapidly and skillfully repeated until the trachea has been cleared and further resuscitation can commence. Repeated suctioning is rarely necessary. The presence of meconium in the trachea does not imply subsequent respiratory problems. Gregory et al.[16] reported that while meconium was aspirated from the trachea of 56% of all infants who were born covered with meconium, only half of these had abnormal radiographic changes, and one third became sick. None of the infants without meconium in the trachea became sick, although some did have radiographic changes. In another study of meconium-stained infants, a significant decrease in neonatal mortality was observed in the group that received endotracheal suctioning at birth. However, a recent study suggests that endotracheal suctioning in meconium-stained infants without evidence of prenatal asphyxia may be unnecessary.[18] At the present time, we recommend that the oropharynx be suctioned after delivery of the infant's head, but prior to delivery of the body. In addition, after delivery is completed, the trachea should be intubated and cleared of meconium by direct aspiration.

Two overlapping clinical presentations have been observed in symptomatic infants who pass meconium before birth. Some infants in whom pneumonitis secondary to aspirated meconium predominates develop respiratory distress with tachypnea, patchy infiltrates on radiographic examination, and an oxygen requirement. Pulmonary air leaks are a common complication in infants with *meconium aspiration pneumonia*. Meconium is thought to obstruct the distal airways and act as a ball valve that allows air to enter during inspiration but obstructs air outflow during expiration. This may contribute to air trapping and alveolar rupture. Although an inflammatory process occurs, there is no place for systemic glucocorticoids in the management of pneumonitis that accompanies this disorder.[19]

In contrast, a second group of infants presents primarily with severe hypoxemia, frequently out of proportion to the degree of disease seen on chest radiographs. The term *persistent fetal circulation* (PFC) has been coined for this clinical presentation, but as discussed later, this entity has many other underlying etiologies in addition to meconium aspiration.

## CONGENITAL PNEUMONIA

Congenital pneumonia is another common cause of respiratory distress in the first days of life. Frequently, signs of respiratory distress, especially grunting, are accompanied by temperature instability, apnea, hypotension, and other signs of sepsis. Laboratory studies may show evidence of infection, including high or low white blood cell count, increased numbers of immature neutrophils, and marked metabolic acidosis. Group B streptococcal pneumonia, a frequent cause of bacterial pneumonia in neonates, may present soon after birth with radiographic evidence of patchy infiltrates or a diffuse granular process indistinguishable from RDS. This has prompted administration of antibiotics to many neonates with respiratory distress until a bacterial etiology can be excluded. *Listeria monocytogenes* pneumonia may have the same clinical presentation as streptococcal pneumonia. Gram-negative bacilli, especially *Escherichia coli* and *Klebsiella*, also are occasionally acquired prenatally or intrapartum and manifest during the first 3 days of life. *Pseudomonas aeruginosa* is a common pathogen when prolonged respiratory therapy has been required. Fungal pneumonia, especially due to *Candida albicans*, is seen in very low birth weight infants with prolonged hospitalization or antibiotic treatment but may also present at birth when prolonged rupture of the membranes has occurred. Viral pneumonias may be congenital but are most frequently acquired postnatally. Although *chlamydial* infection occurs in the perinatal period, pneumonitis usually presents after the third week of life.

Bacterial pneumonia in the initial neonatal period may be appropriately treated with a penicillin (penicillin or ampicillin) together with an aminoglycoside (gentamicin or kanamycin) until the pathogen is identified. Later, the possibility of other pathogens, such as *Staphylococcus epidermidis* and *C. albicans*, may necessitate modification of this antibiotic therapy.

## PNEUMOTHORAX AND OTHER AIR LEAK SYNDROMES

An *asymptomatic pneumothorax* is found in about 1% of all routine newborn chest radiographic examinations. Considering the very high intrathoracic pressures that occur during the first minutes of life, it is surprising that pneumothorax is not a more frequent occurrence. Pneumothorax and other air leak syndromes are common complications in infants with RDS occurring in as many as one third of those requiring assisted ventilation. In infants with meconium aspiration syndrome, the incidence of air leaks may be even higher.

Macklin[20] described the path of the air after rupture: air from the ruptured alveolus dissects up the vascular sheath into the mediastinum and from there may continue into the pleural or pericardial cavities. In some series, as many as half of the patients symptomatic with a pneumothorax had aspirated meconium or blood. This suggests that obstruction with a ball-valve action may be the basis for the rupture.

*Pneumothorax* should be suspected in any newborn with respiratory distress, or in a baby whose condition suddenly worsens while on a respirator. Cyanosis, tachypnea, grunting, and flaring of the nares are often observed. Percussion of the chest is sometimes helpful, but a shift of the apical impulse is usually more easily noted. Auscultation may be misleading because of the wide referral of breath sounds. Hypotension may be present. The sudden onset of a tense, distended abdomen is often a useful clinical feature signifying a *pneumoperitoneum*, which may accompany a pneumothorax.

If the pneumothorax is asymptomatic and the infant is free of underlying respiratory disease, no specific therapy is necessary; however, color, heart rate, respiratory rate, and blood pressure should be closely observed. If respiratory distress is noted, a thoracostomy tube should be placed in the mid axillary or anterior axillary line. Effective evacuation of a pneumothorax depends on achieving anterior placement of the tip of the thoracostomy tube as free air will rise anteriorly in a supine infant (see Chapter 5). Lung perforation, a major complication of thoracostomy, may occur in as many as 25% of treated infants and can be prevented in part, by careful insertion technique, without the use of a trocar. Partial obstruction of the thoracic aorta may be observed when a posterior chest tube pushes on mediastinal structures. Obstruction may be suspected when tachycardia, along with decreased lower extremity pulses are seen soon after chest tube placement.

*Pulmonary interstitial emphysema* and *pneumomediastinum* do not require evacuation but should alert the clinician to the possibility of other subsequent air leaks, and efforts should be aimed at reducing barotrauma. Selective bronchial intubation of the nonemphysematous side has been performed in the treatment of interstitial emphysema.[21] *Pneumopericardium*, on the other hand, has specific clinical manifestations including hypotension, muffled heart sounds, and decreased pulse pressure. Evacuation is required to prevent impaired cardiac output. Massive *air embolism* into the vascular system usually presents with rapid cardiopulmonary deterioration, and air bubbles may be observed in blood obtained from indwelling arterial catheters in patients ventilated at extremely high pressures. Inspired oxygen concentration should be increased to 1.0 as oxygen can be absorbed faster than nitrogen. However, there is no specific treatment, and death usually occurs during the episode.

Use of a high-intensity transilluminating light with a fiberoptic probe is especially helpful in quickly diagnosing a pneumothorax. If the infant's clinical condition is relatively stable, it is wise to confirm the diagnosis radiographically prior to treatment.

## PERSISTENT FETAL CIRCULATION

Persistent fetal circulation (PFC) is a condition that manifests as severe reversible hypoxemia secondary to pulmonary artery hypertension with right-to-left shunting in the absence of structural heart disease. Persistent pulmonary hypertension of the newborn (PPHN) is an alternative name for this condition. Persistent fetal circulation can be associated with pulmonary diseases such as pneumonia, meconium aspiration or hypoplastic lungs; with metabolic disturbances such as hypoglycemia, hypocalcemia, or polycythemia; with sepsis, congenital heart disease or birth asphyxia. The common underlying pathophysiologic process involves an abnormal elevation of pulmonary vascular resistance with consequent extrapulmonary right-to-left shunt through the foramen ovale and the ductus arteriosus. Recently, increased muscularization of the pulmonary vessels has been observed in infants with PFC who died very early in the neonatal period, implying that the process started prenatally.[22]

The diagnosis of PFC may be supported by echocardiography with the observation of an increased ratio of systolic pre-ejection period to ejection time of the pulmonary valve, and the finding of right-to-left shunt at the foramen ovale.[23] An echocardiogram is also useful to exclude structural heart disease. Nonetheless, similar findings may be observed in other neonatal respiratory disorders such as RDS in which pulmonary hypertension may be present. A gradient between preductal and postductal $PaO_2$ can be observed by transcutaneous monitoring when the right-to-left shunt is occurring at the ductus arteriosus and by this means progression of the disease can be followed. Marked fluctuations of $Pa_{O_2}$ even in the absence of this preductal to postductal gradient suggest a variable shunt and exclude a fixed anatomical lesion of the heart.

Some mildly ill infants respond to supplemental oxygen but most patients with PFC require assisted ventilation. Respiratory or metabolic alkalosis decreases pulmonary vascular resistance, and hyperventilation may be beneficial in the infant with a poor response to conventional assisted ventilation. *Hyperventilation* to the point at which the $Pa_{CO_2}$ is decreased to 20 to 25 mm Hg and the pH is increased to 7.55 to 7.6 may be required, but the potential risk of decreased cerebral perfusion must be considered.[24] Sodium bicarbonate is a useful adjunct for achieving sufficient *alkalinization* without severe hyperventilation and barotrauma.[25] Deafness has recently been reported to be a side effect in patients receiving prolonged hyperventilation together with furosemide therapy.[26] Nonetheless, long-term outlook in these patients probably depends to a large extent on the severity of the initial asphyxial insult.[27]

*Vasodilator therapy* (e.g., tolazoline) has been effective in some intractable cases. Tolazoline may be used as a rapid infusion of 1 to 2 mg/kg followed by a maintenance infusion of 1 to 2 mg/kg/hour.[26] Continuous $Pa_{O_2}$ monitoring must be employed. Improved oxygenation is sometimes seen immediately after tolazoline is given, but many infants develop hypotension and hemorrhagic manifestations. Impaired renal function is also common. Selective pulmonary vasodilators such as prostaglandin $I_2$ and $D_2$ are presently under evaluation to determine their usefulness in PFC. Sodium nitroprusside, a systemic vasodilator, may also reduce pulmonary artery resistance and increase $Pa_{O_2}$ in some infants with PFC.[28] Recently, the use of *inotropic agents* (e.g., dopamine) has been proposed to increase systemic vascular resistance and to reduce the right-to-left shunting.[26] *High-frequency ventilation* has been found to be of no benefit in an animal model of meconium aspiration, but insufficient human data are presently available (see Chapter 14). In a recent clinical study, term infants with intractable respiratory failure, in some cases secondary to PFC, were successfully treated with *extracorporeal membrane oxygenation*[29] (see Chapter 15).

During the first hours and days of life, there is marked lability of oxygenation. During this period, aggressive therapy, in particular alkalinization, is required and cautious weaning of the ventilatory support is recommended. However, at around 2 to 6 days of life, oxygenation becomes more stable, and only small changes in $Pa_{O_2}$ occur in response to reduction of hyperventilation.[30] After this *transitional phase*, the infant should be weaned from ventilatory support to prevent lung injury. A higher partial pressure of $CO_2$ in arterial blood ($Pa_{CO_2}$) is frequently well tolerated by the patients. However, mortality remains up to 50% despite aggressive treatment. Recently in two uncontrolled studies, a conservative ventilatory approach to the treatment of infants with PFC has been reported to be very successful.[31, 32] These investigators reported 100% survival by maintaining a Pa$O_2$ of 50 to 70 mm Hg and allowing the Pa$_{CO_2}$ to increase up to 60 mm Hg. Further studies are certainly needed to determine the strategies of ventilatory care that optimize gas exchange in patients with PFC.

## OTHER CAUSES OF RESPIRATORY DISTRESS

The vast majority of admissions to a neonatal intensive care unit are prompted by respiratory difficulties. Most of these infants will prove ultimately to have pulmonary parenchymal disease. However, a small number will have respiratory embarrassment resulting from extrapulmonary disorders. Failure to recognize the possibility of nonpulmonary causes of respiratory distress may lead to serious therapeutic errors.

The exchange of gases that occur at the alveolar capillary interface is only a small component of the numerous steps needed to ensure adequate oxygen delivery to peripheral tissues. Neural signals generated in the central nervous system must travel over intact peripheral nerves to activate the musculature of the chest wall and diaphragm. The bony thorax structure must be mobile and of normal configuration before airflow occurs via unobstructed upper airways. Following gas exchange, sufficient hemoglobin of a normal structure must be available to bind oxygen for transport. Finally, the heart must be structurally and functionally capable of adequate output to ensure oxygen delivery to peripheral tissues. A failure in any of these systems may present as respiratory embarrassment. Fanaroff and Martin have proposed a schema for evaluation of extrapulmonary causes of respiratory distress (Table 10–6).

### Central Nervous System

Respiratory difficulties due to intracranial pathology are related usually to *perinatal asphyxia* or to *intracranial hemorrhage*. Infants suffering from perinatal asphyxia frequently are at term gestation or post-term while infants with intracerebral hemorrhage are more often preterm. A history of difficult labor, fetal distress, meconium-stained amniotic fluid, and low Apgar scores may be obtained. The infants present with a wide range of respiratory symptoms including apnea, periodic breathing, and tachypnea. Abnormal respiratory patterns are seen in more severely affected infants, while infants who are mildly ill may only show tachypnea. The chest x-ray is normal. Arterial blood gas analysis demonstrates a primary respiratory alkalosis. In infants with hemorrhage that is sufficiently large to lead to intravascular hypovolemia, a metabolic acidosis may also be present. Radiographic studies of the brain, either ultrasound or computerized tomographic scan, will confirm the diagnosis.

*Central nervous system depression* leading to apnea may result from transplacental passage of medications administered to the mother. A thorough review of the maternal history should be obtained in all depressed infants. Magnesium sulfate and opiate analgesics are the most frequently encountered respiratory depressants in the delivery suite. Naloxone (0.01 mg/kg per dose) may reverse the respiratory depression induced by narcotics. However, its half-life is shorter than that of morphine, and therefore repeated administration of naloxone or respiratory support with mechanical assisted ventilation may be needed until the morphine is fully metabolized. Infants born to mothers who are addicted to narcotics rarely exhibit respiratory depression. When withdrawal begins, respiratory symptoms of tachypnea, yawning, and sneezing predominate.

**TABLE 10–6.**
Extrapulmonary Causes of Respiratory Distress

Neuromuscular disorders
   Central nervous system disorders
   Spinal cord injury
   Motor end-plate disease
   Muscle disease
Hematologic disorders
   Anemia
   Polycythemia
   Methemoglobinemia
Disorders of the respiratory apparatus
   Upper airway anomalies
   Rib cage abnormalities
   Diaphragmatic dysfunction
Cardiovascular
   Congenital structural heart disease
   Congestive heart failure

Adapted from Fanaroff AA, Martin RJ: Extrapulmonary causes of respiratory distress, in Stern L (ed): *Diagnosis and Management of Respiratory Disorders in the Newborn.* Menlo Park, Calif, Addison-Wesley Publishing, 1983.

## Spinal Cord Disease

The most common disorder of the spinal cord seen in infants is injury that occurs following excessive traction or torsion of the spine. Seventy-five percent of recognized neonatal *spinal injuries* are associated with breech deliveries. Usually an audible "snap" has been heard at delivery. The lesion is most commonly found in the lower cervical or high thoracic area. Cephalic deliveries may also be associated with cord injuries, particularly following extreme rotational maneuvers such as rotation of the head with forceps. This is usually associated with injury in the high or midcervical spine. The cord may be *edematous* and *hemorrhagic* or may be *completely transected*.

The clinical presentation of the infant varies with the level of the lesion. Frequently the infant is depressed at birth, often with delayed or absent respiratory effort. Lower lesions may lead to feeble respiratory efforts, associated with phrenic nerve paralysis and elevation of the abdomen on inspiration. If unsupported, this may lead to death in the first days of life. Death may be delayed by mechanical ventilation leading to major ethical dilemmas.

## Lower Motor Neuron Disease

Disorders affecting the lower motor neuron are the most frequent causes of severe hypotonia and weakness in the neonatal period. The major disorders in this group that present with respiratory symptoms include Werdnig-Hoffmann disease, Pompe's disease, and neonatal poliomyelitis.[33] *Werdnig-Hoffmann disease* is the most common and most important. The disorder is an autosomal recessively inherited form of severe, infantile anterior horn cell degeneration. Respiratory distress is apparent at birth or within the first 2 months of life. Frequently, the infant's mother will report decreased and weak fetal movements. The infants are hypotonic and areflexic. The clinical course is characterized by inexorable deterioration and death; 60% die within 1 year and 80% by 4 years.[34] Infants with *Pompe's disease* also present with weakness and progressive respiratory complications, but usually become ill later in the neonatal period. The presence of cardiac involvement, a large tongue, and prominent skeletal muscles due to glycogen deposition distinguish it from Werdnig-Hoffmann's disease. Infection with *poliomyelitis* in utero may lead to the birth of an affected infant. Patients present with diffuse flaccid paralysis and respiratory failure. The diagnosis is made by isolation of the virus from the stool. Frequently cerebral spinal fluid shows pleocytosis.

## Disorders of the Neuromuscular Junction

Disorders of the neuromuscular junction are infrequent causes of neonatal hypotonia and weakness. However, these disorders are critical to recognize as therapeutic intervention may be lifesaving. Included in this group of disorders is congenital myasthenia gravis, transient neonatal myasthenia gravis, and infantile botulism. *Congenital myasthenia gravis* results from inherited, nonreversible defects of neuromuscular transmission. *Transient myasthenia gravis* occurs in 10% to 15% of infants born to myasthenic mothers in which anti-acetylcholine receptor antibody has traversed the placenta. Onset of weakness and hypotonia occurs within hours of birth in two out of three cases. The diagnosis can be made at the bedside by administration of neostigmine, 0.1 mg/kg, intramuscularly, with maximal improvement within 30 minutes. Most infants will require anticholinesterase therapy. The mean duration of illness is 18 days.[35]

*Infantile botulinum* is the result of intestinal infection with *Clostridium botulinum* in contrast to adult forms of the disorder in which ingestion of preformed toxin is the usual cause. Ingestion of honey that harbors *C. botulinum* spores is a common cause. Most cases described have occurred after the neonatal period, but some have presented in the first month. Feeding difficulties and constipation are the presenting problems, followed by a progressive cephalocaudal paralysis. Most infants require mechanical ventilator support for a number of months. No specific therapy is available.

## Muscle Disorders

A large number of different disorders of muscle account for a substantial number of infants with hypotonia and weakness. *Myotonic dystrophy*, an inherited defect transmitted by the mother, is the most frequently observed disorder. Occasionally, the mother is unaware that she has the disease, but the alert clinician may recognize typical facies characterized by wasting of the masseter and temporalis muscles, ptosis, and a straight stiff smile. Polyhydramnios, due to impaired swallowing of amniotic fluid, is frequently seen prenatally. Respiratory compromise may be so marked that the infant fails to establish effective respiration at birth. The resultant asphyxia may mask the myotonic dystrophy. Approximately 50% of severely affected infants die in the neonatal period; less severely affected neonates may present later in the first year of life and survive into young adulthood. There is no laboratory test that is diagnostic, and electromyographic changes may be difficult to detect in the neonatal period. Several other myopathies can also lead to respiratory failure in the neonatal period including nemaline myopathy, myotubular myopathy, and infantile cytochrome c oxidase deficiency.

## Disorders of the Respiratory Apparatus

### Obstruction of the Upper Airway

These occur infrequently but can present dramatically and cause significant respiratory distress (see Chapter 4).

### Rib Cage Abnormalities

This group of rare conditions may cause respiratory distress by causing hypoplasia of the ribs leading to restriction of thoracic volume.[36] Diseases associated with hypoplasia of the ribs include *asphyxiating thoracic dystrophy* (Jeune's syndrome), *thanatophoric dwarfism, achondrogenesis, achondroplasia, osteogenesis imperfecta, Ellis-van Creveld syndrome,* and *hypophosphatasia.* Asphyxia and respiratory distress are present from birth. The infants are cyanotic, tachypneic, and in marked respiratory distress. Physical examination reveals extreme narrowing of the thorax, short ribs, and a characteristically immobile chest wall. Jeune's syndrome, thanatophoric dwarfism, and achondroplasia are associated with short limb dwarfism. Infants with osteogenesis imperfecta or hypophosphatasia have demineralized bones and multiple fractures present on skeletal radiographs.

### Diaphragmatic Disorders

Diaphragmatic disorders may result from *phrenic nerve injury* that most frequently occurs in the setting of difficult obstetric deliveries of large infants, or those in breech presentation. An associated brachial plexus injury occurs in 80% of affected newborns. Fractures of the humerus or clavicle may further testify to the traumatic nature of the birth. Lateral traction of the neck may lead to avulsion or partial disruption of cervical nerve roots 3 to 5. Phrenic nerve injury may be unilateral or bilateral. In unilateral lesions, mortality is approximately 10%; most of these can be prevented with prompt supportive care. Most infants recover in the first 12 months of life. In infants with bilateral lesions, mortality is nearly 50%.[37] Infants typically present with tachypnea, hypoxia, and hypercapnia in the first hours after birth, and with supplemental oxygen and ventilator support, they gradually improve. The diagnosis of diaphragmatic paralysis may be missed on radiographic exams as elevation of the hemidiaphragm may not be present early in the course.

Compromise of diaphragmatic motion may also occur when marked *abdominal distention* occurs in the setting of hydrops fetalis, ascites, or necrotizing enterocolitis. Paracentesis may improve respiratory function if a fluid collection is present. Significant respiratory impairment may occur following repair of a diaphragmatic hernia, gastroschisis, or omphalocele as abdominal distention is created when the visceral contents are returned to the abdominal cavity. Orogastric tubes that maintain gastric decompression may minimize these problems.

**Hematologic Disorders**

Both *anemia* and *polycythemia* can lead to respiratory difficulties in the neonate. Infants who suffer acute blood loss may present with classic signs of shock: tachycardia, pallor, poor perfusion, as well as signs of respiratory distress. Immediate blood transfusion is indicated. Chronic blood loss may occur so slowly that adequate intravascular volume is maintained. These infants will have pallor but minimal respiratory symptoms. Transfusion in these circumstances is less urgent.

*Polycythemia*, a central venous hematocrit in excess of 65%, may be associated with many undesirable symptoms in the newborn infant. Infants may present with cyanosis, irritability, seizures, feeding intolerance, and signs of respiratory distress. Symptoms are thought to relate to hyperviscosity associated with the elevated hematocrit and therefore poor blood flow in microcirculations. Cyanosis may occur in the face of normal oxygen tension, as even a normal saturation may lead to more than 3 gm of desaturated hemoglobin, the level at which cyanosis may first be clinically detectable. Symptomatic infants with central venous hematocrits greater than 65% may be treated with a partial exchange transfusion with the goal of reducing the hematocrit to approximately 55%. Dramatic resolution of symptoms is noted after reduction of the hematocrit.

A rare hematologic cause of neonatal respiratory distress is *methemoglobinemia*, which is an otherwise normal hemoglobin in which the iron is oxidized and therefore unable to carry oxygen. This may occur as a congenital enzyme defect or as the result of exposure to oxidant stresses that increase the levels of methemoglobin. When greater than 10% of hemoglobin is present as methemoglobin, the skin becomes dusky, and the blood is a brown color; no improvement is seen with high concentrations of oxygen. A bedside diagnosis can be made by placing a drop of the infant's blood and that of a normal control on filter paper that is exposed to room air. Normal hemoglobin should turn red, while blood with high levels of methemoglobin remains brown. Treatment requires elimination of sources of oxidant stress and administration of methylene blue, 1 to 2 mg/kg intravenously. Improvement occurs within 1 to 2 hours. Failure of response suggests the presence of abnormal hemoglobins, which can be confirmed by electrophoresis.

**Cardiovascular Disorders**

The problem of differentiating lung and heart disease occurs frequently in the neonate. Congenital structural cardiac defects that cause cyanosis and respiratory distress may be classified as having inadequate or torrential pulmonary blood flow. The most common lesions associated with a right-to-left shunt and *inadequate pulmonary blood flow* include tetralogy of Fallot, pulmonary atresia or stenosis, and tricuspid atresia or stenosis. Lesions associated with cyanosis in the face of *torrential pulmonary blood flow* include transposition of the great vessels, hypoplastic left heart syndrome, critical coarctation of the aorta, total anomalous pulmonary venous return, truncus arteriosus, and atrioventricular canal. In the first group of lesions the $PaO_2$ does not improve when the infant breathes 100% oxygen, while in the second group mild improvement may occur. Two-dimensional echocardiography can rapidly distinguish between these lesions.

Two commonly seen noncyanotic lesions with left-to-right shunt, patent ductus arteriosus (PDA) and ventricular septal defects (VSD), may be associated with cyanosis. Patent ductus arteriosus can occur at anytime in the neonatal period and usually manifests with respiratory distress but without cyanosis. However, infants with VSD present with respiratory distress but no cyanosis late in the neonatal period when pulmonary resistance falls and blood shunts left to right. When pulmonary hypertension is present, blood is shunted right to left through these lesions, and cyanosis occurs.

Respiratory distress may also occur in neonates who have structurally normal but functionally abnormal hearts that are failing. This may occur with *viral or bacterial myocarditis, endocardial fibroelastosis,* or *glycogen storage disease.* A variety of arrythmias may also precipitate heart failure; the most common are *congenital heart block* and *prolonged supraventricular tachycardia.* Neonates who may undergo severe *asphyxia* may also present with congestive heart failure due to hypoxic-ischemic damage to the myocardium. Clinically, infants with a failing heart appear lethargic, mottled, and diaphoretic with rapid shallow respirations. The peripheral pulses are barely palpable. The liver is usually massively enlarged, as may be the spleen. On chest x-ray, massive cardiomegaly indicates the diagnosis of congestive heart failure. Prompt and aggressive respiratory and cardiotonic support is needed. Even with this support, mortality is high.

## APNEA

Neonates commonly experience pauses in their breathing of variable duration. Short respiratory pauses (less than 5 to 10 seconds) are usually benign. Short pauses recurring repetitively in a regular pattern are called periodic breathing. This breathing, normal in neonates, is not accompanied by signs of clinical deterioration and requires no treatment. Periods of absent respiration of more than 10 to 15 seconds are generally defined as apneas, particularly if accompanied by bradycardia or cyanosis. Infants under 1,000 gm at birth have apnea during the neonatal period.[38] These infants experience repeated pauses in respiration longer than 10 seconds duration which, when prolonged, are accompanied by a fall in heart rate to less than 100 beats per minute. Significant hypoxia and hypercapnia are associated with prolonged apnea (longer than 15 seconds), necessitating active medical intervention to decrease both the apnea frequency and duration.

Apnea may be associated with such diverse conditions as sepsis, hypoglycemia, intraventricular hemorrhage, hypoxemia, anemia, and maternal drug ingestion (Table 10–7). When such underlying causes are not present, the apnea is presumed to be due to a primary transient disorder of respiratory control (apnea of prematurity) that occurs predominantly during rapid eye movement (REM) sleep. In premature infants, 91% of apneas are characterized by obstruction to airflow at the level of the pharynx.[39] This pharyngeal obstruction may occur at the beginning or end of the apnea (mixed apnea), throughout the apnea (obstructive apnea), or not at all (central apnea).

Apnea in infants may be conveniently detected by continuous car-

**TABLE 10–7.**
Common Problems That May Cause Apnea

| | |
|---|---|
| CNS disorders | Decreased oxygen delivery |
|     Asphyxia/cerebral edema |     Hypoxemia |
|     Hemorrhage |     Anemia |
|     Seizure |     Shock |
|     Malformations | Drugs |
| Metabolic disorders |     Maternal |
|     Hypoglycemia |     Fetal |
|     Hypocalcemia | Infection |
|     Hyponatremia |     Septicemia |
|     Hyperammonemia |     Meningitis |
| Thermal instability |     Pneumonia |
|     Hyperthermia |     Necrotizing enterocolitis |
|     Hypothermia | |
|     Temperature changes | |

diorespiratory impedance monitoring[40] (see Chapter 3). The diagnosis of apnea of prematurity is made only after carefully excluding the specific conditions associated with apnea that were mentioned above. Treatment directed at these underlying conditions results in prompt resolution of apneic episodes.

Several alternative methods for treatment of recurrent apnea of prematurity are currently available. Irregularly oscillating water beds have been found to reduce the frequency of apnea.[41] Theophylline and caffeine are effective respiratory stimulants that may be given either orally or by an intravenous route. Theophylline and its derivatives decrease the number of apneas an infant experiences[42] probably by stimulation of the medullary respiratory control center. In addition, low pressure CPAP (4 to 6 cm $H_2O$) by nasal prongs or endotracheal tube also can reduce the number of apneas with an obstructive component probably by splinting open the pharyngeal airway and preventing its collapse. Treatment for idiopathic apnea of prematurity depends on the severity of the clinical presentation. The occasional occurrence of a short apnea with spontaneous recovery does not require medical intervention. However, when apnea is prolonged, hypoxic depression of the infant's brain may occur, and resuscitative efforts are needed. Tactile stimulation or water beds may be adequate for infants with infrequent or short duration apneas but nasal CPAP of 4 to 5 cm $H_2O$ or theophylline therapy at a serum level of 5 to 10 mg/dl may be required for sicker ones. While CPAP has been shown to preferentially resolve obstructive apnea, theophylline is beneficial for all types of apnea. Severe apneic episodes may require intervention with endotracheal intubation and assisted ventilation.

Fortunately, both the incidence and severity of apneic episodes in premature infants spontaneously decrease with advancing postconceptional age. Rarely will apneic episodes persist in premature infants beyond 37 weeks' postconceptional age.[43] This type of patient may require theophylline therapy as well as home apnea monitoring after discharge from the hospital.

## REFERENCES

1. Lees MH: Cyanosis of the newborn infant. *J Pediatr* 1970; 77:484.
2. Carlo WA, Martin RJ, Florens GA, et al: The effect of respiratory distress syndrome on chest wall movements and respiratory pauses in preterm infants. *Am Rev Respir Dis* 1982; 126:103.
3. Carlo WA, Martin RJ, Bruce EN, et al: Alae nasi activation (nasal flaring) decreases nasal resistance in preterm infants. *Pediatrics* 1983; 72:338.
4. Harrison VC, Hesse H deV, Klein M: The significance of grunting in hyaline membrane disease. *Pediatrics* 1968; 41:549.

5. Berman LS, Fox WW, Rapkally RC, et al: Optimum level of CPAP for tracheal extubation of newborn infants. J Pediatr 1976; 89:109.
6. Perelman RH, Farrell PM: Analysis of causes of neonatal death in the United States with specific emphasis on fatal hyaline membrane disease. Pediatrics 1982; 70:570.
7. Nicks J, Schram M, Schumacher R: Continuous end tidal $CO_2$ monitoring reflects disease severity in newborn RDS. Pediatr Res 1987; 21:461A.
8. Ikegami M, Adams FH, Towers B, et al: The quantity of natural surfactant necessary to prevent the respiratory distress syndrome in premature lambs. Pediatr Res 1980; 14:1082.
9. Enhorning G, Shennan A, Possmayer F, et al: Prevention of neonatal respiratory distress syndrome by tracheal instillation of surfactant: A randomized clinical trial. Pediatrics 1985; 76:145.
10. Hallman M, Merritt TA, Jarvenpaa AL, et al: Exogenous human surfactant for treatment of severe respiratory distress syndrome: A randomized prospective clinical trial. J Pediatr 1985; 106:963.
11. Kwong MS, Egan EA, Notter RH, et al: Double-blind clinical trial of calf lung surfactant extract for the prevention of hyaline membrane disease in extremely premature infants. Pediatrics 1985; 76:585.
12. Gitlin JD, Soil RF, Parad RB, et al: Randomized controlled trial of exogenous surfactant for the treatment of hyaline membrane disease. Pediatrics 1987; 79:31.
13. Merritt TA, Hallman M, Bloom BT, et al: Prophylactic treatment of very premature infants with human surfactant. N Engl J Med 1986; 315:785.
14. Danford DA, Miske S, Headley J, et al: Effects of routine care procedures on transcutaneous oxygen in neonates. Arch Dis Child 1983; 58:20.
15. Carson BS, Losey RW, Bowes WA, et al: Combined obstetric and pediatric approach to prevent meconium aspiration syndrome. Am J Obstet Gynecol 1976; 126:712.
16. Gregory GA, Gooding, CA, Phibbs RH, et al: Meconium aspiration in infants: A prospective study. J Pediatr 1974; 85:848.
17. Ting P, Brady JP: Tracheal suction in meconium aspiration. Am J Obstet Gynecol 1975; 122:767.
18. Linder N, Aranda JV, Tzur M, et al: Is endotracheal intubation and lavage required in meconium-stained neonates? Pediatr Res 1987; 21:458A.
19. Yeh TF, Srinivasan G, Harris V, et al: Hydrocortisone therapy in meconium aspiration syndrome: A controlled study. J Pediatr 1977; 90:140.
20. Macklin CC: Transport of air along sheaths of pulmonic blood vessels from alveoli to mediastinum. Arch Intern Med 1939; 64:913.
21. Brooks JG, Koops BL, Hilton S, et al: Selective bronchial intubation for the treatment of severe localized interstitial emphysema. Pediatr Res 1976; 10:458.
22. Murphy JD, Rabinovitch M, Goldstein JD, et al: The structural basis of persistent pulmonary hypertension of the newborn infant. J Pediatr 1981; 98:962.

23. Riggs T, Hirschfeld S, Fanaroff A, et al: Persistence of fetal circulation syndrome: An echocardiographic study. *J Pediatr* 1977; 91:626.
24. Drummond WH, Gregory GA, Heymann MA, et al: The independent effects of hyperventilation, tolazoline, and dopamine on infants with persistent pulmonary hypertension. *J Pediatr* 1981; 98:603.
25. Lyrene RK, Welch KA, Godoy G, et al: Alkalosis attenuates hypoxic pulmonary vasoconstriction in neonatal lambs. *Pediatr Res* 1985; 19:1268.
26. Hendricks-Munoz K, Walton JP: Hearing loss in infants with PPHN. *Pediatr Res* 1986; 20:379A.
27. Ferrara B, Johnson DE, Change PN, et al: Efficacy and neurologic outcome of profound hypocapneic alkalosis for the treatment of PPHN in infancy. *J Pediatr* 1984; 105:457.
28. Benitz WE, Malachowski N, Cohen RS, et al: Use of sodium nitroprusside in neonates: Efficacy and safety. *J Pediatr* 1985; 106:102.
29. Bartlett RH, Roloff DW, Cornell RG, et al: Extracorporeal circulation in neonatal respiratory failure: A prospective randomized study. *Pediatrics* 1985; 76:479.
30. Sosulki R, Fox WW: Transition phase during hyperventilation therapy for persistent pulmonary hypertension of the neonate. *Crit Care Med* 1985; 13:715.
31. Wung JT, James S, Kilchevsky E, et al: Management of infants with severe respiratory failure and persistence of the fetal circulation, without hyperventilation. *Pediatrics* 1985; 76:488.
32. Dworetz AR, Moya FR, Sabo B, et al: Survival in infants with persistent pulmonary hypertension without extracorporeal membrane oxygenation. *Pediatr Res* 1987; 21:360A.
33. Volpe JJ: *Neurology of the Newborn*, ed 2. WB Saunders Co, Philadelphia, Penn, 1987.
34. Brandt S: *Werdnig-Hoffmann's Progressive Muscular Atrophy*. Ejnar Munksgaard, Copenhagen, 1950.
35. Namba T, Brown SB, Grob D: Neonatal myasthenia gravis: Report of two cases and review of the literature. *Pediatrics* 1970; 45:488.
36. Yang SS, Heidelberger IU, Brough AJ, et al: Lethal short limbed chondrodysplasia in early infancy, in Rosenberg HS, Bolande RP (eds): *Perspectives in Pediatric Pathology*. Year Book Medical Publishers, Chicago, 1976.
37. Yasuda R, Nishoka T, Fukumasu H, et al: Bilateral phrenic nerve palsy in the newborn infant. *J Pediatr* 1976; 89:986.
38. Alden ER, Mandelhorn T, Woodrum DE, et al: Morbidity and mortality of infants weighing less than 1,000 grams in an intensive care nursery. *Pediatrics* 1972; 50:40.
39. Miller MJ, Carlo WA, Martin RJ: Continuous positive pressure selectively reduces obstruction apnea in preterm infants. *J Pediatr* 1985; 106:91.
40. Stein JM, Shannon DC: The pediatric pneumogram: A new method for detecting and quantitating apnea in infants. *Pediatrics* 1975; 55:599.
41. Korner AF, Kraemer HC, Haffner ME, et al.: Effects of waterbed flotation on premature infants: A pilot study. *Pediatrics* 1975; 56:361.

42. Kuzemko JA, Paala J: Apnoeic attacks in the newborn treated with aminophylline. Arch Dis Child 1973; 48:404.

# 11

# Radiologic Findings of Newborn Respiratory Diseases

Stuart C. Morrison, M.B., Ch.B., M.R.C.P.

## BASIC RADIOGRAPHIC CONCEPTS

Radiographs (x-rays) are produced in the x-ray or cathode ray tube by bombardment of a metallic (usually tungsten) anode with electrons. The x-ray beam is then narrowed or collimated to the size of the anatomical area to be x-rayed. A film inside a cassette is placed behind the patient, exposed, and then developed chemically to provide a permanent record.

The film obtained is a photographic negative. Intensifying screens are also present within the cassette that holds the film. The function of the intensifying screens is to convert the x-rays to light. The light then exposes the film in a manner similar to the principle of a camera. By using intensifying screens that produce greater amounts of light, the amount of x-rays used can be decreased. Newer rare earth screens can convert x-rays to more light photons and reduce the dose to the patient further.

The number of x-ray photons produced by the x-ray tube is governed by the amount of *current* flowing through the tube. This is measured in milliamperes. The higher the milliamperes, the greater the number of x-ray photons produced with a corresponding increase in the film density. Another way to increase film density is to have a longer exposure time, but any motion will produce a blurred image. For infants whose respiratory rates may well reach 100 breaths per minute, this means that the *exposure time* must be very short. The energy of the x-ray photons is determined by the *kilovoltage* applied across the x-ray or cathode-ray tube. This is measured as the peak kilovoltage (kVp). The higher this value, the more energetic the x-ray photons and the more penetrating they become. Neonates, because of their small size and the large amount of air in the lungs that attenuates the x-rays very little, need low peak kilovoltage such as 55 or 60 kVp. A typical exposure time is 10 msec, but the portable x-ray machine always combines the exposure time with the milliamperes so that a typical exposure for a neonatal chest would be 1 mamp-sec.

The routine frontal chest x-ray in neonates is always obtained with the x-ray beam entering the anterior surface of the chest and exiting posteriorly to expose the posteriorly positioned film. This projection is commonly referred to as anteroposterior (AP) position. As the neonate is supine, the x-ray beam is in a vertical orientation or at right angles to the ground. A right or left lateral view of the chest refers to the position of the film (which is enclosed within the cassette). A left lateral projection has the film on the left side of the chest. With this projection, the x-ray beam is parallel to the floor or ground. This view is also sometimes called a cross-table lateral view. For a decubitus view, the infant has to be turned onto its side. With a left lateral decubitus view, the left lateral chest wall is dependent or on the inferior surface closest to the ground. This view is especially helpful to demonstrate or show changes in position of pleural air or pleural fluid.

Infants can easily be x-rayed without being moved from the incubator. The Plexiglas or Lucite of the incubator is not visible on the x-ray. Occasionally, a hole in the incubator can produce an artifact on the x-ray film, and this very round lucency should never be mistaken for an abnormal gas collection of extraventilatory air. Scatter of x-rays to personnel in the nursery can be reduced substantially by increasing the distance from the x-ray tube.[1] For example, doubling the distance from an x-ray tube will reduce the dose to one quarter. If an infant needs to be restrained, then a lead apron and glove must be worn. The dosage to the infant can be reduced by proper collimation of the x-ray beam to the area of concern and a fast recording system that includes fast film and intensifying screens. Most importantly, there should be a clear indication for the x-ray and the possibility of altering patient management according to the radiographic finding. Routine lateral films of infants are not necessary and should not be obtained.

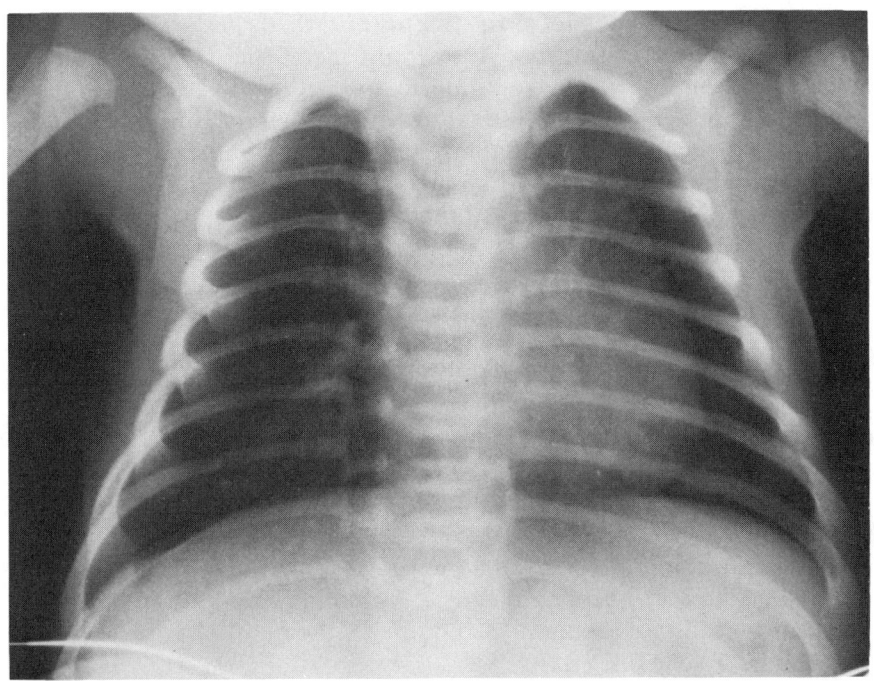

**FIG 11–1.**
Normal AP view of chest. Note wavy contour of left lobe of the thymus.

## NORMAL CHEST RADIOGRAPH (INCLUDING A STEP-BY-STEP INTERPRETATION PROCEDURE)

A systematic approach to interpretation of the chest x-ray will help prevent errors. Such an approach is described below.

**Correct Positioning of the Infant.**—To assess for rotation, check the anterior ends of ribs, which should be an equal distance from the midline as judged by the spine. An adequate inspiration has been obtained when at least six ribs are identified anteriorly above the diaphragm (Fig 11–1).

**Check All Tubes and Catheters.**—All tubing must be radiopaque for easy identification on an x-ray film. Follow each tube and catheter from start to finish. The endotracheal tube tip should be above the carina and below the vocal cords. An ideal position would be to have the tip of the endotracheal tube at the level of the clavicles with the infants head in a neutral position. A high umbilical artery catheter tip should be beneath the level of the ductus arteriosus and above the level of origin of the celiac artery. This would mean that its tip should be between T-6 and T-10. A low umbilical artery catheter tip should be between L-3 and L-4. An umbilical venous catheter should have its tip in the inferior vena cava or right atrium. Thoracostomy tubes for drainage of a pneumothorax should be positioned correctly on both the AP and lateral views. Most pneumothoraces are anterior in supine infants, and anterior positioning of the tip of the thoracostomy tube is optimal.

**Soft Tissues and Bones.**—Check for any ossification centers in the proximal humerus that would suggest that the infant is full-term. Rib fractures may be the first sign of rickets[2] in infants who are on prolonged hyperalimentation. Infants of diabetic mothers tend to have increased amounts of subcutaneous fat.

**Position of Tracheal Air Column.**—The trachea in neonates is a redundant and easily mobile structure. A left aortic arch will displace the trachea to the right, and a right aortic arch will displace the trachea to the left. The aortic arch and central pulmonary arteries are not identified individually as separate structures.

**Cardiothymic Silhouette.**—The heart and the thymus are of similar water density on the x-ray and cannot be distinguished from each other. The thymus is a soft pliable structure and will often show a wavy lateral border. This represents the indentations of the thymus between the ribs and intercostal spaces. A sharp lower border of the thymus is sometimes seen especially on the right side when the right lobe of the thymus may be compared to the sail of a yacht. On the lateral view, the thymus is identified anteriorly and behind the sternum. Infants with stress from sepsis or intrauterine growth retardation for example, will often have a small thymus. Steroid administration will produce a similar effect. A lack of visualization of the thymus occurs as part of the rare diGeorge syndrome (absent parathyroids and thymus).

The normal cardiothymic silhouette should not be greater than 60% of the transverse diameter of the thorax. Enlargements past this level represent cardiomegaly. Specific cardiac chamber enlargement can rarely be distinguished on the chest x-ray.

**Lungs.**—The major bronchi and trachea can be seen normally in an infant. More peripherally the air passages are not seen, and the lung markings represent pulmonary vessels. Pathologic processes in the lung can be divided into alveolar and interstitial. Interstitial patterns produce lines and nodules in the lung parenchyma. Examples of these would be the increased fluid in the interstitial compartment of the lungs identified with transient tachypnea of the newborn and heart failure. Alveolar diseases produce larger, confluent, poorly defined densities within the lungs with the peripheral bronchi occasionally visible. This identification of the previously invisible peripheral bronchi is called an air bronchogram. This pattern is also sometimes described as a "ground glass" appearance of the lungs and is seen, for example, with respiratory distress syndrome.

**Pulmonary Vascularity.**—Normal pulmonary vascularity tapers smoothly as the vessels are followed from the mediastinum peripherally. The assessment of increased or decreased pulmonary vascularity is difficult and often subjective. An objective method to improve this situation is a comparison of the right pulmonary artery with the tracheal air column. If the right pulmonary artery is larger than the width of the tracheal air column, then increased pulmonary vascularity exists. Seeing many vessels as circles or "end on" in the peripheral lungs is also another sign of increased pulmonary vascularity. The vessel margins should be sharp; hazy or indistinct vessel margins are an early sign of interstitial pulmonary edema.

**Diaphragm and Abdomen.**—The position of the diaphragm should be checked not only for an adequate inspiration, but also for its shape and contour. The costophrenic angles should be sharp with no evidence of pleural fluid. The right hemidiaphragm is normally slightly higher than the left due to the liver, but abnormal positions of the diaphragm may be related to diaphragmatic paralysis, perhaps secondary to birth trauma.

The upper abdomen is often included on a chest x-ray and should be examined carefully. Calcifications in the upper abdomen may be due to renal calculi from furosemide treatment[3] or to gallstones from hyperalimentation.

## RESPIRATORY DISTRESS SYNDROME

Respiratory distress syndrome, a common lung disease of prematurity, gives a characteristic and usually diagnostic radiographic appearance. This consists of a decrease in lung volume, a *granular appearance* to the lungs, and the extension of air *bronchograms* more peripherally into the lung parenchyma (Fig 11–2).

The *underinflation* of the lungs is usually uniform and symmetrical but may not be so obvious when infants are on artificial ventilation.

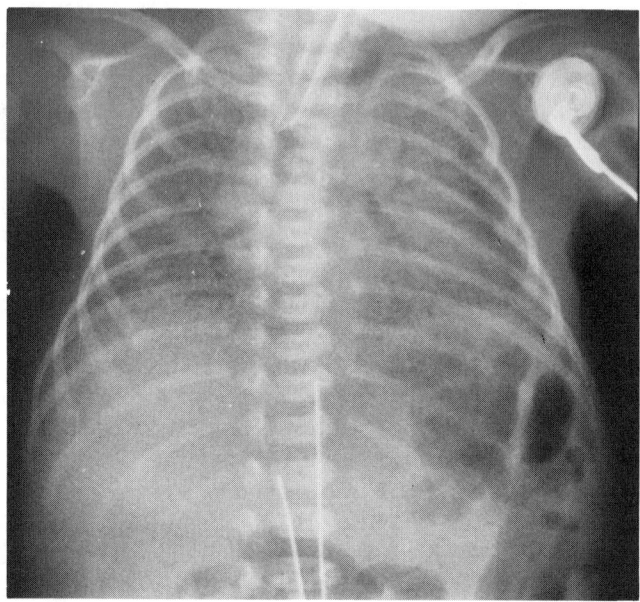

**FIG 11–2.**
Respiratory distress syndrome. Decreased lung volume, together with a "ground glass" appearance to the lung parenchyma, and air bronchograms are identified in this premature infant with respiratory distress syndrome.

The granular appearance of the lung parenchyma and the prominent air bronchograms all represent the radiographic appearance of underinflation and peripheral collapse. No pleural fluid is seen on the x-ray.

Usually these x-ray findings are present within the first few hours of life. Occasionally there is a lag when the clinical picture shows some deterioration, but the radiograph may appear normal. Usually, however, radiographic changes have occurred by 12 hours and at the latest by 24 hours from birth.

More severe disease appears radiographically earlier and also clears more slowly. A grading system is presented below.

*Grade 1:* The air bronchograms are confined to lie within the borders of the cardiothymic silhouette. The outlines of this silhouette remain sharp. The granularity of the lungs is very fine and difficult to appreciate.

*Grade 2:* Air bronchograms now project beyond the cardiothymic borders. The typical ground glass or granular appearance of the lung parenchyma is now obvious.

*Grade 3:* There is an increase in the overall opacification of the lung with more confluence of the abnormal granular pattern. The outline of the cardiothymic silhouette is slightly blurred.

*Grade 4:* Complete opacification of the lung has now occurred with no air bronchograms present. The distinction between the cardiothymic silhouettes, diaphragm, and lung parenchyma is lost.

## TRANSIENT TACHYPNEA OF THE NEWBORN

Another name used to describe transient tachypnea of the newborn syndrome is "wet lung." Both these titles are accurate descriptions of what is seen clinically and radiographically. A prolonged slow clearance of the intrauterine fluid from the lungs by the normal physiological process of removal causes this syndrome. It represents an exaggeration of a normal process rather than a disease.

These infants present with tachypnea within the first few hours of life. The chest x-ray obtained soon after birth may appear alarmingly abnormal, with fluid even present in the alveolar spaces of the lung parenchyma producing a diffuse opacification to the segments of lung involved. However, this pattern is uncommon, and the typical chest x-ray shows increased fluid in the interstitial spaces of the lung. The fluid can be identified radiating from the hilus of the lung bilaterally as well as producing a haziness to the vessels around the hilus (Fig 11-3). Small pleural fluid collections are frequently present, with fluid in the right minor fissure especially common. While the radiographic appearance is usually symmetrical, occasionally the right side can be more severely involved. The heart size is normal or slightly enlarged. The lung volume is normal or slightly increased.

The radiographic and clinical findings are usually in step with one another, and as the child rapidly improves in the first 24 to 48 hours of life so the x-ray shows complete resolution, usually by 24 hours and certainly by 48 hours.

This rapid clearance, clinically and radiographically, helps confirm the diagnosis and exclude more serious diseases such as neonatal pneumonia, respiratory distress syndrome, and heart failure.

## PNEUMONIA

While pneumonia is usually bacterial in origin, other causes such as viral and fungal pneumonia do occur in this age group. The most common bacterial pneumonia is due to group B *Streptococcus*. In low birth weight infants, this gives a radiographic appearance that is diffuse and bilateral (Fig 11-4). The appearance is often similar to that of respiratory distress syndrome. The radiologist, therefore, may be unable

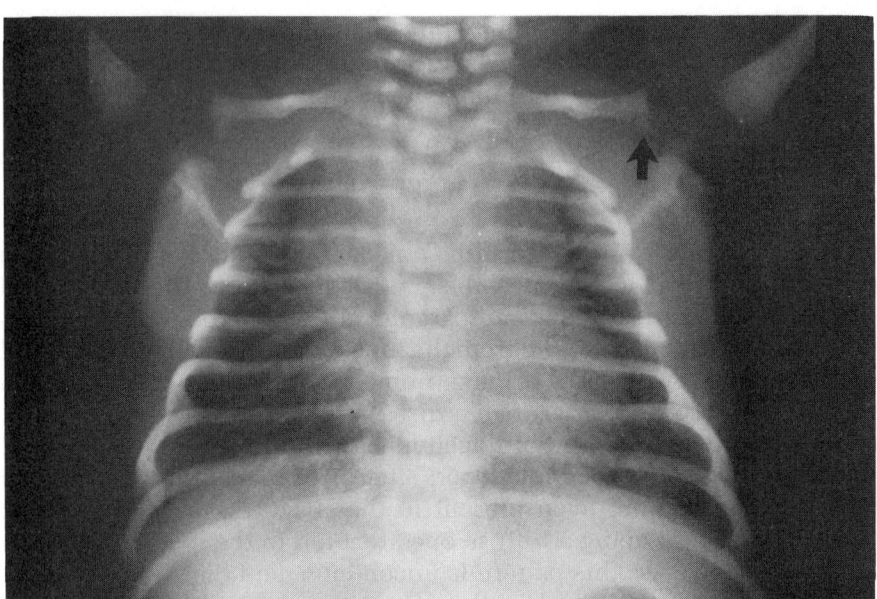

**FIG 11-3.**
Transient tachypnea of the newborn. Linear radiating densities represent interstitial fluid. Note the good lung volume. Ossification centers in the proximal humerus and coracoid *(arrow)* confirm that this is a full-term infant.

to distinguish these two common clinical problems. The presence of pleural fluid, if seen, is very helpful to point toward the diagnosis of bacterial pneumonia. Rarely, other bacterial pneumonias can give a similar radiographic appearance.

Lobar consolidation alone from a bacterial pneumonia is extremely rare in neonates. One autopsy-proved series of neonatal pneumonias[4] showed the commonest radiographic appearance to consist of bilateral extensive diffuse alveolar densities. However, 17% of this series showed a radiographic appearance consistent with transient tachypnea of the newborn, and 13% showed an appearance identical to respiratory distress syndrome.

Fungal infection of the lung, especially as an embolic form from indwelling catheters, is being recognized more frequently. *Candida* pneumonia unfortunately does not have a characteristic radiographic appearance.[5]

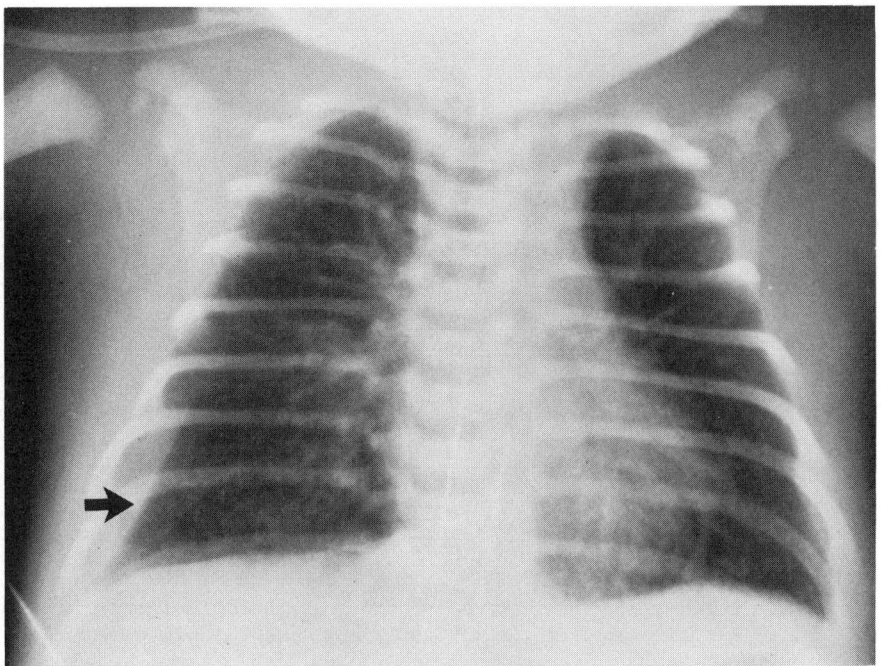

**FIG 11–4.**
Pneumonia. Bilateral increased densities are identified symmetrically throughout the lungs in this full-term infant with streptococcal pneumonia. Note the right pleural fluid collection (arrow).

## PLEURAL EFFUSION

Pleural fluid will collect in the most dependent parts of the pleural space. With changes in position, the fluid will move, and small amounts of fluid can be best shown by a lateral decubitus chest x-ray. The free fluid will layer on the dependent side (side closest to the ground). Fluid can also be well shown by ultrasound. Larger amounts of fluid produce a complete opacification of that hemithorax with mediastinal shift to the opposite side (Fig 11–5).

Chylothorax (accumulation of chyle in the thorax) is more commonly found on the right side. An underlying hypoplastic lung is occasionally seen so that when pleural fluid is removed, air leak problems such as a pneumothorax or pneumomediastinum may occur. However, the x-ray cannot distinguish between the several causes of fluid in the pleural space. A chylothorax (milk-like fluid) cannot be distinguished radiographically from hydrothorax (straw-colored fluid), hemothorax (blood), or empyema (pus). Babies who have been fed milk may dem-

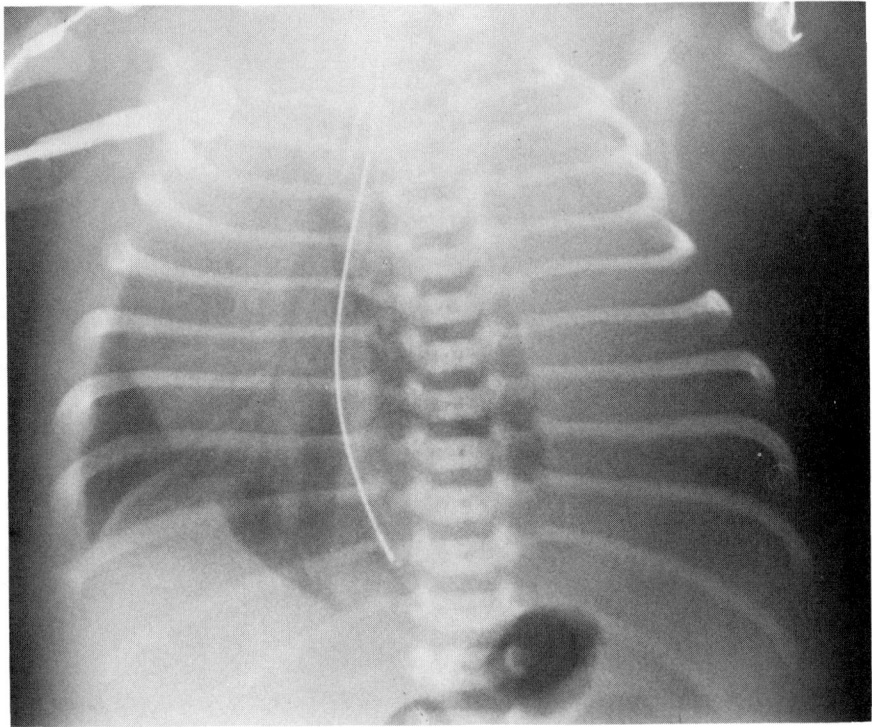

**FIG 11-5.**
Chylothorax. A large left chylothorax has caused displacement of the mediastinal structures toward the right. There is complete opacification of the left hemithorax by this abnormal fluid collection. Note the displacement of the endotracheal tube and nasogastric tube.

onstrate a chylothorax that will change in character and become straw-colored when milk is withdrawn and that is then often thought mistakenly to represent a simple hydrothorax.

Pleural fluid collections are also seen in infants with immune and nonimmune hydrops, transient tachypnea of the newborn, and occasionally with streptococcal pneumonia.

## MECONIUM ASPIRATION

The definition of meconium aspiration is the finding of meconium beneath the level of the vocal cords. The chest x-ray appearance may vary from normal in mild cases to grossly abnormal, with bilateral infiltrates and air trapping in severe cases (Fig 11–6). Meconium passage does not occur in fetuses less than 34 weeks' gestation, and there-

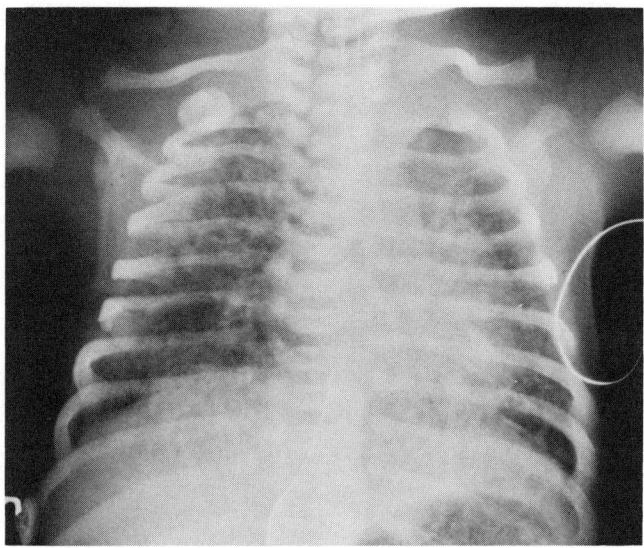

**FIG 11-6.**
Meconium aspiration. Bilateral diffuse infiltrates are present in lungs of normal volume secondary to meconium aspiration.

fore, meconium aspiration occurs predominantly in mature and postmature babies. Fetal distress possibly related to asphyxia results in passage of meconium that gives a chemical pneumonitis if sufficient amounts are aspirated into the airways and lung parenchyma. The chest x-ray shows overaeration with air trapping in a mature infant. Asymmetrical infiltrates are identified that have a variable pattern due to different degrees of severity of the associated chemical pneumonitis. Extraventilatory air, such as a pneumomediastinum and even a pneumothorax, is associated with air trapping. Persistent fetal circulation, a common problem in these infants, cannot be identified on the chest x-ray. Over a period of several days to a week, the infiltrates and overinflation of the lungs gradually return to normal.

## CHRONIC PULMONARY SYNDROMES

### Bronchopulmonary Dysplasia

This complication of neonatal respiratory distress syndrome was first radiographically described in 1967.[6] This original description divided the disease into four stages. The first stage, which occurred 2 to 3 days after delivery, is identical to respiratory distress syndrome. Stage II represents increasing pulmonary opacification. This can be difficult

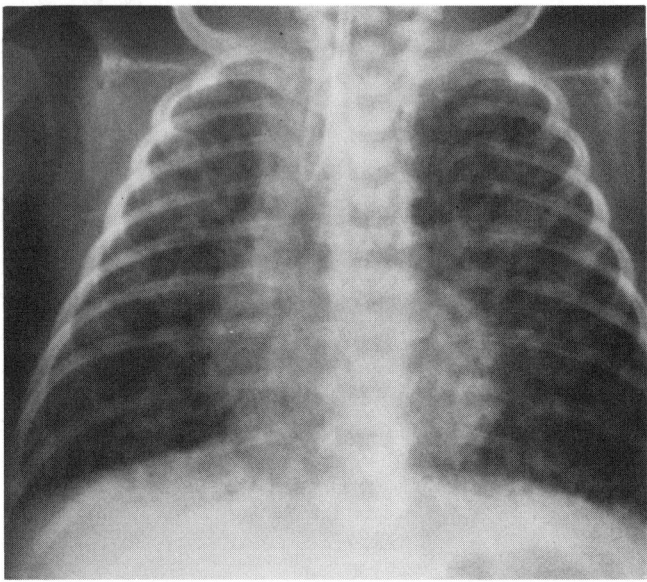

**FIG 11–7.**
Bronchopulmonary dysplasia, stage III. Multiple cyst-like lucencies are present in both lungs.

to distinguish from the pulmonary edema of a patent ductus arteriosus. Stage III is the more classical picture of bronchopulmonary dysplasia with small cyst-like lucencies representing focal emphysema identified on the chest x-ray (Fig 11–7). The x-ray is a mixture of areas of atelectasis and these bubbly cyst-like lucencies. Stage IV is identified as an increase in lung volume with linear densities scattered throughout the lungs in an asymmetrical distribution (Fig 11–8). These radiographic changes again are thought to represent areas of atelectasis alternating with irregular emphysematous foci. Uneven lung perfusion may be diagnosed with a perfusion scan (Fig 11–9). Often the heart is enlarged, and cor pulmonale is present. The lung may slowly and gradually return to normal, or the child dies because of irreversible cor pulmonale and severe lung disease.

The problem with the above described and original classification is that few children follow this chronological order. Stage I disease is now thought to be part of respiratory distress syndrome, and Stage III disease can be difficult to distinguish from pulmonary interstitial emphysema.

The clinical and radiographic appearance of bronchopulmonary dysplasia has changed since its original description. More recently, a more satisfactory definition of the disease combines clinical and ra-

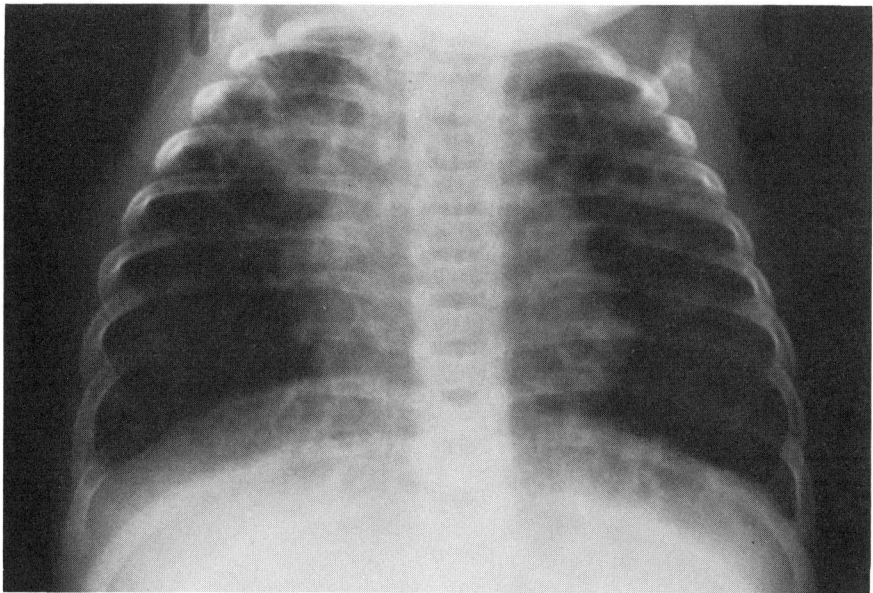

**FIG 11–8.**
Bronchopulmonary dysplasia, stage IV. The lungs are more overinflated with emphysematous changes particularly obvious in the upper lobes. Cystic areas are more obvious in the left upper lung with densities of atelectasis in the right upper lobe.

diographic findings. Any infant with persistent radiographic abnormalities and with a previous history of pulmonary disease and who still requires oxygen after 28 days of age is now defined as having bronchopulmonary dysplasia.

One other cause of an enlarged emphysematous area to the lung is acquired lobar emphysema.[7] This usually occurs on the right side from frequent suctioning with catheters. This irritation and trauma to the airway produces granulation tissue that partially occludes the bronchi. This granulation tissue acts as a check-valve mechanism with obstruction to the airway distally producing the overinflated emphysematous lobe. This is an important consideration as this iatrogenic disease may be cured by removal of the granulation tissue.

**Wilson-Mikity Syndrome**

Wilson-Mikity syndrome is now recognized as a very rare neonatal lung problem. These infants are asymptomatic at birth and, by definition, must have not required intubation or oxygen supplementation during the first few days of life. Initial chest x-rays are normal; later,

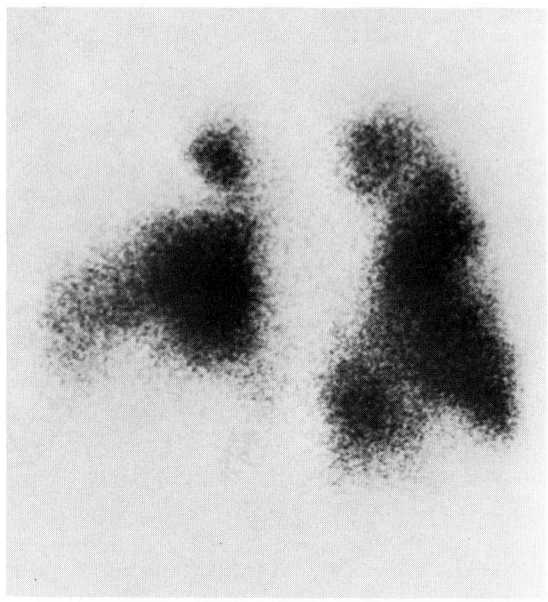

**FIG 11–9.**
A lung perfusion scan performed on a child with bronchopulmonary dysplasia shows the abnormal and uneven areas of perfusion with large segments, especially of the right lung, not being perfused.

symptoms and radiographic abnormalities indistinguishable from bronchopulmonary dysplasia appear (Fig 11–10).

### Chronic Pulmonary Insufficiency of the Premature Infant

Very small infants weighing less than 1,000 gm seem to often escape the severe radiographic and clinical abnormalities that are classically associated with respiratory distress syndrome. Some of these infants will develop a picture that is similar, but not identical, to respiratory distress syndrome. The lungs show a granular appearance, but air bronchograms are usually absent, and the lung volume for the size of the infant is maintained. It is unknown why these very small neonates develop this different radiographic and clinical disease.

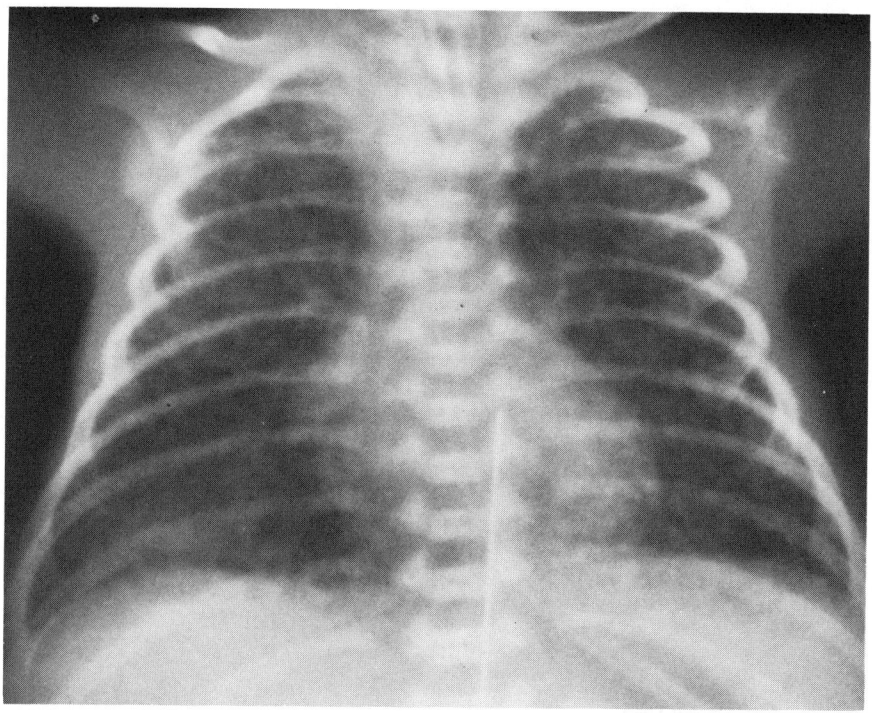

**FIG 11-10.**
Wilson-Mikity syndrome. Overinflated lungs are identified with cystic changes that radiographically appear identical to bronchopulmonary dysplasia. While this infant later had to be intubated, initially no oxygen or intubation occurred.

## CONGENITAL MALFORMATION OF THE RESPIRATORY TRACT

### Lung Hypoplasia

The small size of the lungs in pulmonary hypoplasia is often surprisingly hard to judge on a chest x-ray, and the main clinical presentation of these infants is with extraventilatory air. The classification of lung hypoplasia by Swischuk et al.[8] is a logical approach and includes extrathoracic compression, intrathoracic compression, and bony dysplasia.

*Extrathoracic Compression*

Oligohydramnios (decreased amniotic fluid volume) from whatever cause will produce lung hypoplasia. The commonest cause of oligohydramnios is a renal abnormality that must be bilateral and severe. Examples would include renal agenesis, posterior urethral valves, and

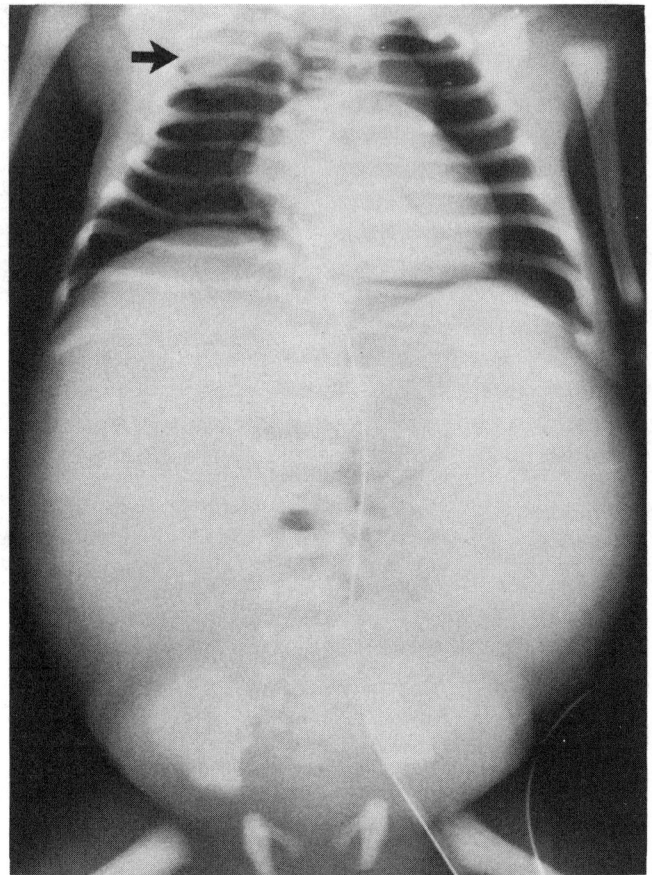

**FIG 11–11.**
Hypoplastic lungs. *Bilateral pneumothoraces* and a *pneumomediastinum* are present. The thymus has been elevated *(arrow)* by the pneumomediastinum. The sharp outline of the cardiac silhouette is secondary to the bilateral pneumothoraces. Huge bilateral abdominal masses, which represent infantile polycystic kidneys, are present.

infantile polycystic kidneys (Fig 11–11). Prolonged rupture of membranes may produce a similar degree of oligohydramnios and lung hypoplasia. The clinical syndrome of decreased amniotic fluid secondary to renal agenesis, lung hypoplasia, and limb and facial abnormalities is called Potter's syndrome.

### Intrathoracic Compression

Any intrathoracic mass in utero will produce compression of the adjacent lung and result in pulmonary hypoplasia. Diaphragmatic herniation of bowel contents into the thorax will produce ipsilateral, and often also contralateral, lung hypoplasia. Other mediastinal or lung masses are less common causes of intrathoracic compression. Chylothorax may produce some degree of pulmonary hypoplasia, but this event often occurs later in gestation and therefore causes less damage to the lungs. Hydrops also will produce milder forms of lung hypoplasia, again presumably because this is a later gestational event.

### Bony Dysplasias

Bony dysplasias are the easiest type of lung hypoplasia to recognize on the chest x-ray because of the very small rib cage due to the bony dysplasia. Examples of pulmonary hypoplasia secondary to rib and bony anomalies include asphyxiating thoracic dystrophy, thanatophoric dwarfism, and osteogenesis imperfecta.

### Primary Pulmonary Hypoplasia

Primary pulmonary hypoplasia occurs when the other three major causes of lung hypoplasia can be excluded. As mentioned, the presentation in these infants is with repeated collections of extraventilatory air. An exaggeration of the normal bell-shaped chest on the chest x-ray suggests pulmonary hypoplasia.

## AIR LEAK SYNDROMES

### Pneumothorax

When air collects in the pleural space, a lucency is identified in the pleural space with displacement of the lung away from the chest wall. A lateral pneumothorax shows an absence of lung markings (lung markings actually represent pulmonary blood vessels) together with a sharp white line of visceral pleura medially (see Fig 11–14).

A tension pneumothorax will displace compliant structures. The mediastinum is pushed away from the side of the tension pneumothorax, the diaphragm may be everted, and the pleura can occasionally be identified bulging at the intercostal spaces. Such a finding is an emergency that requires immediate insertion of a thoracostomy tube. A cross-table lateral chest x-ray is often helpful before insertion of a tube and is obligatory following the insertion of a thoracostomy tube, especially if the result is suboptimal. The thoracostomy tube may not have reached the pneumothorax. For example, the tip of the thoracostomy tube may be pointing posteriorly in the thorax when the pneumothorax lies anteriorly. This is a common cause of failure to drain a pneumothorax following insertion of a thoracostomy tube. Occasionally, a thoracostomy tube may be inadvertently positioned in the lung parenchyma, resulting in a continuous bubbling of the drainage apparatus but failure to resolve the pneumothorax.

Occasionally, it is difficult to distinguish a pneumothorax from other abnormal air collections, and a lateral decubitus view will show on the nondependent side the free intrapleural air of a pneumothorax. A skin fold may be mistaken for a pneumothorax. Usually a skin fold can be traced outside the pleural space into the soft tissues or abdomen. Also, the orientation of a skin fold is completely different from that of a pneumothorax.

In a supine infant, free air in the pleural space will commonly collect anteriorly, and the radiographic appearance of this anterior pneumothorax can be misleading.[9] Large anterior pneumothoraces can even displace adjacent lung laterally. The sharpness of the edge of the mediastinal contours together with an increased lucency are the best indicators of an anterior pneumothorax (Fig 11–12). A sharp line suggests that extraventilatory air is interfacing with the soft tissues of the heart and mediastinum.

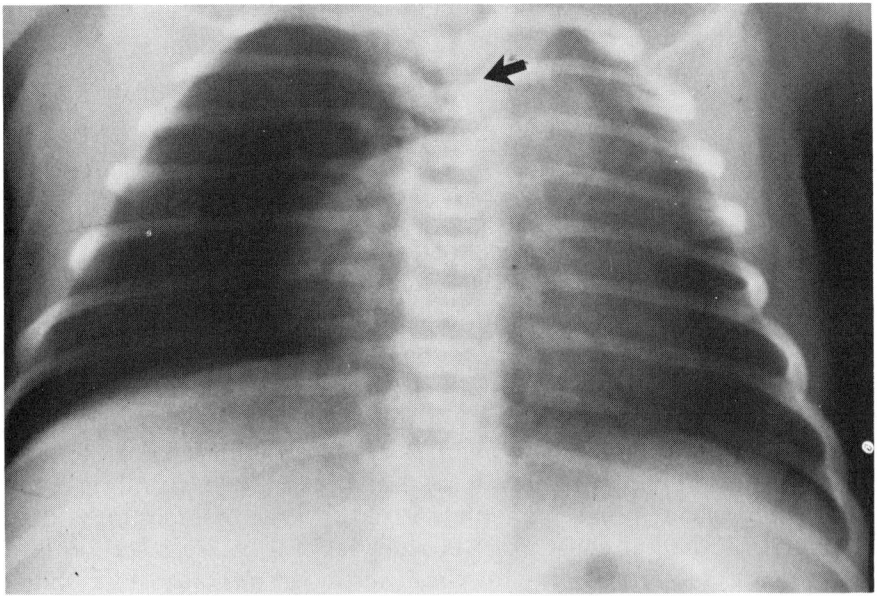

**FIG 11–12.**
Anterior pneumothorax. A right-sided anterior pneumothorax that has produced increased lucency in the right midlung and a sharpness to the right heart border is identified. Also note the herniation of right lung across the midline superiorly *(arrow)*.

## Pneumomediastinum

Unlike air collections in the pleural space, collections of air in the mediastinal space are rarely symptomatic. The main problems are in interpretation and distinguishing them from the more dangerous pneumothorax. Collections of air in the mediastinum will commonly outline the thymus (Fig 11–13). Identification of the thymus confirms the diagnosis of a pneumomediastinum. The thymus may be completely surrounded by air on either the AP or lateral view, or less commonly, its inferior surface is surrounded by air, and the thymus is elevated into the superior mediastinum. The complete outlining of a thymus by air is often called a spinnaker sign since the outline resembles a windblown sail. Subcutaneous emphysema in the neck often accompanies a pneumomediastinum but not a pneumothorax. Decubitus views of the chest fail to show a change in position of the mediastinal air unlike that of a pneumothorax.

Occasionally, mediastinal air collections can be confusing and collect in areas not usually thought of as the mediastinum. Oval or circular lucencies around the hilar region are sometimes called pseudocysts.[10] These represent mediastinal air collections. Another confusing area in

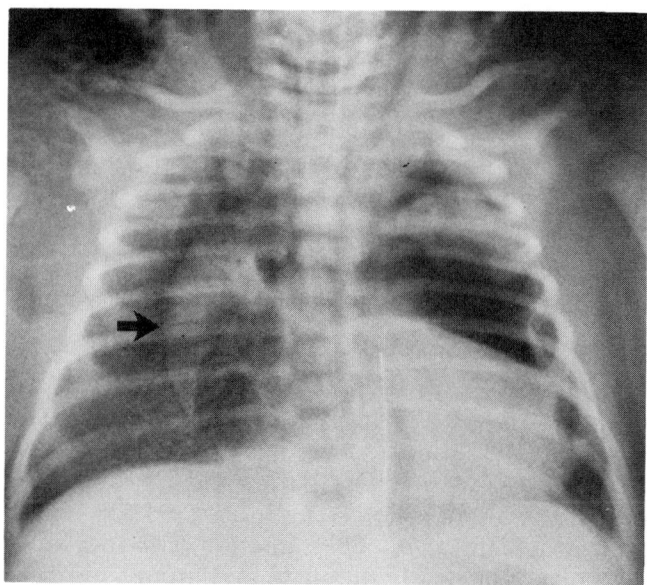

**FIG 11–13.**
Pneumomediastinum. The right lobe of the thymus is outlined by air secondary to a pneumomediastinum *(arrow)*. This appearance is likened to a spinnaker. Also note the subcutaneous air in the neck and shoulders, and left anterior pneumothorax.

which mediastinal air collects is within the inferior pulmonary ligament.[11] This is a fold of pleura that extends from the hila of the lungs down to the diaphragm. Air collections in this mediastinal space have a characteristic oval or triangular shape.

### Pneumopericardium

Air within the pericardial space almost completely encircles the heart on the chest x-ray, an appearance sometimes likened to a "halo" around the heart.[12] This distinguishes pneumopericardium from other abnormal air collections that are often bilateral but that outline only part of the cardiac silhouette. Superiorly, a complete encirclement of the cardiac silhouette is not visualized as the pericardium blends into the adventitial lining of the great vessels. The air in a pneumopericardium, however, should be able to be traced all the way around the two lateral and inferior borders of the heart seen on the AP view (see Fig 13–2). The size of the cardiac silhouette within the pericardium must be carefully observed, as tamponade from the air in the pericardial space can occur and be diagnosed radiographically.

### Pulmonary Interstitial Emphysema

The origin of the air for all the air-leak syndromes is a tear at the level of the alveolus. This air then tracks through the interstitial spaces to obtain access to either the mediastinum (pneumomediastinum), pleural space (pneumothorax), pericardial space (pneumopericardium), and less commonly the soft tissues of the neck and skin (subcutaneous emphysema; see Fig 11–13), and even occasionally into the peritoneal cavity (pneumoperitoneum; see Fig 11–16). Air within the interstitial space of the lung produces a characteristic radiographic appearance called pulmonary interstitial emphysema. The site of the alveolar leak is never discerned by x-ray. Pulmonary interstitial emphysema is located within dilated lymphatics.[13] The demonstration of pulmonary interstitial emphysema will often appear rapidly and may just as rapidly disappear. The lucent collections of air in the interstitial space splint the involved lung segment in overinflation and may give a false impression of normally ventilated lung. The interstitial air appears tubular, circular, or oval depending on its orientation with respect to the x-ray beam (Fig 11–14). It is clearly defined, of relatively uniform size, and nonbranching. Pulmonary interstitial emphysema air does not change in shape or position with decubitus views. In fact, a decubitus position is often used initially for the treatment of pulmonary interstitial emphysema. Other possible treatments include conservative management

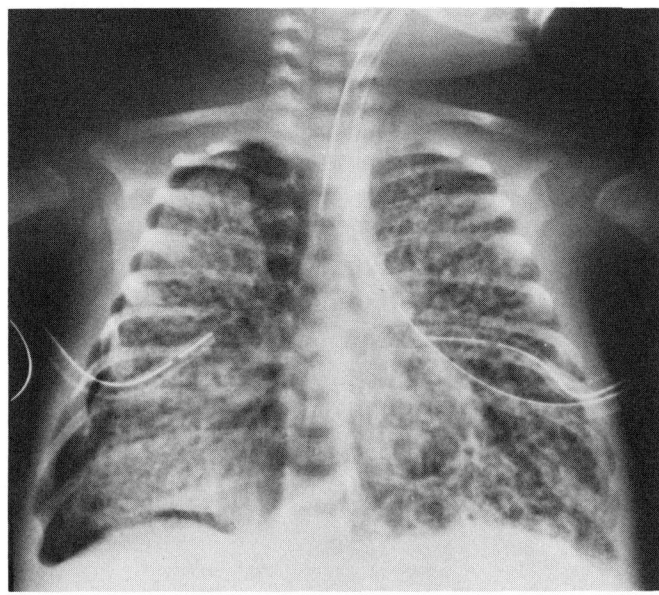

**FIG 11–14.**
Pulmonary interstitial emphysema. Bilateral pulmonary interstitial emphysema can be identified as circular and tubular lucencies extending throughout both lungs. A right pneumothorax is also present.

and selective intubation of an involved lobe with the endotracheal tube or with a balloon catheter.[14]

Occasionally, these interstitial air collections become more chronic, and the initially tubular or circular shape of the interstitial air collections changes to that of a more cystic collection with larger air spaces. At this stage, it can be difficult to distinguish the cysts of bronchopulmonary dysplasia from pulmonary interstitial emphysema. The sequence of events and the more localized collection favors a diagnosis of pulmonary interstitial emphysema.

### Subcutaneous Air

Once in the mediastinum, the abnormal air collection can track in various ways following anatomical pathways. Tracking of air into the subcutaneous tissues of the neck, axilla, and chest wall is easily observed on x-ray (see Fig 11–13) and physical examination.

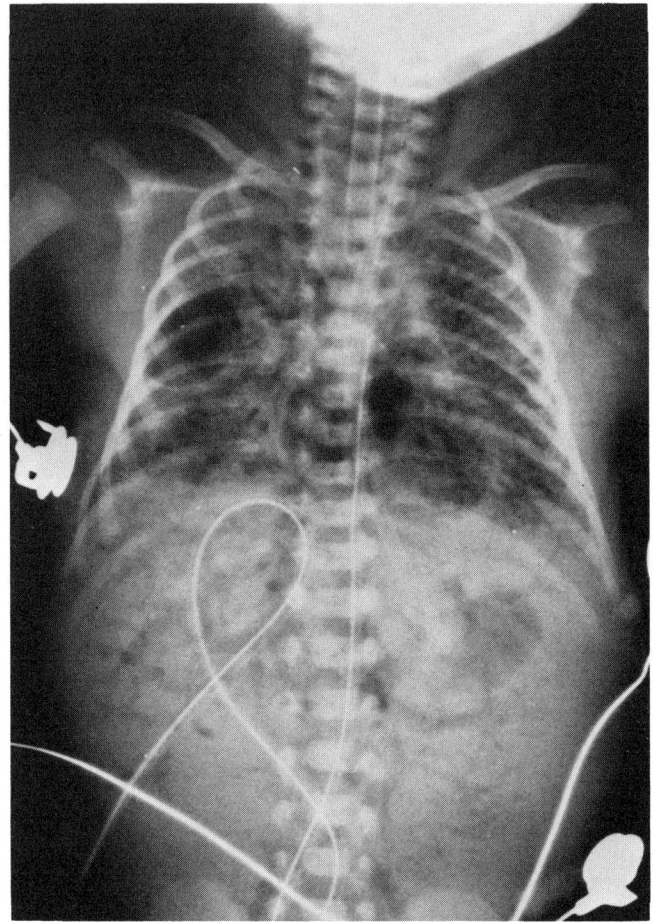

**FIG 11-15.**
Air embolism. Air can be identified in the vessels in the neck, axilla, and abdomen, as well as inside the heart. Bilateral pulmonary interstitial emphysema is also present.

### Air Embolism

Rarely, the interstitial air may gain access to the vascular system, and air embolism is produced (Fig 11–15). Air is identified not only within the heart but within all the major vessels of the thorax, abdomen, and extremities.

### Pneumoperitoneum

Air may also dissect down through the diaphragm resulting in a pneumoperitoneum (Fig 11–16).

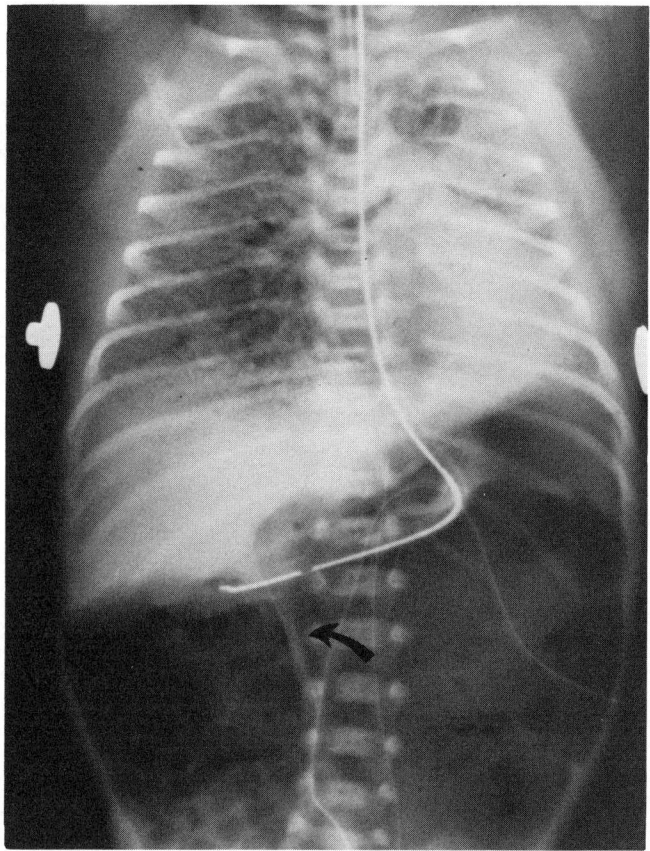

**FIG 11–16.**
Pneumoperitoneum. A large air collection is identified in the peritoneal cavity. This has dissected down from the pneumomediastinum. Pulmonary interstitial emphysema is present in the right lung with collapse of the left lung. The falciform ligament *(arrow)* is outlined by the free intraperitoneal air.

## DIAPHRAGMATIC HERNIA

A failure of closure of the pleuroperitoneal canal, which is one of the major components that forms the diaphragm, results in a posterolateral defect of the diaphragm or foramen of Bochdalek. This defect more commonly occurs on the left side. Bowel and rarely other abdominal viscera (such as liver and spleen) can herniate through this hole in the diaphragm into the thorax.

The earlier in gestation this event occurs, the more severe the damage to the lungs. The mediastinum is displaced away from the side of the hernia. The abdomen is therefore relatively "empty." This diagnosis

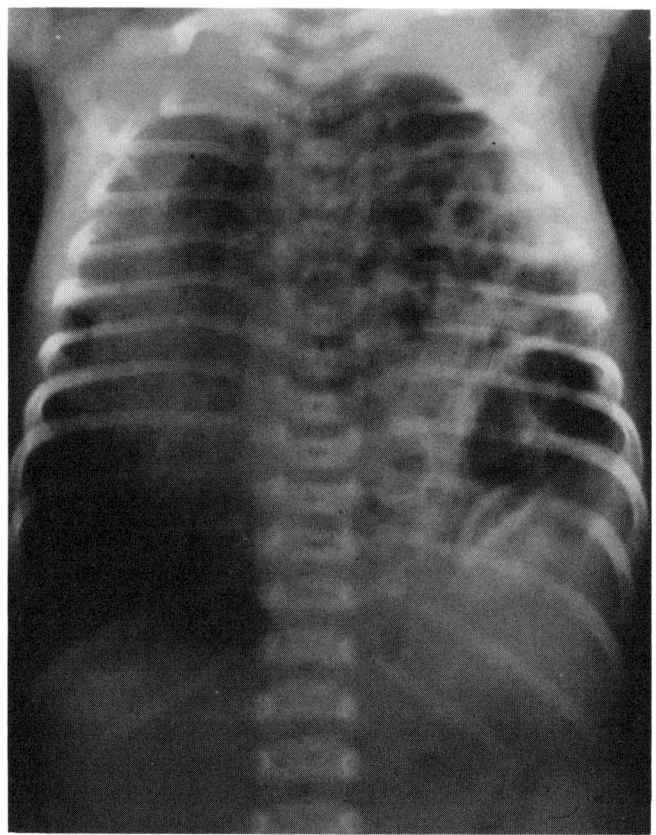

**FIG 11–17.**
Diaphragmatic hernia. Loops of bowel are identified in the left side of the thorax. They are displacing the mediastinum toward the right.

can now be made in utero by ultrasound and would theoretically be an excellent example of corrective in utero surgery. The herniation could be surgically repaired and the pregnancy continued to term. At present, unfortunately, this is not yet feasible.

These children usually have respiratory distress in the immediate newborn period, and chest x-ray shows the displaced mediastinum and loops of bowel in the thorax (Fig 11–17). If the loops of bowel are air-filled, the diagnosis is relatively easy. Fluid-filled loops of bowel may, however, be harder to recognize and the abnormal position of a nasogastric tube will confirm that the stomach is in the chest. Following surgery to repair the diaphragmatic hernia, the main postoperative problems are the underlying lung hypoplasia and persistent fetal circulation that frequently accompany this condition.

## PULMONARY HEMORRHAGE

Bleeding into the alveoli and interstitium produces opacification of the respective compartment. Radiographically, pulmonary hemorrhage cannot be distinguished from other fluid collections in the alveolar or interstitial compartments. The clinical finding of blood from the endotracheal tube or mouth suggests the correct interpretation of the x-ray.

## PULMONARY EDEMA

Fluid initially accumulates in the interstitial spaces of the lung and later in the alveolar spaces. This progression of the accumulation of fluid is often not appreciated on chest x-rays. Fluid in the interstitial spaces can be identified as an indistinctness and haziness to the pulmonary vascularity. This may be the earliest radiographic sign of a patent ductus arteriosus. Fluid in the interstitial spaces is also identified in the lymphatics and interlobular septa. This is identified on the x-rays as linear densities that appear to radiate from the hila. Transient tachypnea of the newborn characteristically shows these changes (see Fig 11–3).

Alveolar pulmonary edema presents as increased parenchymal densities in the lungs, usually bilaterally (see Fig 11–19). These densities can be hard to distinguish from other lung processes that also produce fluid in the alveolar spaces. Often a diagnosis of pulmonary edema is only made in retrospect following the rapid clearance of lung densities after fluid restriction or administration of diuretics.

## SELECTED CONGENITAL HEART DISEASES

Enlargement of the cardiac silhouette is a nonspecific finding found in many conditions besides congenital heart disease. Some examples of noncardiac causes of cardiomegaly include hypervolemia that may be associated with excessive umbilical cord stripping, a maternal-fetal transfusion, or a twin-twin transfusion. Metabolic causes of an enlarged cardiac silhouette include hypoglycemia and hypocalcemia. Neonatal asphyxia produces a mild enlargement of the cardiac silhouette. Arrhythmias such as supraventricular tachycardia, paroxysmal atrial tachycardia, and complete heart block may all produce an enlarged cardiac silhouette. Arteriovenous malformations such as a vein of Galen aneurysm or an hepatic hemangioendothelioma may also produce a large heart by their increased blood flow.

Heart failure with pulmonary venous congestion (seen on the chest x-ray as indistinctness of the pulmonary vascularity and edema) is most commonly due to a hypoplastic left heart in the first week of life, followed by coarctation (Fig 11–18) as the most common cause later in the neonatal period. Despite the name of a hypoplastic left heart, the cardiac silhouette is enlarged on chest x-ray.

A complete transposition may present with normal heart size and pulmonary vascularity in the first few days of life because the persistent fetal pulmonary artery hypertension prevents an increase in vascular flow to the lung. Soon the chest x-ray shows congestive failure with increased pulmonary vascularity. Clinically, these infants are profoundly cyanotic.

Left-to-right shunts in the absence of congestive heart failure are frequently not identified in the newborn period except for the occasional presentation of an endocardial cushion defect. The raised pulmonary artery pressure of the neonate prevents left-to-right shunting in the newborn period. Tetralogy of Fallot, unless very severe, also does not commonly present in the newborn period.

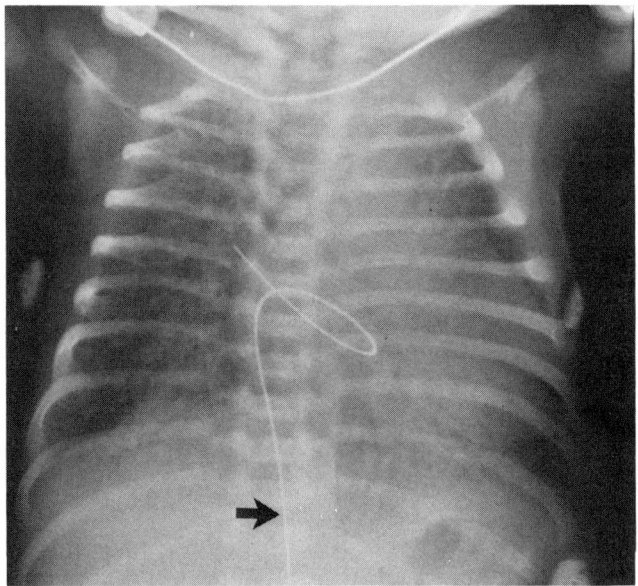

**FIG 11–18.**
Pulmonary edema. There is indistinctness to the pulmonary vascularity together with increased interstitial lines in the lung parenchyma. These are all related to pulmonary edema in this infant with a coarctation. Note the enlarged heart. An umbilical venous catheter *(arrow)* is extending from the right atrium through a patent foramen ovale into the left atrium and then turning up into a right pulmonary vein.

Total anomalous pulmonary venous return, which drains below the level of the heart into the inferior vena cava or portal vein, will produce severe obstruction to the venous return of the heart. Severe pulmonary edema and congestion is present on the chest x-ray of a cyanotic infant, but the heart size is normal. This combination of findings should suggest the diagnosis.

## CONGESTIVE HEART FAILURE

Enlargement of the cardiac silhouette with vascular engorgement and pulmonary edema are the radiographic findings of a patent ductus arteriosus (Fig 11–19). These findings of congestive heart failure are usually superimposed on the radiographic appearance of respiratory distress syndrome. Comparison with old films is mandatory to appreciate the enlargement of the heart size and the change in the lung pattern. The increased haziness of the lung parenchyma due to pulmonary edema, together with the engorgement and haziness of the

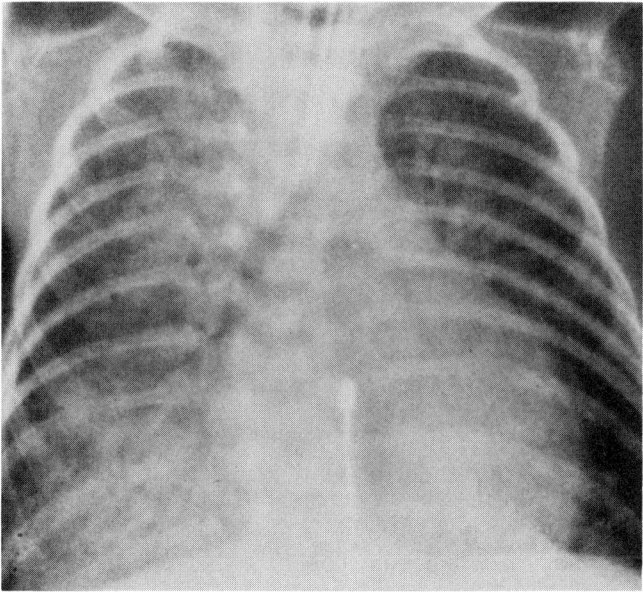

**FIG 11–19.**
Congestive heart failure—patent ductus arteriosus. Bilateral lung consolidation is present, greater on the right than the left. This pulmonary edema is producing an alveolar pattern on the right side. The cardiac silhouette had enlarged from earlier films, and this represents congestive heart failure secondary to a patent ductus arteriosus in a premature infant with respiratory distress syndrome.

pulmonary vessels, must be distinguished from the underlying pattern of respiratory distress syndrome.

The radiographic changes of congestive heart failure secondary to a patent ductus arteriosus can be difficult to identify, and echocardiography with direct visualization of the patent ductus and Doppler studies to assess flow are more specific. Increase in heart size may be hard to determine if the infant is on a positive end-expiratory pressure ventilator. These sick children are regularly having x-rays, and the interpretation of congestive failure is often first made by recognizing these subtle radiographic findings.[15] Occasionally, the x-ray will even be positive before a murmur is detected. This may especially occur if the shunt is large, and there is, therefore, less turbulence to produce a murmur.

## RADIOGRAPHIC EVIDENCE OF MATURATION (OSSIFICATION CENTERS)

Obstetric ultrasound is most accurate at predicting gestational age in the first trimester between 7 and 13 weeks. Later in pregnancy the accuracy is less, and in the last trimester, accuracy is only plus or minus 3 weeks of the measured gestational age. The diagnosis of intrauterine growth retardation, which is a disease of the last trimester, is difficult unless there has been accurate dating in the first trimester. Practically, this is a major problem unless routine obstetric ultrasound scanning is performed in the first trimester.

The appearance of the ossification centers of the distal femur and proximal tibia have traditionally provided an estimate of gestational age. These ossification centers can also be identified on ultrasound in utero and provide similar evidence of maturation. The range of appearance of these ossification centers means that in isolation they do not provide an accurate estimate of gestational age. The distal femoral ossification center appears between the 31st week (5th percentile) and the 39th week (95th percentile). The mean appearance is at 36 weeks. The proximal tibial ossification center appears later at the 34th week (5th percentile) and has a mean appearance of 38 weeks. The 95th percentile is reached 2 to 5 weeks postnatally. Neonatal hypothyroidism produces gross delay in the appearance of the ossification centers.

The proximal femoral ossification center is usually not seen in the newborn period, which makes x-ray of the hips for the diagnosis of congenital dislocation of the hips difficult to interpret. This is an area in which ultrasound may become the best imaging test.[16] The proximal humeral epiphysis, if seen on a chest x-ray, confirms that the infant is full-term (see Fig 11–3) This may be a helpful finding, for example, to help exclude a diagnosis of respiratory distress syndrome that only occurs in immature infants.

The molar teeth are frequently included on the chest film and can provide helpful information for assessing maturity. The appearance of the first molar deciduous teeth occurs at approximately 33 weeks. The second deciduous molar is radiographically visible at approximately 36 weeks.

## RADIOLOGIC EVALUATION OF THE UPPER AIRWAY

A lateral film of the upper airway and nasopharynx combined with an AP view of the tracheal air column is recommended for evaluation of the upper airway. Neonates do not have radiographically visible adenoids. The trachea is very mobile in neonates and young infants and, on a lateral film not taken in full inspiration, may give the false appearance of a mass in the prevertebral soft tissues. The lateral film of the neck must be obtained with the neck extended and the mouth closed. If the infant is crying during the exposure or the film is obtained with the neck flexed and the mouth open, a false impression of a retropharyngeal mass is obtained.

Fluoroscopy has been recommended for the diagnosis of laryngomalacia, although usually this can be diagnosed clinically. Vocal cord paralysis can also be appreciated fluoroscopically but is rarely necessary.

Lymphangiomas and hemangiomas can occur in the neck and obstruct the upper airway. Hemangiomas characteristically produce a posterior eccentric subglottic narrowing. Laryngeal stenosis, which may be congenital or related to previous intubation, can be recognized on good quality films of the airway.

## ULTRASOUND

Ultrasound uses high-frequency sound waves to image structures. It produces no harmful biological effects. Air or gas produces a total reflection of sound waves, which makes visualization of the lung impossible by ultrasound. However, there are still some uses for ultrasound in the neonatal chest.[17] The confirmation and diagnosis of pleural fluid is easily accomplished with ultrasound. A site for possible thoracocentesis can be safely located under ultrasound guidance. The diaphragm is easily seen on ultrasound, and diaphragmatic motion or paralysis can be confirmed. The relationship of the abdominal viscera to the diaphragm can be easily identified. Subphrenic fluid is also well seen on ultrasound.

Echocardiography uses the same principles of ultrasound examination to identify the heart and great vessels. Catheters in the abdominal and thoracic aorta can be identified.[18] Complications of poor position and catheter-associated thrombi can also be identified.[19] Thrombi associated with aortic catheters are presumed to represent a common cause of neonatal hypertension.

**Acknowledgment**

I would like to thank Rayna Lipscomb for help in preparation of the manuscript and Joe Molter for photographic work.

## REFERENCES

1. Sabau MN, Radkowski MA, Vyborny CJ: Radiation exposure due to scatter in neonatal radiographic procedures. AJR 1985; 144:811–814.
2. Gefter WB, Epstein DM, Anday EK, et al: Rickets presenting as multiple fractures in premature infants on hyperalimentation. Radiology 1982; 142:371.
3. Gilsanz V, Fernal W, Reid BS, et al: Nephrolithiasis in premature infants. Radiology 1985; 154:107.
4. Haney PJ, Bohlman M, Sun CCJ: Radiographic findings in neonatal pneumonia. AJR 1984; 143:23.
5. Kassner EG, Kauffman SL, Yoon JJ, et al: Pulmonary candidiasis in infants: Clinical, radiologic, and pathologic features. AJR 1981; 137:707.
6. Northway WH, Rosan RC, Porter DY: Pulmonary disease following respirator therapy of hyaline membrane disease: Bronchopulmonary dysplasia. N Engl J Med 1967; 276:357.
7. Miller KE, Edwards DK, Hilton S, et al: Acquired lobar emphysema in premature infants with bronchopulmonary dysplasia: An iatrogenic disease? Radiology 1981; 138:589.
8. Swischuk LE, Richardson CJ, Nichols MM, et al: Bilateral pulmonary hypoplasia in the neonate. AJR 1979; 133:1057.
9. Moskowitz PS, Griscom T: The medial pneumothorax. Radiology 1976; 120:143.
10. Clarke TA, Edwards DK: Pulmonary pseudocysts in newborn infants with respiratory distress syndrome. AJR 1979; 133:417.
11. Volberg FM Jr, Everett CJ, Brill PW: Radiologic features of inferior pulmonary ligament air collections in neonates with respiratory distress. Radiology 1979; 130:357.
12. Burt TB, Lester PD: Neonatal pneumopericardium. Radiology 1982; 142:81.

13. Wood BP, Anderson VM, Mauk JE, et al: Pulmonary lymphatic air: Locating "pulmonary interstitial emphysema" of the premature infant. *AJR* 1982; 138:809.
14. Mathew OP, Thach BT: Selective bronchial obstruction for treatment of bullous interstitial emphysema. *J Pediatr* 1980; 96:475.
15. Slovis TL, Shankaran S: Patent ductus arteriosus in hyaline membrane disease: Chest radiography. *AJR* 1980; 135:307.
16. Novick G, Ghelman B, Schneider M: Sonography of the neonatal and infant hip. *AJR* 1983; 141:639.
17. Miller JH, Reid BS, Kemberling CR: Water-path ultrasound of chest disease in childhood. *Radiology* 1984; 152:401.
18. Oppenheimer DA, Carroll BA, Garth KE, et al: Sonographic localization of neonatal umbilical catheters. *AJR* 1982; 138:1025.
19. Oppenheimer DA, Carroll BA, Garth KE: Ultrasonic detection of complications following umbilical arterial catheterization in the neonate. *Radiology* 1982; 145:667.

## SUGGESTED READINGS

Swischuk L: *Radiology of the Newborn and Young Infant*, ed 2. Baltimore, Williams & Wilkins Co, 1981.

Stern L (ed): *Hyaline Membrane Disease Pathogenesis and Pathophysiology*. Orlando, Grune & Stratton, 1984.

Poznanski A: *Practical Approaches to Pediatric Radiology*. Chicago, Year Book Medical Publishers, 1976.

# 12

# Assisted Ventilation of the Newborn

Waldemar A. Carlo, M.D.
Robert L. Chatburn, R.R.T.

Assisted ventilation has become an integral part of neonatal intensive care contributing to the increased survival of infants with respiratory distress. The increased survival of critically ill and very low birth weight infants has, however, been accompanied by a high incidence of both acute and chronic complications of assisted ventilation. Pulmonary air leaks occur in approximately 24% of all infants requiring assisted ventilation,[1] and around 20% develop bronchopulmonary dysplasia.[2] Furthermore, respiratory distress syndrome remains the leading cause of neonatal mortality, encompassing about 20% of neonatal deaths.[3] This has generated major impetus toward optimizing ventilatory techniques and strategies to minimize their attendant side effects. The resultant studies have been hampered by the rapidly changing clinical status that characterizes neonatal respiratory disorders. Nonetheless, data from carefully performed clinical studies can be combined with principles of pulmonary mechanics to develop management strategies for patients requiring assisted ventilation. We will first review some basic concepts of pulmonary mechanics and selected clinical studies that are particularly useful in understanding neonatal assisted ventilation. This information will then be integrated to present a rational approach for the use of assisted ventilation in neonatal respiratory disorders.

## APPLIED PULMONARY MECHANICS

A *pressure gradient* between the airway opening and the alveoli must exist to drive the flow of gas during both inspiration and expiration. This airway pressure gradient is required to overcome the elastic properties of the lung parenchyma and chest wall as well as the resistance to airflow.

### Compliance

*Compliance* describes the property of elasticity or distensibility of the lungs and chest wall and is expressed as the change in volume per unit change in pressure:

$$\text{compliance (L/cm H}_2\text{O)} = \frac{\Delta \text{ volume (L)}}{\Delta \text{ pressure (cm H}_2\text{O)}}$$

In neonates the chest wall is very distensible and does not contribute a substantial elastic load when compared to the lungs. Compliance of the total respiratory system (both chest wall and lungs) in infants with normal lungs ranges from 0.003 to 0.006 L/cm $H_2O$. The most striking abnormality of pulmonary mechanics in neonates with respiratory distress syndrome (RDS) is decreased lung compliance. Their total respiratory system compliance ranges from 0.0005 to 0.001 L/cm $H_2O$ (Fig 12–1).

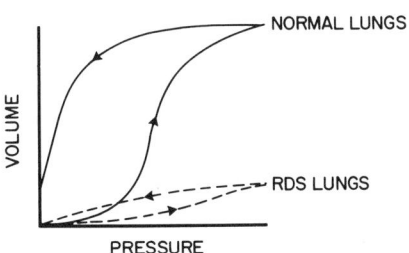

**FIG 12–1.**
Schematic pressure-volume relationship of the lungs of a normal infant and one with respiratory distress syndrome (RDS). The slope of this relationship is the compliance. The decreased lung compliance of the infant with RDS manifests as a decreased volume change for the same change in pressure. (From Carlo WA, Martin RJ: Principles of assisted ventilation. *Pediatr Clin North Am* 1986; 33:221. Adapted from Gribetz I, Frank NR, Avery ME: Static volume-pressure relations of excised lungs of infants with hyaline membrane disease, newborn and stillborn infants. *J Clin Invest* 1959; 38:2168.)

## Resistance

In addition to the pressure required to overcome the elasticity of the respiratory system, pressure is needed to force gas through the airways (airway resistance) and exceed the viscous resistance of the lung tissue (tissue resistance). *Resistance* is a property of the inherent capacity of the lungs to resist airflow and is expressed as the change in pressure per unit change in flow.

$$\text{Resistance (cm H}_2\text{O/L/second)} = \frac{\Delta \text{ pressure (cm H}_2\text{O)}}{\Delta \text{ flow (L/second)}}$$

Total (both airway and tissue) pulmonary resistance values for normal newborn infants are generally in the range of 20 to 40 cm $H_2O$/L/second and are not markedly affected in infants by the presence of RDS. Since the endotracheal tube adds a resistance, values of total pulmonary resistance for intubated infants range from approximately 50 to 150 cm $H_2O$/L/second.[4]

## Time Constant

Compliance and resistance can be used to describe the time necessary for an instantaneous or step change in airway pressure (e.g., square pressure waveform during pressure-limited ventilation) to equilibrate throughout the lungs. Once pressure is equilibrated throughout the lungs, there will be no airflow and thus no further volume changes. The *time constant* of the respiratory system is a measure of the time necessary for the alveolar pressure to reach 63% of the change in airway pressure and is defined as the product of resistance and compliance.

Time constant (seconds)
= resistance (cm $H_2O$/L/second) × compliance (L/cm $H_2O$)

Thus, if inspiration lasts a time equal to one time constant, 63% of the pressure difference between airway opening and alveoli will be equilibrated, and a volume proportional to this pressure equilibration will be delivered. The longer the duration allowed for equilibration, the higher the percentage of equilibration that will occur (Fig 12–2). With more time for pressure equilibration, 63% of the remaining pressure difference will be equilibrated and consequently 63% of the remaining potential volume delivered. This process continues with each extra time constant. As can be seen from the shape of the curve in Figure 12–2, little further pressure equilibration occurs beyond three to five time constants. For practical purposes, volume delivery is also complete after five time constants. The application of this concept to assisted ventilation becomes particularly important when either inspiratory or expiratory time are so short that they may be insufficient for pressure equilibration and thus completion of inspiration or expiration. It should be noted that since values of compliance and resistance may differ slightly between inspiration and expiration, inspiratory and expiratory time constants of the respiratory system may be different.

Therefore, the time necessary for the lungs to inflate and deflate will depend on their mechanical characteristics, specifically resistance and compliance. For example, in a healthy infant with a resistance of 30 cm $H_2O$/L/second and a compliance of 0.004 L/cm $H_2O$, one time constant will be 0.12 seconds. For a fairly complete equilibration of pressure (five time constants or 5 × 0.12 seconds), an inspiratory or expiratory phase of 0.6 seconds will be necessary (if the time constant remains the same during inspiration and expiration). In contrast, since infants with RDS typically have a decreased compliance, their time constant and corresponding time for pressure equilibration will be shorter. Therefore, lungs with decreased compliance will complete inflation and deflation in a shorter time than normal lungs.

If inspiratory time is less than five time constants for a given step change in airway pressure, an incomplete tidal volume may be delivered.[5] If expiratory time is insufficient, expiration may not be complete, leading to an increase in functional residual capacity and inadvertent positive end-expiratory pressure (PEEP).[6,7] Because infants with RDS have decreased time constants, short inspiratory and expiratory times may be appropriate during the period of peak severity of their disease but insufficient after recovery from RDS (or in infants with normal lungs) when compliance is much higher. Furthermore, the time con-

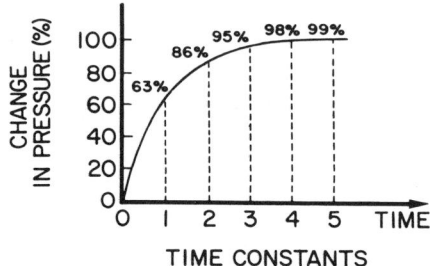

**FIG 12–2.**
Percentage change in pressure in relation to the time (in time constants) allowed for equilibration. As a longer time is allowed for equilibration, a higher percentage change in pressure will occur. The same rules govern the equilibration for step changes in volume. (From Carlo WA, Martin RJ: Principles of assisted ventilation. *Pediatr Clin North Am* 1986; 33:221. Used by permission.)

stant of the ventilator and delivery system has to be considered,[8] and as discussed later, at high frequencies limitation in delivery of an adequate tidal volume may occur.[9]

In summary, it is important to consider the mechanical characteristics of the respiratory system to better understand the physiologic rationale for the blood gas responses that occur after ventilator setting changes. This is especially true in neonates with RDS whose disease is characterized by rapidly changing pulmonary mechanics and in whom rapid ventilatory frequencies are being increasingly employed.

## RESPIRATORY GAS EXCHANGE

The aim of assisted ventilation is ultimately to accomplish effective gas exchange. Although impairments of carbon dioxide ($CO_2$) elimination and oxygen ($O_2$) uptake frequently occur simultaneously, this section will review individually the strategies that may be employed to accomplish $CO_2$ or $O_2$ exchange focusing primarily on assisted ventilation of infants with RDS.

### Carbon Dioxide Elimination

As $CO_2$ diffuses readily from the blood into the alveoli, $CO_2$ elimination depends largely on the total amount of air that passes in and out of the alveoli.[10, 11] Since some of the tidal volume is distributed to parts of the lungs, such as the airways, that are not involved in gas exchange (dead space), *alveolar ventilation* is calculated as follows:

Alveolar ventilation = (tidal volume − dead space) × frequency

where frequency is the number of breaths per minute. Since dead space stays relatively constant, increases in tidal volume or frequency increase alveolar ventilation, enhance $CO_2$ elimination, and reduce the partial pressure of $CO_2$ in arterial blood ($Pa_{CO_2}$).[9, 11, 12] With a volume ventilator, the delivered volume is preset, although some of this volume will be lost, depending on the mechanics of the respiratory system and delivery circuit as well as air leaks around the uncuffed endotracheal tube. With a pressure ventilator, tidal volume depends on lung compliance and the pressure gradient (pressure difference between airway pressure and alveolar pressure) or peak inspiratory pressure (PIP) minus PEEP. The inspiratory duration may, under special circumstances, partially determine tidal volume.[5, 9] For example, depending on the time constant of the respiratory system (and the endotracheal tube and ventilator), a very short inspiratory time may reduce the tidal volume at a given pressure gradient.[5, 9] Frequency is the other major determinant of alveolar ventilation. In addition to the frequency set on the ventilator, the infant may take spontaneous breaths since modern neonatal ventilators provide a continuous flow of gas during the expiratory phase. Figure 12–3 illustrates these interrelationships between ventilator controls, pulmonary mechanics, and ventilation.[13]

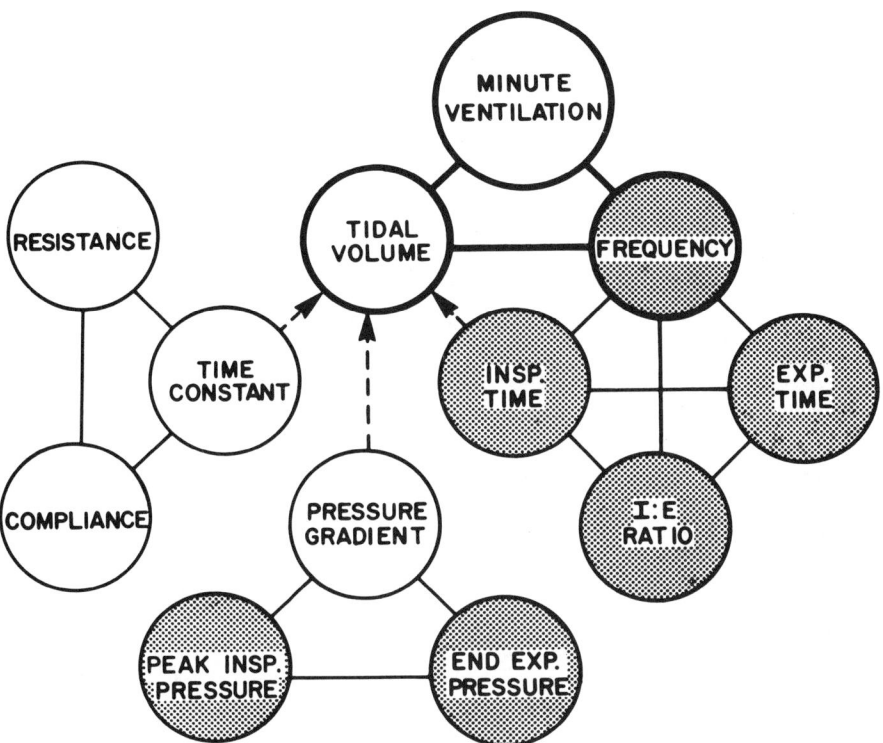

**FIG 12–3.**
Relationship between ventilator-controlled variables *(shaded circles)* and pulmonary mechanics *(unshaded circles)* in determining minute ventilation during pressure-limited time-cycled ventilation. The relation between the circles that are joined by solid lines is described by simple mathematical equations. Thus, simple mathematical equations determine the time constant of the lungs, the pressure gradient, and inspiratory time. These in turn determine the delivered tidal volume, which when multiplied by the respiratory frequency gives the minute ventilation. Alveolar ventilation may be calculated from the product of tidal volume and frequency when dead space is subtracted from the former. (Adapted from Chatburn RL, Lough MD: Mechanical ventilation, in Lough MD, Doershuk D, Stern R (eds): *Pediatric Respiratory Therapy,* ed 3. Chicago, Year Book Medical Publishers, 1985, p 161.)

## Oxygen Uptake

Several studies in infants, mostly with RDS, have concluded that oxygenation depends on *mean airway pressure* ($\overline{P}aw$) (Fig 12–4).[10, 12, 14–19] Mean airway pressure is a measure of the average pressure to which the lungs are exposed during the respiratory cycle and may be calculated by dividing the area under the airway pressure curve by the duration of the cycle, or from the following equation:

$$\overline{P}aw = K(PIP - PEEP)(T_I/[T_I + T_E]) + PEEP$$

where K is a constant that depends on the rate of rise of the airway pressure curve, $T_I$ is inspiratory time, and $T_E$ is expiratory time.[20] Therefore, $\overline{P}aw$ will be augmented by increasing any of the following (Fig 12–5):

1. Inspiratory flow (will increase K)
2. PIP
3. Ratio of inspiratory time to expiratory time (I:E ratio)
4. PEEP

It is unclear precisely why $\overline{P}aw$ determines oxygenation, but it probably relates to prevention of atelectasis, optimization of lung volume, and

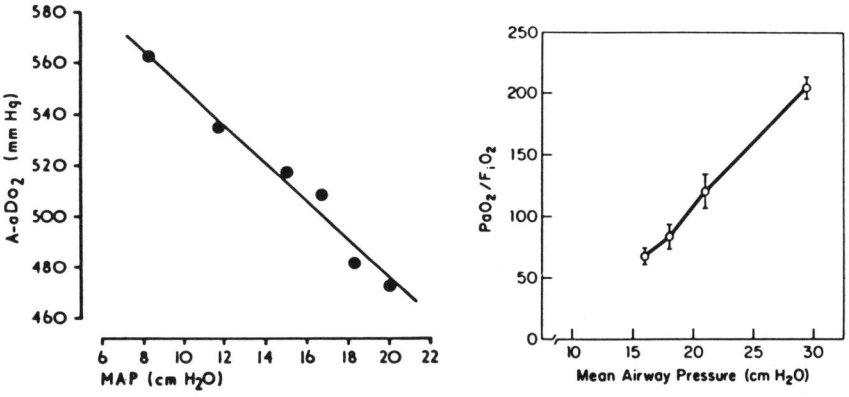

**FIG 12–4.**
Changes in the alveolar to arterial oxygen gradient (A-a$DO_2$) *(left)* and $Pa_{O_2}/Fi_{O_2}$ *(right)* are correlated with changes in mean airway pressure. There is a direct relationship between changes in oxygenation and mean airway pressure. *(Left* from Herman S, Reynolds EOR: Methods for improving oxygenation in infants mechanically ventilated for severe hyaline membrane disease. *Arch Dis Child* 1973; 48:612–617. *Right* from Boros SJ: Variations in inspiratory:expiratory ratio and airway pressure waveform during mechanical ventilation: The significance of mean airway pressure. *J Pediatr* 1979; 94:114–117.)

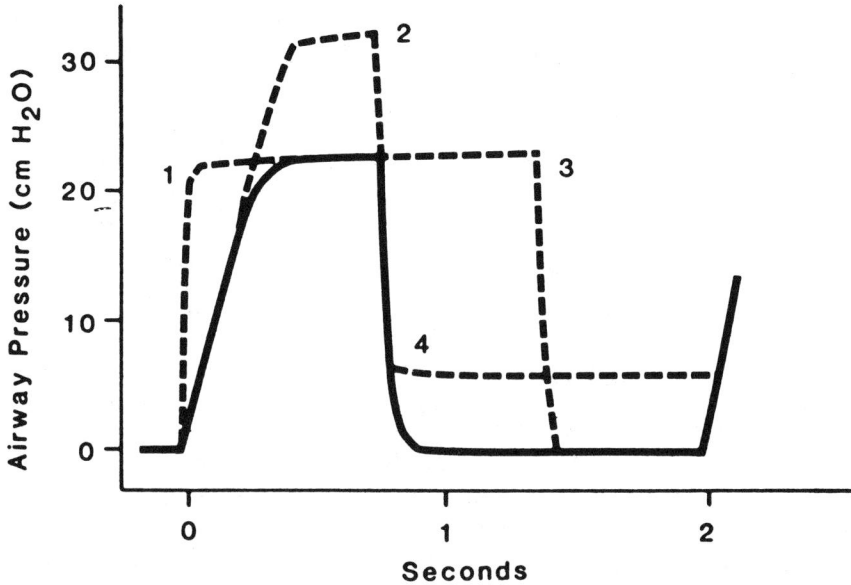

**FIG 12–5.**
Four different ventilator-setting increases that augment mean airway pressure: 1, inspiratory flow; 2, peak inspiratory pressure; 3, I:E ratio; and 4, positive end-expiratory pressure. (From Harris TR: Physiological principles, in Goldsmith JP, Karotkin EH (eds): *Assisted Ventilation of the Neonate*. Philadelphia, WB Saunders Co, 1981, p 43. Used by permission.)

improved ventilation-perfusion relationships. Although a direct relationship between $\bar{P}_{aw}$ and oxygenation exists, there are several limitations:

1. For the same change in $\bar{P}_{aw}$, increases in PIP and PEEP enhance oxygenation more than do changes in I:E ratio.[18]
2. Changes in PEEP are not as effective once an elevated level ($>$ 5–6 cm $H_2O$) is reached and may, in fact, not alter oxygenation at all.[21]
3. Very high $\bar{P}_{aw}$ may cause overdistention of alveoli leading to right-to-left shunting of blood in the lungs.
4. If a very high $\bar{P}_{aw}$ is transmitted to the intrathoracic structures, cardiac output may decrease, and thus, despite adequate oxygenation, oxygen transport (arterial oxygen content $\times$ cardiac output) may decrease.

## METHODS FOR ASSISTING VENTILATION

Depending on the infant's clinical condition one of the techniques for assisting ventilation described below may be the treatment of choice.

When the need for artificial ventilation is transient (e.g., for resuscitation of a newborn) bag-and-mask bagging is usually sufficient. Infants with mild RDS will respond well to continuous distending pressure with or without endotracheal intubation, while infants with severe respiratory failure will require mechanical ventilation with endotracheal intubation.

## Bag-and-Mask Ventilation

Bag and face masks of various sizes are essential pieces of equipment in the care of ill infants. These should be readily available in delivery rooms and on resuscitation trays, as well as at the bedside of critically ill infants. When there is a temporary need for assisted ventilation, a bag and mask will in most cases be sufficient to maintain adequate gas exchange. Two types of bags may be used. *Flow-inflating* bags require a flow of gas to inflate, while *self-inflating bags* become distended due to their recoil pressure. Self-inflating bags are necessary when a source of gas flow is unavailable. A pressure manometer should be used to facilitate consistent pressure delivery. Use of inappropriately high peak inspiratory pressure or inadvertent positive end-expiratory pressure should be avoided. Some bags have a pressure relief or "pop-off" valve for extra safety. If the bag has a "pop-off" valve, it should always be partially open to prevent delivery of excessively high pressures. In addition, a small leak between the mask and the infant's face will minimize the development of high pressures and $CO_2$ retention.

## Continuous Distending Pressure

When oxygen supplementation is not sufficient to maintain adequate oxygenation or when a high inspired oxygen concentration is required, *continuous distending pressure* (CDP) may improve gas exchange in infants with RDS.[22] Continuous distending pressure may be applied either as a *continuous positive airway pressure* (CPAP) or as a *continuous negative pressure* (CNP). Continuous positive airway pressure may be delivered via nasal prongs, endotracheal tube, nasopharyngeal tube, or face mask, while a CNP is given by applying a negative pressure around the thorax. There is no consensus as to the most effective method of CDP delivery, but application of CPAP is clinically easier and most frequently used. Access to the infant is markedly limited when CNP is applied. The application of CDP throughout the respiratory cycle constituted a major breakthrough in the treatment of severe RDS. The studies of Gregory et al.[22] demonstrated that gas exchange in RDS can be improved significantly by applying a constant positive pressure to the airway.[22] Continuous distending pressure is the first method that should be used to support ventilation of most infants with RDS. However, small infants may need endotracheal intubation and mechanical ventilation soon after birth.

Infants with RDS have alveolar instability secondary to surfactant deficiency with resultant collapse of alveolar and diffuse microatelectasis. Maintenance of a CDP prevents alveolar collapse. Furthermore, the increase in functional residual capacity that accompanies the application of CDP is thought to decrease intrapulmonary shunting and thus improve ventilation-perfusion relationship. However, if overdistention occurs, lung compliance will be decreased. Because of the Hering-Breuer reflex and the increase in functional residual capacity that accompanies the application of CDP, expiratory time is lengthened and respiratory rate decreases.

The technique for applying CPAP was developed primarily by Gregory and his colleagues,[22] and a modification is shown in Figure 12–6. A suitable air/$O_2$ mixture (total flow not exceeding 5 L/minute) passes through a humidifier. Gas passes to the elbow, which is attached to an

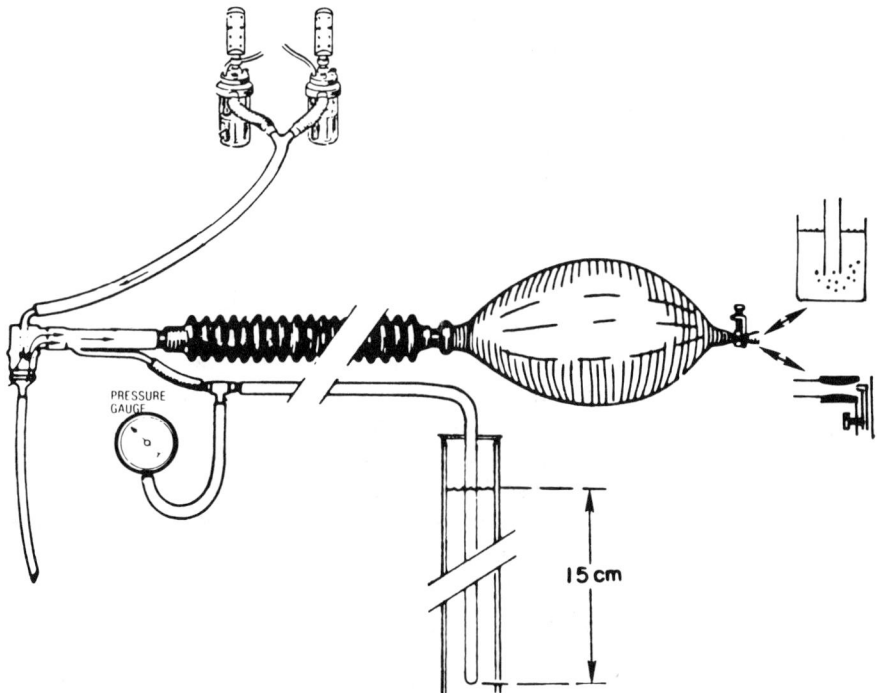

**FIG 12–6.**
System for applying continuous positive airway pressure (CPAP) through an endotracheal tube during spontaneous breathing.

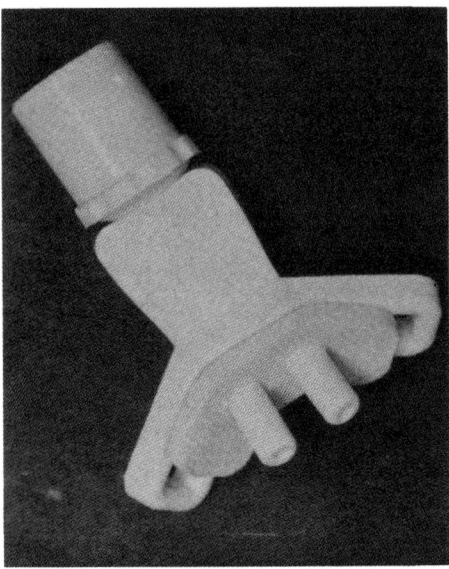

**FIG 12–7.**
Silastic prongs for administration of nasal CPAP.

endotracheal tube. The screw clamp on the reservoir bag is used to control the flow of gas and maintain a constant positive pressure within the system, as indicated on the pressure manometer. The side arm ends under a 15-cm column of water and acts as a safety valve. Applying CPAP with an endotracheal tube was most successful initially, but alternative methods that have been developed avoid the risks of intubation. We administer CPAP with nasal prongs, an apparatus that cannulates both nares for the administration of CPAP (Fig 12–7). This apparatus is strapped to the infant's head in the same manner as oxygen prongs are used in older children. During nasal CPAP, the infant is easily accessible without interruption of therapy. With the exception of substitution of the CPAP nasal cannula for the endotracheal tube and the need for an orogastric tube, the rest of the apparatus is essentially identical with that described by Gregory et al.[22]

We initiate CPAP whenever more than 70% oxygen is needed to maintain a partial pressure of oxygen in arterial blood ($Pa_{O_2}$) greater than 50 to 60 mm Hg, although others prefer an even earlier use.[23] A pressure of 6 to 8 cm $H_2O$ is used to initiate therapy. If this fails to improve oxygenation, 10 or even 20 cm $H_2O$ may be tried. These positive pressures at the airways are not transmitted completely to the pleural space because of the severely reduced lung compliance. Hence, venous return and cardiac output are usually not compromised. How-

**TABLE 12-1.**
Effects of Ventilator Setting Changes on Blood Gases*

| Ventilator Setting Changes | Effects on Blood Gases | |
|---|---|---|
| | $Pa_{CO_2}$ | $Pa_{O_2}$ |
| ↑ PIP | ↓ | ↑ |
| ↑ PEEP | ↑ | ↑ |
| ↑ Frequency | ↓ | ± ↑ |
| ↑ I:E ratio | — | ↑ |
| ↑ $FI_{O_2}$ | — | ↑ |
| ↑ Flow | ± ↓ | ± ↑ |

*↑ = increase; ↓ = decrease; ± = minimal effect; — = no consistent effect; $FI_{O_2}$ = fraction of $O_2$ in dry inspired air.

ever, in infants with normal lungs, CPAP is more likely to result in complications such as pulmonary air leaks, air trapping, impairment of venous return, and even decreased lung compliance. An increase in $Pa_{CO_2}$, as CPAP is augmented, may indicate a reduction in lung compliance. Because CPAP has a variable effect on $Pa_{CO_2}$, blood gases should be monitored closely. If severe respiratory acidosis ensues, assisted ventilation with endotracheal intubation will be necessary. The use of CPAP during weaning from assisted ventilation is discussed later.

## Mechanical Ventilation

The ensuing discussion will focus on the effect that specific ventilator-setting changes have on blood gases. There is much confusion regarding the specific blood gas responses to each type of setting change. A summary of the major effects of ventilator setting changes on blood gases appears in Table 12–1. While effects may vary, and trial and error may be used at times, certain basic principles should serve as guidelines. We will review these principles with a focus on the complex interrelationship between the ventilator and the mechanical characteristics of the respiratory system.

### *Peak Inspiratory Pressure*

Changes in PIP (or tidal volume with volume ventilators) will, in part, determine the pressure gradient ($\Delta P$) that occurs between onset and end of inspiration. For a given compliance of the respiratory system, the delivered tidal volume will be proportional to this pressure gradient. Thus, since $\Delta P$ equals PIP minus positive end-expiratory pressure, changes in PIP will affect delivered tidal volume and thus in part determine alveolar ventilation. Therefore, an increase in PIP will increase tidal volume, increase $CO_2$ elimination, and decrease $Pa_{CO_2}$.[9, 18] Furthermore, increases in PIP will raise $\bar{P}aw$ and thus improve oxygenation.[12, 18] Use of an elevated PIP increases the risk of barotrauma with resultant air leaks,[24] bronchopulmonary dysplasia,[25] and impaired cardiac function; and thus, caution must be exercised when high levels of PIP are used.

### *Positive End-Expiratory Pressure*

An adequate PEEP prevents alveolar collapse, maintains lung volume at end expiration, and improves ventilation/perfusion relationships. Because changes in PEEP alter the pressure gradient between inspiration and expiration, $CO_2$ elimination may be affected.[14] Thus, elevation of PEEP may decrease tidal volume and $CO_2$ elimination, and therefore increase $Pa_{CO_2}$.[9, 14, 18] Furthermore, the use of high PEEP (>5 to 6 cm $H_2O$) may decrease lung compliance,[5, 26] which will manifest as decreased tidal volume on a pressure-limited time-cycled ventilator or as increased PIP on a volume ventilator. Thus, alveolar hypoventilation could occur with a corresponding increase in $Pa_{CO_2}$. Increases in PEEP will raise $\bar{P}aw$ and thus improve oxygenation.[14, 18] Nonetheless, as mentioned above, use of a very elevated PEEP does not benefit oxygenation substantially.[21] It is important to note that although increases in PIP and PEEP both increase $\bar{P}aw$ and thus oxygenation, they usually have different effects on $CO_2$ elimination. In addition, use of very high PEEP may impair venous return, decrease cardiac output, and decrease oxygen transport. The differential effect of PIP and PEEP on $CO_2$ elimination may be helpful when deciding the most appropriate ventilator setting changes at a particular time. A minimum PEEP of 2 to 3 cm $H_2O$ is recommended since endotracheal intubation eliminates the active maintenance of functional residual capacity that infants accomplish by vocal cord adduction.

### *Frequency (or Rate)*

Frequency changes will substantially alter alveolar ventilation and thus $Pa_{CO_2}$.[9, 11, 12] Use of moderately high frequencies (up to 60 breaths per minute) has allowed the use of a lower PIP and reduced the incidence of pneumothorax.[24] Contrary to earlier observations,[10, 12] recent studies suggest that adequate oxygenation can be maintained at relatively high frequencies.[11, 24] Nonetheless, it appears that the incidence of chronic lung disease or mortality is not altered by ventilation at these moderately high frequencies.[24] When very high frequencies are used, inspiratory time ($T_I$) is shortened and resultant tidal volume may decrease.[5, 9] Using a mechanical lung model, it has been demonstrated that with some pressure-preset ventilators, minute ventilation reaches a plateau or decreases at rates higher than 75 per minute when an I:E ratio of 1:2 is used due to a reduction in the tidal volume.[9] In infants with RDS ventilated with pressure-limited time-cycled ventilators, tidal volume delivery is maintained fairly constant as long as $T_I$ is longer than 0.4 seconds.[5] Furthermore, if a very short expiratory time ($T_E$) is employed during high frequencies, expiration may be incomplete.[6] The gas trapped in the lungs would increase functional residual capacity and place the infant on the flat part of the pressure-volume curve, thus decreasing lung compliance.[6] As discussed for PEEP, the gas trapping, also known as inadvertent PEEP, that may accompany the use of a very short $T_E$ would result in reduction of the effective pressure gradient and elevation of $Pa_{CO_2}$.

It is important to note that frequency changes alone (with a constant I:E ratio) usually do not alter $\overline{P}aw$ and do not substantially affect $Pa_{O_2}$. Nonetheless, because it takes a certain time for a pressure plateau to be reached, changes in $T_I$ that accompany frequency adjustments may affect the airway pressure waveform and thus $\overline{P}aw$. Therefore, the decreased oxygenation observed by some investigators when high frequencies are employed is likely due to an inadvertent reduction in $\overline{P}aw$.[10] In addition, a small increase in $Pa_{O_2}$ may be expected as frequency is increased due to a reduction of alveolar carbon dioxide tension ($PA_{CO_2}$) and corresponding increase in alveolar oxygen tension ($PA_{O_2}$). If pulmonary artery hypertension and right-to-left shunting are prominent, the increased pH and reduced $Pa_{CO_2}$ that accompany the use of high frequencies may reduce shunting and markedly increase $Pa_{O_2}$ in the absence of any increase in $\overline{P}aw$.

### Ratio of Inspiratory to Expiratory Time (I:E Ratio)

The major effect of changes in I:E ratio is on $\overline{P}aw$ and thus oxygenation.[12, 14, 15] Reversed I:E ratios (longer $T_I$ than $T_E$) of as high as 4:1 have been shown effective in increasing $Pa_{O_2}$.[12, 14] Although a retrospective study suggested a decreased incidence of bronchopulmonary dysplasia with the use of reversed I:E ratios,[25] a large well-controlled, randomized clinical trial has revealed only a reduction in the duration of high inspired $O_2$ concentration and PEEP exposure with reversed I:E ratios but no difference in morbidity or mortality.[17] Furthermore, when corrected for $\overline{P}aw$, I:E ratio changes are not as effective in increasing oxygenation as changes in PIP or PEEP.[18] Caution should be exercised when employing very long $T_I$ since this practice may increase the risk of air leaks[27] and impede venous return. Changes in I:E ratio do not usually alter tidal volume, unless $T_I$ or $T_E$ become too short,[10] that is, less than three to five time constants. Thus, $CO_2$ elimination is usually not altered by I:E ratio changes.[12, 14, 15, 17, 18]

### *Inspired Oxygen Concentration ($FI_{O_2}$)*

Changes in inspired oxygen concentration ($FI_{O_2}$) alter alveolar oxygen tension and thus oxygenation. Since $FI_{O_2}$ and $\bar{P}aw$ both determine oxygenation, we attempt to balance them as follows:

1. During increasing support, $FI_{O_2}$ is first increased (until around 60% to 70%) when additional increases in $\bar{P}aw$ are warranted.
2. During weaning, $FI_{O_2}$ is first decreased (to around 40% to 70%) before $\bar{P}aw$ is reduced since maintenance of an appropriate $\bar{P}aw$ may allow a substantial reduction in $FI_{O_2}$. $\bar{P}aw$ should be reduced before a very low $FI_{O_2}$ is reached. A higher incidence of air leaks has been observed when distending pressures are not weaned until a low $FI_{O_2}$ is reached.[28]

However, insufficient data on oxygen vs. pressure-related lung injury are available.

### *Flow*

Flow changes have not been well studied in infants but probably affect arterial blood gases minimally as long as a sufficient flow is used. To maintain a square pressure waveform and adequate tidal volume, high inspiratory flows are needed when inspiratory time is shortened.

## Volume vs. Pressure Ventilators

Ventilators may be classified according to the way gas delivery during inspiration is controlled. Thus *pressure* ventilators control the peak inspiratory pressure applied to the airways during inspiration, whereas *volume* ventilators control the delivered volume. In addition to controlling pressure or volume, the inspiratory cycle may be terminated after a certain preset time or volume is reached. These ventilators are thus time- or volume-cycled, respectively. For safety purposes, some ventilators may also be made to cycle when a preset PIP is reached independently of their time- or volume-cycling mechanisms. Because of ease of use, most neonatal ventilators are pressure-limited time-cycled ventilators commonly called pressure ventilators. Volume ventilators are less frequently used, primarily for economic and technological reasons. Controversial data are presently available regarding differences in outcome of infants treated with volume vs. pressure ventilators. Using a volume-cycled machine, one presets the tidal volume (generally 7 to 10 cc/kg) delivered to the patient and adjusts the flow rate to determine the time over which it is delivered, thus determining the I:E ratio. It must be recognized, however, that such ventilators will deliver these volumes irrespective of the pressure generated unless overriding pressure limits are set. This assumes increasing importance in infants with severe RDS in whom compliance is so markedly diminished that delivery of a "normal" tidal volume requires a tremendous PIP. Furthermore, the high flow rates limit the adjustment of the I:E ratio. The alternative is the use of a pressure ventilator, wherein flow is delivered to the patient until the predetermined PIP is reached. At this point, the pressure may be immediately allowed to return to end-expiratory levels, producing a sawtooth pressure curve, or it may be maintained at peak levels for some time before the expiratory phase begins, producing a pressure curve with plateaus. Thus the pressure ventilator used in this way is really time-cycled and pressure-limited.

In this chapter, we have presented principles of pulmonary mechanics and gas exchange that are pertinent regardless of the brand of ventilator used. The reader is referred to other texts that review the specific ventilators. Chapter 13 reviews the complications secondary to assisted ventilation. New modes to assist ventilation and gas exchange are discussed in Chapters 14 and 15.

## PRACTICAL HINTS FOR ASSISTED VENTILATION

### Respiratory Distress Syndrome

**Indications for Assisted Ventilation.**—We recommend initiation of assisted ventilation if any of the following are present:

1. Respiratory acidosis with a pH less than 7.20 to 7.25
2. Severe hypoxemia ($Pa_{O_2}$ less than 50 to 60 torr) despite a high $FI_{O_2}$ (70% to 100%)
3. Apnea complicating the clinical course of RDS

Although a controversial practice, elective intubation has been shown in a prospective randomized trial to increase survival of very low birth weight infants.[29]

**Initial Ventilator Settings.**—One approach for selecting initial ventilator settings is the use of manual mask-and-bag ventilation by an experienced person while the pressures required to inflate the lungs and maintain normal blood gases are measured. Caution must be exercised because estimation of ventilating pressure is frequently inaccurate unless a pressure manometer is used. We have found that the ventilator settings in Table 12-2 are frequently adequate to start assisted ventilation during the first hours of life.

**Suggested Limits of Blood Gases and pH.**—We attempt to maintain a $Pa_{O_2}$ of 50 to 80 torr. pH is maintained between 7.25 and 7.45, which is usually achieved by keeping $Pa_{CO_2}$ between 35 and 50 torr during the acute stage of RDS. With increasing postnatal age and resolution of RDS, metabolic compensation permits an even higher $Pa_{CO_2}$ to be tolerated, as long as pH is above 7.25. At that time an even lower $Pa_{O_2}$ range may be acceptable.

**Weaning From the Ventilator.**—Termination of ventilatory support may be attempted when the ventilation provided by the ventilator is relatively minimal compared to the infant's spontaneous ventilation. Mean airway pressure and $F_{I_{O_2}}$ should also be relatively low. In infants with resolving RDS, weaning of assisted ventilation can usually proceed when the following settings have been achieved: PIP less than 18 cm $H_2O$, frequency less than 10 breaths per minute, and $F_{I_{O_2}}$ less than 40%. We administer CPAP through the endotracheal tube at the same pressure that has been used for PEEP, but increase $F_{I_{O_2}}$ by 5% to 10%. If adequate oxygenation and ventilation occur, endotracheal CPAP may be either weaned gradually to around 2 to 3 cm $H_2O$ before extubation, or alternatively, nasal CPAP may be initiated. A minimum endotracheal CPAP of 2 to 3 cm $H_2O$ should be used to maintain lung volume since tracheal intubation eliminates laryngeal mechanisms that control expiratory airflow and lung volume.[30] We prefer to restrict the use of nasal CPAP to preterm infants with resolving RDS who are at risk for atelectasis and apnea. Because very small endotracheal tubes add a high resistive load,[4] assisted ventilation is continued until even lower settings are achieved in patients intubated with a 2.5-mm tube, and endotracheal CPAP is only used for a short period before extubation. Infants with apnea, bronchopulmonary dysplasia, or extreme immaturity typically require a much slower weaning process that may last many days to weeks. In small infants, a low backup rate of assisted

**TABLE 12-2.**
Suggested Initial Ventilator Settings

|  | Infants With Normal Lungs | Infants With RDS |
| --- | --- | --- |
| PIP | 12–18 cm $H_2O$ | 20–25 cm $H_2O$ |
| PEEP | 2–3 cm $H_2O$ | 4–5 cm $H_2O$ |
| Frequency | 10–20/min | 20–40/min |
| I:E ratio | 1:2 to 1:10 | 1:1 to 1:3 |

ventilation elevates functional residual capacity.[31] In some infants, increasing respiratory drive with xanthines, such as theophylline, may facilitate weaning.[32]

## ALGORITHM FOR VENTILATORY MANAGEMENT OF INFANTS WITH RDS

Based on the physiologic principles and clinical studies discussed, we have developed a complex flowchart (Fig 12–8) that considers possible ventilatory maneuvers that may be performed with neonatal ventilators.[33] This algorithm has been based on blood gas results since that is how fine adjustment of ventilator settings is made by most clinicians. This approach should provide a rapid, logical, and consistent means of arriving at ventilator management decisions. The strategies of this algorithm are based largely on clinical studies of infants with respiratory failure usually due to RDS[5, 13, 41] and on the common practice including that of our institution. Major concepts of gas exchange included in the algorithm are that oxygenation is directly related to $\bar{P}_{aw}$ and that $CO_2$ elimination will depend on minute ventilation. Since the complexity of this algorithm limits its practical use, we have adapted it into an interactive user-friendly computer program. While the use of artificial intelligence is very new in patient management, it is possible that such a standardized approach may facilitate teaching, as well as improve patient care.

The flowchart illustrated in Figure 12–8 is composed of two types of symbols, diamonds, and squares. Diamond-shaped symbols indicate that a decision must be made about a specific condition. One or two lines enter each diamond, or decision symbol, and two lines emerge from it. Emerging lines are labeled with decisions, such as "yes" or "no". These lines indicate the direction to be taken, based on the decision made. Square symbols indicate the type and direction of a particular ventilator setting change. The magnitude of each suggested ventilator change is not indicated but will depend on how much the patient's blood gas tensions deviate from the normal range. Table 12–3 lists other symbols and abbreviations used in the flowchart and in the text.

We make several assumptions concerning use of the algorithm: (1) that mechanical ventilation is being employed at appropriate settings; (2) that significant metabolic acidosis has been corrected; (3) that complications such as pneumothorax and endotracheal tube misplacement or obstruction have been ruled out; (4) that the infant has uncomplicated RDS without significant components of persistent pulmonary hyper-

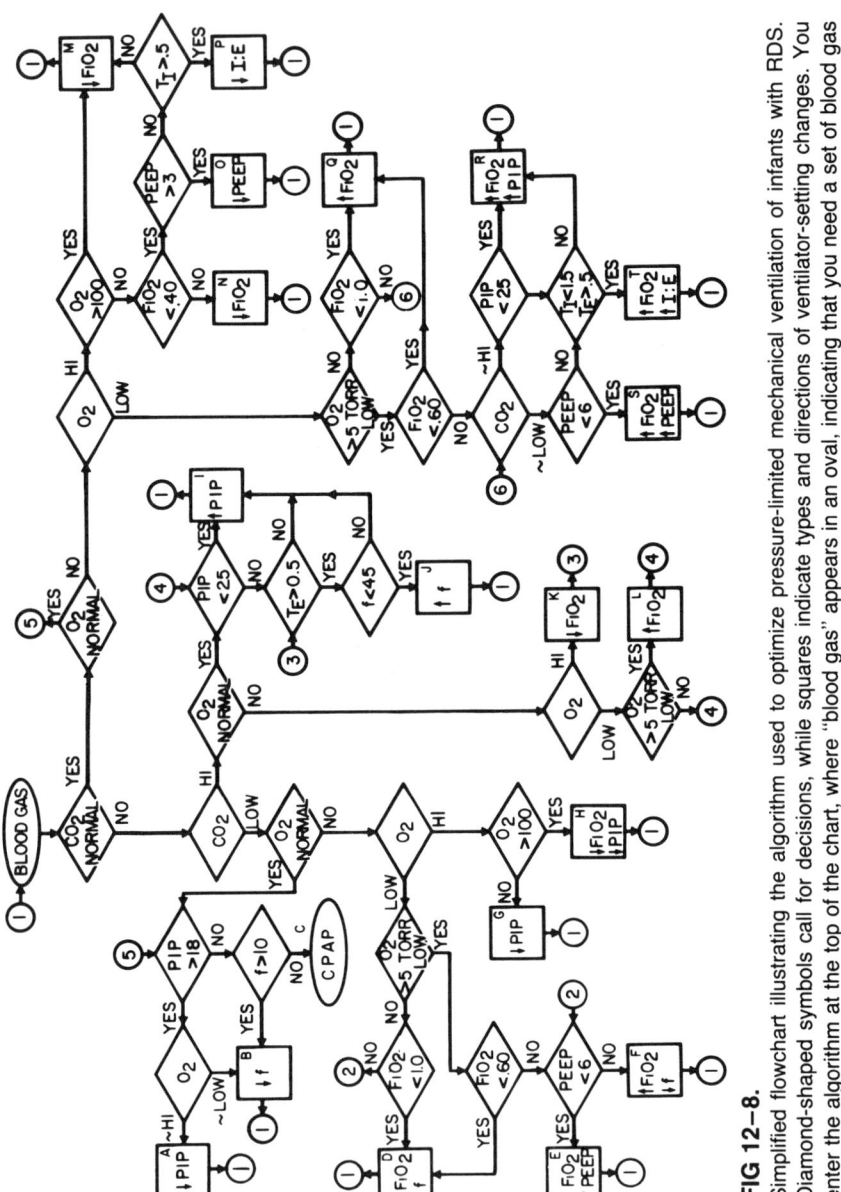

**FIG 12–8.**
Simplified flowchart illustrating the algorithm used to optimize pressure-limited mechanical ventilation of infants with RDS. Diamond-shaped symbols call for decisions, while squares indicate types and directions of ventilator-setting changes. You enter the algorithm at the top of the chart, where "blood gas" appears in an oval, indicating that you need a set of blood gas values to get started. Follow the flowchart until a square is reached. If a number other than 1 is reached, reenter the algorithm as appropriate. Rationales for the recommended ventilator-setting changes are included in the text. (From Chatburn RL, Carlo WA, Lough MD: Clinical algorithm for pressure-limited ventilation of neonates with respiratory distress syndrome. *Resp Care* 1983; 28:1579. Used by permission.)

**TABLE 12–3.**
Abbreviations and Symbols Used in the Flowchart in Figure 12–8

| | |
|---|---|
| $CO_2$ | Arterial carbon dioxide tension (mm Hg) |
| $O_2$ | Arterial oxygen tension (mm Hg) |
| $FI_{O_2}$ | Fraction of inspired oxygen |
| PIP | Peak inspiratory pressure (cm $H_2O$) |
| $\bar{P}aw$ | Mean airway pressure (cm $H_2O$) |
| PEEP | Positive end-expiratory pressure (cm $H_2O$) |
| CPAP | Continuous positive airway pressure without mechanical ventilation (cm $H_2O$) |
| I:E | Ratio of inspiratory to expiratory time |
| f | Ventilator frequency (breaths/min). Unless otherwise specified, a change in frequency should be accompanied by a change in I:E to maintain the same $T_I$, so that tidal volume remains constant |
| $T_I$ | Inspiratory time (sec) |
| $T_E$ | Expiratory time (sec) |
| HI | The variable in the decision symbol is above normal range |
| LOW | The variable in the decision symbol is below normal range |
| ≈HI | The variable in the decision symbol is at the high end of normal |
| ≈LOW | The variable in the decision symbol is at the low end of normal |
| ↑ | Increase |
| ↓ | Decrease |
| > | Greater than |
| < | Less than |
| Torr | Unit of pressure; 1 torr = 1 mm Hg |

tension, sepsis or other problems; (5) that other observations, such as chest movement and breath sounds, are being made continuously and are being integrated into clinical decisions.

It should be remembered that many uncontrollable features may influence ventilation and perfusion and the resulting gas exchange of a neonate, and that a given maneuver sometimes produces an unexpected and difficult-to-explain result. Therefore, the algorithm, though based on sound reasoning, can give less than optimal results in certain situations. At such times, the clinician must rely on personal experience and intuition in the absence of other relevant clinical data.

### Rationales for This Algorithm

In this flowchart each square symbol, which contains a recommended ventilator change, is labeled with a letter in the upper right-hand corner. The letter corresponds to a specific line of reasoning that justifies the change. We prefer to limit ventilator changes to no more than one per blood gas result. When two simultaneous changes have been recommended, one relates to $FI_{O_2}$. The limits for the ventilator settings in this algorithm (e.g., f up to about 45 breaths/minute, PEEP up to about 6 cm $H_2O$) represent our usual clinical practice in the management of the uncomplicated patient, but may have to be changed according to other protocols in the management of some complicated patients. The following is an explanation of the specific rationale corresponding to each square-symbol letter:

A. Decreasing PIP will decrease tidal volume and should increase $Pa_{CO_2}$. If you have arrived here or at B via 5, then the ventilator changes represent weaning procedures, with the hope that the infant's spontaneous respirations will help maintain normal gas exchange. It should be noted that infant ventilators are designed to be used primarily in the intermittent mandatory ventilation (IMV) mode. Changes in $\bar{P}aw$ have been shown to be directly related to oxygenation. The reduction in $\bar{P}aw$ caused by the lowering of PIP is appropriate, as $Pa_{O_2}$ is relatively high.

B. Ventilation is reduced by a decrease in frequency. Compared to a decrease in PIP, the decrease in frequency should have less potential for lowering $Pa_{O_2}$ because it has little or no effect on lung volume.

C. When the ventilator settings have been reduced to PIP less than 18 cm $H_2O$ and f less than 10/minute, the infant may be given a trial of CPAP with the ventilator through the endotracheal tube. The $F_{I_{O_2}}$ may be raised slightly to help compensate for the increased work of breathing when IMV is stopped.

D. Ventilation is decreased by a decrease in frequency rather than a decrease in PIP, for the same reason as in B. However, the low oxygenation necessitates a concomitant increase in $F_{I_{O_2}}$.

E. If the $F_{I_{O_2}}$ is greater than 60% and $Pa_{O_2}$ is very low (more than 5 mm Hg below the lowest acceptable value), it is better to make a ventilator setting change that substantially increases $\bar{P}aw$. Therefore, if PEEP is less than 6 cm $H_2O$, it can be increased, and a concomitant temporary increase in $F_{I_{O_2}}$ may be in order. Increasing PEEP in this situation has two effects: first, it increases $\bar{P}aw$, which should improve oxygenation; second, it should reduce the tidal volume and increase $Pa_{CO_2}$.

F. Ventilation is decreased by a frequency decrease, rather than a decrease in PIP, as explained in B. In contrast to D, here the reduction in frequency should be made while the I:E is maintained or slightly increased (as long as $T_I$ is less than 1.5 seconds). If the I:E is held constant, $\bar{P}aw$ and hence oxygenation will not decrease along with the frequency. On the other hand, an increase in $\bar{P}aw$ achieved by increasing the I:E may improve oxygenation. As in E, a temporary increase in $F_{I_{O_2}}$ might be necessary to assure adequate oxygenation.

G. Lowering PIP will decrease tidal volume and should increase $Pa_{CO_2}$. This, in conjunction with the decrease in $\bar{P}aw$, should decrease $Pa_{O_2}$. Note: if the PIP is relatively low (less than 23 cm $H_2O$) compared to f (more than 20/minute), it would probably be better to decrease f instead, as in H, to prevent atelectasis.

H. PIP is decreased for the same reason as in G. In addition, the $F_{I_{O_2}}$ should be immediately reduced, as a high $Pa_{O_2}$ has been implicated in the etiology of retrolental fibroplasia.

I. Increasing PIP increases the tidal volume and should decrease $Pa_{CO_2}$. A change in PIP rather than in frequency at this point illustrates our philosophy that this form of ventilation is truly IMV, favoring relatively large tidal volumes and low rates. We have arbitrarily set an upper limit of 25 cm $H_2O$ on PIP (and thus limited tidal volume), although at times we are forced to exceed this limit (see J and T). The increase in $\overline{P}_{aw}$ consequent to increasing PIP could also increase oxygenation.

J. Once the upper limit of PIP has been reached, ventilation is increased by means of frequency. However, an arbitrary limit on frequency has been set at 45 breaths/minute. When this limit has been reached, further increases in ventilation should be made by raising PIP above 25 cm $H_2O$. Notice that a further limitation of frequency is that $T_E$ must be at least 0.5 second because time constants for the lungs of preterm infants may range approximately from 0.05 to 0.14 second. This means that lung pressure may require as much as 0.5 to 0.7 second to equilibrate with mouth pressure. Maintaining $T_E$ at 0.5 second reduces the risk of alveolar gas trapping.

K. The $F_{I_{O_2}}$ is reduced because of the high $Pa_{O_2}$. At the same time, either PIP or frequency is increased based on decisions starting with an evaluation of $T_E$. An alternative approach at this point would be simply to decrease the PEEP, assuming it is greater than 3 or 4 cm $H_2O$. This would at once increase the tidal volume (decreasing $Pa_{CO_2}$) and decrease $\overline{P}_{aw}$ (decreasing $Pa_{O_2}$). If the $Pa_{O_2}$ is much greater than 100 mm Hg, a concomitant decrease in $F_{I_{O_2}}$ may be necessary to avoid the risk of retrolental fibroplasia.

L. Increasing $F_{I_{O_2}}$ is probably the surest way to increase $Pa_{O_2}$. In addition, since $Pa_{O_2}$ is more than 5 mm Hg below normal and $Pa_{CO_2}$ is above normal, a change in PIP or f is indicated. If $Pa_{O_2}$ is less than 5 mm Hg below normal, however, a change in ventilation only, especially by an increase in PIP, might bring oxygenation into the normal range.

M. If the $Pa_{O_2}$ is too high, the $F_{I_{O_2}}$ should be immediately reduced, as in H.

N. The $F_{I_{O_2}}$ is reduced before PEEP is lowered, as maintenance of PEEP might also allow a substantial reduction in $F_{I_{O_2}}$. The upper limit of PEEP is 6 cm $H_2O$, so the algorithm would not lead to an instance in which the $F_{I_{O_2}}$ is too low while the PEEP is too high.

O. Given that the $F_{I_{O_2}}$ is relatively low, the next consideration should be given to PEEP. This block allows for the reduction of PEEP, the lower limit of which we have set at 3 cm $H_2O$. In addition to decreasing $\overline{P}aw$ and thus, it is hoped, $Pa_{O_2}$, this maneuver may increase the tidal volume, which would eventually allow a reduction of PIP.

P. If PEEP has already been reduced, $\overline{P}aw$ may be lowered by decreasing the I:E. Maintaining $T_I$ at 0.5 second helps to ensure delivery of adequate tidal volume.

Q. When oxygenation is low, an $F_{I_{O_2}}$ increase is the most direct way of increasing $Pa_{O_2}$. If $F_{I_{O_2}}$ is greater than 60% and $Pa_{O_2}$ is very low, an increase in $\overline{P}aw$ is indicated (R,S,T).

R. An increase in PIP is recommended because it should improve ventilation as well as oxygenation. A concomitant increase in $F_{I_{O_2}}$ might be necessary if the $Pa_{O_2}$ is too low.

S. If PEEP is relatively low, it may be increased independently of PIP to improve oxygenation. The possible slight decrease in tidal volume should not be a problem, as the $Pa_{CO_2}$ is in the low range of normal. As in R, a concomitant increase in $F_{I_{O_2}}$ might be necessary.

T. Once PIP is at 25 cm $H_2O$, an increase in the I:E may be used to increase $\overline{P}aw$ and consequently improve oxygenation. Note that an I:E increase should be considered only when $T_I$ is less than 1.5 seconds and $T_E$ is greater than 0.5 second. If one of these conditions is not met, it would be better to increase PIP above 25 cm $H_2O$, our recommended upper limit, as well as to increase $F_{I_{O_2}}$ if it is less than 1.0.

Readers should remember that the flowchart represents our own philosophy of ventilator management, which is by no means universally accepted. For example, some researchers advocate higher frequency and lower pressures to prevent barotrauma. Until long-term controlled studies show an advantage of high-frequency ventilation over conventional techniques, we prefer to use rates lower than 60 breaths/minute. We believe that this algorithm represents what can be considered "conventional" therapy for preterm neonates.

## Validation of This Algorithm

Although this algorithm is based on previous clinical studies, its evaluation in clinical use is necessary. To determine the effectiveness of the computer program, we evaluated the correction of deranged arterial blood gases in three groups of neonates: a retrospective control group, a prospective control group, and a computer-assisted management group in which patients were managed after consultation with the computer program.[34] We observed that arterial blood gases improved more frequently in the neonates managed with computer con-

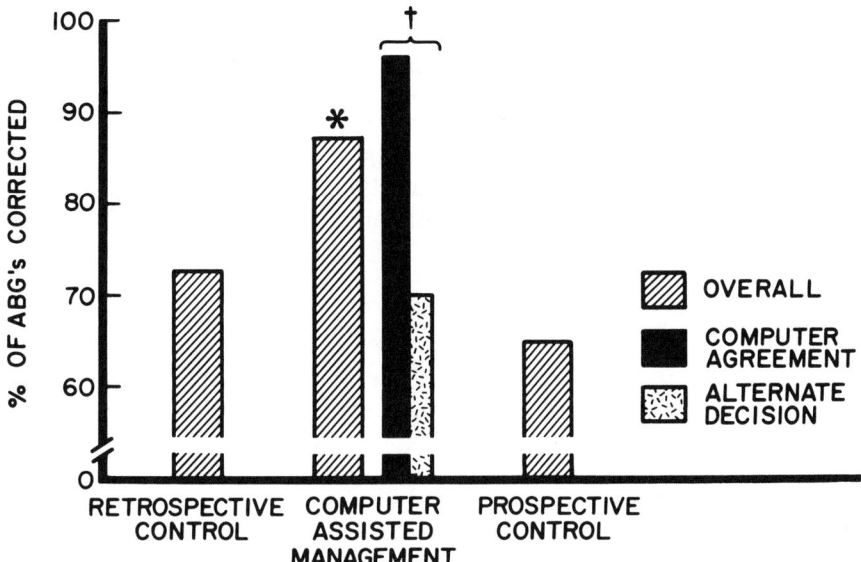

**FIG 12-9.**
Percentage correction of arterial blood gas derangements in three groups of patients with RDS. In the computer-assisted management group, arterial blood gases were corrected more frequently when computer recommendations were followed than when alternate decisions were implemented (†$P<.05$). Arterial blood gases were more frequently corrected in the computer-assisted management group (*) than in either retrospective ($P<.05$) or prospective control groups ($P<.005$). From Carlo WA et al: Efficacy of computer-assisted management of respiratory failure in neonates. *Pediatrics* 1986; 78:139. Used by permission.)

sultation than in both control groups (Fig 12-9). Because rationales are included for each recommended ventilator setting change, the algorithm may also be used as a didactic tool, particularly for those inexperienced in neonatal assisted ventilation. This logical approach will provide consistent care that is important in clinical studies on assisted ventilation.

## DISEASES OTHER THAN RESPIRATORY DISTRESS SYNDROME

### Persistent Fetal Circulation

In diseases such as meconium aspiration syndrome, asphyxia and congenital diaphragmatic hernia, in which extrapulmonary shunting dominates the clinical picture, hyperventilation to reduce $Pa_{CO_2}$ to 20 torr (or even lower) may be necessary. The accompanying alkalosis and hypocapnia reduce pulmonary vascular resistance and right-to-left shunting. Patients with persistent fetal circulation are less likely to increase their oxygenation in response to elevation in $\bar{P}_{aw}$, but rather improve when shunting is reduced. Since lung compliance is not markedly decreased in these infants, high frequencies (up to 80/minute) rather than high PIP are usually safer. Caution must be exercised when a short $T_E$ is employed in these infants, who usually have a normal lung compliance and a relatively long time constant, because gas trapping may occur. The use of low PEEP is also recommended in these infants.

**Apnea**

Infants that need assisted ventilation for apnea usually have normal lungs and can be ventilated with relatively low ventilator settings (see Table 12–2).

## SUMMARY

Based on the current knowledge of pulmonary mechanics and results of clinical studies, we have reviewed principles that govern gas exchange during assisted ventilation in infants with RDS. Guidelines for changes in ventilator settings have been presented with respect to their specific effects on $CO_2$ elimination and $O_2$ uptake. In addition, their possible mechanisms of action and potential side effects have been addressed. While general strategies have been presented, they must be employed with caution. All infants will not exhibit the expected response to ventilator-setting changes, and thus their ventilatory management, as well as their general medical care, will need to be individualized.

## REFERENCES

1. Modansky DL, Lawson EE, Chernick V, et al: Pneumothorax and other forms of pulmonary air leaks in newborns. Am Rev Resp Dis 1979; 120:729–737.
2. Edwards DK, Dyer WM, Northway WH: Twelve years experience with bronchopulmonary dysplasia. Pediatrics 1977; 59:839–846.
3. Perelman RH, Farrell PM: Analysis of causes of neonatal death in the United States with specific emphasis on fatal hyaline membrane disease. Pediatrics 1982; 70:570–575.
4. LeSouef PN, England SJ, Bryan AC: Total resistance of the respiratory system in preterm infants with and without an endotracheal tube. J Pediatr 1984; 104:108–111.

5. Field D, Milner AD, Hopkin IE: Inspiratory time and tidal volume during intermittent positive pressure ventilation. *Arch Dis Child* 1985: 60:259–261.
6. Cartwright DW, Willis MM, Gregory GA: Functional residual capacity and lung mechanics at different levels of mechanical ventilation. *Crit Care Med* 1984; 12:422–427.
7. Gonzalez F, Richardson P, Carlstrom J: Effect of rapid rate ventilation on pulmonary function in an animal model of respiratory distress syndrome. *Am Rev Respir Dis* 1984; 129:A108.
8. Simbruner G, Gregory GA: Performance of neonatal ventilators: The effects of changes in resistance and compliance. *Crit Care Med* 1981; 9:509–514.
9. Boros SJ, Bing DR, Mammel MC, et al: Using conventional infant ventilators at unconventional rates. *Pediatrics* 1984; 74:487–492.
10. Boros SJ, Campbell K: A comparison of the effects of high frequency-low tidal volume and low frequency-high tidal volume mechanical ventilation. *J Pediatr* 1980; 97:108–112.
11. Field D, Milner AD, Hopkin IE: High and conventional rates of positive pressure ventilation. *Arch Dis Child* 1984; 59:1151–1154.
12. Reynolds EOR: Effect of alterations in mechanical ventilator settings on pulmonary gas exchange in hyaline membrane disease. *Arch Dis Child* 1971; 46:152–158.
13. Chatburn RL, Lough MD: Mechanical ventilation, in Lough MD, Doershuk C, Stern R (eds): *Pediatric Respiratory Therapy*, ed 3. Year Book Medical Publishers, Chicago, 1985, pp 148–191.
14. Herman, S, Reynolds EOR: Methods for improving oxygenation in infants mechanically ventilated for severe hyaline membrane disease. *Arch Dis Child* 1973; 48:612–617.
15. Boros SJ: Variations in inspiratory:expiratory ratio and airway pressure wave form during mechanical ventilation: The significance of mean airway pressure. *J Pediatr* 1979; 94:114–117.
16. Ciszek TA, Modanlou HD, Owings D, et al: Mean airway pressure: Significance during mechanical ventilation in neonates. *J Pediatr* 1981; 99:121–126.
17. Spahr RC, Klein AM, Brown DR, et al: Hyaline membrane disease: A controlled study of inspiratory to expiratory ratio in its management by ventilator. *Am J Dis Child* 1980; 134:373–376.
18. Stewart AR, Finer NN, Peters KL: Effects of alterations of inspiratory and expiratory pressures and inspiratory/expiratory ratios on mean airway pressure, blood gases, and intracranial pressure. *Pediatrics* 1981; 67:474–481.
19. Ratner I, Hernandez J, Accurso F: Low peak inspiratory pressures for ventilation of infants with hyaline membrane disease. *J Pediatr* 1982; 100:802–804.
20. Chatburn RL, Primiano FP, Lough MD: Mechanical ventilation, in Lough MD, Chatburn RL, Schrock WA (eds): *Handbook of Respiratory Care*. Year Book Medical Publishers, Chicago, 1983, p 75.

21. Fox WW, Gewitz MH, Berman LS, et al: The $Pa_{O_2}$ response to changes in end expiratory pressure in the newborn respiratory distress syndrome. Crit Care Med 1977; 5:226–229.
22. Gregory GA, Kitterman JA, Phibbs RH, et al: Treatment of the idiopathic respiratory distress syndrome with continuous positive airway pressure. N Engl J Med 1971; 284:1333.
23. Avery ME, Tooley WH, Keller JB, et al: Is chronic lung disease in low birth weight infants preventable? A survey of eight centers. Pediatrics 1987; 79:26–30.
24. Heicher DA, Kasting DS, Harrod JR: Prospective clinical comparison of two methods for mechanical ventilation of neonates: Rapid rate and short inspiratory time versus slow rate and long inspiratory time. J Pediatr 1981; 98:957–961.
25. Reynolds EOR, Taghizadeh A: Improved prognosis of infants mechanically ventilated for hyaline membrane disease. Arch Dis Child 1974; 49:505–515.
26. Philips JB III, Beale EF, Howard JE, et al: Effect of positive end-expiratory pressure on dynamic respiratory compliance in neonates. Biol Neonate 1980; 38:270–275.
27. Primhak RA: Factors associated with pulmonary air leak in premature infants receiving mechanical ventilation. J Pediatr 1983; 102:764–768.
28. Hall RT, Rhodes PG: Pneumothorax and pneumomediastinum in infants with idiopathic respiratory distress syndrome receiving continuous positive airway pressure. Pediatrics 1975; 55:493–496.
29. Drew JH: Immediate intubation at birth of the very-low-birth-weight infant: Effect on survival. Am J Dis Child 1982; 136:207–210.
30. Fox WW, Berman LS, Dinwiddie R, et al: Tracheal extubation of the neonate at 2–3 centimeters $H_2O$ continuous positive airway pressure. Pediatrics 1977; 59:257–261.
31. Shutack JG, Fox WW, Shaffer TH, et al: Effect of low-rate intermittent mandatory ventilation on pulmonary function of low-birth-weight infants. J Pediatr 1982; 100:799–802.
32. Harris MC, Baumgart S, Rooklin AR, et al: Successful extubation of infants with respiratory distress syndrome using aminophylline. J Pediatr 1983; 103:303–305.
33. Chatburn RL, Carlo WA, Lough MD: Clinical algorithm for pressure-limited ventilation of neonates with respiratory distress syndrome. Resp Care 1983; 28:1579–1585.
34. Carlo WA, Pacifico L, Chatburn RL, et al: Efficacy of computer-assisted management of respiratory failure in neonates. Pediatrics 1986; 78:139–143.

# 13

# Complications of Neonatal Respiratory Care

Richard J. Martin, M.D.
Avroy A. Fanaroff, M.B., F.R.C.P.E.

As the population of low birth weight infants requiring assisted ventilation has dramatically increased, so has the incidence of acute complications of their ventilatory care. Of equal concern is the large number of preterm infants who develop chronic lung injury. This process commonly referred to as bronchopulmonary dysplasia (BPD) is a symptom complex typically associated with prolonged ventilator and oxygen therapy, although controversy reigns regarding the individual contributions of oxygen, endotracheal intubation, and ventilatory pressure to this clinicopathologic process. While the various components of assisted ventilation may potentially compromise all the infant's developing organ systems, we will focus primarily on the impact of respiratory care on the maturing cardiorespiratory and central nervous systems.

## ACUTE AND SUBACUTE COMPLICATIONS

The acute complications of neonatal respiratory care range from instantaneous, potentially life-threatening events, such as a tension pneumothorax, to more subacute complications, such as a patent ductus arteriosus (PDA) that may in turn predispose to the development of chronic lung disease. The complications of neonatal assisted ventilation are summarized in Table 13–1, and the major ones not addressed in other chapters will be reviewed in greater detail.

**TABLE 13–1.**
Complications of Assisted Ventilation

| | |
|---|---|
| Air leaks | Pneumothorax, pneumomediastinum, pneumopericardium, pulmonary interstitial emphysema (PIE), pulmonary venous air embolism |
| Endotracheal tube | Dislodgement, extubation, atelectasis, occlusion |
| Hyperinflation | Air trapping, increased dead space, impaired cardiac output |
| Infection | Pneumonia, septicemia, meningitis |
| Airway injury | Erosion, granuloma, palatal groove, subglottic stenosis, necrotizing tracheobronchitis |
| Chronic lung disease | Bronchopulmonary dysplasia (BPD) |
| Miscellaneous | Intracranial hemorrhage, patent ductus arteriosus (PDA), retinopathy of prematurity |

## Air Leaks

Pulmonary air leaks comprise a clinical spectrum that includes *pneumothorax, pneumomediastinum, pneumopericardium, pulmonary interstitial emphysema* (PIE), and *pulmonary venous air embolism*.[1, 2] If significant morbidity and even mortality are to be minimized with these conditions, particularly tension pneumothorax, a high index of suspicion is essential to initiate early diagnosis and aggressive management.

Infants without underlying lung disease may spontaneously develop a small pneumothorax, but many of these air leaks are asymptomatic and go undetected. The risk of pulmonary air leaks is dramatically increased by vigorous resuscitation (i.e., manual ventilation) at birth, respiratory distress syndrome (RDS), meconium aspiration syndrome, and pulmonary hypoplasia. In infants treated with assisted ventilation, the incidence of pneumothorax and other air leaks is further increased, depending in part on the ventilatory technique employed (Fig 13–1).[2, 3] At our institution there has been a relatively high incidence of air leaks in infants with respiratory disease and who weigh less than 1.5 kg, a majority of whom have RDS (Table 13–2). In term infants with meconium aspiration syndrome, the incidence of air leaks is reported to range from 20% to 50%, often occurring early in the course of the disease. Infants with *hypoplastic lungs* accompanying renal agenesis (Potter's syndrome), other forms of renal dysplasia, or congenital diaphragmatic hernia are at highest risk for air leaks during assisted ventilation.

*Uneven alveolar ventilation* and *air trapping* both appear to figure in the pathophysiology of the air-leak syndromes. Nonhomogeneity of ventilation is a result of both atelectatic alveoli in RDS and small airway plugs in meconium aspiration syndrome. When relatively more com-

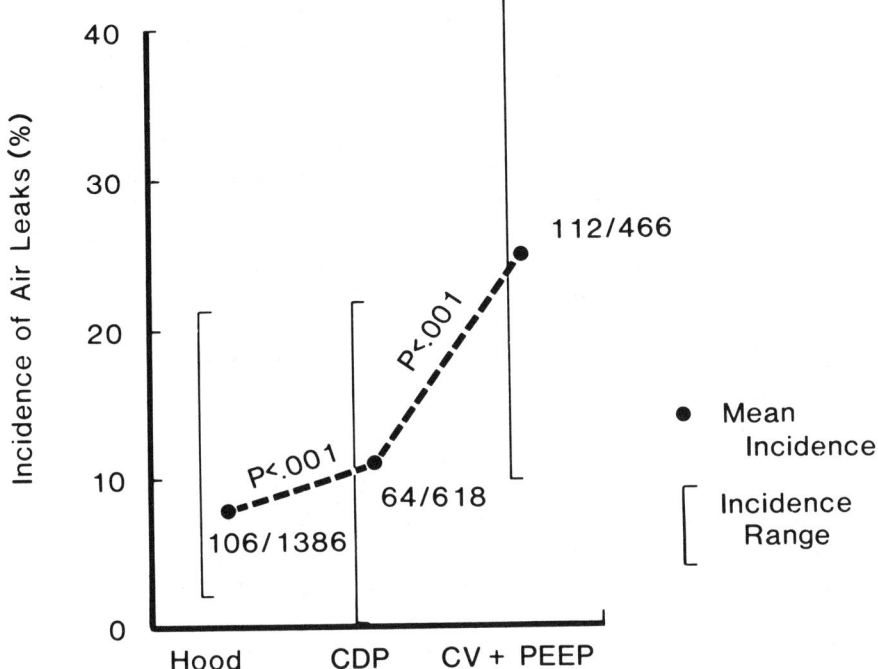

**FIG 13–1.**
The effect of type of ventilatory support on the incidence of air leaks in neonates. Ranges are incidence reported in different studies. The increased incidence of air leaks with continuous distending pressure *(CDP)* is accounted for by studies in which the distending pressure was applied endotracheally. Nasal CDP was not accompanied by an increase in air leaks. CV = conventional ventilation; PEEP = positive end-expiratory pressure; CDP = continuous distending pressure. (Adapted from Madansky DL, Lawson EE, Chernick V, et al: Pneumothorax and other forms of pulmonary air leaks in newborns. *Am Rev Respir Dis* 1979; 120:729.)

pliant areas of the lung are subjected to high transpulmonary pressures, overdistention leading to an increased risk of alveolar rupture may occur. Furthermore, during partial airway obstruction, full expiration is prevented, and with subsequent inspirations, accumulation of air

**TABLE 13–2.**
Incidence of Air Leaks in Infants With Respiratory Disease and Birth Weight Less Than 1.5 kg*

|  | Lived, % (n = 104) | Died, % (n = 44) | Total, % (n = 148) |
|---|---|---|---|
| Pneumothorax | 18 | 32 | 22 |
| PIE | 22 | 45 | 29 |
| Pneumomediastinum | 1 | 2 | 1 |
| Pneumopericardium | 1 | 4 | 2 |

*Data from Rainbow Babies and Childrens Hospital, 1985.

may rupture the alveolar space. The high incidence of air leaks during assisted ventilation has been attributed to barotrauma secondary to either high levels of peak inspiratory pressure or excessive positive end-expiratory pressure and resultant air trapping[3] (see Chapter 12). While optimal ventilator regimens need to be clarified, excessive prolongation of inspiratory time during conventional ventilation may be the major risk factor in the pathogenesis of air leaks.[3]

Extrapulmonary air should be suspected in any infant with respiratory disease whose condition suddenly deteriorates. Tachypnea is a uniform finding and may be accompanied by grunting and increasing pallor or cyanosis. If there is a unilateral pneumothorax, the cardiac apex may be shifted away from the affected side and breath sounds decreased. Some infants may develop abdominal distention from downward displacement of the diaphragm. Signs of shock may be present because of compression of the great veins and decreased cardiac output especially with a pneumopericardium. Hypoxemia results from both decreased alveolar ventilation and right-to-left shunting of pulmonary blood flow through the atelectatic areas.

*Transillumination* of the chest is extremely useful for immediate diagnosis of pneumothorax and is invariably positive for a large, unilateral pneumothorax. Transillumination is a technique in which a fiberoptic probe conducting a high-intensity light is placed against the chest. Normal lung tissue diffuses the light but large pockets of intrathoracic air show up as bright spots. The principal benefit of transillumination is to quickly detect sudden life-threatening air leaks that require immediate therapy prior to obtaining a definitive diagnosis with a *chest radiograph*. When there are questionable areas of abnormal transillumination and the infant's condition is stable, radiologic confirmation is indicated prior to therapeutic intervention. This will allow precise localization of the pneumothorax and differentiation from other causes of air leaks (see Chapter 11). Figure 13–2 is a chest radiograph that illustrates some of the air leaks that complicate assisted ventilation.

In infants with moderate to severe lung disease, the presence of a pneumothorax accentuates the respiratory difficulty and requires prompt if not urgent intervention. This consists of the placement of a large-bore, multiple-hole chest tube into the pleural space, preferably anterior to the lung. Anterior placement in the pleural space is best achieved by insertion of the tube into the chest at or just lateral to the anterior axillary line. This should be connected to an underwater seal at a suction pressure of 10 to 20 cm $H_2O$, since reaccumulation of air may occur if suction is not applied. Suction should be maintained until active bubbling has ceased. Once this has been observed, the tube should be clamped and removed within 24 hours if there has been no reac-

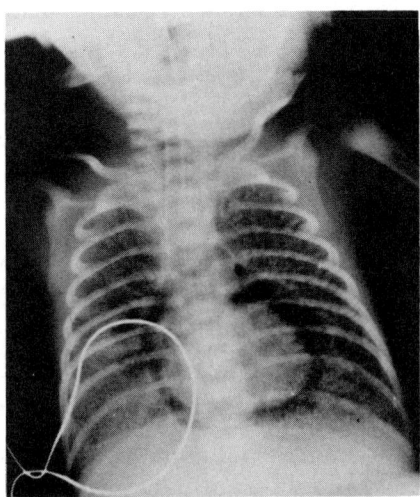

**FIG 13–2.**
Radiologic appearance of a pneumopericardium in a 1-week-old preterm infant with diffuse pulmonary interstitial emphysema.

cumulation of air in the pleural cavity. Lung perforation has been observed at autopsy in infants who required pleural drainage for pneumothorax, particularly when a trocar is employed during insertion. Infants with a large pneumomediastinum rarely benefit from decompression via an anteriorly placed chest tube. Pneumopericardium frequently presents with an overwhelming cardiorespiratory embarrassment, and pericardiocentesis may be lifesaving. Conservative therapy may be followed in cases of pneumothorax and pneumopericardium if there is no accompanying respiratory and hemodynamic compromise.

There appears to be an association between the occurrence of a pneumothorax and intraventricular hemorrhage in preterm infants.[4] Development of a pneumothorax seems to cause a marked increase in anterior cerebral artery blood flow followed by hemorrhage. Thus, it is proposed that a pneumothorax may increase the risk of intraventricular hemorrhage by impairing venous return to the heart and increasing cerebral arterial blood flow secondary to hypercapnia and raised systemic diastolic pressure.

Pulmonary interstitial emphysema, primarily a radiologic and pathologic diagnosis, occurs when air ruptures from alveoli or small airways into the perivascular tissues of the lung. Pulmonary interstitial emphysema is seen predominantly in preterm infants who require prolonged or intensive use of assisted ventilation. It may result in a vicious cycle by causing compression atelectasis of the adjacent lung, necessitating a further increase in ventilatory pressure and permitting still more escape of air into the interstitial tissues. The infants with PIE at highest risk for mortality are those of lowest birth weight and gestational age in whom PIE appears within the first 24 hours of life. In this population, the subsequent incidence of BPD may exceed 50%. During management of *diffuse PIE*, every attempt must be made to maintain mechanical ventilatory pressures at a safe minimum. High frequency ventilation shows real promise as a means of alleviating or even eliminating PIE in some cases. Conservative management of *localized PIE* is initially recommended as is positioning the infant such that the emphysematous lung is dependent. This may lead to clinical and radiologic improvement within 48 hours.

### Endotracheal Tube Complications and Airway Injury

Accidental *dislodgment* of an endotracheal tube into a main-stem bronchus, the pharynx, or esophagus is a well-recognized and extremely hazardous complication of mechanical ventilation. Intubation of the right main-stem bronchus usually results in atelectasis of the right upper lobe and hyperinflation of the remainder of the right side and the left lung. This is clinically characterized by deterioration in the patient's condition, often with cyanosis. Sudden deterioration from tube displacement must be differentiated from a pneumothorax. For example, esophageal intubation is characterized by loss of breath sounds and chest rise during assisted ventilation with air leaking from a gastric tube during inspiration and bubbling sounds heard from the stomach area. Auscultation of the chest may suggest if these complications are present, but radiologic studies may be needed to resolve the issue. It may also be necessary to quickly determine whether there is any mechanical failure of the ventilator by assuming manual ventilation with a bag. Similarly, accidental *extubation* usually is accompanied by sudden deterioration with cyanosis, bradycardia, and respiratory failure. Endotracheal-tube *occlusion* secondary to thick or impacted secretions can be minimized by adequate humidification during assisted ventilation. This complication is primarily detected by loss of breath sounds and chest rise and an inability to pass a suction catheter.

Postextubation *atelectasis*, most frequently involving the right upper lobe, may occur frequently during resolution of lung disease. The infants demonstrate increased respiratory difficulty with hypoxemia and hypercapnia. The approach to treatment comprises physiotherapy with postural drainage, CPAP, or endotracheal suctioning. Flexible fiberoptic bronchoscopy may allow removal of mucus plugs or even bronchial casts if present, resulting in prompt clinical and radiologic improvement. In patients with intractable atelectasis, reintubation and assisted ventilation may be necessary.

Prolonged use of orotracheal tubes has been associated with *palatal groove* formation, although subsequent growth and remodeling of the palate probably repair any early deformation.[5] Gross and histologic evidence of *inflammation* and epithelial *erosions* of the trachea have been noted at postmortem examination of infants dying after prolonged endotracheal intubation. Furthermore, fiberoptic inspection of the airways of infants who have been intubated for a prolonged period will reveal some pearly lesions below the cords, although most of these prove to be clinically insignificant. During assisted ventilation, use of a small endotracheal tube that ensures the presence of an air leak when the tube is in place is recommended to reduce the likelihood of tracheal damage (see Chapter 4). *Subglottic stenosis* has been noted in approximately 1% of survivors of mechanical ventilation with birth weights less than 1.5 kg.[7] Tracheostomy may be necessary for this small group of infants. Whether severe complication of endotracheal tubes can be reduced by performing earlier tracheostomy in some infants remains to be proven.

Necrotizing tracheobronchitis is a newly described lesion that has been reported at autopsy (or less frequently at bronchoscopy) in some ventilated infants.[6] Airway obstruction is caused by necrosis and detachment of epithelium, with airway injury extending into the submucosal tissues. The most common mode of clinical presentation appears to be sudden severe hypercapnia with decreased air entry that may require bronchoscopy to remove obstructing necrotic debris from the airway. This entity appears to represent iatrogenic injury, and inadequate humidification during either conventional or high-frequency ventilation has been implicated (although not proven) as the major etiologic factor.

**Infection**

The lungs represent a common site for the establishment of sepsis in the neonate. Bacterial, viral, or fungal infection may be acquired prior to delivery, at the time of birth, or in the postnatal period. Sepsis carries a substantial mortality in the neonate, and an extremely high index of suspicion must be maintained in infants requiring assisted ventilation and indwelling arterial or venous lines, since their risk for infection is increased. Apart from respiratory deterioration, other alerting features include thermal instability, apneic spells, abdominal distention, jaundice, or a metabolic acidosis. Full sepsis workup should be supplemented by white blood cell count with differential, platelet count, and Gram stain of tracheal aspirate, although the latter may not differentiate overt pulmonary infection from early colonization.

Antibiotic treatment almost invariably is instituted prior to identification of the pathogenic organism and determination of its antibiotic sensitivities. Broad-spectrum coverage, including a penicillin and an aminoglycoside, is the initial line of treatment, although for infections of later onset, agents specific for staphylococcal infection should be added and antifungal therapy considered. Periodic surveillance cultures should keep track of the predominant bacterial and fungal organisms to which these infants are predisposed in the intensive care unit.

## Intracranial Hemorrhage

*Subependymal* and *intraventricular hemorrhage* (IVH) occur in up to 50% of very immature infants with severe pulmonary disease. Numerous causes for IVH have been proposed, including neonatal asphyxia with hypotension, rapid volume expansion, changes in serum osmolarity resulting from excessive bicarbonate administration, coagulation abnormalities, hypoxemia, and hypercapnia. Intraventricular hemorrhage has been further correlated with mechanical ventilation employing high peak inflation pressures, prolonged inspiratory times, and especially the development of alveolar rupture and air leaks, all of which would be expected to alter cerebral blood flow or volume by impairing venous return. There is considerable interest in the roles of sedation and muscle paralysis for prevention of IVH during assisted ventilation. Unfortunately, widespread prophylactic use of phenobarbital does not appear to decrease the incidence of intraventricular hemorrhage in ventilated preterm infants,[8] while only selected infants with marked cerebral blood flow velocity fluctuations may benefit from paralysis with pancuronium bromide.[9]

## Patent Ductus Arteriosus

Congestive heart failure of varying severity is quite common in very low birth weight infants, and a PDA should be suspected when there is a delay in clinical improvement from RDS and the infant has persistent ventilator or oxygen dependency. Aggressive management is indicated if a PDA is clinically apparent and left-to-right shunting is confirmed by echocardiography. Therapy includes fluid restriction, medical management of congestive heart failure, and either surgical or pharmacologic (indomethacin) closure of the ductus. Persistence of a PDA has been implicated in the cause of BPD because it prolongs the duration of ventilatory assistance. Excess fluid intake has been associated with both entities. A multicenter collaborative trial has studied the efficacy of indomethacin therapy for preterm infants with a hemodynamically significant PDA.[10] A ductal closure rate of approximately 70% was achieved when indomethacin was given either concurrently with, or after failure of, usual medical therapy, without adverse effects when either strategy was used. Birth weight, gestational age, or age at time of drug administration did not significantly modify drug efficacy, and there was a reopening rate of approximately 25%, although in most situations the PDA subsequently closed without need for surgery.

## CHRONIC LUNG DISEASE

### Diagnostic Criteria

The increasing incidence of chronic respiratory disease can be directly related to the more aggressive respiratory management and increased survival of small preterm infants. While most infants with acute pulmonary disease in the first days of life make a rapid and complete recovery and subsequently have normal lungs, nonetheless, a substantial number of survivors are left with persistent pulmonary sequelae. *Bronchopulmonary dysplasia* (BPD) is the major form of chronic pulmonary disease in neonates. In 1967 Northway et al.[11] introduced the term BPD to describe chronic pulmonary insufficiency following severe RDS in infants who had been treated with artificial ventilation and prolonged high oxygen concentrations. Subsequent reports have described a similar disorder after prolonged assisted ventilation for meconium aspiration syndrome, persistent fetal circulation, and various forms of congenital cardiopulmonary disease.

Most centers have now adopted a more liberal definition of BPD and include all patients that, after requiring mechanical ventilation during the first week of life, remain oxygen dependent for more than 28 days and have persistent increased densities on chest radiographs. This disease is frequently referred to as chronic lung disease rather than BPD.[12, 13] Both incidence and severity vary widely, depending on precise diagnostic criteria and the neonatal population examined. The overall incidence varies from about 15% to 50% of infants weighing less than 1,500 gm and requiring assisted ventilation (Table 13–3).

The development of BPD often is suspected when substantial ventilator and oxygen dependence extends beyond 7 days. Nonetheless, definitive radiologic features (see Chapter 11) do not typically develop until later in the course, usually around the third week of life. The progression of BPD through the sequence of the four stages originally

**TABLE 13-3.**
Course of Respiratory Support in *Surviving* Infants Less Than 1.5 kg*†

| | Oxygen Supplementation, % | Ventilatory Assistance, %‡ |
|---|---|---|
| ≤6 days | 18 | 32 |
| 7-27 days | 29 | 32 |
| ≥28 days | 53 | 28 |

*Data from Rainbow Babies and Childrens Hospital, 1985.
†N = 104.
‡Not all infants received ventilatory assistance.

described by Northway et al.[11] and resulting in hyperinflation and cystic changes (Table 13-4) (for unknown reasons) is no longer commonly seen. Thus, a radiologic picture showing nonspecific chronic pulmonary involvement such as linear streaks, infiltrates, or residual haziness plus a clinical course that is compatible with BPD allows one to make this diagnosis with some degree of consistency. Of all the differential

**TABLE 13-4.**
Classification of Bronchopulmonary Dysplasia*

| | Postnatal Age | Radiographic Findings† | Pathological Findings |
|---|---|---|---|
| Stage I | 2-3 days | Identical to RDS | Hyaline membranes; atelectasis; metaplasia and necrosis of bronchiolar mucosa; loss of ciliated cells; lymphatic dilation |
| Stage II | 4-10 days | Increased pulmonary opacification | Thickening of basement membrane; necrosis and repair of bronchial and alveolar epithelium; start of emphysematous changes |
| Stage III | 10-20 days | Small cyst-like radiolucent areas | Alveolar coalescence; focal emphysematous changes; bronchial mucosal metaplasia and hyperplasia with increased mucus; atelectasis |
| Stage IV | >1 mo | Decrease in lung volume; strands of increased density | Group of emphysematous alveoli; atelectasis; increased collagen |

*Adapted from Northway WH, Rosan RC, Porter DY: Pulmonary disease following respirator therapy of hyaline membrane disease: Bronchopulmonary dysplasia. *N Engl J Med* 1967; 276:357.
†Many patients who do not show these sequential radiographic evolutions also develop changes typical of Stage IV BPD. Also, many patients develop radiographic findings consistent with Stages II or III BPD that clear within a few days evolving into chronic pulmonary disease.

diagnostic possibilities, Wilson-Mikity syndrome has probably engendered the greatest confusion with BPD. The radiologic similarities have caused some investigators to associate the two conditions, although differences appear to exist in their clinical course. Patients with Wilson-Mikity syndrome generally have an initially benign course, frequently with normal early chest radiographs and an insidious onset of respiratory difficulty. In contrast, patients who develop BPD tend to initially have severe respiratory disease (usually RDS) and a need for high inspired oxygen concentrations and assisted ventilation. For unknown reasons, there has been a decline in the incidence of the Wilson-Mikity syndrome in recent years, and in its typical form, this entity is rarely seen. It may be that the diagnosis of Wilson-Mikity syndrome has become irrelevant as the spectrum of disease incorporating BPD has broadened.

**Pathophysiologic Features**

The term bronchopulmonary dysplasia implies a disorder of growth accompanied by abnormal histologic features. During resolution of RDS, intra-alveolar exudate may be absorbed into the alveolar wall, resulting in *interstitial fibrosis*, or organized so that there is an obliteration of the alveolar space. Parts of the lung also may become airless and solid because of simple alveolar collapse. In either case, these regions of the lung are not contributing to gas exchange. Nonaerated regions may reaerate or, if they continue to be airless, will form scars of condensed lung tissue and become fibrotic. The bronchiolar mucosa is markedly abnormal with *dysplasia* and *peribronchiolar inflammation*. There is *bronchiolar muscular hypertrophy* and fibrosis of structural portions of the pulmonary lobule. Arterioles are variably hypertrophic, and there is significant involvement of lymphatic and perilymphatic areas. The typical macroscopic appearance in BPD is a coarse pattern of scarring mixed with regions of *emphysema*.

*Pulmonary function* testing has revealed severe maldistribution of ventilation in these infants.[14] Minute ventilation tends to be normal in infants with BPD, with increased respiratory frequency, decreased tidal volume, and hypercapnia. Infants with BPD characteristically have a marked increase in airway resistance (Table 13–5), a decreased dynamic compliance, and a large increase in the work of breathing. Static compliance has been found to be normal or increased indicating that the decrease in dynamic compliance is mainly due to nonhomogeneity of mechanical properties (time constants) among different lung regions. Functional residual capacity (FRC) may be decreased, normal, or increased, depending on the severity and stage of the pulmonary involvement.

**TABLE 13–5.**
Mechanisms of Airway Obstruction in Chronic Lung Disease*

Bronchiolar epithelial hyperplasia and metaplasia
Increased mucus
Mucosal edema (inflammation, fluid)
Bronchoconstriction
Small-airway closure

*Adapted from Bancalari E, Gerhardt T: Bronchopulmonary dysplasia. *Pediatr Clin North Am* 1986; 33:1.

## Etiology

It has become generally accepted that *barotrauma* resulting from high pressures used in assisted ventilation is the major factor in the development of BPD. Nonetheless, pulmonary *oxygen toxicity* related to high levels of inspired oxygen and immaturity of the respiratory system itself are key etiologic components (Fig 13–3). Furthermore, the role of the endotracheal tube itself may be substantial; endotracheal tubes hinder the drainage of tracheal secretions and increase both dead space and resistance to airflow. Airway resistance appears to be increased after 3 to 5 days in infants mechanically ventilated for RDS who subsequently develop BPD.[15] Increased airway resistance could result in air-trapping and air-leak syndromes.

Although peak inspiratory pressure during assisted ventilation has been implicated in causing BPD, it is difficult to determine whether the high pressures have a causal effect on the chronic lung damage or

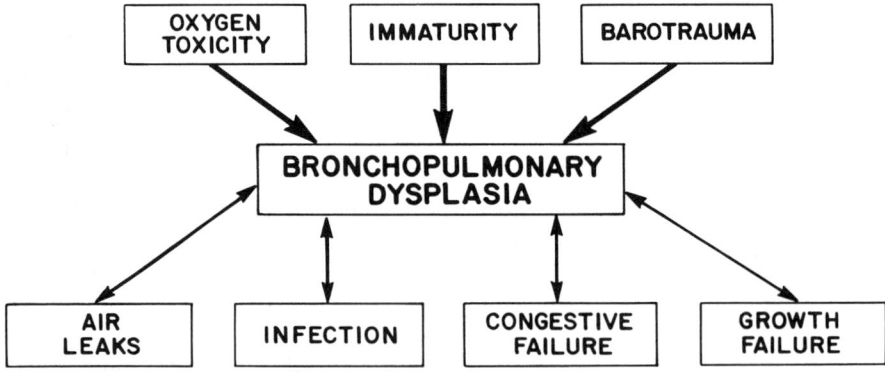

**FIG 13–3.**
A schematic representation of the pathophysiologic events that contribute to the progressive development of chronic lung injury. (From Fox WW, Morray JP, Martin RJ: Chronic neonatal lung disease, in Fanaroff AA, Martin RJ (ed): *Neonatal-Perinatal Medicine,* ed 4, CV Mosby Co, St Louis, 1987, p 634.)

whether these high settings are required after lung damage is already established. No prospective study controlling for other variables that may influence the development of BPD has shown a relationship between peak or mean airway pressure and BPD. The advent of high-frequency ventilation has raised hopes that these techniques may decrease the incidence of BPD primarily by achieving gas exchange at reduced airway pressures (see Chapter 14).

Clinical and experimental evidence have suggested that pulmonary oxygen toxicity is a major factor in the cause of BPD. Although many body tissues can be injured by high oxygen concentrations, the lung is exposed directly to the highest partial pressure of inspired oxygen. The precise concentration of oxygen that is toxic to the lung probably depends on a large number of variables, including maturation, nutritional and endocrine status, and duration of exposure to oxygen and other oxidants. The contribution of the alveolar macrophage to pathologic effects in the lung is not clear. Continued exposure to high oxygen is accompanied by an influx of polymorphonuclear leukocytes containing proteolytic enzymes. Therefore, proteolytic damage of structural elements in alveolar walls may be an important pathogenetic factor.[16]

Although the cellular basis for oxygen toxicity has not been completely elucidated, the principal mechanisms involve the univalent reduction of molecular oxygen and formation of free-radical intermediates. The latter can react with intracellular constituents and membrane lipids, thus initiating chain reactions that may result in tissue destruction.[17] To resist the detrimental effects of oxygen toxicity, the body has evolved various antioxidant enzymes, such as superoxide dismutase, which eliminate the superoxide radical, whereas other compounds such as vitamin E and selenium also may offer endogenous antioxidant protection. Controlled studies designed to enhance antioxidant protection in the neonate by the administration of high doses of vitamin E, however, have failed to demonstrate any beneficial effect.[18, 19]

The role of *infection* in the origin of BPD is not clear. Pneumatoceles and cystic lung disease occur in neonatal lungs secondary to infections by various bacteria. If these infections are chronic, they might result in bronchitis or small-airway disease. Recurrent infections appear, on the other hand, to be a common complication of long-term BPD.

The precise relationship between *fluid therapy*, PDA, and BPD has also not yet been completely established. Evidence suggests that presence of a PDA complicating the course of RDS increases the risk of BPD.[20] Increased pulmonary blood flow due to a PDA and the resulting increase in interstitial fluid cause a decrease in pulmonary compliance and an increase in airway resistance. These two changes may prolong the need for mechanical ventilation with higher ventilatory pressures and oxygen concentrations increasing the risk for BPD.

## Management

Successful treatment of severe BPD may require a long-term multidisciplinary commitment, since some infants require care for many years. Respiratory support may utilize intermittent mandatory ventilation (IMV), a form of assisted ventilation that allows the infant to breathe spontaneously between a set number of mechanical breaths per minute. This technique is of particular value in infants with BPD who may require prolonged ventilatory support. An IMV rate is selected that allows the partial pressure of $CO_2$ in arterial blood ($Pa_{CO_2}$) to be maintained in a high normal range. An increased inspired oxygen concentration is required to maintain a partial pressure of $O_2$ in arterial blood ($Pa_{O_2}$) in the 50 to 70 mm Hg range and prevent the pulmonary artery hypertension that occurs secondary to hypoxemia. The oxygen requirement decreases gradually as the disease process improves, but increases during feeding, physical activity, or during episodes of pulmonary infection or edema. Adequacy of gas exchange should be monitored by arterial blood gases at intervals dictated by the child's clinical condition. During times of stability, transcutaneous $Po_2$ measurements are satisfactory, although they underestimate $Pa_{O_2}$ by approximately 15 mm Hg in infants with BPD beyond 2 to 3 months of age.[21] Oxygen saturation monitors appear not to be influenced by advancing postnatal age, and arterial saturations in the range of 88% to 92% are clinically acceptable. Transcutaneous carbon dioxide tension ($TcPco_2$) can also be used to estimate $Pa_{CO_2}$, or capillary and venous blood samples can be used alternatively. The latter two techniques give values that overestimate (approximately by 5 mm Hg) $Pa_{CO_2}$.

Long-term mechanical ventilation requires the presence of a secure airway. If the use of such support is for 1 to 2 months or less, a well-secured endotracheal tube is sufficient, provided that attention is given to fit. If no leak occurs, the endotracheal tube is too large and should be replaced with a smaller tube. If mechanical ventilation is required for more than 1 to 2 months, tracheostomy may be a more appropriate form of airway control. Prolonged use of oversized endotracheal tubes may result in a high incidence of *subglottic stenosis* (see Chapter 4).

Inspired gases must be humidified to prevent damage to the respiratory tract mucosa by exposure to dry gas. Chest physiotherapy is performed at variable intervals (depending on secretions) in an attempt to prevent atelectasis and the pooling of secretions. Meanwhile, every effort should be made to keep the inspired oxygen concentration and ventilator pressures as low as possible to prevent further pulmonary damage. Intercurrent illnesses such as upper or lower respiratory tract infections, bronchospasm, congestive heart failure, or pulmonary artery hypertension may interrupt the weaning process and should be treated aggressively. Weaning from oxygen should progress concurrently and with even greater caution. Reduction in inspired oxygen of as little as 2% may result in a profound change in the infant's clinical condition and requires constant reassessment.

Adequate nutrition is a key aspect of care for the infant with BPD, who may have a 25% increase in resting $O_2$ consumption over controls, partially contributed by the elevated work of breathing.[22] Malnutrition will delay somatic growth and the development of new alveoli, making weaning from mechanical ventilation almost impossible. The malnourished patient is also more prone to infection. For these reasons, an aggressive approach should be taken toward supplying a parenteral or oral caloric intake that is adequate for growth. High-calorie formulas and supplements may be used to maximize the intake of calories while fluid intake is restricted to prevent congestive heart failure. Extra calcium and vitamin D intake may be indicated.

Infants with BPD are particularly susceptible to cor pulmonale, congestive failure, and pulmonary edema. Fluids are restricted as much as possible, considering the need for a high caloric intake, and chronic diuretic therapy is instituted. Parameters that need frequent monitoring include intake and output, electrolytes, and urine specific gravity. Physical examination with particular attention to body weight, rales, peripheral edema, and liver enlargement is necessary. The use of diuretics in these infants is associated with a rapid improvement in lung compliance and decrease in resistance, while blood gases may also show significant improvement.[23]

Even though many types of infection can have serious consequences for the child with BPD, bacterial and fungal sepsis generally result in the most profound setback. As a result, the child needs to be closely watched for early evidence of infection. Tracheal secretions are obtained biweekly for culture and Gram stain, or more often if a change in the quality and quantity of secretions indicates possible infection. Although it is difficult to distinguish between colonization of the airway and true infection, this distinction is important because overtreatment with antibiotics may result in the emergence of more virulent organisms. Selection of antibiotics is based on the sensitivity of the implicated organism, and treatment is continued for a minimum of 1 week or until the infection has been controlled. Clinical measures to prevent pulmonary superinfection are important. These include changing tracheostomy tubes twice weekly and careful hand washing prior to handling the infant.

Infants with both subacute and chronic forms of BPD may exhibit clinical elements of bronchospasm. Theophylline therapy tends to decrease pulmonary resistance and increase dynamic compliance.[24] Inhalation bronchodilators are also used in patients with BPD, and a decrease in airway resistance follows their use. Administration of dexamethasone may transiently improve lung function, but the increased risk of major infection and hypertension may not justify steroid administration.

Finally, as the infant with severe BPD may be ventilator dependent for many months and is thus deprived of normal parental stimulation, a well-organized program of infant stimulation may help the infant achieve maximum potential. Such a program will instruct the caretakers in helping the infant with various social, language, cognitive, and motor skills. Parental support groups may also offer a valuable resource for these families.

Infants with BPD are being increasingly discharged from the hospital prior to weaning from supplemental inspired oxygen or even assisted ventilation. While the cost effectiveness and psychologic benefits of home management are clearly enormous, it places considerable responsibility in the hands of parents or other caretakers, and the physician team who must frequently monitor the infant's well-being. Equipment failure and medication errors must be guarded against. Clinic visits must ensure that congestive heart failure is well controlled, weight gain and nutritional support are appropriate, and that oxygenation is adequate. Furthermore, infants with resolving BPD do appear to be at increased risk for sudden infant death. Thus parents must be instructed in suctioning techniques and cardiopulmonary resuscitation, and must be well prepared, capable, and willing to accept the responsibilities to which they will be exposed.

## LONG-TERM OUTCOME OF NEONATAL RESPIRATORY CARE

The neurodevelopmental follow-up of high-risk neonates, many of whom have received assisted ventilation, should comprise evaluations for growth, intellectual development, vision, and hearing. Major factors influencing outcome include variable mixtures of inborn and transported infants, socioeconomic factors, ranges of birth weight and gestational age, varying degrees of asphyxia, as well as differing indications and techniques of ventilation. The current developmental outcome for infants with mild or moderate RDS is probably comparable to that of infants without RDS. Birth weight and gestational age have a much stronger influence on mental and motor developmental scores of preterm infants at 2 years than either the presence or severity of RDS. Factors associated with poor outcome include a neonatal history of seizures, extensive IVH, other severe neurologic sequelae, and severe BPD.

Overall, a normal *neurodevelopmental outcome* can be anticipated in approximately 80% to 85% of low birth weight infants less than 1.5 kg at birth.[26] A less favorable neurodevelopmental outcome has been reported for ventilated vs. nonventilated infants weighing less than 1.0 kg at birth.[27] Such an association may, however, have little to do with respiratory disease per se, as indications for prolonged assisted ventilation in these very low birth weight infants are multifactorial and may vary between centers. For infants weighing less than 1.5 kg at birth, infants with BPD have more neurodevelopmental sequelae at 2 years when compared to comparable control groups.[25] While data from longer-term studies are not yet available, it is apparent that neurodevelopmental prognosis will depend on the diagnostic criteria used to define chronic lung disease in neonates.

*Pulmonary sequelae* occur in some infants with BPD, and there is some evidence that late abnormalities of pulmonary function are detectable, although in the absence of progression to BPD in infancy, this has not been a clinical problem in childhood. Lower respiratory tract infections are common during the first year of life in patients with BPD, although their exact incidence is difficult to ascertain from the literature. Frequently no specific organisms are isolated, and the disease resolves with broad-spectrum antibiotic therapy. Among survivors of BPD, hospitalization for episodes of wheezing suggestive of bronchiolitis or asthma is common during the first 2 years of life. Pulmonary function studies of infants with a history of BPD indicate that pulmonary function may be impaired beyond 2 years in many cases, with an increased incidence of obstructive airway disease.[28] Recent data indicate that infants who have radiologic evidence of pulmonary abnormalities at discharge are at increased risk for subsequent respiratory illness.[29] Data on longer-term follow-up studies of pulmonary function in larger numbers of these infants are currently unavailable, although these clearly will be very important to ascertain in the future.

*Retinopathy of prematurity (retrolental fibroplasia)* may develop in the incompletely vascularized retina of premature infants, leading to a wide range of outcomes from normal vision and myopia to total visual loss in extreme cases. In the 1950s, a randomized multicenter trial linked oxygen to this disease when it showed that the practice of administering over 50% inspired oxygen for greater than 4 weeks resulted in an increased incidence of severe retinopathy in survivors under 1,500 gm birth weight. In the era that followed, oxygen use was severely restricted, resulting in an increased cerebral palsy and mortality rate, but nearly eliminating retinopathy for a time. The current resurgence of retinopathy is believed to result from the increased survival of infants with retinas so immature at birth that current cautious use of oxygen is not always sufficient to prevent the problem and other etiologies may be responsible.

## REFERENCES

1. Carlo WA, Martin RJ, Fanaroff AA: Assisted ventilation and the complications of respiratory distress, Fanaroff AA, Martin RJ (eds): in Neonatal-Perinatal Medicine, ed 4. St Louis, CV Mosby Co, 1987.
2. Madansky DL, Lawson EE, Chernick V, et al: Pneumothorax and other forms of pulmonary air leaks in newborns. Am Rev Respir Dis 1979; 120:729.
3. Primhak RA: Factors associated with pulmonary air leak in premature infants receiving mechanical ventilation. J Pediatr 1983; 102:764.
4. Hill A, Perlman JM, Volpe JJ: Relationship of pneumothorax to occurrence of intraventricular hemorrhage in the premature newborn. Pediatrics 1982; 69:144.
5. Erenberg A, Nowak AJ: Palatal groove formation in neonates and infants with orotracheal tubes. Am J Dis Child 1984; 138:974.
6. Kirpalani H, Higa T, Perlman M, et al: Diagnosis and therapy of necrotizing tracheobronchitis in ventilated neonates. Crit Care Med 1985; 13:792.
7. Ratner I, Whitfield J: Acquired subglottic stenosis in the very low birth weight infant. Am J Dis Child 1983; 137:40.
8. Kuban KCK, Leviton A, Krishnamoorthy KS, et al: Neonatal intracranial hemorrhage and phenobarbital. Pediatrics 1986; 77:443.
9. Perlman JM, Goodman S, Kreusser KL, et al: Reduction in intraventricular hemorrhage by elimination of fluctuating cerebral blood-flow velocity in preterm infants with respiratory distress syndrome. N Engl J Med 1985; 312:1353.
10. Gersony WM, Peckham GJ, Ellison RC, et al: Effects of indomethacin in premature infants with patent ductus arteriosus: Results of a national collaborative study. J Pediatr 1983; 102:895.
11. Northway WH, Jr, Rosan RC, Porter DY: Pulmonary disease following respirator therapy of hyaline membrane disease: Bronchopulmonary dysplasia. N Engl J Med 1967; 276:357.
12. Bancalari E, Gerhardt T: Bronchopulmonary dysplasia. Pediatr Clin North Am 1986; 33:1.
13. Bronchopulmonary Dysplasia and Related Chronic Respiratory Disorders, report of the Ninetieth Ross Conference on Pediatric Research. Columbus, Ohio, Ross Laboratories, March 1986.

14. Watts JL, Ariagno RL, Brady JP: Chronic pulmonary disease in neonates after artificial ventilation: Distribution of ventilation and pulmonary interstitial emphysema. Pediatrics 1977; 60:273.
15. Goldman SL, Gerhardt T, Sonni R, et al: Early prediction of chronic lung disease by pulmonary function testing. J Pediatr 1983; 102:613.
16. Bruce M, Boat TF, Martin RJ, et al: Proteinase inhibitors and inhibitor inactivation in neonatal airway secretions. Chest 1982; 81:44S.
17. Deneke SM, Fanburg BL: Normobaric oxygen toxicity of the lung. N Engl J Med 1980; 303:76.
18. Ehrenkranz R, Ablow RC, Warshaw JB: Prevention of BPD with vitamin E administration during acute stages of RDS. J Pediatr 1979; 95:873.
19. Saldanha R, Cepeda EE, Poland RL: The effect of vitamin E prophylaxis on the incidence and severity of BPD. J Pediatr 1983; 101:89.
20. Brown ER, Stark A, Sosenko I, et al: Bronchopulmonary dysplasia: Possible relationship to pulmonary edema. J Pediatr 1978; 92:982.
21. Rome ES, Stork EK, Carlo WA, et al: Limitations of transcutaneous $PO_2$ and $PCO_2$ monitoring in infants with bronchopulmonary dysplasia. Pediatrics 1984; 74:217.
22. Weinstein MR, Oh W: Oxygen consumption in infants with bronchopulmonary dysplasia. J Pediatr 1981; 99:958.
23. Kao LC, Warburton D, Sargent CW, et al: Furosemide acutely decreases airways resistance in chronic bronchopulmonary dysplasia. J Pediatr 1983; 103:642.
24. Rooklin AR, Moomjian AS, Shutack JG, et al: Theophylline therapy in bronchopulmonary dysplasia. J Pediatr 1979; 95:882.
25. Vohr BR, Bell EF, Oh W: Infants with bronchopulmonary dysplasia: Growth pattern and neurologic and developmental outcome. Am J Dis Child 1982; 136:443.
26. Hack M, Fanaroff AA, Merkatz IR: The low birth weight infant: Evolution of a changing outlook. N Engl J Med 1979; 301:1152.
27. Rothberg AD, Maisels MJ, Bagnato S, et al: Infants weighing 1,000 grams or less at birth: Developmental outcome for ventilated and nonventilated infants. Pediatrics 1983; 71:599.
28. Smyth JA, Tabachnik E, Duncan WJ, et al: Pulmonary function and bronchial hyperactivity in long-term survivors of bronchopulmonary dysplasia. Pediatrics 1981; 68:336.
29. Myers MG, McGuinness GA, Lachenbruch PA, et al: Respiratory illnesses in survivors of infant respiratory distress syndrome. Am Rev Respir Dis 1986; 133:1011.

# 14

# High-Frequency Ventilation

Waldemar A. Carlo, M.D.
Robert L. Chatburn, R.R.T.

Since the widespread introduction of assisted ventilation over the last 20 years, the survival rates of infants with pulmonary disorders have steadily improved. Unfortunately, this has been accompanied by a concurrent increase in the number of infants manifesting lung injury, including both air leak syndromes (pneumothorax, interstitial pulmonary emphysema, pneumomediastinum) and/or bronchopulmonary dysplasia (BPD). Pulmonary air leaks occur in 24% of all infants requiring assisted ventilation,[1] while BPD occurs in about 25% of very low birth weight infants who survive.[2] These complications are thought to result, in part, from prolonged exposure of the airways and pulmonary parenchyma to high inflating pressures. Furthermore, some infants still die with intractable respiratory failure despite the use of presently available conventional ventilators.

Conventional ventilation (CV) has been applied in a manner whereby adequate minute ventilation is maintained by means of low rates and high tidal volumes that correspond to those of healthy infants during spontaneous ventilation. Delivery of these volumes to noncompliant lungs necessitates excessively high inflating pressures. To diminish this problem, various systems capable of delivering high-frequency ventilation (HFV) have been developed. With these ventilators, adequate gas exchange may be maintained at high ventilatory frequencies despite greatly reduced delivered volumes. If accompanied by decreased inflating pressures, HFV could result in a reduction of barotrauma. Recent data from our own and other institutions indicate that, when compared to CV, short-term HFV maintains adequate gas exchange in critically ill neonates, usually at lower airway pressures.[3-21] However, before HFV becomes an accepted therapy, further large controlled clinical trials of prolonged study periods must be performed in critically ill neonates to determine the advantages of this new mode of assisted ventilation.

## HISTORICAL PERSPECTIVES

Despite the wide acceptance that tidal volumes larger than dead space are needed to achieve ventilation, data from as early as the last century suggest that gas exchange also occurs with very small tidal volumes. However, early in this century the field of assisted ventilation was in its infancy, and the use of large tidal volumes became standard practice. In 1959, Jack Emerson,[22] an inventor of medical equipment, patented a device that vibrated air into the patient's lungs. His original purpose was to facilitate chest physiotherapy, but he postulated that the vibrations would also enhance gas mixing. In the late 1960s Sjöstrand and co-workers[23] modified standard ventilators with low-compliance tubing and connectors in an effort to reduce the cardiovascular depression that occurred with assisted ventilation. This modification allowed adequate gas exchange at moderately high frequencies (60 to 120/minute or 1 to 2 Hz) and small tidal volumes. Other workers using extremely high frequencies (up to 2,400/minute) reported that, in apneic animals, normal blood gases were maintained using very small tidal volumes.[24] Development of new ventilators and many in vitro, animal, and human studies soon followed. In 1974 Heijman and Sjöstrand[3] first reported the application of HFV to neonates with respiratory distress syndrome (RDS), and since then, other investigators have evaluated various types of high-frequency ventilators in this patient population.

## CLASSIFICATION OF HIGH-FREQUENCY VENTILATORS

Multiple ventilators capable of delivering small volumes at high frequencies have been developed. It is not surprising that each group of inventors or developers has made its ventilator unique and that a simple classification is not an easy task. Circuits and delivery-system designs also vary, and these may have major impact on the functioning of a high-frequency ventilator. Furthermore, the strategies employed with a high-frequency ventilator may also affect its functioning. Needless to say, considerable overlap also exists between the various high-frequency ventilators presently used (Fig 14–1).[25] Nonetheless, for the

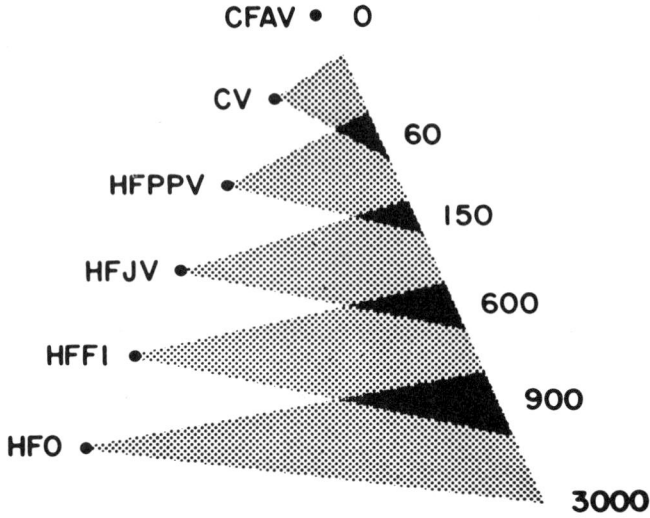

**FIG 14–1.**
Frequency spectrum for assisted ventilation of neonates. The numbers represent approximate ranges of cycles per minute since strict limits of frequency for each mode of ventilation do not exist and overlap of the frequencies is common. Continuous flow apneic ventilation (CFAV) is discussed in Chapter 15. (From Carlo WA, Martin RJ: Principles of neonatal assisted ventilation. *Pediatr Clin North Am* 1986; 33:221. Used by permission.)

purpose of simplicity, we have attempted to classify and characterize the principle techniques presently employed to deliver HFV (Table 14–1).

### High-Frequency Positive-Pressure Ventilation

High-frequency positive-pressure ventilation (HFPPV) employs ventilators with low-compliance tubing and connectors so that an ad-

**TABLE 14–1.**
Techniques for High-Frequency Ventilation

|  | HFPPV* | Jet Ventilation | Flow Interruption | Oscillation |
|---|---|---|---|---|
| Tidal volume | >Dead space | >or <Dead space | >or <Dead space | <Dead space |
| Expiration | Passive | Passive | Passive | Active |
| Airway pressure waveform | Variable | Triangular | Triangular | Sine wave |
| Entrainment | None | Possible | None | None |
| Frequency | 60–150/min | 60–600/min | 300–900/min | 300–3,000/min |

*HFPPV = high-frequency positive-pressure ventilation.

equate tidal volume may be delivered despite very short inspiratory times. The tidal volume delivered is smaller than during CV but larger than dead space. As with CV, expiration is passive. The pressure waveform may be square-like if pressure-limited ventilation or inspiratory hold is used but will tend to become triangular, particularly at the higher frequencies. Frequencies of 60 to 150/minute may be used during HFPPV, but ventilator and circuit design as well as pulmonary mechanics of the patient may limit this range. This technique was developed by Sjöstrand and co-workers[23] in an effort to reduce cardiac side effects from assisted ventilation but was found effective in achieving normal blood gases at reduced airway pressures. Today most neonatal ventilators have been modified to deliver rates of up to 150/minute. However, as the frequency is increased, tidal-volume delivery may be so compromised that actual minute ventilation can even decrease at the higher frequencies.[26]

### High-Frequency Jet Ventilation

With high-frequency jet ventilation (HFJV), a high-pressure source is allowed to deliver a volume of gas through a small-bore injector cannula (Fig 14–2). Delivered tidal volumes may be large, but volumes

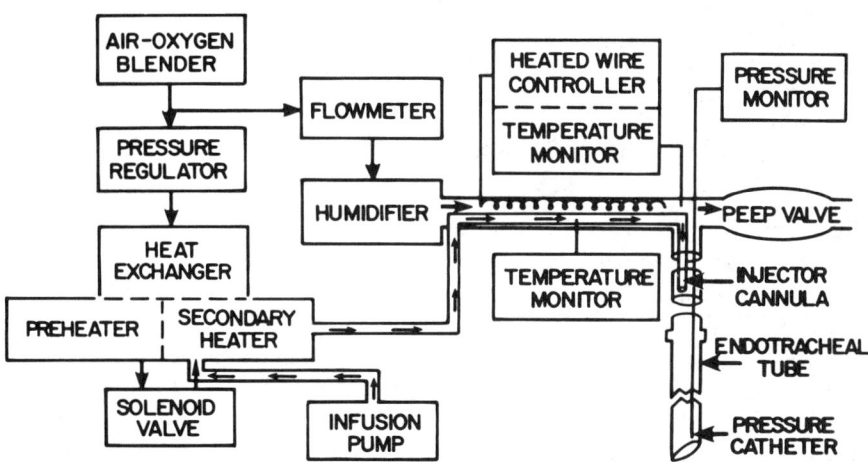

**FIG 14–2.**
Schematic diagram of the high-frequency jet ventilator with the heating and humidification system used at our institution. With this setup, air and oxygen are blended and then delivered by a pressure regulator. The gas is heated before it reaches the solenoid valve. The gas is then humidified and reheated, and the temperature is subsequently maintained by passing the gas within a heated circuit. The gas is delivered to the proximal end of the endotracheal tube by means of an injector cannula. Airway pressures are monitored at the distal tip of the endotracheal tube.

smaller than dead space can maintain normal $CO_2$ elimination.[27] Gas entrainment (the addition of gas from areas surrounding the jet injector cannula to that intrinsically delivered by the jet ventilator) is an important characteristic of jet ventilators. Entrainment occurs because of the viscous shearing force that exists between moving and static layers of gas causing the nonmoving gas to be dragged into the moving stream.[28] It is also possible that entrainment occurs when areas of relative negative pressure develop near the injector as gas with a high flow rate is delivered to the patient.[29] However, gas entrainment may only occur at ventilator settings and circuit and patient characteristics that allow high rates of flow without significant back pressure.[29,30] Thus humidification of bias-flow gases alone is not always sufficient.

During jet ventilation, humidification of gases is particularly difficult, and inadequate humidification may cause tracheal lesions (see "Problems During HFV"). Most jet ventilators operate like a constant-flow time-cycled ventilator, and the pressure waveform typically is triangular. However, one commercially available jet ventilator, the Bunnell Life-Pulse Jet Ventilator, is pressure-servocontrolled and tends to achieve a square pressure waveform. Expiration during HFJV is completely passive. Frequencies used vary widely and range from about 60 to 600/minute. Jet ventilation was first introduced by Smith and coworkers,[31] and since then it has undergone extensive testing. There is an abundant literature of successful applications of HFJV in various laboratory preparations and patient populations.

## High-Frequency Flow Interruption

Like jet ventilation, high-frequency flow interruption (HFFI) employs small volumes delivered at high frequencies by interrupting a flow or high-pressure source.[8] However, in contrast to jet ventilation, there is no injector cannula and no gas entrainment. As with jet ventilation, tidal volumes may be smaller or larger than dead space; expiration is passive; and the pressure waveform is triangular. Frequencies used are in the range of 300 to 900/minute. There is limited clinical experience and animal research using HFFI, although other nomenclatures (including HFV and high-frequency oscillation) have been used for this technique (Fig 14–3).

## High-Frequency Oscillatory Ventilation

High-frequency oscillatory ventilation (HFOV), also called high-frequency oscillation (HFO), is a unique form of high-frequency ventilation because, in contrast to all other techniques, expiration is active

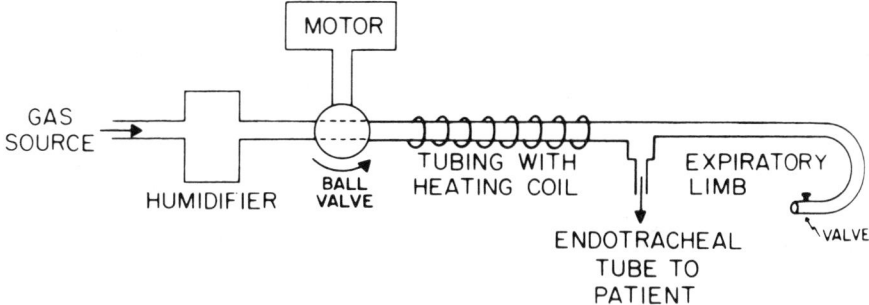

**FIG 14–3.**
Schematic diagram of Emerson high-frequency flow interrupter. Desired air-oxygen mixture is heated and humidified, and bias gas flow is interrupted by a motor-driven ball valve. Continuous distending pressure is determined by a screw valve at the end of circuit. The length of the expiratory limb is chosen to have higher impedance than that of the infant's respiratory system. (From Frantz ID III, Werthammer J, Stark AR: High-frequency ventilation in premature infants with lung disease: Adequate gas exchange at low tracheal pressures. *Pediatrics* 1983; 71:483. Used by permission.)

(Fig 14–4).[7] Delivered volumes are usually very small (even less than dead space) and frequencies very high (up to 3,000/minute). Volume delivery and active expiration are achieved by a piston pump or acoustic speaker. Since expiration is active, shorter expiratory times may be used, and air trapping is less of a problem (see "Gas Trapping"). Bryan and co-workers pioneered with HFOV during the late 1970s. Since then extensive laboratory research has been performed using HFOV, but more controlled clinical trials are presently needed.

Delivery of HFV has been modified by applying the pressure changes

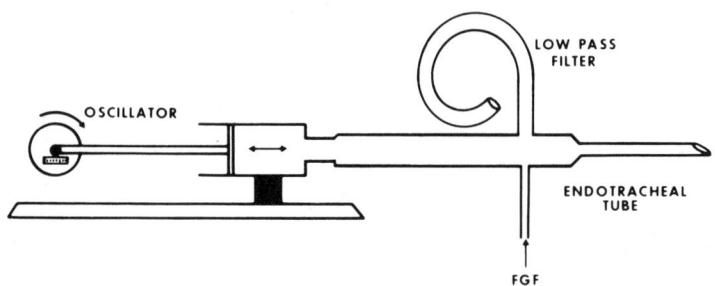

**FIG 14–4.**
Diagram of circuit used for high-frequency oscillatory ventilation (HFOV). The piston's stroke volume is adjusted by positioning the shaft along a vernier scale on an eccentric cam. Fresh gases enter the system just proximal to the endotracheal tube *(FGF)*. Excess fresh gas and mixed gases that are oscillated out of the lung exit via the low pass filter. (From Marchak BE, Thompson WK, Duffy P, et al: Treatment of RDS by high-frequency oscillatory ventilation: A preliminary report. *J Pediatr* 1981; 99:298. Used by permission.)

externally to the chest wall. These techniques are attractive particularly because they may eliminate endotracheal intubation and could prevent upper airway and parenchymal damage associated with this procedure.[32] Initial studies utilizing various techniques to deliver HFV to the chest wall in normal animals demonstrated the potential of this application of HFV. Hayek and co-workers[32] have shown that external high-frequency oscillations improve blood gases in normal and surfactant-deficient adult cats. Their system employed a thoracoabdominal chamber connected to a vacuum source that maintained lung volume by controlling the negative pressure. Oscillation in pressures above and below this level were then applied to the chest wall. This technique is reminiscent of the negative-pressure ventilators that were successfully used in neonates with RDS in the past. New modifications may facilitate effective ventilation through the application of pressure changes to the chest wall without previously encountered problems (frequent interruptions, leaks). However, no neonatal human studies have been reported.

Few reports of comparisons of the various types of high-frequency ventilators are available. An in vitro evaluation of eight commercially manufactured neonatal high-frequency ventilators, including HFJV, HFFI, and HFOV, revealed that independent of the ventilator type, delivered tidal volume decreased with increasing ventilatory frequencies or decreasing endotracheal tube size. However, tidal volume delivery was relatively insensitive to lung compliance.[33]

## GAS EXCHANGE DURING HIGH-FREQUENCY VENTILATION

The primary aim of assisted ventilation is ultimately to accomplish effective gas exchange. Although impairment of carbon dioxide ($CO_2$) elimination and oxygen ($O_2$) uptake frequently occur simultaneously, strategies to correct $CO_2$ or $O_2$ derangements may vary widely and will be reviewed separately. However, because adequate gas exchange may occur at tidal volumes smaller than dead space, mechanisms other than bulk (convective gas transport) have to be involved (Fig 14–5).

### Mechanisms of Gas Exchange

Gas transport by *convection* will occur during HFV if tidal volumes larger than dead space are employed. However, alveoli close to the airway get *direct ventilation* at tidal volumes smaller than dead space.[34] Direct ventilation is not restricted to HFV, as it is well known that some

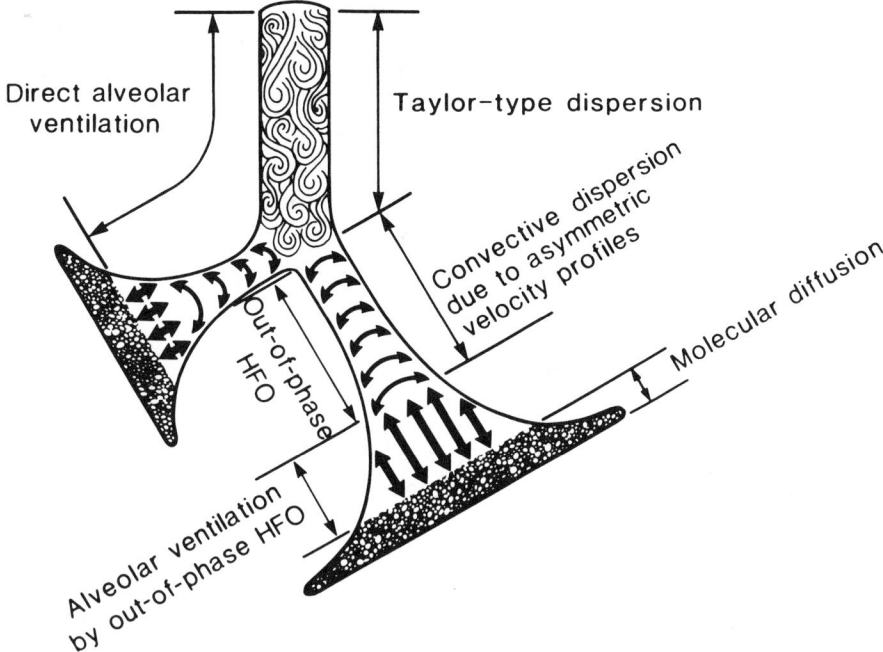

**FIG 14–5.**
Modes of gas transport during high-frequency ventilation (HFV) and tentative sketch of their zones of dominance. These modes of transport are not mutually exclusive and may interact to achieve efficiency observed in animal or patient studies. HFO = high-frequency oscillation. (From Chang HK: Mechanisms of gas transport during ventilation by high-frequency oscillation. *J Appl Physiol* 1984; 56:553. Used by permission.)

$CO_2$ elimination occurs during spontaneous breathing at very small tidal volumes. This is due to the fact that alveoli have different dead space volumes and that the reported dead space in any subject is just an average value.

Gas transport may occur between gas exchanging units as some alveoli may fill or empty faster than others. This mechanism is called *pendelluft* and will occur when there is a nonhomogeneous distribution of mechanical properties (i.e., time constants) in the lungs in the presence of relatively short inspiratory or expiratory times. Photographic[35] and asymmetric alveolar pressure data[36] support the existence of this mechanism of gas exchange during HFV.

Other mechanisms may theoretically explain the enhanced gas exchange that occurs during HFV, but less evidence for them is available. Velocity profiles of gases in the airways are probably faster in the center than in the periphery and differ during inspiration and expiration. This convective mechanism, called *streaming*, will effectively reduce dead space as air in the center of the airways will be preferentially advanced forward for gas exchange, while the marginated dead-space volume will show a net backward movement. *Turbulence* due to high-frequency velocity fluctuations and *augmented diffusion* or intermingling of gas molecules may also enhance gas exchange during HFV. It is unclear which of the above mechanisms of gas exchange occur with each of the modes of HFV. The relative role that these mechanisms have in improving gas transport is also unknown.

## Carbon Dioxide Elimination

The most consistent observation about gas exchange during HFV is that $CO_2$ elimination is usually very easily accomplished. This is, in part, due to the increased minute ventilation that HFV allows. In addition, tidal volumes smaller than dead space may be sufficient for adequate gas exchange to occur during HFJV[27] and HFOV.[37, 38] However, $CO_2$ elimination during both HFJV[37] and HFOV[39] is more dependent on tidal volume than on frequency. Since it is usually difficult to measure tidal volume during HFV, practically it is better to relate $CO_2$ elimination to the difference between peak inspiratory and end-expiratory pressures. The partial pressure of $CO_2$ in arterial blood ($Pa_{CO_2}$) decreases with increases in the airway pressure gradient (Fig 14–6). While $CO_2$ elimination is easily accomplished with most forms of HFV, caution

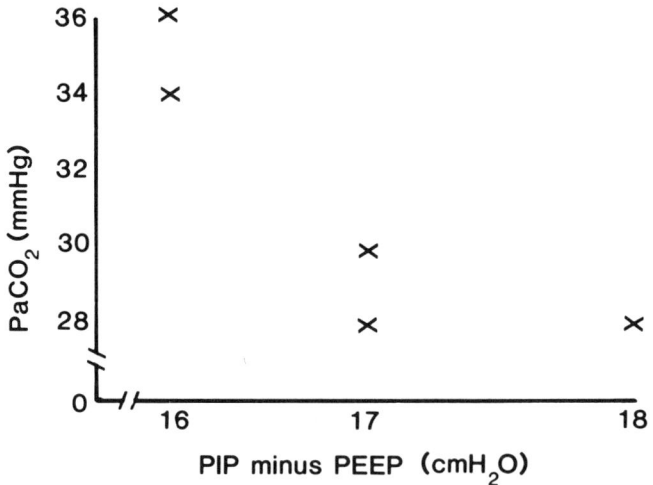

**FIG 14–6.**
The effect of pressure amplitude (difference between peak inspiratory pressure [PIP] and positive end-expiratory pressure [PEEP]) on $Pa_{CO_2}$ in one infant with RDS during HFJV. Pressure changes were performed in random order. As pressure amplitude was increased, $Pa_{CO_2}$ decreased.

should be exercised to prevent air trapping since this will cause $CO_2$ retention.[27]

## Oxygen Uptake

Unfortunately, unlike $CO_2$ elimination, reports on the efficacy of oxygenation during HFV are mixed. Increases, decreases, or no change in oxygenation has been reported during HFV. However, initial studies paid little attention to mean lung volume and mean airway pressure. As with CV, studies have shown that during HFV, oxygenation is largely determined by mean airway pressure (Fig 14–7) and the maintenance of an adequate lung volume.[7] Accordingly, maneuvers that recruit lung volume will also improve oxygenation. However, overdistention and air trapping (for example, with very high mean airway pressures) will cause ventilation-perfusion mismatch and impair oxygenation.

## CLINICAL APPLICATIONS OF HFV

### Neonatal Experience

#### High-Frequency Positive-Pressure Ventilation

Heijman and Sjöstrand,[3] pioneers in the field of HFV, developed the first prototype system of HFPPV for neonates. Using frequencies of 60 to 90/minute, they successfully ventilated three out of six neonates

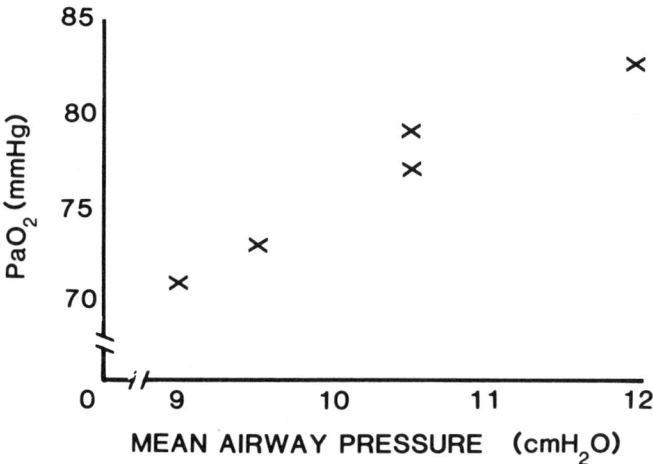

**FIG 14–7.**
The effect of mean airway pressure on $Pa_{O_2}$ during high-frequency jet ventilation (HFJV) on the same infant as in Figure 14–6. Pressure changes were performed in random order. As mean airway pressure was increased $Pa_{O_2}$ improved.

that had RDS. Subsequently Bland et al.[4] modified conventional pressure- or volume-limited ventilators to attain rates of 60 to 110/minute and adequately ventilated 24 preterm infants (average birth weight of 1,244 gm) throughout the period that they required assisted ventilation. Despite the low birth weight and immaturity of these infants, a high percentage (92%) of them survived. Concurrently, Boros and Campbell[5] performed a controlled crossover study comparing HFPPV at rates of 66 ± 10/minute vs. "low-frequency, high-tidal volume" in 10 neonates with severe lung disease, mostly RDS. Although these investigators observed a fall in the partial pressure of $O_2$ in arterial blood $Pa_{O_2}$ during HFPPV, they noticed that an inadvertent reduction in mean airway pressure had occurred. In a large controlled trial of neonates with RDS or pneumonia, Heicher et al.[6] demonstrated that HFPPV markedly decreased the incidence of pneumothorax. Other studies have more recently confirmed that adequate gas exchange may be achieved with HFPPV in critically ill neonates with RDS.[12, 13, 19] It should be noted that many neonatal studies have reported the use of conventional ventilators at rates beyond 60/minute but have not used the term HFPPV.

### *High-Frequency Jet Ventilation*

Pokora et al.[9] reported in 1983 the first use of HFJV in 10 neonates with respiratory failure. These investigators employed rates of 260 ± 50/minute and observed a reduction in the alveolar-arterial $PO_2$ gradient and $Pa_{CO_2}$ during HFJV as compared to CV. However, their success was adversely affected by the development of necrotizing tracheobronchitis and fatal tracheal obstruction. In a larger group of patients treated by this group of investigators, 44% of the infants developed tracheobronchitis.[14, 40]

We used a crossover design to study 12 preterm infants with RDS and compared control periods of CV to a 1– to 3–hour period of HFJV.[10] A rate of 250/minute was employed at an I:E ratio of 1:3 to 1:4. The $Pa_{CO_2}$ decreased at lower peak inspiratory and mean airway pressures during HFJV, while $Pa_{O_2}$, positive end-expiratory pressure, and cardiovascular parameters did not change. Measurements of chest impedance suggested that air trapping was not present (Fig 14–8). The short-term effects of HFJV on gas exchange have been confirmed by others.[15, 16] To further compare HFJV with pressure-limited time-cycled conventional ventilation, we randomized 41 infants with RDS during the first day of life to receive either HFJV for 48 hours or conventional therapy.[18] Despite comparable oxygenation in both groups, infants treated with HFJV had lower $Pa_{CO_2}$ and mean airway pressure (Fig 14–9). Furthermore, bronchoscopies did not reveal evidence of necrotizing tracheobronchitis. Gonzalez et al.[20] using HFJV have confirmed these

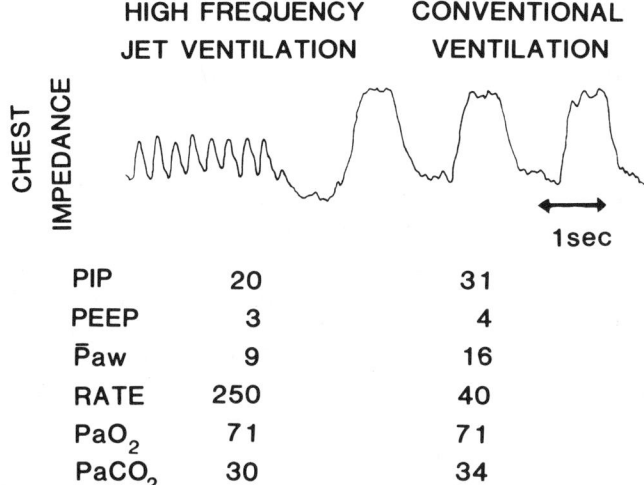

**FIG 14–8.**
Chest impedance during HFJV and CV in one infant with RDS. The comparable baseline chest impedance during end expiration suggests that gas trapping did not occur during HFJV.

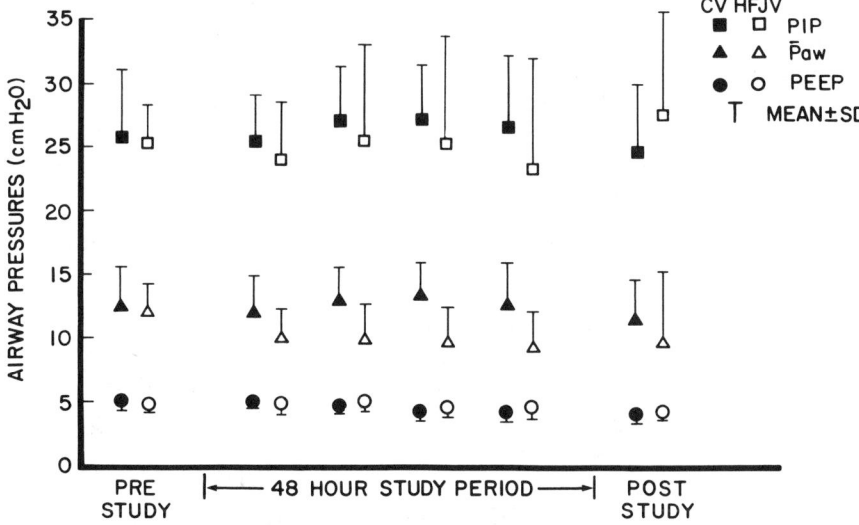

**FIG 14–9.**
Airway pressures (mean ± SD) during both control and four 12-hour study periods for infants with RDS treated with CV and HFJV. Airway pressures were comparable in prestudy and poststudy periods. Analysis of variance of airway pressures revealed that mean airway pressures ($\bar{P}aw$) were lower ($P<.001$) in the HFJV group, but peak inspiratory pressures (PIP) and positive end-expiratory pressures (PEEP) were comparable. (From Carlo WA, Chatburn RL, Martin RJ: Randomized trial of high-frequency jet ventilation versus conventional ventilation in respiratory distress syndrome. *J Pediatr* 1987; 110:275. Used by permission.)

observations in neonates with a persistent gas leak through thoracotomy tubes. They also demonstrated that the flow rate of the air leak decreased markedly at the same time that HFJV allowed a reduction in the mean airway pressure.

### High-Frequency Flow Interrupter

Frantz and co-workers[8] reported in 1983 the application of HFFI at frequencies of 300 to 1200/minute in 10 neonates with RDS and 5 with pulmonary interstitial emphysema. Gas exchange (both $Pa_{O_2}$ and $Pa_{CO_2}$) was improved during HFFI at lower peak inspiratory pressures but mean airway pressures could not be decreased. Even though this was an uncontrolled study, resolution of RDS and emphysema occurred in most infants.

### High-Frequency Oscillatory Ventilation

In 1981, Marchak and co-workers[7] reported a crossover controlled study in eight neonates with RDS using HFOV at rates of 480 to 1200/minute for 1- to 4-hour periods. Oxygenation was improved during HFOV, but in three infants in whom airway pressure was measured, the increase in $Pa_{O_2}$ was found to be dependent on increases in mean airway pressure. A multicenter collaborative trial employing HFOV in premature infants weighing less than 2,000 gm has recently been completed. Preliminary results indicate that HFOV at rates of 900 cycles per minute did not reduce the incidence of BPD, air leaks, or mortality. However, the incidence of intracranial hemorrhage was increased in the HFOV group. Long-term follow-up of survivors is still in progress.[40a]

## Combined High-Frequency Ventilation/Conventional Ventilation

Recently, several investigators have successfully combined HFV and intermittent mandatory ventilation in patients with severe respiratory failure. Boynton et al.[11] used an oscillator at a frequency of 1,200/minute combined with intermittent mandatory ventilation as a rescue in 12 neonates with respiratory failure despite CV. Oxygenation and $CO_2$ elimination were markedly improved with combined HFOV despite a reduction in mean airway pressure and CV rate. Gaylord et al.[20] used a modification of HFFI combined with CV in nine preterm infants with severe PIE and also demonstrated improved gas exchange at lower mean airway pressures and rates. HFJV (rates 300 to 450/minute) was combined with CV in 11 preterm infants by Donn et al.[15] Adequate blood gases were maintained also at lower mean airway pressures than with CV. Combining HFV with intermittent mandatory ventilation consistently improves gas exchange and prevents a reduction in mean airway pressure. The rationale behind the role of intermittent inflations is that they may prevent or resolve atelectasis that sometimes complicates prolonged periods of HFV, especially when very small tidal volumes are employed.

**Animal Models of Neonatal Diseases**

Studies using animal models of RDS have compared high-frequency to conventional ventilators. Truog et al.[41] using HFOV at rates of 600/minute, ventilated five preterm monkeys with RDS for short periods, during which mean airway pressure was matched between periods of HFOV and CV. They observed a lowering of $Pa_{CO_2}$ despite a marked reduction in peak inspiratory pressure, but there was no significant improvement in oxygenation. Keuhl et al.[42] ventilated nine preterm baboons with RDS during alternating 2-hour periods with either HFOV or CV. Blood gases tended to improve with HFOV as compared with the conventional ventilator, but again mean airway pressure was not reduced. Subsequent attempts to continue HFOV for 24 hours resulted in significant cardiopulmonary deterioration and were thus unsuccessful.

Hamilton et al.[43] noted that in adult rabbits with lung injury induced by lung lavage, HFOV improved oxygenation at mean airway pressure comparable to CV. Further observations in rabbits indicate that optimally administered HFOV requires mean airway pressures in excess of closing pressure and/or sustained lung inflation to minimize further lung damage[44] and improve oxygenation and lung compliance.[45] These data and those of Wright et al.[46] suggest that the beneficial effect of HFOV may be enhanced by periodic hyperinflation to prevent atelectasis.

Another potential benefit of HFOV has been reported in dogs with bronchopleural fistula. High-frequency oscillatory ventilation was found to be superior to CV in achieving adequate blood gas exchange.[47] This is consistent with the findings of Frantz et al.[8] who observed resolution of pulmonary interstitial emphysema in neonates with RDS during HFFI. However, studies in premature baboons with RDS have shown that interstitial emphysema may develop during HFFI.[48]

Animal models of meconium aspiration have also been studied to elucidate the role of HFV in this disease. In cats with experimental meconium aspiration syndrome, CV produced better oxygenation than HFPPV.[49] Similar results were reported by Mammel and co-workers using HFJV.[50] In the cats treated with HFJV, the later investigators also reported an increase in pulmonary vascular resistance, a side effect that potentially could be detrimental to infants with meconium aspiration who occasionally develop pulmonary artery hypertension. In contrast,

Trindade et al.,[51] who also used HFJV, reported that comparable blood gases, but lower peak and mean airway pressures, occurred during HFV. However, a major limitation in these animal studies of meconium aspiration syndrome is that most likely the experimental postnatal aspiration does not strictly mimic the insult that some meconium-stained babies undergo.

Reservations concerning the use of very high ventilatory rates have stimulated the design of protocols to evaluate possible adverse effects of such therapeutic modalities. Animal and human adult studies have provided necessary information otherwise unavailable from clinical trials in infants or neonatal animal models. Lung fluid balance, surfactant content, and light and electron microscopy findings have been largely unaffected by HFOV.[41, 52-55] Measurements of radioactive label clearance from lung airways during HFOV in dogs suggest a possible disturbance of mucociliary function.[56] Furthermore, thick secretions and tracheal lesions have been a major problem during clinical application of some jet ventilators.[40] Evaluations of intracranial pressure in animals made during various modes of HFV have revealed stable levels of baseline intracranial pressure and decreased amplitude in the pressure fluctuations that might offer protection against the development of intracranial hemorrhage.[57, 58] This wide range of studies suggests that HFV with appropriate humidification is safe, does not appear to produce parenchymal lung injury,[59] and may be of therapeutic benefit for specific clinical situations.

The effects of HFV on respiratory regulation have been actively studied. In anesthetized dogs, HFOV appears to inhibit spontaneous respiratory efforts and leads to apnea, an effect that is vagally mediated,[60, 61] reversed by vagotomy,[61] and not directly related to alterations in lung volume or blood gas states.

## Other Potential Clinical Uses of HFV

### Bronchopleural Fistula/Pneumothorax

Pneumothorax is a frequent occurrence in neonatal ventilatory therapy. A recent study by Gonzalez et al.[20] used HFJV in six infants who had severe pulmonary disease and persistent air leaks via thoracotomy tubes placed for pneumothoraces. When infants were treated with HFJV, the flow through the bronchopleural fistula decreased. Simultaneously, peak and mean airway pressures were decreased during HFJV while adequate gas exchange was maintained. This well-designed study confirms previous case reports describing similar observations in animals and adult patients. However, no data exist to indicate that HFV can prevent the development of air leaks.

## Impaired Cardiac Function

Although several authors have reported worsening cardiac hemodynamics during HFV, the increased mean airway pressure employed in those studies may have accounted for the adverse cardiac effects. Recent animal studies in which mean airway pressure was comparable during HFV and CV have shown no change in cardiac output. Following cardiac surgery in infants and children, cardiac output either improved or remained unchanged during periods of either HFFI[62] or HFJV.[63] Interestingly, cardiac output improved during HFJV in those infants who initially had poor cardiac output during CV. Regardless of the ventilatory mode, cardiac output was dependent on mean airway pressure (Fig 14–10). It is likely that the lower mean airway pressure used during HFJV may reduce the cardiovascular side effects of transpulmonary pressures.

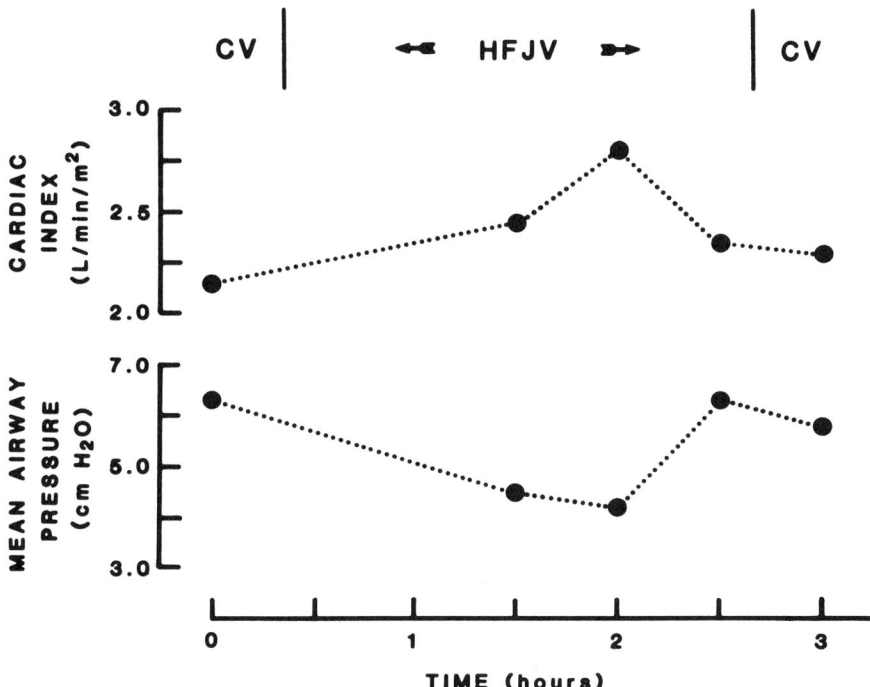

**FIG 14–10.**
A comparison of mean airway pressure and cardiac index during HFJV and control periods of CV in one child after open heart surgery. HFJV allowed a significant reduction of mean airway pressure that was accompanied by corresponding increases in cardiac index. (From Weiner JH, Chatburn RL, Carlo WA: Ventilatory and hemodynamic effects of high-frequency jet ventilation following cardiac surgery. *Respir Care* 1987; 32:332. Used by permission.)

### Bronchoscopy and Airway and Thoracic Surgery

Because HFV allows adequate gas exchange with small tidal volumes, it reduces airway and thoracic structure movement that may facilitate surgical procedures. We have devised a system using a combination of jet ventilation and constant air suction, both of which deliver gas through a single interface valve providing active inspiration and expiration through the suction channel of a bronchoscope.[64] When tested in vitro and in rabbits with normal lungs, baseline functional residual capacity remained constant. This system also improved ventilation when performed simultaneously with bronchoscopy. If found to be applicable to neonates, this system will facilitate a safer and more complete visualization of the airways during bronchoscopy. High-frequency ventilation may also facilitate airway and thoracic surgery as excursions during ventilation are decreased.[65] When delivered transtracheally, HFJV may be an alternative mode of ventilation during cardiopulmonary resuscitation.[66]

### Adult Respiratory Distress Syndrome

Although initial enthusiasm occurred with treatment of adult respiratory distress syndrome, a randomized study in which 309 patients received either conventional ventilation or HFJV demonstrated that survival and total duration of intensive care stay was not altered by the ventilatory mode, despite the lower airway pressures required during volume-cycled ventilation.[67] Nonetheless, with their extensive experience, these investigators reported few side effects and safe application of HFV.

## PROBLEMS DURING HFV

### Heating and Humidification

During HFV, inspired gas should ideally be heated and humidified to the same extent as it is during conventional ventilation.[68] However, this is often a difficult goal to accomplish, depending on the form of HFV used. High-frequency positive-pressure ventilation poses few problems as this technique makes use of conventional ventilator humidifiers. Temperature and relative humidity can be maintained at physiologic levels fairly easily as long as the humidifier remains efficient at the relatively high flow rates necessary.

Heating and humidification during HFOV is relatively uncomplicated and is achieved in a way comparable to conventional techniques. The most basic HFOV circuit is simply a continuous positive-airway pressure (CPAP) device with an extra limb attached to a piston pump.

The pump oscillates a portion of the CPAP gas (which is conditioned with any appropriate humidifier) and has little effect on inspired gas temperatures.

High-frequency flow interruption and HFJV introduce some unique problems since two separate sources of gas may be used. For example, with HFJV, one flow of gas comes from the jet ventilator and one from a continuous flow CPAP circuit. The CPAP circuit gas can be conditioned by conventional means. However, the gas from the jet ventilator is difficult to heat and humidify with conventional devices since it is under high pressure (5 to 45 psi). In addition, since the jet ventilator circuit must have an extremely low compressible volume to maintain a useful pressure waveform, the use of standard humidifiers is not possible. Early researchers experimented with various ways of infusing water into the stream of jet gas. Although this results in the delivery of a cold aerosol to the airways, it was hoped that entrained gases would help warm the jet gas. Unfortunately, entrainment does not always occur,[29, 30] especially in small children and neonates for whom inspired gas temperature is most critical. In small infants, the delivery of a cold aerosol along with inspired gas may contribute to fluid overload, electrolyte imbalance, reduction of body temperature, and necrotizing tracheobronchitis. To avoid these problems, we have developed a heat exchanger that can provide jet gas at physiologic temperatures with relative humidity in excess of 90%.[69] At least one commercial manufacturer has taken a similar approach (Bunnell Life-Pulse Jet Ventilator).

**Necrotizing Tracheobronchitis**

Necrotizing tracheobronchitis (NTB) is a lesion characterized by epithelial erosion, loss of ciliated cells, squamous cell metaplasia, and infiltration of the mucosa by neutrophils. It has been reported as a possible side effect of HFJV by several research groups[14, 40, 70, 71] but has also been observed with HFOV and CV.[72, 73] However, no increased tracheal lesions were observed in premature baboons with RDS treated with HFOV.[74]

The most common site of the lesion is near the distal end of the endotracheal tube.[40] Mucus impaction and granulation tissue formation may result in airway obstruction, lobar emphysema, or atelectasis and impaired gas exchange. One study has reported that NTB was identified at bronchoscopy in 44% of infants surviving HFJV (after prior failure on conventional ventilation). Of the nonsurvivors, up to 83% had autopsy findings of NTB.[14] In contrast, another study in which infants with RDS were randomly assigned to either CV or short-term (48 hours) HFJV, there was no bronchoscopic evidence of NTB or other tracheal damage in survivors of either group. One nonsurvivor in the HFJV group had microscopic evidence at NTB at autopsy.[75]

Although the etiology of NTB is not clear, the most obvious factors relative to its occurrence are the heat and water-vapor content of inspired gas. As mentioned previously, early HFJV systems inadequately humidified the jet gas. Close attention to this aspect of HFJV may reduce the risk of NTB to that comparable to conventional ventilation. However, it should be noted that even conventional humidifiers have been shown to provide inadequate humidity levels,[76] and this condition is aggravated by high ventilatory frequencies and inspiratory flow rates.

**Airway Pressures**

Airway pressure monitoring is crucial in all forms of HFV for at least two reasons. First, the delivered tidal volumes are inconvenient to measure clinically so that the airway pressure waveform must be analyzed to estimate and control the level of ventilation. In general, as the amplitude (the highest point minus the lowest point) of the pressure waveform is increased, the volume change of the lungs increases and $CO_2$ elimination increases. Second, monitoring various parameters of the airway pressure waveform (e.g., peak, mean and baseline pressures) provides a means of detecting life-threatening malfunctions like a patient disconnection or mechanical failure leading to elevated airway pressures. Various commercial devices are available that provide alarm capabilities for each parameter of interest.

The use of high ventilating frequencies introduces a unique problem to the measurement of airway pressures, that of *frequency response*. The frequency response of a measuring system can be defined as the relation between the frequency and the relative accuracy of the measured signal. In general, as the frequency of ventilation increases, the pressure measurement system will have a tendency to distort the pressure waveform due to the system's inherent resistance, compliance, and the inertness of the gas it contains. This distortion can manifest as two types of pressure measurement error, either an overestimation of the airway pressure amplitude,[77] or an underestimation or attenuation of the waveform.[78] Both of these errors are important because they can result in a misleading interpretation of the level of ventilation during HFV and its physiologic effects (e.g., inadvertent PEEP).

Furthermore, the site of pressure measurement during HFV is particularly important as pressure is not equilibrated throughout the airways at high frequencies. Distal endotracheal pressures seem to accurately indicate alveolar pressure measurements at least at moderately high frequencies (Fig 14–11).[18,78] However, pressure measure-

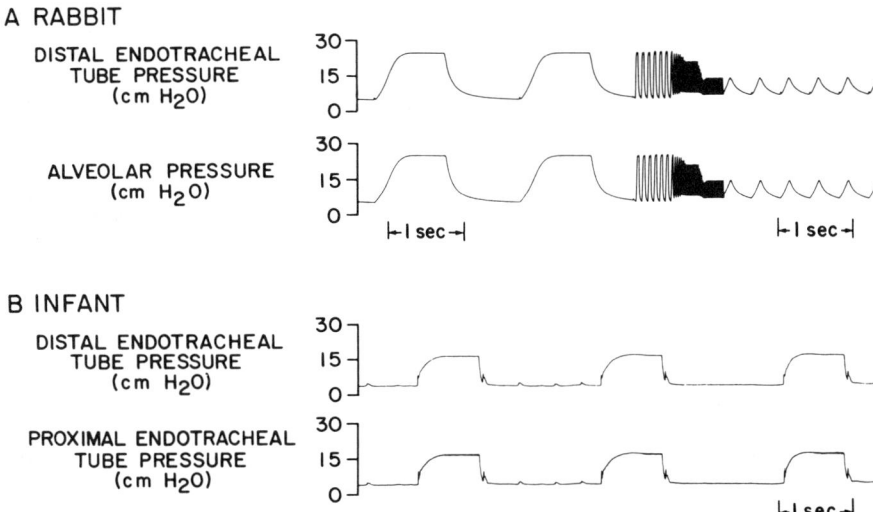

**FIG 14-11.**
Validation of techniques for pressure measurements during HFJV. **A,** distal endotracheal tube and alveolar pressure recordings in an adult rabbit during both CV and HFJV are essentially identical. **B,** distal and proximal endotracheal tube pressures during CV in an infant are also identical. (From Carlo WA, Chatburn RL, Martin RJ: Randomized trial of high-frequency jet ventilation vs. conventional ventilation in respiratory distress syndrome. *J Pediatr* 1987; 110:275. Used by permission.)

ments from the proximal endotracheal tube are usually inaccurate.[79] Before any form of HFV is used, it is important to test the pressure measurement system to assure an adequate frequency response and site of pressure sampling.

### Gas Trapping

As ventilatory frequencies are increased, inspiratory and expiratory times necessarily have to be shortened. Shortening of expiration will increase the likelihood of gas being trapped in the lungs. Gas trapping is more of a problem when expiration is passive (e.g., HFJV) rather than when it is active (e.g., HFOV) during HFV.[80] Furthermore, with larger tidal volumes, shorter expiratory times, and longer expiratory time-constants, the problem is compounded.[27, 30, 79] It should be recalled that gas trapping may decrease lung compliance. In addition, gas trapping will cause $CO_2$ retention[27] and partly explains why $CO_2$ elimination may decrease as very high tidal volumes are used with short expiratory times (Fig 14–12). Increases in mean airway pressure during HFV may

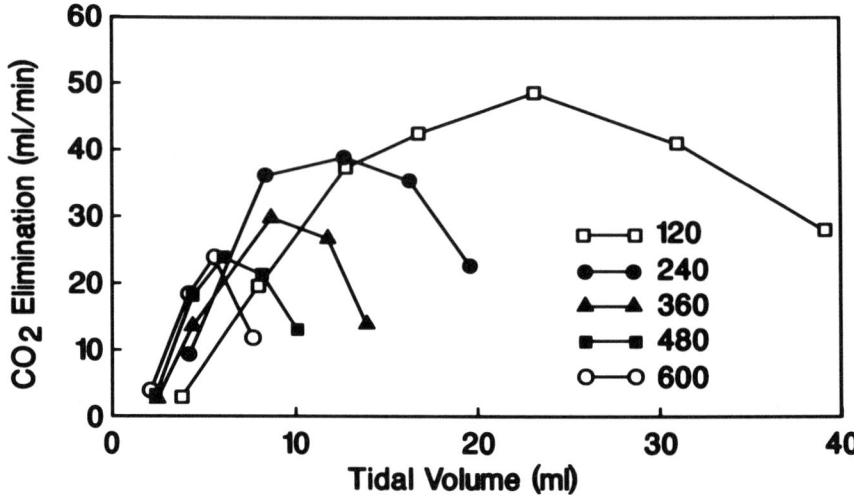

**FIG 14–12.**
Relationship between tidal volume and $CO_2$ elimination when PEEP is not controlled during HFJV in adult rabbits with normal lungs. Each frequency has a significant ($P<.01$ to .001) tidal volume effect on $CO_2$ elimination. At higher tidal volume levels, $CO_2$ elimination is decreased (SD not shown. Symbols represent frequencies used in cycles per minute). (From Korvenranta H, Carlo WA, Goldthwait DA, et al: Carbon dioxide elimination during high-frequency jet ventilation. *J Pediatr* 1987; 111:107. Used by permission.)

also impair $CO_2$ elimination in part due to an increased volume of the conducting airway.[81]

Although HFJV may reduce barotrauma, the optimal ventilator settings at which complications such as air trapping are minimized have not been determined. To develop ventilator strategies applicable to the human infant during HFJV, we studied six rabbits before and after lung lavage.[30] Changes in functional residual capacity and airway pressure gradient (peak inspiratory pressure minus positive end-expiratory pressure) were measured while inspiratory time and expiratory time were varied. Frequencies of 120, 240, and 480 cycles per minute and I:E ratios of 1:1, 1:3, 1:5, and 1:9 resulted in inspiratory times that varied from 12 to 250 milliseconds and expiratory times from 62 to 450 milliseconds. Analysis of variance demonstrated that as inspiratory time was shortened, a higher airway pressure gradient was necessary to maintain a constant tidal volume (Fig 14–13). As expiratory time was shortened, air trapping, as determined from both inadvertent positive end-expiratory pressure and an increase in functional residual capacity, increased (Fig 14–14). Lung lavage reduced air trapping as would be expected with the decrease in time constant of the respiratory system as compliance is decreased. From these observations, we concluded

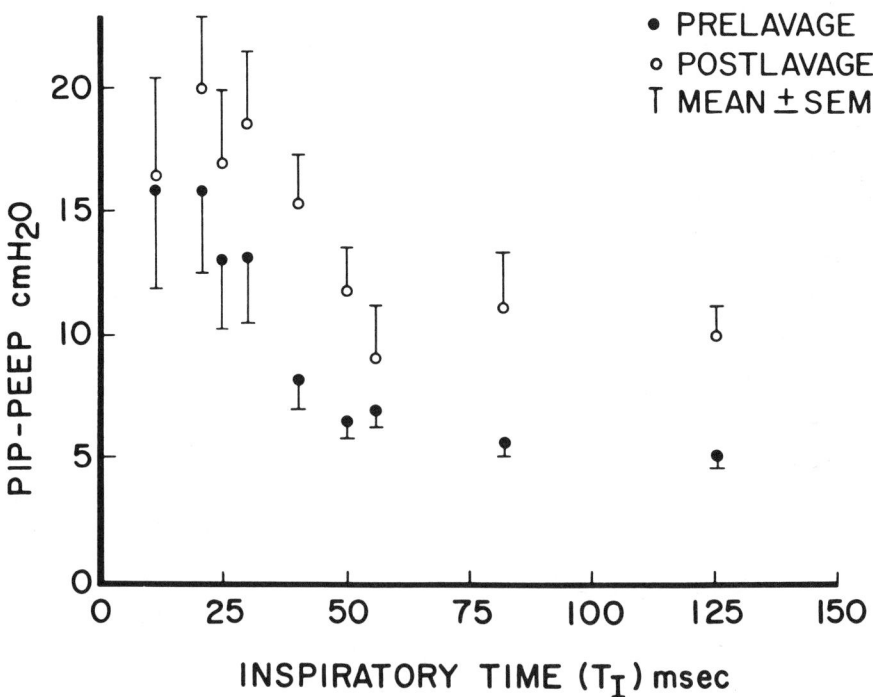

**FIG 14–13.**
Relationship between inspiratory time and distal airway pressure gradient (PIP-PEEP) needed to maintain constant tidal volume during high-frequency jet ventilation before and after lung lavage in rabbits. Shortening inspiratory time caused a significant increase in airway pressure gradient. (From Weisberger SA, Carlo WA, Chatburn RL, et al: Effect of varying inspiratory and expiratory times during high-frequency jet ventilation. *J Pediatr* 1986; 108:596. Used by permission.)

that a relatively narrow range of inspiratory and expiratory times may be necessary for optimal use of HFJV to reduce airway pressures and minimize the risk of air trapping. These results have led us to employ even lower frequencies 150 to 250/minute when ventilating patients with relatively long time constants of the respiratory system such as subjects with high compliance, increased resistance, or large lungs.

Much work has been done with HFV, and space limitation has restricted this review. However, further work is still necessary to answer vital questions, particularly related to benefit to risk ratio and cost considerations. Until then, HFV should be considered an experimental therapy.

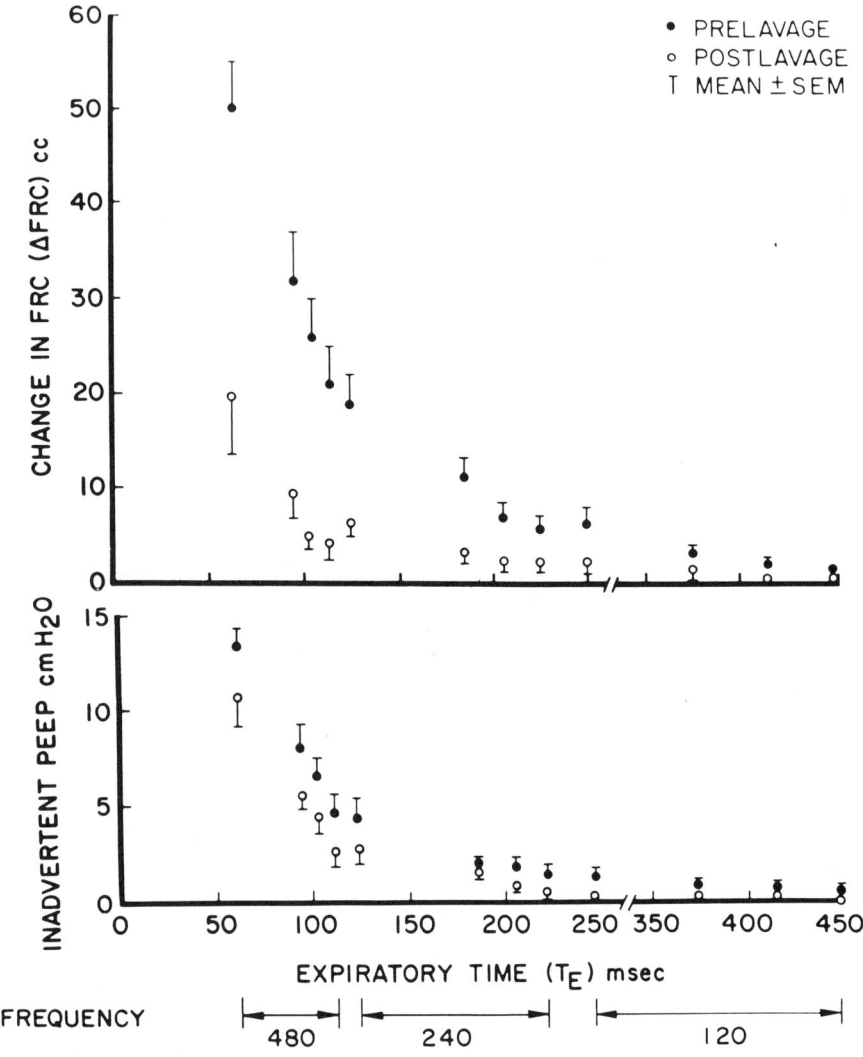

**FIG 14-14.**
Relationship between expiratory time and both change in functional residual capacity (Δ FRC) and inadvertent positive end-expiratory pressure (PEEP) before and after lung lavage in the same rabbits as in Figure 14–13. Shortening expiratory time caused air trapping as demonstrated by a significant increase in both FRC and inadvertent PEEP. (From Weisberger SA, Carlo WA, Chatburn RL, et al: Effect of varying inspiratory and expiratory times during high-frequency jet ventilation. *J Pediatr* 1986; 108:596. Used by permission.)

# REFERENCES

1. Madansky DL, Lawson EE, Chernick V, et al: Pneumothorax and other forms of pulmonary air leaks in newborns. Am Rev Respir Dis 1979; 120:729.
2. Avery ME, Tooley WH, Keller JB, et al: Is chronic lung disease in low birthweight infants preventable? A survey of eight centers. Pediatrics 1987; 79:26.
3. Heijman K, Sjöstrand U: Treatment of the respiratory distress syndrome: Preliminary report. Opusc Med 1974; 19:235.
4. Bland RD, Kim MH, Light MJ, et al: High frequency mechanical ventilation in severe hyaline membrane disease: An alternative treatment? Crit Care Med 1980; 8:275.
5. Boros SJ, Campbell K: A comparison of the effects of high frequency-low tidal volume and low frequency-high tidal volume mechanical ventilation. J Pediatr 1980; 97:108.
6. Heicher DA, Kasting DS, Harrod JR: Prospective clinical comparison of two methods for mechanical ventilation of neonates: Rapid rate and short inspiratory time versus slow rate and long inspiratory time. J Pediatr 1981; 98:957.
7. Marchak BE, Thompson WK, Duffy P, et al: Treatment of RDS by high-frequency oscillatory ventilation: A preliminary report. J Pediatr 1981; 99:298.
8. Frantz ID III, Werthammer J, Stark AR: High-frequency ventilation in premature infants with lung disease: Adequate gas exchange at low tracheal pressures. Pediatrics 1983; 71:483.
9. Pokora T, Bing D, Mammer M, et al: Neonatal high-frequency jet ventilation. Pediatrics 1983; 72:27.
10. Carlo WA, Chatburn RL, Martin RJ, et al: Decrease in airway pressure during high-frequency jet ventilation in infants with respiratory distress syndrome. J Pediatr 1984; 104:101.
11. Boynton BR, Mannino FL, Davis RF, et al: Combined high-frequency oscillatory ventilation and intermittent mandatory ventilation in critically ill neonates. J Pediatr 1984; 105:297.
12. Field D, Milner AD, Hopkin IE: High and conventional rates of positive pressure ventilation. Arch Dis Child 1984; 59:1151.
13. Eyal FG, Arad ID, Godder K, et al: High-frequency positive-pressure ventilation in neonates. Crit Care Med 1984; 12:793.
14. Boros SJ, Mammel MC, Coleman JM, et al: Neonatal high-frequency jet ventilation: Four years' experience. Pediatrics 1985; 75:657.
15. Donn SM, Nicks JJ, Bandy KP, et al: Proximal high-frequency jet ventilation of the newborn. Pediatr Pulmonol 1985; 1:267.
16. Pagani G, Rezzonico R, Marini A: Trials of high frequency jet ventilation in preterm infants with severe respiratory disease. Acta Paediatr Scand 1985; 74:681.
17. Menset A, Fromentin C, Simonin B, et al: High-frequency positive-pressure respiration in newborn infants. Ann Pediatr (Paris) 1985; 32:607.

18. Carlo WA, Chatburn RL, Martin RJ: Randomized trial of high-frequency jet ventilation versus conventional ventilation in respiratory distress syndrome. J Pediatr 1987; 110:275.
19. Sedin G: Positive-pressure ventilation at moderately high frequency in newborn infants with respiratory distress syndrome (IRDS). Acta Anaesthesiol Scand 1986; 30:515.
20. Gonzalez F, Harris T, Black P, et al: Decreased gas flow through pneumothoraces in neonates receiving high-frequency jet versus conventional ventilation. J Pediatr 1987; 110:464.
21. Gaylord MS, Quissell BJ, Lair ME: High-frequency ventilation in the treatment of infants weighing less than 1,500 grams with pulmonary interstitial emphysema: A pilot study. Pediatrics 1987; 79:915.
22. Emerson JM: Apparatus for vibrating portions of a patient's airway. US patent 2,918,917; 1959.
23. Sjöstrand U: High-frequency positive-pressure ventilation (HFPPV): A review. Crit Care Med 1980; 8:345.
24. Lunkenheimer PP, Raffllenbeul W, Keller H, et al: Application of transtracheal pressure oscillations as a modification of "diffusion respiration." Br J Anaesth 1972; 44:627.
25. Carlo WA, Martin RJ: Principles of neonatal assisted ventilation. Pediatr Clin North Am 1986; 33:221.
26. Boros SJ, Bing DR, Mammel MC, et al: Using conventional infant ventilators at unconventional rates. Pediatrics 1984; 74:487.
27. Korvenranta H, Carlo WA, Goldthwait DA, et al: Carbon dioxide elimination during high-frequency jet ventilation. J Pediatr 1987; 111:107.
28. Scacci R: Air entrainment masks: Jet mixing is how they work; the Bernoulli and Venturi principles are how they don't. Respir Care 1979; 24:928.
29. Hamilton LH, Londino JM, Linehan JH, et al: Pediatric endotracheal tube designed for high-frequency ventilation. Crit Care Med 1984; 12:988.
30. Weisberger SA, Carlo WA, Chatburn R, et al: Effect of varying inspiratory and expiratory times during high-frequency jet ventilation. J Pediatr 1986; 108:596.
31. Klain M, Smith B: High-frequency percutaneous transtracheal jet ventilation. Crit Care Med 1977; 5:280.
32. Hayek Z, Peliowski A, Ryan CA, et al: External high frequency oscillation in cats. Am Rev Respir Dis 1986; 133:630.
33. Fredberg JJ, Glass GM, Boynton BR, et al: Factors influencing mechanical performance of neonatal high-frequency ventilators. J Appl Physiol 1987; 62:2485.
34. Chang HK: Mechanisms of gas transport during ventilation by high-frequency oscillation. J Appl Physiol 1984; 56:553.
35. Lehr JL, Butler JP, Westerman PA, et al: Photographic measurement of pleural surface motion during lung oscillation. J Appl Physiol 1985; 59:623.
36. Fredberg JJ, Keefe DH, Glass GM, et al: Alveolar pressure inhomogeneity during small amplitude high frequency oscillation. J Appl Physiol 1985; 57:788.

37. Bohn DJ, Miyasaka K, Marchak BE, et al: Ventilation by high-frequency oscillation. *J Appl Physiol* 1980; 48:710.
38. Wright K, Lyrene RK, Truog WE, et al: Ventilation by high-frequency oscillation in rabbits with oleic acid lung disease. *J Appl Physiol* 1981; 50:1056.
39. Slutsky AS, Kamm RD, Rossing RH: Effects of frequency, tidal volume and lung volume on $CO_2$ elimination in dogs by high frequency (2–30 Hz), low tidal volume ventilation. *J Clin Invest* 1981; 68:1475.
40. Boros SJ, Mammel MC, Lewallen PK, et al: Necrotizing tracheobronchitis: A complication of high-frequency ventilation. *J Pediatr* 1986; 109:95.
40a. The HIFI Study Group and the Division of Lung Diseases: *A Collaborative Randomized Trial of High Frequency Oscillatory Ventilation in the Treatment of Respiratory Failure in Preterm Infants*, in press 1988.
41. Truog WE, Standaert TA, Murphy J, et al: Effect of high-frequency oscillation on gas exchange and pulmonary phospholipids in experimental hyaline membrane disease. *Am Rev Respir Dis* 1983; 127:585.
42. Kuehl T, Meredit K, Ackerman N, et al: High vs low frequency ventilation in the premature baboon with RDS (abstract). *Pediatr Res* 1982; 16:295A.
43. Hamilton PP, Onayeim A, Smyth JA, et al: Comparison of conventional and high-frequency ventilation: Oxygenation and lung pathology. *J Appl Physiol* 1983; 55:131.
44. Kolton M, Cattran CB, Kent G, et al: Oxygenation during high frequency ventilation compared with conventional mechanical ventilation in two models of lung injury. *Anesth Analg* 1982; 61:323.
45. Walsh MC, Carlo WA: Sustained inflation during high-frequency oscillatory ventilation improves pulmonary mechanics and oxygenation, *J Appl Physiol* in press, 1988.
46. Wright K, Lyrene RK, Truog WE, et al: Ventilation by high-frequency oscillation in rabbits with oleic acid lung disease. *J Appl Physiol* 1981; 50:1056.
47. Hoff BH, Wilson E, Smith RB, et al: Intermittent positive pressure ventilation and high frequency ventilation in dogs with experimental bronchopleural fistulae. *Crit Care Med* 1983; 11:598.
48. Ackerman NB, Coalson JJ, Kuehl TJ, et al: Pulmonary interstitial emphysema in the premature baboon with hyaline membrane disease. *Crit Care Med* 1984; 12:512.
49. Karlson KH, Du Rant RH: High frequency positive pressure ventilation in experimental meconium aspiration syndrome. *Am J Med Sci* 1986; 229:92.
50. Mammel MC, Gordon MJ, Connett JE, et al: Comparison of high-frequency jet ventilation and conventional mechanical ventilation in a meconium aspiration model. *J Pediatr* 1983; 103:630.
51. Trindade O, Goldberg RN, Bancalari E, et al: Conventional vs high-frequency jet ventilation in a piglet model of meconium aspiration: Comparison of pulmonary and hemodynamic effects. *J Pediatr* 1985; 107:115.

52. Frantz ID, Stark AR, Davis JM, et al: High frequency ventilation does not affect pulmonary surfactant, liquid or morphologic features in normal cats. Am Rev Respir Dis 1982; 126:909.
53. Raj JU, Goldberg RB, Bland RD: Vibratory ventilation decreases filtration of fluid in the lungs of newborn lambs. Circ Res 1983; 53:456.
54. Mannino FL, McEvoy RD, Hallman M: Surfactant turnover in high frequency oscillatory ventilation (HFOV) (abstract). Pediatr Res 1982; 16:356A.
55. Rehder K, Schmid ER, Knopp TJ: Long term high-frequency ventilation in dogs. Am Rev Respir Dis 1983; 128:476.
56. McEvoy RD, Davies NJH, Hedenstierna G, et al: Lung mucociliary transport during high-frequency ventilation. Am Rev Respir Dis 1982; 126:452.
57. Raju TNK, Braverman B, Nadkarny U, et al: Intracranial pressure and cardiac output remain stable during high frequency oscillation. Crit Care Med 1983; 11:856.
58. Todd M, Toutant M, Shapiro M: The effects of high-frequency positive pressure ventilation on intracranial pressure and brain surface movement in cats. Anesthesiology 1981; 54:496.
59. Keszler M, Klein R, McClellan L, et al: Effects of conventional and high frequency jet ventilation on lung parenchyma. Crit Care Med 1982; 10:514.
60. Man GCW, Man SFP, Kappagoda CT: Effects of high-frequency oscillatory ventilation on vagal and phrenic nerve activities. J Appl Physiol 1983; 54:502.
61. Thompson WK, Marchak BE, Bryan AC, et al: Vagotomy reverses apnea induced by high-frequency oscillatory ventilation. J Appl Physiol 1981; 51:1484.
62. Vincent RN, Stark AR, Lang P, et al: Hemodynamic response to high-frequency ventilation in infants following cardiac surgery. Pediatrics 1984; 73:426.
63. Weiner JH, Chatburn RL, Carlo WA: Ventilatory and hemodynamic effects of high-frequency jet ventilation following cardiac surgery. Respir Care 1987; 32:332.
64. Nutman J, Carlo WA, Chatburn RL: Low frequency oscillatory ventilation through the suction channel of a pediatric bronchoscope increases the safety and utility of bronchoscopy. Ann Otol Rhinol Laryngol, in press, 1988.
65. El-Baz N, Holinger L, El-Ganzouri A, et al: High-frequency positive pressure ventilation for tracheal reconstruction supported by tracheal T-tube. Anesth Analg 1982; 61:796.
66. Klain M, Keszler H, Brader E: High frequency jet ventilation in CPR. Crit Care Med 1981; 9:421.
67. Carlon GC, Howland WS, Ray C, et al: High-frequency jet ventilation: A prospective randomized evaluation. Chest 1983; 84:551.
68. Chatburn RL, Primiano FP Jr: A rational basis for humidity therapy. Respir Care 1987; 32:249.

69. Chatburn RL, McClellan LD: A heat and humidification system for high-frequency jet ventilation. *Respir Care* 1982; 27:1386.
70. Carlon GC, Kohn RC, Howland WS, et al: Clinical experience with high frequency jet ventilation. *Crit Care Med* 1981; 9:1.
71. Harris TR, Gooch WM, Wilson JF, et al: Necrotizing tracheobronchitis associated with high-frequency jet ventilation in neonates. *Clin Res* 1984; 32:132A.
72. Kirpalani H, High T, Perlman M, et al: Diagnosis and therapy of necrotizing tracheobronchitis in ventilated neonates. *Crit Care Med* 1985; 12:792.
73. Fox WW, Spitzer AR, Musci M, et al: Tracheal secretion impaction during hyperventilation for persistent pulmonary hypertension of the neonate. *Pediatr Res* 1984; 18:323A.
74. Clark RH, Wiswell TE, Null DM, et al: Tracheal and bronchial injury in high-frequency oscillatory ventilation compared with conventional positive pressure ventilation. *J Pediatr* 1987; 111:114.
75. Kercsmar CM, Martin RJ, Chatburn RL, et al: Bronchoscopic findings in infants treated with high-frequency jet ventilation versus conventional ventilation. *Pediatrics*, in press, 1988.
76. Tarnow-Mordi WO, Sutton P, Fletcher M, et al: Evidence of inadequate humidification of inspired gas during artificial ventilation of newborn babies in the British Isles. *Lancet* 1986; 1:909.
77. Boynton BR, Mannino FL, Meathe EA, et al: Airway pressure measurement during high-frequency oscillatory ventilation. *Crit Care Med* 1984; 12:39.
78. Chatburn RL, Carlo WA, Primiano FP Jr: Airway-pressure measurement during high-frequency ventilation. *Respir Care* 1985; 30:750.
79. Frantz ID III, Close RH: Elevated lung volume and alveolar pressure during jet ventilation of rabbits. *Am Rev Respir Dis* 1985; 131:134.
80. Bancalari A, Gerhardt T, Bancalari E, et al: Gas trapping with high-frequency ventilation: Jet versus oscillatory ventilation. *J Pediatr* 1987; 110:617.
81. Yamada Y, Venegas JG, Strieder DJ, et al: Effects of mean airway pressure on gas transport during high-frequency ventilation in dogs. *J Appl Physiol* 1986; 61:1896.

# 15

# Extracorporeal Membrane Oxygenation and Other New Modes of Gas Exchange

## 15A      Extracorporeal Membrane Oxygenation

Joanne J. Nicks, R.R.T.
Robert H. Bartlett, M.D.

For the past 20 years, mechanical ventilation has played a major role in the management of acute respiratory failure associated with respiratory distress syndrome, meconium aspiration syndrome, persistent pulmonary hypertension, congenital diaphragmatic hernia, and sepsis in infants. While conventional ventilation is usually a successful treatment, a small percentage of these infants (5%–10%) are unresponsive and die of respiratory failure. Complications of vigorous mechanical ventilation, including barotrauma and bronchopulmonary dysplasia associated with the use of high pressures and oxygen concentrations, occur frequently in infants.[1] As a result, technological advancements have lead to the development of alternative modes of therapy including high-frequency ventilation and extracorporeal membrane oxygenation (ECMO).[2, 3]

## DEVELOPMENT OF ECMO

Extracorporeal membrane oxygenation is a process that allows for prolonged *extracorporeal circulation* (ECC). Venous drainage from the infant is pumped through a membrane oxygenator where diffusion of carbon dioxide and oxygen occur, and oxygenated blood is returned to the body.

The capability of applying ECMO to neonates would not be possible without the pioneer work of many individual investigators, including the development of ECC itself by Gibbon in 1937. This development paved the way to the introduction of the heart-lung machine used for open heart surgery in the 1950s. The modifications necessary for the long-term application of ECC were developed in the 1960s and included the refinement of a membrane oxygenator and elimination of a large blood reservoir that required total anticoagulation. Whereas the bubble oxygenator directly exposed the blood to oxygen molecules causing cellular damage within hours, the membrane oxygenator allowed for safe delivery of oxygen and removal of carbon dioxide to and from the tissues through a semipermeable membrane, similar to the lung itself, for a period of days or weeks.[4] Clinical application of ECMO began in 1970 when White et al.[5] treated three infants with respiratory failure who did not survive, but who demonstrated satisfactory gas exchange. In 1972 Hill et al.[6] successfully treated the first adult patient with ECMO. However, a randomized study of the use of ECMO in adults with acute respiratory failure showed a survival of only 9.5% in treated patients vs. 8.3% in the controls.[6] Our group began treating infants with ECMO in 1973—first in Irvine at the University of California and now in Ann Arbor at the University of Michigan Medical Center. ECMO has progressed greatly over the past years with over 100 infants having been treated in our group and over 700 infants treated nationally at 18 other centers.[7,8]

## INDICATIONS FOR ECMO

Indications for the use of ECMO have evolved continuously, resulting in a more successful treatment modality. Initially ECMO was applied as a rescue technique in dying newborns who were thought to have reversible respiratory disorders. Early contraindications included infants who were less than 1 kg and/or had evidence of a bulging fontanelle. Screening techniques have improved dramatically, and infants are now evaluated with ultrasonography for intracranial hemorrhage and cyanotic congenital heart disease. Currently, to be considered for ECMO, an infant must be greater than 34 weeks' gestation with no evidence of intracranial hemorrhage, bleeding disorders, or congenital anomalies incompatible with quality life. Quality-of-life potential following ECMO therapy is an important consideration since the majority of treated infants will survive. Only disorders with short-term reversibility should be treated with ECMO. Bronchopulmonary dysplasia results in chronic lung disease that is not easily reversed; therefore ECMO is reserved for infants receiving less than 10 days of mechanical ventilation. Parental permission must be obtained prior to initiating ECMO.[9]

Selection criteria for the application of ECMO is determined by retrospective analysis of infants treated in a particular institution and estimated to have a greater than 80% mortality (Table 15A–1). Many ECMO centers have followed the alveolar-arterial oxygen gradient

**TABLE 15A–1.**
Selection Criteria for the Application of ECMO

1. Newborn pulmonary insufficiency index (NPII).—The NPII score assesses the severity of respiratory distress in the neonate. It is calculated by plotting the fraction of oxygen in dry inspired air ($F_{I_{O_2}}$) and the pH during the infant's first 24 hr of life. The NPII score was used during the early phases of ECMO to assess mortality risk (80% to 100%) but is no longer applicable since the advent of hyperventilation to treat persistent pulmonary hypertension of the newborn (PPHN).[9, 10]
2. Alveolar-arterial oxygen difference (A−a$DO_2$)

$$A-aDO_2 = (F_{I_{O_2}})(P_B - P_{H_2O}\text{ vapor}) - Pa_{O_2} - Pa_{CO_2}$$

when $F_{I_{O_2}}$ = 100%. An A−a$DO_2$ greater than 620 mm Hg for 12 consecutive hours usually correlates with 80% mortality. $P_B$ = barometric pressure; $P_{H_2O}$ vapor = water vapor pressure; $Pa_{O_2}$ = partial pressure of $O_2$ in arterial blood; $Pa_{CO_2}$ = partial pressure of $CO_2$ in arterial blood.
3. Oxygenation index (OI)

$$OI = \frac{\overline{P}_{aw} \times F_{I_{O_2}}}{Pa_{O_2}} \times 100$$

where $\overline{P}_{AW}$ is mean airway pressure; an OI of 40 or greater for 3 of 5 blood gases correlates with over 80% mortality; an OI of 25 or greater correlates with over 50% mortality.[7, 9]
4. Acute deterioration with a $Pa_{O_2}$ of less than 40 mm Hg or pH less than 7.15 for 2 hr qualified an infant for ECMO during phase II.[12]
5. Lack of response to treatment of persistent pulmonary hypertension qualified an infant for ECMO if the $Pa_{O_2}$ was less than 55 mm Hg or the pH was less than 7.40 or if persistent hypotension was present (two of the above for 3 hr).[12]
6. Presence of any four of the following barotrauma criteria qualified an infant for ECMO:
    Interstitial emphysema
    Pneumothorax
    Pneumoperitoneum
    Pneumopericardium
    Subcutaneous emphysema
    Persistent air leak for 24 hr
    Mean airway pressure >15 cm $H_2O$[12]
7. Infants with congenital diaphragmatic hernia qualified for ECMO if their $Pa_{O_2}$ was less than 80 mm Hg on an $F_{I_{O_2}}$ of over 0.80 at twenty-four hours after surgery.[12]

($A - aDO_2$), treating infants with an $A - aDO_2$ greater than 620 mm Hg for 12 hours.[10]

## CLINICAL EXPERIENCE

At the University of Michigan, supported by a National Institute of Health grant, application of ECMO has passed through three phases, with different objectives and criteria for each phase. In phase I, infants who had failed all conventional forms of treatment available at that time, and who had a newborn pulmonary insufficiency index (NPII) indicating 100% mortality, were selected by neonatologists for ECMO. The objectives were to determine the safety and efficacy of ECMO as a rescue treatment for dying infants.[11] The phase II trial was designed to evaluate outcome of these infants. A complex set of criteria that selected patients with greater than 80% predicted mortality was developed. These criteria included the NPII, acute respiratory deterioration, unresponsiveness to treatment for persistent pulmonary hypertension, severe barotrauma, and respiratory failure with congenital diaphragmatic hernia. The phase II trial also included a controlled randomized study of 12 infants who were entered based on the above criteria. This study used a randomized "play-the-winner" statistical method. With this design, infants were randomly assigned to a specific treatment, i.e., ECMO or conventional therapy. The success of that therapy influenced the odds of obtaining that treatment in the next random assignment so that the patient had a greater chance of being assigned to the more successful therapy. This study design was chosen to minimize the chance of withholding a potentially life-saving treatment for a dying infant. Eleven infants were assigned to ECMO and survived; one infant was assigned to conventional treatment and died. This study suggested that ECMO was more successful in treating infants with severe respiratory failure than was the conventional approach. However, the limited number of control patients treated conventionally has caused criticism and raised questions that will only be answered with further randomized clinical trials.[12,13] Currently the phase III protocol for the ECMO project is being implemented. Selection criteria are being based on the oxygenation index with early randomization of patients with a predicted 50% to 80% mortality. The objective is to address the issue of morbidity and medical costs in the infants treated with ECMO as compared to conventional treatment.[7]

## TECHNIQUES FOR PERFUSION

The most common method of ECMO perfusion is *venoarterial (VA) ECMO*, which requires cannulation of the right internal jugular vein and the right common carotid artery. Venous blood from the right atrium is drained through the internal jugular vein. Oxygenated blood is returned to the aortic arch through the right common carotid artery (Fig 15A–1). Venoarterial ECMO is capable of providing excellent support of the heart and lungs with initial flows of 100 to 120 ml/kg. This results in minimal perfusion to the pulmonary circulation and approximately 80% cardiopulmonary bypass. Oxygenated blood from the extracorporeal circuit provides adequate delivery of oxygen to the myocardium and systemic circulation. Although little blood flows through the heart, conduction and contraction continues. To achieve adequate flows, the patient must have an adequate circulation volume. The advantages of venoarterial ECMO include reduction of mechanical ventilation to minimal settings and elimination of life-threatening hypoxia. The major risks associated with venoarterial bypass include potential infusion of air or clots into the arterial circulation and potential reduction in cerebral perfusion with carotid artery ligation.[9, 14]

*Venovenous (VV) ECMO* has been applied in 16 infants treated at the University of Michigan. This route employs cannulation of the internal jugular vein, which drains venous blood from the right atrium, with return of oxygenated blood to the femoral vein (Fig 15A–2). This method eliminates the need for carotid artery ligation and minimizes the risks of emboli formation as only the venous circulation is affected.

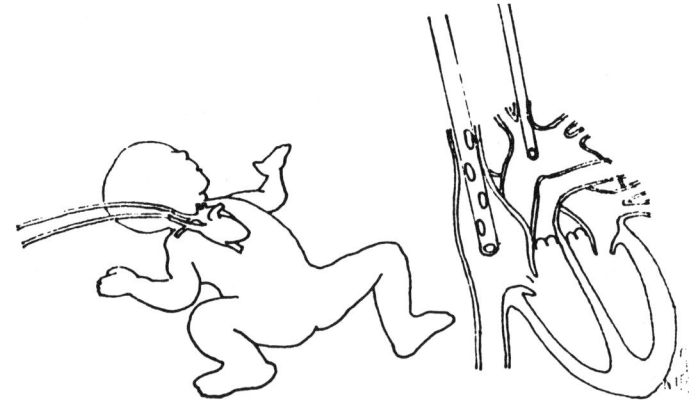

**FIG 15A–1.**
Catheter placement for venoarterial ECMO. Blood is drained from the venous catheter placed in the superior vena cava/right atrium through the internal jugular vein. Oxygenated blood from the ECMO circuit is returned to the aortic arch through the right carotid artery.

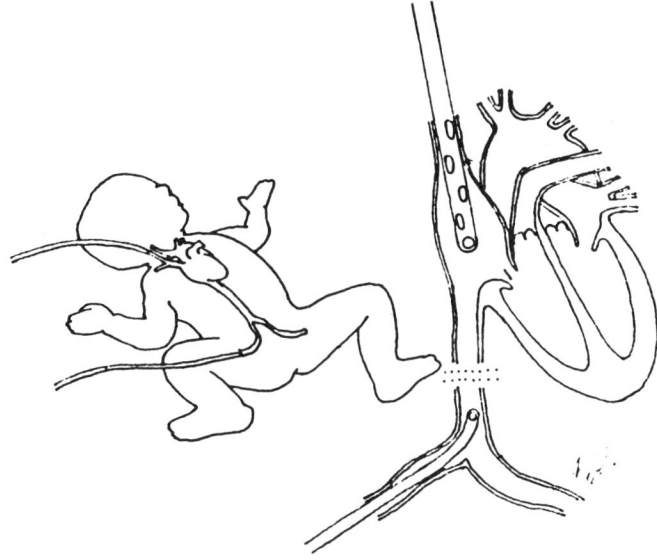

**FIG 15A–2.**
Catheter placement for venovenous ECMO. Blood is drained from a venous catheter placed in the superior vena cava/right atrium through the internal jugular vein. Oxygenated blood from the ECMO circuit is returned to the inferior vena cava through the femoral vein.

However, with venovenous bypass two surgical dissections are necessary, lengthening the cannulation procedure. Venovenous bypass does not provide cardiac support and therefore requires good myocardial function, which may be a problem in the asphyxiated infant. Due to recirculation of arterial blood into the venous circulation, higher pump flows and ventilatory support are necessary to achieve adequate respiratory function. Initial stabilization on ECMO took an average of 5 hours with venovenous bypass and less than 2 hours with venoarterial support. Complications associated with femoral vein cannulation include infection and insufficient venous flow to the leg.[15]

The single-catheter approach to venovenous bypass allows for a single cannulation site and still eliminates the need for carotid artery ligation. Two methods are being developed; one uses a double-lumen catheter with venous drainage and arterial perfusion occurring through one catheter in the jugular vein; the other method uses synchronized pneumatic valves that allow drainage of blood in one direction and reinfusion in another through a single-lumen catheter.[16] Currently, while feasible, the advantages of venovenous ECMO do not outweigh the disadvantages, but single-catheter venovenous ECMO may become more prominent in the future.

## CIRCUIT COMPONENTS

The ECMO circuit consists of cannulas, polyvinylchloride tubing with Luer-Lok connectors and stopcocks, a silicone bladder, bladder-box assembly, polyurethane raceway, roller pump, membrane oxygenator, heat exchanger, infusion pump, and activated clotting time (ACT) monitor[9, 14] (Fig 15A–3).

The *cannulas* sometimes used for ECMO are Argyle chest tubes; however, new catheters designed for ECMO are now available for cannulation in sizes 8 to 16 (Elecath, Gesco). The catheter must have the largest internal diameter possible to achieve adequate flow rates for total heart-lung support. Prior to cannulation, a loading dose of 100 units/kg of heparin is given. In addition, the infant is paralyzed to

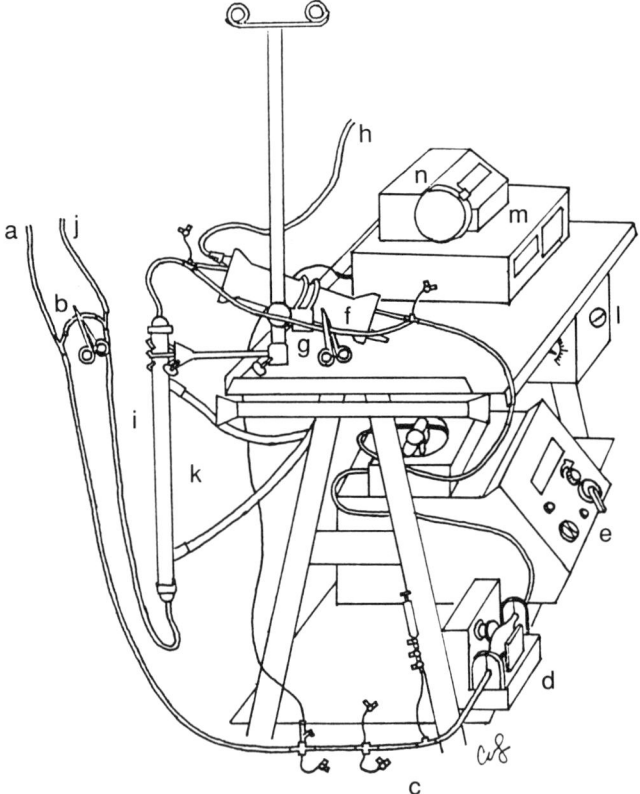

**FIG 15A–3.**
Components of the ECMO circuit: *a*, venous line; *b*, patient bridge; *c*, infusion sites; *d*, bladder assembly; *e*, ECMO pump; *f*, oxygenator; *g*, oxygenator bridge; *h*, gas inlet; *i*, heat exchanger; *j*, arterial line; *k*, water heater/heat exchanger lines; *l*, water heater; *m*, venous saturation oximeter; *n*, ACT machine.

prevent aspiration of air into the internal jugular vein during venous cannulation.⁹, ¹⁴

The *tubing and connectors* of the ECMO circuit provide access sites for fluid administration and sampling. Infusion sites are usually located before the bladder since the bladder functions as an air trap. Hyperalimentation, heparin, blood products, and medications are infused through separate sites. Samples of blood for pump venous blood gases, laboratory analysis, and activated clotting times are drawn just before the oxygenator. Samples of blood for pump arterial blood gases are drawn after the oxygenator; platelets are also infused after the oxygenator to prevent aggregation. Contamination is avoided by having separate sites for withdrawals and infusions. The complete circuit volume is 350 ml. Prior to initiating ECMO, this circuit is primed, flushing it completely with carbon dioxide that aids in removing air from the system and therefore minimizing the risk of air embolism. Following the carbon dioxide flush, the pump is primed with Plasmalyte solution, which is then displaced with packed red blood cells to which calcium and heparin have been added. The pH correction with tris(hydroxymethyl)aminomethane (THAM) or sodium bicarbonate may be necessary.⁹, ¹⁴

The *bladder-box* assembly consists of a silicone bladder that is placed in line proximal to the oxygenator and pump. Blood draining from the venous catheter fills the reservoir prior to entering the pump. The bladder contacts a microswitch sensor that detects collapse or expansion of the bladder. The sensor controls the pump via a relay switch. If pump flow rate exceeds venous return, the bladder collapses; this collapse activates the microswitch and simultaneously inactivates the pump and sounds an alarm.⁹, ¹⁴

The *ECMO pump* currently used is a roller pump that moves blood by compression and displacement. The output of the pump is dependent on the size of the tubing, the occlusion setting, and the revolutions per minute of the rollers regulated by the pump controller. A microprocessor converts revolutions per minute to circuit flow in cubic centimeters per minute.⁹, ¹⁴

The *oxygenator* consists of blood and gas compartments separated by a semipermeable membrane. Oxygenation and ventilation occur by diffusion. Oxygen transfer is related to the membrane surface area, pump flow rate, and degree of desaturation of the blood entering the oxygenator. Carbon dioxide elimination is regulated by adjusting the gas flow rate. The diffusion of carbon dioxide is much greater than that of oxygen, resulting in the need for additional carbon dioxide to be added to the gas flow (5% Carbogen).⁹, ¹⁴

The *heat exchanger* maintains the temperature of the blood through warm-water recirculation. Blood and water paths are separated by a metal surface through which heat passes. The heat exchanger is positioned distal to the oxygenator to counteract the heat loss caused by the gas flow rate and condensation within the oxygenator.[9,14]

An *infusion pump* delivers heparin to the ECMO circuit to prevent clot formation. Prior to cannulation, the infant is given a heparin loading dose of 100 units/kg. Anticoagulation therapy is continued by a heparin maintenance dose of 20 to 50 units/kg/hour to the ECMO circuit. Heparin delivery is adjusted to maintain an activated clotting time of two to three times normal (220 to 250 seconds); the activated clotting time is monitored every hour with an ACT monitor.[9,14]

## MANAGEMENT OF AN INFANT ON ECMO

When a moribund infant is placed on ECMO, the transformation is quite dramatic. Prior to the initiation of ECMO, patient management often includes hyperventilation with high pressures and subsequent barotrauma. In addition, pharmacologic support with high doses of vasopressors, alkalizing agents, paralyzing agents, and sedatives are frequently needed. Large amounts of fluids are often necessary to maintain the mean arterial blood pressure.[17] Despite this support, some babies deteriorate and are difficult to oxygenate. Usually, upon *initiation of ECMO* the improvement is immediate. On an initial ECMO flow of 100 to 120 cc/kg/min, the baby's heart and lungs are completely supported resulting in dramatically improved oxygenation and color. All vasopressor substances and muscle relaxants are discontinued. Ventilator parameters are adjusted to "rest" settings (fraction of oxygen in dry inspired air [$FI_{O_2}$], 0.30; rate, 10 per minute; peak pressure, 20 cm $H_2O$; and positive end-expiratory pressure (PEEP), 4 cm $H_2O$). The baby is allowed to move about and breathe spontaneously.[9,12,14]

*Maintenance on ECMO* requires extensive monitoring and frequent adjustments in therapy to optimize oxygenation, ventilation, and blood pressure. ECMO support is adjusted to maintain normal blood gas values (pH, 7.35 to 7.45; partial pressure of $CO_2$ in arterial blood [$Pa_{CO_2}$], 40 to 45; partial pressure of oxygen in arterial blood [$Pa_{O_2}$], 60 to 80). In addition, monitoring of the infant's arterial saturation and the circuit's venous oxygen saturation provides valuable continuous monitoring of oxygen content and delivery. Heparin requirements will vary from hour to hour, depending on the urine output and platelet consumption. Careful monitoring and adjustment of heparin with measurement of an activated clotting time every hour is critical to prevent bleeding or clotting. Blood products may be transfused into the circuit to replace red blood cells and platelets as necessary. The hematocrit is maintained between 45% and 50% and the platelet count at greater than 70,000 cells/cu mm. Platelet consumption often increases on ECMO due to blood-surface interactions. Fluid and electrolytes are monitored and adjusted as necessary to maintain adequate mean arterial blood pressure and urine output, and intake and output are closely balanced. Diuretics are indicated for decreased urine output from the initial hypoxic insult or for interstitial edema from pre-ECMO fluid resuscitation. If urine output continues to be inadequate, a hemofilter (Amicon minifilter) may be added to correct hypervolemia. Hypovolemia can also be a problem with ECMO; therefore, volume must be replaced for adequate circulating volume to achieve the necessary flow rates. Lung function is usually very poor during the first 24 to 48 hours of ECMO. The chest x-ray may show complete atelectasis with whiteout of the lung fields. Pulmonary function tests show a marked decrease in compliance. To facilitate lung expansion and removal of secretions, postural drainage, percussion, and suctioning are performed every hour. Following suctioning, lungs are "conditioned" with manual ventilation using increased pressures and inflation hold. Within 48 to 72 hours, breath sounds improve; the chest x-ray shows increased aeration; and pulmonary function studies show increased compliance. As a result, oxygenation often improves allowing weaning from ECMO.[9,12,14]

*Weaning from ECMO* is accomplished by decreasing the flow rate in small increments of 10 to 20 ml. Continuous monitoring of arterial and venous saturation helps determine when weaning is possible and how it is tolerated. Arterial and venous oxygen saturation are maintained at greater than 90% and 65%, respectively. As ECMO flow rate through the membrane lung is decreased, pulmonary blood flow in the infant will increase. Evidence of adequate saturation values indicates that the infant's lungs are now able to support some gas exchange. ECMO is discontinued when pump flow rates have been decreased to 25 to 50 ml/kg. To determine an infant's ability to maintain oxygenation and ventilation independent of ECMO, the venous and arterial lines are clamped for a trial period. Ventilator settings are adjusted by monitoring arterial saturation and blood gases. If the baby is able to maintain adequate oxygenation and ventilation with a mean airway pressure lower than 10 cm $H_2O$ and $FI_{O_2}$ less than 0.50, decannulation is performed. On removal of the cannulas, the vessels are ligated rather than repaired to prevent dislodgment of emboli. The usual duration of ECMO is 3 to 7 days.[9,14]

*Complications during ECMO* may be related to the patient's primary disease process or to technical aspects of the circuit. Due to the severity of the infant's initial disease, multiple organ problems may become apparent while ECMO is in progress (Table 15A−2). Careful monitoring, anticipation, prevention, and treatment of these clinical complications is vital. Mechanical problems related to the ECMO circuit are often critical and necessitate emergent corrective actions. These technical complications include tubing rupture, air in the circuit, oxygenator failure, power failure, and decannulation. Because the infant is dependent on ECMO, urgent recognition and correction of any technical problems requires the skills of highly trained ECMO specialists.[7, 9, 14]

Treating a patient with ECMO requires an extensive support system. This system begins at the referral hospital with timely recognition of a potential ECMO candidate, arrangements to transfer while the patient is stable enough to tolerate the transport, and cooperation with the referring ECMO center for transport arrangements. At the ECMO center, the services of many departments outside of the direct patient-care area, including the blood bank, radiology, cardiology, neurology, and surgery, are also necessary. Within the patient-care area, this intensively challenging infant requires the skills and teamwork of many highly trained professionals including neonatologists, neonatal intensive care nurses, neonatal respiratory therapists, and ECMO specialists. The neonatology staff provides bedside intensive care of these infants, evaluating and treating them with aggressive medical management and assessing their qualifications for ECMO. The neonatal intensive-care nursing staff must arrange coverage to provide one-on-one management

**TABLE 15A−2.**
Complications Seen in Patients Treated with ECMO

| System | Complications From Primary Illness | Complications Related to ECMO |
|---|---|---|
| Central nervous | Seizures, edema, intracranial hemorrhage | Emboli, infarction, intracranial hemorrhage |
| Respiratory | Barotrauma, extraventilatory air leaks, necrotizing tracheobronchitis, pulmonary edema | Pulmonary edema, release of vasoactive substances by platelet-membrane interaction, hemothorax |
| Cardiovascular | Hypoxic cardiomyopathy, hypervolemia, patent ductus arteriosus | Hypervolemia, hypovolemia, hypertension, hemopericardium |
| Renal | Acute tubular necrosis, oliguria, hypervolemia, electrolyte disorders | Alteration of renin-angiotensin-aldosterone axis by nonpulsatile perfusion |
| Hematologic | Anemia, leukopenia, thrombocytopenia | Consumption of blood components by membrane surface that results in anemia, leukopenia, and thrombocytopenia; hemorrhage |

of this extremely demanding infant. The neonatal respiratory therapists provide the latest technological equipment and intensive management and monitoring of the cardiopulmonary status of these infants. The ECMO specialist is a nurse, respiratory therapist, perfusionist, or physician who has completed an extensive training program consisting of classroom, laboratory, and clinical instruction. Responsibilities of the ECMO specialist include maintaining and monitoring the ECMO circuit, assessing the infant, monitoring and maintaining cardiopulmonary and hematologic parameters (e.g., oxygenation, mean arterial blood pressure, hematocrit, platelet count, and activated clotting time), assisting with nursing care, and responding to technical emergencies. One nurse is always available to provide intensive nursing management including clinical assessment, blood gas sampling, preparation of medications, suctioning and postural drainage, monitoring fluid administration, and assisting the ECMO specialist as needed. Bedside medical management of the patient is provided by the ECMO specialist who is a surgery or neonatology fellow participating in specialty training for ECMO. They are responsible for patient selection, cannulation and decannulation, and management of the infant during the ECMO course. The team approach to ECMO management fosters excellent cooperation between all medical services, provides specific responsibilities for each individual, and results in the most complete, errorless care of the infant.[9, 14]

Enthusiasm over ECMO is very high because of reports showing dramatic reduction in mortality in this population of infants with predicted 80% to 90% mortality risk. The number of centers providing neonatal ECMO or contemplating starting programs is increasing rapidly. An ECMO registry has been developed to keep records for all ECMO treatment centers. Currently there are 26 centers internationally including one in West Germany and one in Japan. Our institution offers an annual ECMO training seminar to assist with the establishment of new programs in other centers.

*Outcome* of patients treated with ECMO has been improving as experience and knowledge increase. Currently over 700 patients have been treated with ECMO with 81% survival.[8] Our group treated 100 infants between 1973 and 1986. With improved technology and development of extensive qualifying criteria, our survival rate has increased from 54% with the first 50 infants to 90% with the following 50 infants for an overall survival of 72% (Table 15A–3). Seven infants who survived ECMO died at a later date. Most of these infants surviving ECMO are functioning normally; however, 17% had moderate to severe neurologic dysfunction, and 8% had severe residual pulmonary dysfunction. The major complication seen was intracranial bleeding that

**TABLE 15A–3.**
Diagnosis and Outcome of the First 100 Patients Treated by Bartlett et al.*

| Diagnosis[†] | Phase I[‡] | Phase II[‡] | Phase III[‡] | Overall[‡] |
|---|---|---|---|---|
| MAS | 24 (17) | 12 (12) | 8 ( 8) | 44 (37) |
| RDS | 16 ( 6) | 7 ( 5) | 3 ( 2) | 26 (13) |
| PPH | 2 ( 2) | 4 ( 4) | 4 ( 4) | 10 (10) |
| CDH | 3 ( 1) | 3 ( 3) | 3 ( 3) | 9 ( 7) |
| Sepsis | 4 ( 1) | 2 ( 1) | 2 ( 1) | 8 ( 3) |
| Other | 1 ( 0) | 2 ( 2) | 0 ( 0) | 3 ( 2) |
| Overall | 50 (27) | 30 (27) | 20 (18) | 100 (72) |

*From Bartlett RH, Gazzaniga AB, Toomasian JM, et al: Extracorporeal membrane oxygenation (ECMO) in neonatal respiratory failure: 100 cases. *Ann Surg* 1986; 204:236.
[†]MAS = meconium aspiration syndrome; RDS = respiratory distress syndrome; PPH = persistent pulmonary hypertension; CDH = congenital diaphragmatic hernia.
[‡]Numbers in parentheses denote survivors.

occurred in 89% of premature infants less than 35 weeks' gestation, as compared to 15% of full-term infants. Neurologic impairment may be related to pre-ECMO events since many of these treated infants had suffered from birth asphyxia, prolonged hypoxia, acidosis, and cardiac arrest. These events increase the risk of abnormal neurologic sequelae, but they are not totally reliable outcome predictors since some infants considered to be high risk had a normal neurologic outcome.[7] There is some evidence that right carotid artery ligation is not without its risks. Recent reports indicate that following ECMO there is an increased incidence of right-sided brain lesions detected by computed tomographic (CT) scans of the head and by electroencephalogram. However, with retrospective analysis of asphyxiated infants not treated with ECMO, predominance of left-sided lesions was noted.[18] Extensive follow-up of infants treated with ECMO is imperative, and centers offering ECMO must carefully weigh the benefits against the risks.

Extracorporeal membrane oxygenation has been recognized as a lifesaving treatment for infants with severe cardiopulmonary disease who fail conventional management, but future advances are necessary. Current randomized trials address the morbidity and cost-effectiveness of ECMO when used early in the course of infant respiratory failure. The utilization of ECMO continues to be of interest for the management of children and adults with respiratory and cardiac failure and as a bridge to organ transplant. Although the history of adult ECMO has been bleak, a spark of hope has resurfaced with a recent study reporting 50% survival in 43 adults treated with a modified ECMO procedure for severe acute respiratory failure.[19] Development of heparin-bonded circuits that eliminate the need for systemic anticoagulation may allow treatment of premature infants. Ability to apply venovenous ECMO through a double-lumen, one-catheter system may result in more extensive use of ECMO without complications and concerns associated with carotid artery ligation. Technical refinements being developed include computerized, servocontrolled pumps and automated monitoring to simplify the ECMO procedure. The complications associated with heparinization, carotid ligation, and blood-membrane interactions should be eliminated with a more advanced procedure and improved equipment. In the future, preterm and nonmoribund infants, children, and adults may be treated with ECMO.[7, 20]

## REFERENCES

1. Phillips AGS: Oxygen plus pressure plus time: The etiology of bronchopulmonary dysplasia. Pediatrics 1975; 55:44.
2. Carlo WA, Chatburn RL, Martin RJ, et al: Decrease in airway pressure during high-frequency jet ventilation in infants with respiratory distress syndrome. J Pediatr 1984; 104:101.
3. Donn SM, Nicks JJ, Bandy KP, et al: Proximal high-frequency jet ventilation of the newborn. Pediatr Pulmonol 1985; 1:227.
4. Lillehei CW: A personalized history of extracorporeal circulation. Trans Am Soc Artif Intern Organs 1982; 28:5.
5. White JJ, Andrews HG, Risemberg H, et al: Prolonged respiratory support in newborn infants with a membrane oxygenator. Surgery 1971; 70:288.
6. Zapol WM, Snider MT, Hill JD, et al: Extracorporeal membrane oxygenation in severe acute respiratory failure: A randomized prospective study. JAMA 1979; 242:2193.
7. Bartlett RH, Gazzaniga AB, Toomasian JM, et al: Extracorporeal membrane oxygenation (ECMO) in neonatal respiratory failure: 100 cases. Ann Surg 1986; 204:236.
8. Toomasian JM, Snedecor SM, Cornell RD, et al: National experience with extracorporeal membrane oxygenation (ECMO) for newborn respiratory failure: Data from 715 cases. University of Michigan, ECMO Data Registry, Department of Surgery and Biostatistics, 1986.
9. Toomasian JM, Chapman RA, Bartlett RH: Extracorporeal Membrane Oxygenation Technical Specialists Manual. Ann Arbor, University of Michigan Medical Center, 1987.
10. Krummel TM, Greenfield LJ, Kirkpatrick BV, et al: Alveolar-arterial oxygen gradients versus the neonatal pulmonary insufficiency index for prediction of mortality in ECMO candidates. J Pediatr Surg 1984; 19:380.
11. Bartlett RH, Gazzaniga AB, Huxtable RF, et al: Extracorporeal circulation in neonatal respiratory failure. J Thorac Cardiovasc Surg 1977; 74:826.
12. Bartlett RH, Roloff DW, Cornell RG, et al: Extracorporeal circulation in neonatal respiratory failure: A prospective randomized study. Pediatrics 1985; 76:479.

13. Ware JH, Epstein MF: Commentary on extracorporeal circulation in neonatal respiratory failure: A prospective randomized study. *Pediatrics* 1985; 76:849.
14. Nugent J: Extracorporeal membrane oxygenation in the neonate. *Neonatal Network* 1986; 4:27.
15. Andrew AF, Klein MD, Toomasian JM, et al: Venovenous extracorporeal membrane oxygenation for neonates. *J Pediatr Surg* 1983; 18:339.
16. Zwischenberger JB, Toomasian JM, Drake K, et al: Total respiratory support with single cannula venovenous ECMO: Double lumen continuous flow vs single lumen tidal flow. *Trans Am Soc Artif Intern Organs* 1985; 31:610.
17. Fox WW, Duara S: Persistent pulmonary hypertension in the neonate: Diagnosis and management. *J Pediatr* 1983; 103:505.
18. Schumacher RE, Barks JD, Johnston MV, et al: Right-sided brain lesions in infants following unilateral carotid ligation for extracorporeal circulation. *Pediatr Res* 1987; 21:375A.
19. Gattioni L, Pesenti A, Mascheroni D, et al: Low frequency positive pressure ventilation with extracorporeal $CO_2$ removal in severe acute respiratory failure: Clinical results. *JAMA* 1986; 256:881.
20. Bartlett RH: Extracorporeal oxygenation in neonates. *Hospital Prac [Off]* 1984; 19:139.

## 15B — Continuous-Flow Apneic Ventilation*

R. Brian Smith, M.D.

Continuous-flow apneic ventilation (CFAV) is the technique of insufflating oxygen ($O_2$) or air endobronchially in apneic animals or patients. We use the terms diffusion respiration (DR) to describe gas transport in apneic animals with tracheal insufflation of $O_2$ and apneic diffusion oxygenation (ADO) to describe gas transport to apneic patients with tracheal insufflation of oxygen after denitrogenation. Diffusion respiration and ADO have also been used with the insufflating gas introduced through a tracheal stoma or by inserting a needle/catheter through the cricothyroid membrane into the trachea.

## HISTORICAL REVIEW

Since the beginning of the century, multiple studies have indicated that adequate oxygenation may be achieved during apnea. Hirsch in 1905[1] and Volhard in 1908[2] experimented with $O_2$ uptake in rabbits. The animals were paralyzed with curare and given intratracheal $O_2$. Oxygen uptake continued for 1 to 2 hours. However, when air was used in place of $O_2$, the animals died within a few minutes. Volhard is credited with first pointing out that $O_2$ is drawn into the lungs during apnea.

In 1944, Draper and Whitehead[3] described the successful use of DR in dogs. They replaced nitrogen with $O_2$ and observed adequate oxygenation but noted the accumulation of carbon dioxide ($CO_2$) in the alveoli. Comroe and Dripps[4] and Enghoff et al.[5] first reported maintenance of normal oxygenation in apneic patients by administration of $O_2$. However, in this and subsequent investigations respiratory acidosis occurred as $CO_2$ increased at a rate of 3 to 5 torr/minute during apneic oxygenation.[6–10]

We used high flows of $O_2$ in the trachea of dogs in an attempt to "wash out" $CO_2$.[11] Because we had been using percutaneous transtracheal jet ventilation in patients, we decided to use this approach in an experiment on five, anesthetized, paralyzed dogs. A 16-gauge catheter was inserted through the cricothyroid membrane into the trachea and

*Portions of Chapter 15B are modified from Smith RB: Continuous-flow apneic ventilation. *Respir Care* 1987; 32:458–464.

connected to a high-pressure $O_2$ source. A continuous flow of 100% $O_2$ was delivered for 10 minutes at 19, 27, and 33 L/minute through the catheter. During ADO, arterial blood gas samples were analyzed at 20-minute intervals. There was no significant difference in the rise of the partial pressure of $CO_2$ in arterial blood ($Pa_{CO_2}$) at 19, 27, and 33 L/minute, and at all three flow rates, the partial pressure of $O_2$ in arterial blood ($Pa_{O_2}$) was greater than 300 mm Hg. The intratracheal pressures at the three flows (19, 27, and 33 L/minute) were 7, 13, and 18 mm Hg. We concluded that there was no advantage to high-flow delivery because the $Pa_{CO_2}$ remained the same in the dogs.

Recently, Slutsky et al.[12] reported on tracheal insufflation of $O_2$ at low flow rates in dogs. Ten anesthetized, paralyzed dogs were ventilated with conventional mechanical ventilation using room air. When ventilation was stopped, a constant flow of $O_2$ ranging from 0.2 to 3.0 L/minute was inserted through a tracheal stoma to within 1 cm of the carina using a catheter with a 1.0- or 5.0-mm inside diameter (ID). The $Pa_{O_2}$ and $Pa_{CO_2}$ increased at all flow rates. The rate of increase of $Pa_{O_2}$ was greater and that of $Pa_{CO_2}$ was less with increasing flow. In three dogs studied at flow rates of 2.0 to 3.0 L/minute, arterial blood gas values reached a plateau after about 2 hours. Mean values were pH 6.87; $Pa_{CO_2}$, 164 mm Hg; and $Pa_{O_2}$, 353 mm Hg. The authors concluded that tracheal insufflation of $O_2$ at low flow rates can produce sufficient gas exchange to support life in apneic dogs for prolonged periods.

An alternative approach for providing adequate gas exchange and creating conditions conducive to the healing of lung diseases was reported by Hill et al. in 1972.[13] These authors used the Bramson membrane heart-lung machine to provide ventilatory support and lung rest during a severe case of shock lung syndrome. In 1977, Kolobow et al.[14] reported the development of the spiral-coiled membrane lung for $CO_2$ removal. They suggested the possibility of removing $CO_2$ with this device and providing oxygenation with reduced ventilatory rates while providing adequate gas exchange, thus optimizing the chances of lung recovery. Further developments of this technique have shown that ADO can be performed safely for many days when metabolic $CO_2$ is removed by an extracorporeal membrane lung ($ECCO_2R$) and 100% $O_2$ is supplied directly into the trachea, keeping intrapulmonary pressures at 5 cm $H_2O$. Increasing continuous airway pressure to 20 cm $H_2O$ was shown to reduce shunt and improve oxygenation, functional residual capacity, and compliance. In addition, declines in functional residual capacity and compliance occurring after 24 hours with this technique could be reversed with just 5 minutes of manual ventilation. The authors reported a dramatic reduction in the complications associated with assisted ventilation; improvements in $O_2$ transport, renal function, maintenance of functional residual capacity, and compliance; and minimal impairment of cardiovascular function.

More recently $ECCO_2R$ has been used in patients with severe acute respiratory failure of parenchymal origin.[15] Most of the metabolic $CO_2$ production was cleared through a low-flow venovenous bypass. To avoid lung injury from mechanical ventilation, $O_2$ was administered continuously into the trachea (ADO), and 3 to 5 breaths per minute were given at a peak-airway pressure of 35 to 45 cm $H_2O$. The gas exchange of all of these patients was so poor that a mortality of 90% had been expected before $ECCO_2R$ was instituted. Lung function improved in 31 patients (73%), and 21 patients (49%) survived.

## ANIMAL RESEARCH

Successful ventilation of dogs with a continuous flow of air but without respiratory movements was described by Meltzer and Auer in 1909.[16] They noted that it was important to maintain lung inflation and to deliver fresh gas to the lowest part of the trachea.

Lenhert et al.[17] studied continuous-flow air ventilation in apneic dogs. They found that normal blood gas values could be maintained for as long as 2 hours. A correlation between $CO_2$ elimination and total gas flow was found.

We have reported a number of studies on CFAV,[18-22] the first of which evaluated the adequacy of gas exchange during CFAV in dogs. Seventeen dogs (average weight, 23 kg) were placed in one of three experimental groups. Each dog in group 1 (n = 7) was anesthetized, paralyzed, and ventilated with air by intermittent positive-pressure ventilation (IPPV) through a tracheal tube. We then removed the tube and, aided by a fiberoptic bronchoscope, cannulated each main-stem bronchus with a 2.5-mm ID, 4-mm outside diameter OD polyethylene catheter. The tracheal tube was replaced to hold the catheters in place. Heated, humidified air was continuously delivered equally to each catheter. Total flows ranged from 8 to 28 L/minute (0.4 to 1.4 L/kg/minute). Pressure in the trachea did not exceed 2 torr. Adequate gas exchange was found after 30 minutes at flows greater than 16 L/minute. Dogs in group 2 (n = 7) were managed in a similar manner and were insufflated endobronchially with a flow of 1.0 L/kg/minute. Continuous-flow apneic ventilation was continued for 5 hours in all animals. Dogs in group 3 (n = 3) were anesthetized similarly to those in the first two groups, and pulmonary gas distribution in relation to catheter placement was assessed using xenon 133.

The values for $Pa_{O_2}$ differed during CFAV and intermittent positive-pressure ventilation in group 2; however, all animals were adequately oxygenated, and during 5 hours of CFAV, adequate $CO_2$ elimination was achieved in all animals. There was no difference in $Pa_{O_2}$, $Pa_{CO_2}$, and shunt fraction with CFAV at 30 minutes and 5 hours. Differences in heart rate, cardiac output, and systemic vascular resistance at 30 minutes and 5 hours were related to the hypothermia that developed during the course of experimentation. In group 3, with the catheters above the carina, gas-distribution studies demonstrated that insufflated gas was limited to the large airways with no peripheral distribution, resulting in low $Pa_{O_2}$ levels and elevated $Pa_{CO_2}$ levels. On the other hand, endobronchial catheters permitted distribution of insufflated gas to the peripheral airways, and oxygenation and ventilation were normal.

In a subsequent study, we compared $CO_2$ removal during CFAV with both air and oxygen.[19] Normal $Pa_{CO_2}$ levels were obtained with air. However, in the animals in which oxygen was used, $Pa_{CO_2}$ levels rose to 48.5 torr ± 3.2 torr (mean ± SEM). In dogs during thoracotomy, CFAV maintained adequate gas exchange for 5 hours (Table 15B–1).

We also studied the effect of catheter position in the main-stem bronchi on gas exchange during CFAV and found that oxygenation and $CO_2$ elimination improved in dogs with catheter positions approximately 2.0 cm below the carina. Deeper catheter positions did not appear to further enhance gas exchange.[21]

Other investigators have also successfully used CFAV in various animal preparations. Chakrabarti and Whitwam[23] were able to obtain normal gas exchange in six dogs during CFAV delivered via a modified Carlen's tube at a gas flow of 1.0 L/kg/minute. Tallman et al.[24] demonstrated adequate oxygenation with small rises in $Pa_{CO_2}$ using CFAV in an oleic-acid-injury dog model. El Baz et al.[25] used a continuous intratracheal jet insufflation combined with intermittent positive-pressure ventilation in the same dog model and found better oxygenation and $CO_2$ elimination with the combined technique than with intermittent positive-pressure ventilation alone.

## CLINICAL STUDIES

Our group has also used CFAV in five anesthetized patients prior to surgery (Fig 15B–1).[22] Oxygen, instead of air, was used as the ventilating gas to ensure an adequate $Pa_{O_2}$. After 30 minutes of apnea, oxygenation was adequate in all patients—$Pa_{O_2}$, 299 ± 37 (mean ± SEM) (Fig 15B–2). The rise in $Pa_{CO_2}$ was 0.6 torr/minute compared with a rise of 3.8 torr/minute seen with ADO. However, we did not determine if the plateau in $Pa_{CO_2}$ reported in animal studies occurred in patients.[12]

**TABLE 15B-1.**
Continuous-Flow Apneic Ventilation (CFAV) During Thoracotomy*†

| | Control‡ | CFAV, Closed Chest§ | 1 hr | 2 hr | CFAV, Open Chest‖ | 4 hr | 5 hr |
|---|---|---|---|---|---|---|---|
| | | | | | 3 hr | | |
| pH (±SEM) | 7.39 (±0.02) | 7.40 (±0.03) | 7.41 (±0.04) | 7.40 (±0.03) | 7.42 (±0.03) | 7.42 (±0.02) | 7.41 (±0.01) |
| $Pa_{O_2}$ (±SEM) | 93.5 (±1.4) | 146.9# (±7.3) | 126.4# (±9.3) | 138.0# (±5.0) | 136.4# (±7.7) | 140.2# (±10.9) | 138.1# (±11.7) |
| $P\bar{v}_{O_2}$ (±SEM) | 55.5 (±3.1) | 58.0 (±4.1) | 49.1** (±4.2) | 45.7#*** (±4.3) | 42.6#*** (±4.1) | 43.5#*** (±1.6) | 39.9#*** (±3.1) |
| $Pa_{CO_2}$ (±SEM) | 40.8 (±1.9) | 45.2 (±2.8) | 42.2 (±1.0) | 41.3 (±3.0) | 40.0 (±1.8) | 39.0 (±1.8) | 41.8 (±1.9) |

*From Babinski MF, Smith RB, Bunegin L: Continuous flow apneic ventilation during thoracotomy. *Anesthesiology* 1986; 65:399. Used by permission.
†$Pa_{O_2}$ = partial pressure of $O_2$ in arterial blood; $P\bar{v}_{O_2}$ = partial pressure of $O_2$ in mixed venous blood; $Pa_{CO_2}$ = partial pressure of $CO_2$ in arterial blood.
‡Mean values of blood gases during spontaneous respiration ($F_{I_{O_2}}$ 0.21).
§Mean values of blood gases during CFAV with closed chest ($F_{I_{O_2}}$ 0.4).
‖Mean values of blood gases during CFAV with open chest ($F_{I_{O_2}}$ 0.4).
#Significantly different compared with control ($P<.05$).
**Significantly different compared with CFAV with closed chest ($P<.05$).

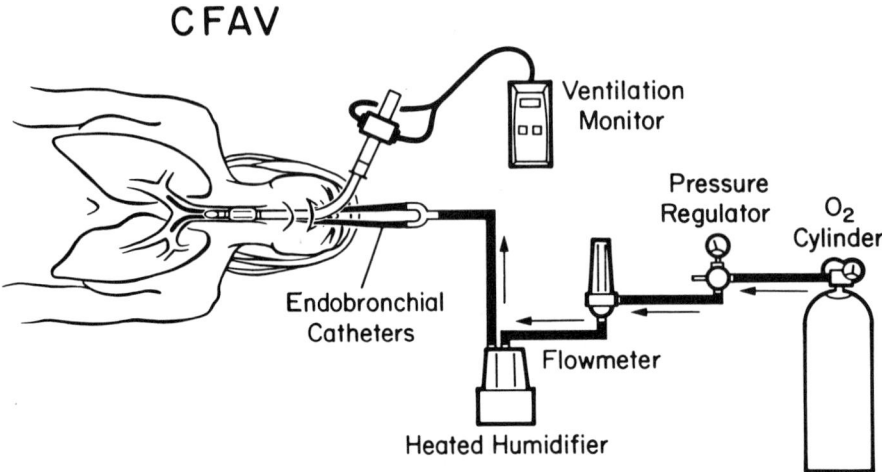

**FIG 15B-1.**
Schematic presentation of the gas delivery system during the clinical application of CFAV. (From Babinski MF, Sierra OG, Smith RB, et al: Clinical application of continuous flow apneic ventilation. *Acta Anesthesiol Scand* 1985; 29:750. Used by permission.)

In one patient, there was no increase in $Pa_{CO_2}$ during 30 minutes of CFAV. The authors concluded that CFAV can maintain blood gas values in a clinically adequate range for as long as 30 minutes, but speculated that the inclusion of some nitrogen in the ventilating gas may result in better $CO_2$ elimination.

Subsequently we began a study of CFAV with an air mixture enriched to 50% $O_2$ in healthy anesthetized patients prior to surgery. The study, approved by our Institutional Review Board, was abandoned after one patient had a rise in $Pa_{CO_2}$ to 73 torr (2.2 torr/minute) with a $Pa_{O_2}$ of 134 torr. Though there were no complications in this patient, the possibility of exposing other patients to such a rise in $Pa_{CO_2}$ was considered to be unjustified.

Breen et al.[26] used endobronchial catheters just below the carina for CFAV in five patients undergoing nonthoracic surgery, with a technique similar to that of Chakrabarti and Whitwam.[23] The insufflating gas was 50% nitrous oxide ($N_2O$) in oxygen at a flow of 1 L/kg/minute. After 30 minutes of CFAV, the $Pa_{CO_2}$ had increased from 35.9 ± 2.9 to 69.2 ± 14.5 torr, a rate of rise of 1.11 torr/minute. The higher rate of rise of $CO_2$ compared to our study[22] may be explained by their more proximal catheter placement.[21] However, the role of nitrogen or $CO_2$ elimination during CFAV is unknown.

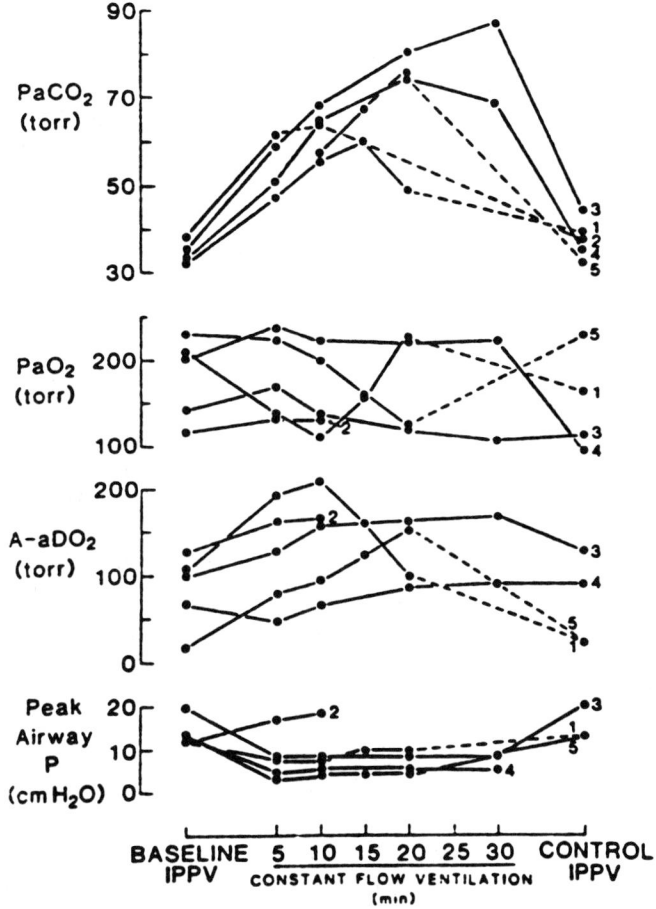

**FIG 15B–2.**
$Pa_{CO_2}$, $Pa_{O_2}$, alveolar-arterial $Po_2$ difference (A–a$Do_2$), and peak airway pressure during CFV and IPPV. Broken lines indicate that CFAV for that patient stopped before 30 minutes. (From Breen PH, Sznajder JF, Morrison P, et al: Constant flow ventilation in anesthetized patients: Efficacy and safety. *Anesth Analg* 1986; 65:1161. Used by permission.)

## SUMMARY

Gas transport during CFAV may be related to convective gas movement, the effects of cardiogenic oscillations, and molecular diffusion. Conceptually, the lungs can be divided into two zones: zone 1, affected by the jet of gas; and zone 2, independent of the jet. Because of the high flow rates used during CFAV, the directional streaming will take place in the area closest to the insufflation jet. Gas will enter and leave the same airway spontaneously. The jet of insufflating gas will generate turbulence below the tips of the catheters, and the turbulent diffusivity will be part of the gas-transport mechanism. The higher the flow of insufflated gas, the further into the periphery of the lungs this turbulence will extend. This may explain in part why patients subjected to CFAV retain $CO_2$ and dogs do not. The flow used in dogs was 1 L/kg/minute, whereas such high flow rates were thought to be dangerous in man, and only 0.6 to 0.7 L/kg/minute was used in the study from our institution.[22]

The effectiveness of cardiogenic oscillation (i.e., pulsation of gas in the airways caused by the heartbeat) in gas transport has support in the literature but is still controversial. West and Hugh-Jones,[27] measuring the air flows in the lobar and segmental bronchi of humans during bronchoscopy, observed that the pulsations clearly augmented the expiratory flow. The authors suggested that the oscillations might enhance mixing between the dead space and the alveolar gas. Studies by Engel et al.[28] suggest that cardiac action and the resulting flow pulsations might increase fivefold the effective diffusion coefficient in the airway. The successful use of CFAV in dogs with open chests does not provide support for the importance of cardiogenic oscillation in gas transport with this technique. Studies by Mackenzie et al.[9-31] in dogs and pigs suggest that cardiogenic oscillation and collateral airways both play a role in gas exchange with CFAV.

A number of questions need to be answered before CFAV can have clinical applicability. Although the optimal catheter position has been found in dogs, it is not known in man. The need to reduce the flow because of risk of barotrauma may be resolved by finding the optimal catheter position. At present, the placement of the catheters requires fiberoptic bronchoscopy—a cumbersome and time-consuming process. A better catheter design that will allow placement without bronchoscopy needs to be developed. In addition, what constitutes an ideal gas mixture and the possible role of nitrogen need elucidation.

Future application for CFAV may be found in major-airway and closed-heart surgery and in nuclear magnetic resonance of the thorax and abdomen—all applications in which a motionless field is desirable. CFAV may play a role in the management of adult respiratory distress syndrome (1) with low-frequency ventilation, (2) with a combination of low-frequency ventilation and low-flow venovenous extracorporeal membrane oxygenation, (3) with conventional mechanical ventilation, or (4) with high-frequency ventilation. Last, it may have an application in resuscitation from respiratory arrest.

# REFERENCES

1. Hirsch H: Uber kunstliche Atmung durch Ventilation der Trachea, dissertation. Giessen, 1905.
2. Volhard F: Uber kunstliche Atmung durch Ventilation der Trachea und ein einfache Vorrichtung zur rhythmischen kunstlichen Atmung. *Muchen Med Wochenschr* 1908; 55:209.
3. Draper WB, Whitehead RW: Diffusion respiration in the dog anesthetized by Pentothal sodium. *Anesthesiology* 1944; 5:262.
4. Comroe JH Jr, Dripps RD: Artificial respiration. *JAMA* 1946; 130:381.
5. Enghoff H, Holmdahl MH, Risholm I: Diffusion respiration in man. *Nature* 1951; 168.
6. Holmdahl MH: Pulmonary uptake of oxygen, acid-base metabolism, and circulation during prolonged apnoea. *Acta Chir Scand* [Suppl] 1956; 212:1.
7. Frumin MJ, Epstein RM, Cohen G: Apneic oxygenation in man. *Anesthesiology* 1959; 20:789.
8. Eger EI, Severinghaus JW: The rate of rise of $PaCO_2$ in the apneic anesthetized patient. *J Anesthesiology* 1961; 22:419.
9. Payne JP: Apnoeic oxygenation in anaesthetized man. *Acta Anaesthesiol Scand* 1962; 6:129.
10. Fraioli RI, Sheffer LA, Steffenson JI: Pulmonary and cardiovascular effects of apneic oxygenation in man. *Anesthesiology* 1973; 39:588.
11. Smith RB, Babinski M: *Transtracheal Apneic Oxygenation Under High Pressure,* abstracts of papers presented at the Sixth World Congress of Anaesthesiology, Mexico City, April 24–30, 1976. New York, Excerpta Medica, series 387, p 161.
12. Slutsky AS, Watson J, Leith DE, et al: Tracheal insufflation of $O_2$ (TRIO) at low flow rates sustains life for several hours. *Anesthesiology* 1985; 63:278.
13. Hill JD, O'Brien TG, Murray JJ, et al: Prolonged extracorporeal oxygenation for acute posttraumatic respiratory failure (shock-lung syndrome). *N Engl J Med* 1972; 286:629.
14. Kolobow T, Gattinoni I, Tomlinson T, et al: The carbon dioxide membrane lung (CDML): A new concept. *Trans Am Soc Artif Intern Organs* 1977; 23:17.
15. Gattinoni L, Pesenti A, Masacheroni D, et al: Low-frequency positive-pressure ventilation with extracorporeal $CO_2$ removal in severe acute respiratory failure. *JAMA* 1986; 256:881.
16. Meltzer SJ, Auer J: Continuous respiration without respiratory movements. *J Exp Med* 1909; 11:622.
17. Lehnert BE, Oberdorster G, Slutsky AS: Constant-flow ventilation of apneic dogs. *J Appl Physiol* 1982; 53:483.
18. Smith RB, Babinski MF, Swartzman S: Continuous flow apneic ventilation (CFAV). *Acta Anaesthesiol Scand* 1984; 28:631.
19. Babinski MF, Smith RB, Bunegin I, et al: Effect of nitrogen on carbon dioxide elimination during continuous flow apneic ventilation in dogs. *Acta Anesthesiol Scand* 1986; 30:357.

20. Babinski MF, Smith RB, Bunegin L: Continuous flow apneic ventilation during thoracotomy. *Anesthesiology* 1986; 65:399.
21. Bunegin L, Gelineau J, Stone E, et al: The effect of endobronchial catheter position on $Pa_{CO_2}$ during continuous flow apneic ventilation. *Crit Care Med* 1986; 14:372.
22. Babinski MF, Sierra OG, Smith RB, et al: Clinical application of continuous flow apneic ventilation. *Acta Anesthesiol Scand* 1985; 29:750.
23. Chakrabarti MK, Whitwam JG: Pulmonary ventilation by continuous flow using a modified Carlen's tube. *Crit Care Med* 1984; 12:354.
24. Tallman RD, Wang YL, Marcolin R: Gas exchange by constant flow ventilation following oleic acid lung injury. *Anesthesiology* 1985; 63:A296.
25. El Baz N, Braverman B, McCarthy R: Continuous jet insufflation combined with IPPV for treatment of induced ARDS: A new technique. *Anesth Analg* 1984; 63:208.
26. Breen PH, Sznajder JF, Morrison P, et al: Constant flow ventilation in anesthetized patients: Efficacy and safety. *Anesth Analg* 1986; 65:1161.
27. West JB, Hugh-Jones P: Pulsative gas flow in bronchi caused by the heart beat. *J Appl Physiol* 1961; 16:697–702.
28. Engel LA, Menkes H, Wood LDH, et al: Gas mixing during breathholding studied by intrapulmonary gas sampling. *J Appl Physiol* 1973; 35:9.
29. Mackenzie CF, Shin B, Takeda J, Harris M, et al: Comparisons of gas exchange during endotracheal insufflation and apneic oxygenation. *Anesthesiology* 1985; 63:A527.
30. Mackenzie CF, Pyne A, Watson RJ, et al: Collateral airway function and gas exchange during endobronchial insufflation. *Crit Care Med* 1986; 14:384.
31. Mackenzie CF, Watson R, Pyne A, et al: Are cardiac oscillations a mechanism of gas exchange with endobronchial insufflation? *Crit Care Med* 1986; 14:384.

# 15C      Liquid Ventilation

## Huda K. Rosen, R.R.T., M.S.

One of the major complications of conventional mechanical ventilation is pulmonary barotrauma, or the overdistention and rupture of pulmonary tissue due to the pressure generated by the ventilator. Often the site of this injury in neonates with RDS is the terminal bronchioles. One reason for this is that the terminal bronchioles are more compliant than either the conducting airways (which have cartilaginous support) or the alveoli (which are often collapsed or thickened due to the formation of hyaline membranes). As a result, they stretch more in response to ventilatory pressure and are prone to rupture.

The compliance of a pulmonary structure actually has two components, one due to the elastic recoil of the tissues and one due to the surface tension generated at the interface of the ventilatory gas with the liquid surface of the tissue. One factor that contributes to the relatively greater compliance of the terminal bronchioles compared to the alveoli is the difference in their geometric configurations. If we assume that the bronchioles are cylindrical and the alveoli are spherical (with no surfactant), then from the law of Laplace it can be shown that the compliance (due to surface tension) of the bronchioles is twice that of the alveoli. Thus, when enough pressure is generated in the lungs to ventilate the alveoli, there is a risk that the terminal airways will be overexpanded.

The experimental approach designed to address this particular problem is liquid ventilation. The use of liquid instead of gas to ventilate the lungs eliminates the gas-liquid interface and therefore reduces the effect of geometry on compliance. The theoretical benefits of using liquid ventilation are reduced ventilatory pressures and hence a decreased incidence of pulmonary barotrauma. However, when liquid replaces gas as the medium in which oxygen and carbon dioxide are transported, several problems arise. These include the oxygen- and carbon dioxide-carrying capacity of the liquid, its viscosity, and the mechanical means of delivery. Fluorocarbon liquids have been found to be particularly useful because they are capable of dissolving large volumes of respiratory gases at atmospheric pressure. For example, under normobaric conditions and at 37°C, a saturated solution contains about 50 vol% oxygen.[1]

Liquid ventilation of mammals has been studied since 1958.[2] Of particular interest have been the effects of liquid ventilation on gas exchange and on lung structure, function, and surface-active properties. In addition, long-term studies have been conducted to determine morphological, biochemical, or histologic evidence of toxicity after ventilation with fluorocarbon liquid.

In 1970 and 1971 Modell et al.[3] after successfully ventilating adult dogs with oxygenated fluorocarbon further studied the long-term effect of liquid ventilation. They conclude that mammals can breathe fluorocarbon liquid for an hour with reconversion to breathing oxygen in gaseous form. However, after liquid ventilation, hypoxemia, bronchiolar inflammatory reaction, and wheezing occurred for several days. These acute changes and the ventilatory difficulty subsided in 10 days. One month later only scattered groups of macrophages were present, and 18 months later the lungs were normal.

Schwieler and Robertson[4] studied liquid ventilation on immature newborn rabbits. They found that oxygenation in the liquid-ventilated rabbits was superior to the gas-ventilated control group. Also, liquid ventilation was less harmful to the bronchiolar epithelium and did not cause the formation of hyaline membrane as in the gas-ventilated ones. They concluded that fluorocarbon liquid ventilation could be a useful therapeutic tool in ventilating animals whose lungs are devoid of surfactant phospholipids. If respiratory acidosis could be avoided, the lungs of such subjects could be temporarily ventilated with oxygenated fluorocarbon while the maturation of the pulmonary surfactant system develops.

Moskowitz et al.[5] developed a demand-regulated liquid breathing system that allowed gas exchange (Fig 15C–1). The liquid breathing system consists of the following elements: gas-operated diaphragm pumps, liquid regenerator with heater, oxygen source, controls, check valves, pressurized gas source, thermal control, transducers, and a standby autocycling regulator. It is a closed-loop system equipped with devices to continuously recharge the liquid with oxygen and remove the carbon dioxide produced. Valves controlling pressurized gas to the pump manifold are regulated by the system fluidics controller that responds to incipient esophageal pressure changes induced by the animal. The animal, therefore, has control over breathing frequency and tidal volume.

The liquid is delivered to and removed from the animal through a cuffed endotracheal tube. The animal and the system are closely monitored (arterial blood gases, heart rate, intrapleural pressures, body and liquid temperatures, pump manifold pressure, and liquid flow rate) throughout the trial. At the end of the trial, the animal is disconnected

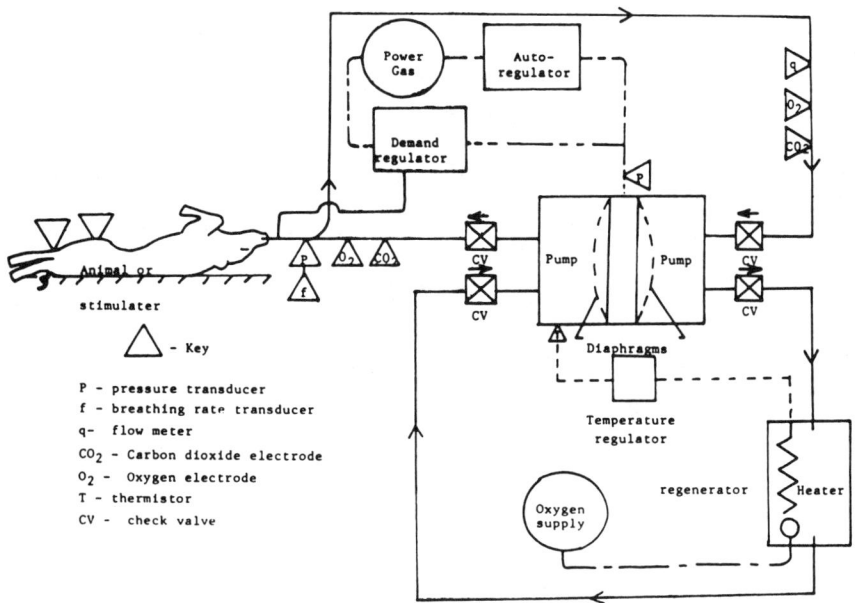

**FIG 15C–1.**
Demand-regulated liquid breathing system. (From Moscowitz GD, Shaffer TH, Dubin SE: Liquid breathing trials and animal studies with a demand-regulated liquid breathing system. *Med Instrum* 1975; 9:28. Used by permission.)

and then tilted up so that the fluorocarbon liquid drains from the lungs.

Shaffer et al.[6] studied gas exchange and acid-base balance in premature lambs during a modification of this system (Fig 15C–2) that had the capability to provide both active delivery and removal of liquid from the lungs thus creating better mixing of alveolar liquid. During this study, premature lambs were successfully oxygenated and mechanically ventilated with fluorocarbon liquid for periods of up to 3 hours. The modified mechanical liquid breathing system effectively eliminated $CO_2$ from the expired liquid. In addition, they observed a significant decrease (about 30%) in peak inspiratory pressure during the recovery period, although inspiratory pressures during liquid ventilation were not measured.

In 1981 Sivieri et al.[7] studied cardiac output during liquid ventilation. They used the liquid breathing system (Fig 15C–3), which was a streamlined and updated version of their previous systems. The new adaptations rendered the system more efficient, easier to use, and less costly.

Although the preliminary results of liquid ventilation experiments are encouraging, its clinical application has been slow. This may be due to several factors including the lack of incentive for commercial

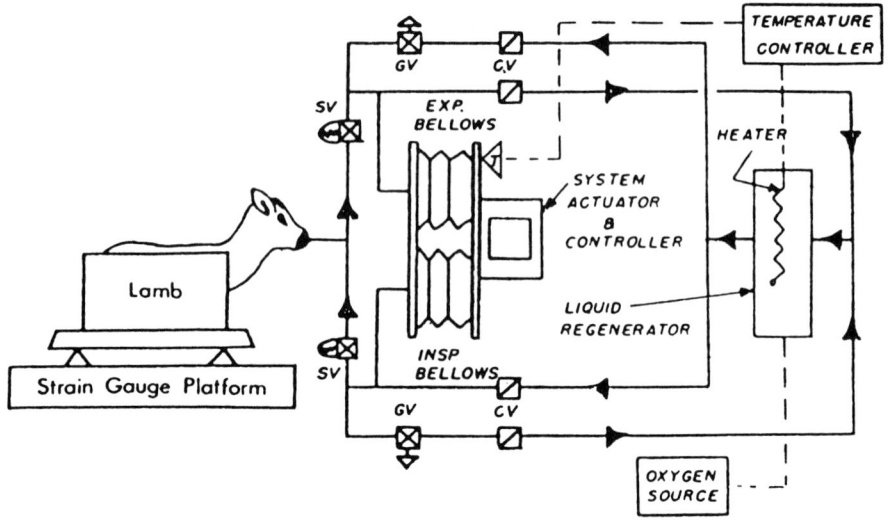

**FIG 15C-2.**
A schematic of the experimental setup for a mechanical liquid breathing system. SV = solenoid valves; GV = gate valves; CV = check valves. (From Shaffer TH, Rubenstein D, Moskowitz GD, et al: Gaseous exchange and acid-base balance in premature lambs during liquid ventilation since birth. *Pediatr Res* 1976; 10:227. Used by permission.)

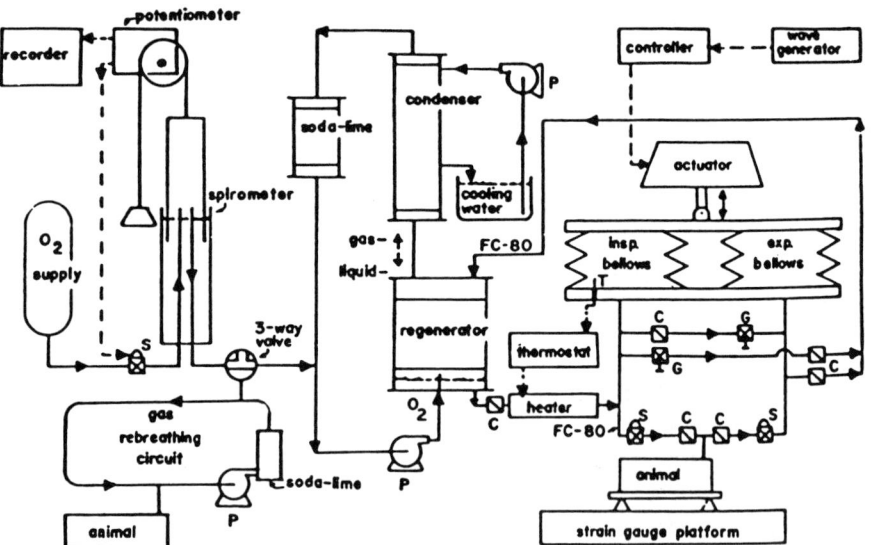

**FIG 15C-3.**
Liquid breathing system with close-looped fluorocarbon oxygenation. P = pump; C = check valve; G = gate valve; S = solenoid valve; FC-80 = fluorocarbon liquid (3M Co., St Paul, Minn). (From Sivieri EM, Moskowitz GD, Shaffer TH: Instrumentation for measuring cardiac output by direct Fick method during liquid ventilation. *Undersea Biomed Res* 1981; 8:75. Used by permission.)

production of a liquid ventilator and competition with alternative strategies, such as high frequency ventilation and ECMO. Nevertheless, this area may provide fruitful research opportunities in the future.

## REFERENCES

1. Sargent JW, Serffi RJ: Properties of perfluoronated liquids. Fed Proc 1970; 29:1699.
2. Kylstra JA; Lavage of the lung. Acta Physiol Pharmacol Neerl 1958; 7:163.
3. Modell JH, Hood CI, Kuck EJ, et al: Oxygenation by ventilation with fluorocarbon liquid (FX80). Anesthesiology 1971; 29:1771.
4. Schweiler GH, Robertson B: Liquid ventilation in immature newborn rabbits. Biol Neonate 1976; 29:343.
5. Moscowitz GD, Shaffer TH, Dubin SE: Liquid breathing trials and animal studies with a demand-regulated liquid breathing system. Med Instrum 1975; 9:28.
6. Shaffer TH, Rubenstein D, Moskowitz GD, et al: Gaseous exchange and acid-base balance in premature lambs during liquid ventilation since birth. Pediatr Res 1976; 10:227.
7. Sivieri EM, Moskowitz GD, Shaffer TH: Instrumentation for measuring cardiac output by direct Fick method during liquid ventilation. Undersea Biomed Res 1981; 8:75.

# Appendix

Bonnie Siner, R.N.
Waldemar A. Carlo, M.D.

## RESPIRATORY SYSTEM

### Growth

**TABLE A-1.**
Respiratory System Dimensions With Growth*

|  | Newborn to 1 mo | Infant |
|---|---|---|
| Chest, diameter, cm | | |
|   Transverse | 10 | 14 |
|   Anteroposterior | 7.5 | 9 |
| Trachea | | |
|   Diameter, mm | 4 | 5 |
|   CSA, sq mm† | 26 | 34 |
| Mainstem bronchi, | | |
|   Diameter, mm | 4 | 4 |
|   CSA, right/left | — | 20/13 |
| Bronchioles, diameter, mm | 0.3 | 0.4 |
|   CSA, sq mm | 0.07 | 0.12 |
| Terminal bronchioles, | | |
|   Diameter, mm | 0.2 | 0.3 |
|   Internal diameter, mm | 0.1 | 0.12 |
|   CSA, sq mm | 0.03 | 0.07 |
| Alveoli, diameter, mm | 0.05 | 0.06–0.07 |
|   Surface area, sq m | 2.8 | 6.5 |
| Body length, cm | 50 | — |
|   Weight, kg | 3.4 | — |
|   Surface area, sq m | 0.21 | 0.3 |
| Lung weight, gm | 50 | 70 |
| Dead space, ml | 7–8 | — |

*From Scarpelli EM (ed): *Pulmonary Physiology of the Fetus, Newborn, and Child.* Philadelphia, Lea & Febiger, 1975, p 168. Used by permission.
†Cross-sectional area.

**TABLE A–2.**
Effect of Age on Lung Size*

|  | Number of Cases Studied | Alveoli ($\times 10^6$) | Respiratory Airways ($\times 10^6$) | Air-Tissue Interface, sq m | Body Surface Area, sq m | Generations of Respiratory Airways |
|---|---|---|---|---|---|---|
| Birth | 1 | 24 | 1.5 | 2.8 | 0.21 | — |
| 3 mo. | 3 | 77 | 2.5 | 7.2 | 0.29 | 21 |
| 7 mo. | 1 | 112 | 3.7 | 8.4 | 0.38 | — |
| 13 mo. | 1 | 129 | 4.5 | 12.2 | 0.45 | 22 |
| 22 mo. | 1 | 160 | 7.1 | 14.2 | 0.50 | — |
| 4 yr | 1 | 257 | 7.9 | 22.2 | 0.67 | — |
| 8 yr | 1 | 280 | 14.0 | 32.0 | 0.92 | 23 |
| Adult |  | 296 | 14.0 | 75.0 | 1.90 | 23 |
| Approximate fold increase, birth to adult | — | 10 | 10 | 21 | 9 | — |

*From Dunnill MS: Postnatal growth of the lung. *Thorax* 1962; 17:329. Used by permission.

**TABLE A–3.**
Airway and Alveolar Dimensions*

|  | Trachea | | Bronchus | | Number of Alveoli |
|---|---|---|---|---|---|
| Age | Length, mm | Diameter, mm | Length, mm | Diameter, mm |  |
| Birth | 40.0 | 6.0 | 9.0 | 5.0 | $24 \times 10^6$ |
| 1 yr | 43.0 | 7.8 | 11.0 | 6.3 | $129 \times 10^6$ |
| 5 yr | 56.0 | 10.0 | 13.5 | 7.5 | $250 \times 10^6$ |
| 10 yr | 63.0 | 11.0 | 14.7 | 8.6 | $280 \times 10^6$ |
| 16 yr | 74.0 | 14.0 | 20.0 | 10.0 | $290 \times 10^6$ |
| Adult | 90.0–150 | 14.0–18.0 | 22.0 | 12.7 | $296 \times 10^6$ |

*From Lough MD, Chatburn RL, Schrock WA: *Handbook of Respiratory Care*. Chicago, Year Book Medical Publishers, 1983, p 245. Used by permission.

## Control of Breathing

### TABLE A–4.
Factors Known to Influence Respiration*

| Stimulants | Depressants |
|---|---|
| *Chemical* | |
| Arterial $P_{CO_2}$ up to about 80 mm Hg | Arterial $P_{CO_2}$ over 80 mm Hg |
| Arterial pH 7.0 to 7.4 | Arterial pH <6.9 or >7.5 |
| Arterial $P_{O_2}$ <about 80 mm Hg (in adults) | Profound hypoxia |
| (Newborn infants with only mild hypoxemia are stimulated by inspired oxygen.) | |
| *Pharmacologic* | |
| Epinephrine | Morphine |
| Lobeline | Barbiturates |
| Nicotine | Chloramphenicol |
| Salicylates | Neomycin |
| Picrotoxin | |
| Nikethamide | |
| Progesterone | |
| *Pulmonary Reflexes* | |
| Deflation receptors (Hering-Breuer reflex) | Stretch receptors in lung |
| Stretch receptors (Head's reflex) | Stretch receptors in aortic arch and carotid sinus |
| *Pressoreceptors* | |
| Decrease in blood pressure | Increase in blood pressure |
| *Bones and Joints* | |
| Stretch receptors in muscles | |
| Tactile responses | |
| *Thermal* | |
| Fever | Hibernation |
| Sudden chilling | |
| *Cortical* | |
| (Voluntary control of breathing is possible within limits.) | |

*From Avery ME, Fletcher BD: *The Lung and its Disorders in the Newborn Infant.* New York, WB Saunders Co, 1981. Used by permission.

## Acid-Base and Blood Gases
### TABLE A–5A.
Blood Gas Values in Full-term Infants*†

|  |  | Umbilical Vein | Umbilical Artery | 5–10 min | 20 min | 30 min | 60 min | 5 hr |
|---|---|---|---|---|---|---|---|---|
| pH | x̄ | 7.320 | 7.242 | 7.207 | 7.263 | 7.297 | 7.332 | 7.339 |
|  | SD | 0.055 | 0.059 | 0.051 | 0.040 | 0.044 | 0.031 | 0.028 |
| $P_{CO_2}$, mm Hg | x̄ | 37.8 | 49.1 | 46.1 | 40.1 | 37.7 | 36.1 | 35.2 |
|  | SD | 5.6 | 5.8 | 7.0 | 6.0 | 5.7 | 4.2 | 3.6 |
| $P_{O_2}$, mm Hg | x̄ | 27.4 | 15.9 | 49.6 | 50.7 | 54.1 | 63.3 | 73.7 |
|  | SD | 5.7 | 3.8 | 9.9 | 11.3 | 11.5 | 11.3 | 12.0 |
| Bicarbonate, mEq/L | x̄ | 20.0 | 18.7 | 16.7 | 17.5 | 18.2 | 19.2 | 19.4 |
|  | SD | 1.4 | 1.8 | 1.6 | 1.3 | 1.5 | 1.2 | 1.2 |
|  |  | 24 hr | 2 Days | 3 Days | 4 Days | 5 Days | 6 Days | 7 Days |
| pH | x̄ | 7.369 | 7.365 | 7.364 | 7.370 | 7.371 | 7.369 | 7.371 |
|  | SD | 0.032 | 0.028 | 0.027 | 0.027 | 0.031 | 0.023 | 0.026 |
| $P_{CO_2}$, mm Hg | x̄ | 33.4 | 33.1 | 33.1 | 34.3 | 34.8 | 34.8 | 35.9 |
|  | SD | 3.1 | 3.3 | 3.4 | 3.8 | 3.5 | 3.6 | 3.1 |
| $P_{O_2}$, mm Hg | x̄ | 72.7 | 73.8 | 75.6 | 73.3 | 72.1 | 69.8 | 73.1 |
|  | SD | 9.5 | 7.7 | 11.5 | 9.3 | 10.5 | 9.5 | 9.7 |
| Bicarbonate, mEq/L | x̄ | 20.2 | 19.8 | 19.7 | 20.4 | 20.6 | 20.6 | 21.8 |
|  | SD | 1.3 | 1.4 | 1.4 | 1.7 | 1.7 | 1.9 | 1.3 |

*From Koch G, Wendel H: Adjustment of arterial blood gases and acid-base balance in the normal newborn infant during the first week of life. *Biol Neonate* 1968; 12:136. Used by permission.
†Blood obtained through umbilical artery line; $P_{O_2}$ and $P_{CO_2}$ measured with Clark and Severinghaus electrodes.

**TABLE A-5B.**
Blood Gas Values in Premature Infants*†

| | | 3–5 hr | 6–12 hr | 13–24 hr | 25–48 hr | 3–4 Days | 5–10 Days | 11–40 Days |
|---|---|---|---|---|---|---|---|---|
| pH | x̄ | 7.329 | 7.425 | 7.464 | 7.434 | 7.425 | 7.378 | 7.425 |
| | SD | 0.038 | 0.072 | 0.064 | 0.054 | 0.044 | 0.043 | 0.033 |
| $P_{CO_2}$, mm Hg | x̄ | 47.3 | 28.2 | 27.2 | 31.3 | 31.7 | 36.4 | 32.9 |
| | SD | 8.5 | 6.9 | 8.4 | 6.7 | 6.7 | 4.2 | 4.0 |
| $P_{O_2}$, mm Hg | x̄ | 59.5 | 69.7 | 67.0 | 72.5 | 77.8 | 80.3 | 77.8 |
| | SD | 7.7 | 11.8 | 15.2 | 20.9 | 16.4 | 12.0 | 9.6 |
| BE, mEq/L | x̄ | −3.7 | −4.7 | −3.0 | −2.3 | −2.9 | −3.5 | −2.1 |
| | SD | 1.5 | 3.1 | 3.3 | 3.0 | 2.3 | 2.3 | 2.2 |

*From Orzalesi MM, Mendicini M, Bucci G, et al: Arterial oxygen studies in premature newborns with and without mild respiratory disorders. *Arch Dis Child* 1967; 42:174. Used by permission.
†Mean birth weight, 1.76 kg; gestational age, 34.5 wk; blood obtained from radial, temporal, or umbilical artery; $P_{O_2}$ measured with Clark electrode and $P_{CO_2}$ calculated using Siggaard-Andersen nomogram. BE = base excess.

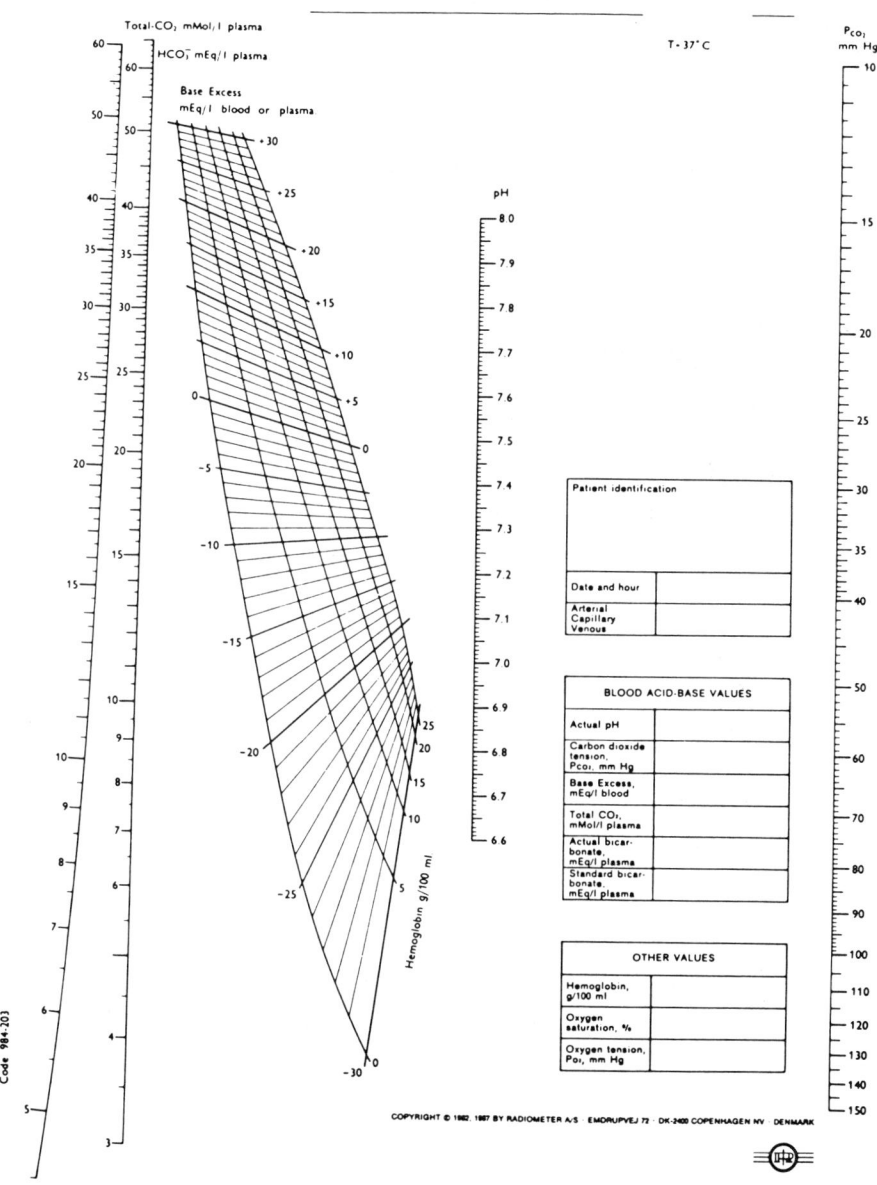

**FIG A–1.**
Siggaard-Andersen nomogram. (From Siggaard-Andersen O: Blood acid-base alignment nomogram. *Scand J Clin Lab Invest* 1963; 15:211. Used by permission.)

**TABLE A–6.**
Mechanisms of Reduced Arterial $P_{O_2}$*

| | Arterial Gas Tensions | | Alveolar-Arterial Oxygen Gradient | |
|---|---|---|---|---|
| | $Pa_{O_2}$ | $Pa_{CO_2}$ | Room Air | 100% Oxygen |
| Reduced atmospheric oxygen (high altitude) | ↓ | ↓ | N† | N |
| Alveolar hypoventilation | ↓ | ↑ | N | N |
| Altered intrapulmonary gas exchange | | | | |
|   Regionally decreased ventilation compared with perfusion | ↓ | ↓ N or ↑ | ↑ | N or ↑ |
|   Intrapulmonary right-to-left shunt | ↓ | N or ↓ | ↑ | ↑ |
|   "Diffusion block" | ↓ | N or ↓ | ↑ | N |
| Anatomical right-to-left shunt (intrapulmonary or intracardiac) | ↓ | N or ↓ | ↑ | ↑ |

*From Guenter CA: Respiratory function of the lungs and blood, in Guenter CA, Welch MH (eds): *Pulmonary Medicine*. JB Lippincott Co, Philadelphia, 1982, p 157. Used by permission.
†N = no effect.

**TABLE A–7.**
Arterial Blood Gas Changes in Different Conditions*†

| Clinical Condition | Functional Alteration | $Pa_{O_2}$ | $Pa_{CO_2}$ | $Pa_{O_2}$ Response to 100% $O_2$ | Response to CPAP |
|---|---|---|---|---|---|
| Neonatal depression | ↓ $\dot{V}_A$ | ↓ | ↑ | (+++) | Worsens |
| Pneumonia | ↓ $C_L$ · ↓ $\dot{V}_A/\dot{Q}$ | ↓ | N or ↑ | (++) | Variable |
| Meconium aspiration | ↑ R · ↓ $C_L$ · ↓ $\dot{V}_A/\dot{Q}$ · ↓ $\dot{V}_A$ | ↓ | N or ↑ | (++) | Variable |
| Hyaline membrane disease | ↓ FRC · ↓ $C_L$ · ↓ $\dot{V}_A/\dot{Q}$ · ↓ $\dot{V}_A$ | ↓ | N or ↑ | (++) | Improves |
| Airway obstruction | ↑ R · ↓ $\dot{V}_A$ | ↓ | ↑ | (+++) | Variable |
| Cyanotic CHD | Right-to-left shunt | ↓ | ↓ or N | (− or +) | Worsens |
| Persistent fetal circulation | ↑ PVR right-to-left shunt | ↓ | ↓ N or ↑ | (− or +++) | Worsens |
| CHD with ↑ PBF | ↓ $C_L$ · ↑ R · ↓ $\dot{V}_A/\dot{Q}$ · ↓ $\dot{V}_A$ | ↓ | ↑ | (++) | May improve |
| Alveolar hyperventilation | CNS irritation, mechanical ventilation | N or ↑ | ↓ | (+++) | No change |

*From Bancalari E: Pulmonary function testing and other diagnostic laboratory procedures, in Thibeault DW, Gregory GA (eds): *Neonatal Pulmonary Care*. East Norwalk, Conn; Appleton-Century-Crofts, 1986, p 223. Used by permission.

†$Pa_{O_2}$ = partial pressure of $O_2$ in arterial blood; $Pa_{CO_2}$ = partial pressure of $CO_2$ in arterial blood; CPAP = continuous positive airway pressure; $\dot{V}_A$ = alveolar ventilation per minute; $C_L$ = lung compliance; $\dot{V}_A/\dot{Q}$ = ventilation-perfusion ratio; FRC = functional residual capacity; R = gas exchange ratio; PVR = pulmonary vascular resistance; CNS = central nervous system; CHD = congenital heart disease; PBF = pulmonary blood flow; N = no effect.

## Ventilation

### TABLE A–8.
Ventilatory Values in Normal Newborns*†

| Reference | Method | Weight, kg | Respiratory Rate | $V_T$, ml | $\dot{V}_E$, ml/min | $\dot{V}_A$, ml/min | $V_D/V_T$ |
|---|---|---|---|---|---|---|---|
| Cook et al. (1955, 1957) | Plethysmography | 3.0 | 38 | 16.0 | — | — | 0.32‡ |
| Swyer et al. (1960) | Pneumotachography | 3.0 | 37 | 20.6 | — | — | — |
| Strang (1961) | Plethysmography | 3.3 | 41 | 18.1 | 750 | 378 | 0.50§ |
| Nelson et al. (1962) | Nonrebreathing valve | 2.2 | 38 | 12.8 | 480 | 309 | 0.25§ |
| Koch (1968) | Nonrebreathing valve | 3.6 | 44 (24 hr) | 16.5 | 703 | 442 | 0.26‡ |
|  |  |  | 39 (7 days) | 16.6 | 632 | 425 | 0.24‡ |
| Bancalari et al. (1970) | Plethysmography | 3.3 | 48 | 18.1 | 868 | — | — |

*From Bancalari E: Pulmonary function testing and other diagnostic laboratory procedures, in Thibeault DW, Gregory GA (eds): *Neonatal Pulmonary Care*. East Norwalk, Conn, Appleton-Century-Crofts, 1986, p 208. Used by permission.
†$V_T$ = tidal volume; $\dot{V}_E$ = expired minute ventilation; $\dot{V}_A$ = alveolar ventilation per minute; $V_D/V_T$ = dead space-tidal volume ratio.
‡Physiologic
§Anatomical

## Lung Volumes

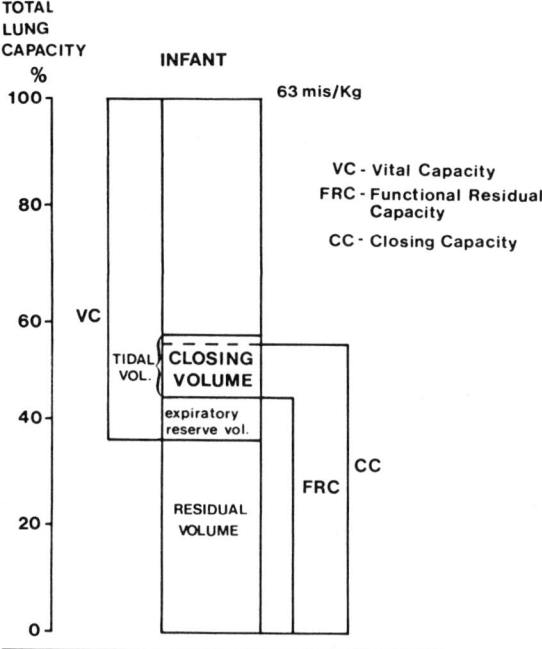

**FIG A–2.**
Lung volumes in the infant. (From Smith CA, Nelson NM: *The Physiology of the Newborn Infant,* ed 4. Springfield, Ill, Charles C. Thomas, Publisher, 1976, p 207. Used by permission.)

## TABLE A-9.
Lung Volume in Full-term and Premature Newborns*

| Reference | Method | Weight, kg | Age | Lung Volume |
|---|---|---|---|---|
| Berglund and Karlberg (1956) | Helium | 2.0–5.0 | 0.5–7 Days | 27 ml/kg |
| Klaus et al. (1962) | Plethysmography | 2.3–4.1 | 11–20 min | 23 ml/kg |
| | | | 30–40 min | 29 ml/kg |
| | | | 25–48 hr | 28 ml/kg |
| | | | >96 hr | 39 ml/kg |
| Nelson et al. (1963) | Plethysmography | 1.3–4.0 | 16 hr–71 Days | 40.6 ml/kg |
| | N₂ washout | 1.3–4.0 | 16 hr–71 Days | 31.3 ml/kg |
| Krauss and Auld (1971) | Plethysmography | >1.75 | <24 hr | 2 ml/cm |
| | Helium | >1.75 | <24 hr | 1.3 ml/cm |
| | Plethysmography | >1.75 | 3–6 Days | 1.8 ml/cm |
| | Helium | >1.75 | 3–6 Days | 1.4 ml/cm |
| | Plethysmography | <1.75 | <24 hr | 1.7 ml/cm |
| | Helium | <1.75 | <24 hr | 0.9 ml/cm |
| | Plethysmography | <1.75 | 12–19 Days | 0.9 ml/cm |
| | Helium | <1.75 | 12–19 Days | 0.8 ml/cm |
| Lacourt and Polgar (1974) | Plethysmography | 0.68–2.65 (prematures) | 1–72 Days | 30.4 ml/kg |
| | | | | 1.12 ml/cm |
| | Plethysmography | 1.5–3.6 (full term) | 1–18 Days | 32.4 ml/kg |
| | | | | 1.72 ml/cm |
| Ronchetti et al. (1975) | Plethysmography | 1.38–2.6 | 4–28 Days | 37.5 ml/kg |
| | Helium | 1.38–2.6 | 4–28 Days | 29.5 ml/kg |
| Hjalmarson et al. (1974) | Plethysmography | 1.31–4.75 | 1–21 Days | 32.5 ml/kg |
| Stocks and Godfrey (1977) | Plethysmography | 1.05–2.66 | 2–67 Days | 35.7 ml/kg |
| | | 2.90–4.00 | 1–14 Days | 35.7 ml/kg |

*From Bancalari E: Pulmonary function testing and other diagnostic laboratory procedures, in Thibeault DW, Gregory GA (eds): Neonatal Pulmonary Care. East Norwalk, Conn, Appleton-Century-Crofts, 1986, p 202. Used by permission.

## Pulmonary Mechanics

**TABLE A–10.**
Compliance and Resistance in Normal Full-term and Premature Newborns*

| Reference | Method | Weight, kg | Age | Compliance, ml/cm H$_2$O | Resistance, cm H$_2$O/L/sec | Work of Breathing, gm × cm/min | Elastic Work, % |
|---|---|---|---|---|---|---|---|
| Cook et al. (1957) | Plethysmography | 2.4–3.8 | 1 hr–6 days | 5.2 | 29 (total) | 1.380 | 70 |
| Swyer et al. (1960) | Pneumotachography | 2.3–3.96 | 2 hr–11 days | 4.9 | 26 (total) | 2.050 | 66 |
| Polgar (1961) | Plethysmography | 1.98–4.55 | 12 hr–17 days | 5.7 | 18.1 (airway) | — | — |
| Karlberg and Koch (1962) | Reverse plethysmography | 1.29–5.3 | 1.5 min–8 days | 1.87 × wt$^{0.843}$ | 3.94 × wt$^{0.379}$ (total) | — | — |
| Drorbaugh et al. (1963) | Reverse plethysmography | 2.6–4.1 | 35 min | 3.22 | — | — | — |
| | | 2.6–4.1 | 5–8 days | 4.7 | | | |
| Chu et al. (1967) | Plethysmography | 2.5–4.3 | <3 hr | 1.5/kg (40/L FRC)† | — | — | — |
| | | 2.5–4.3 | 8 hr–55 days | 2/kg (53/L FRC) | — | | |
| | | 1.13–2.5 | 8 hr–55 days | 1.9/kg (40/L FRC) | | | |
| Polgar and String (1966) | Plethysmography | 3.03–3.85 | 3–60 hr | 6.0 | 34.1 (total) 25.4 (airway) | — | — |
| Doershuk and Mathews (1969) | Plethysmography | 2.2–4.1 | 2 hr–11 days | — | 19.2 (airway) | — | — |
| Wohl et al. (1969) | Forced oscillation | 2.68–4.38 | 3–4 days | — | 69 (total insp.) 97 (total exp.) | — | — |
| Bancalari et al. (1970) | Plethysmography Pneumotachography | 2–4.0 | 2–11 days | 6.6 | 15.4 (total insp.) 21 (total exp.) | 2.928 | 51.8 |
| Lacourt and Polgar (1971) | Pneumotachography | 2.69–3.72 | 10–44 hr | — | 27.3 (total) 9.4 (nasal) | — | — |
| Feather and Russell (1974) | Pneumotachography | 1.83–2.5 | 4–43 hr | 4.1 | — | 2.482 | — |
| Hjalmarson et al. (1974) | Plethysmography + Esophageal balloon | 1.31–4.75 | 1–21 days | 3.7 | 42.0 (total) | — | — |
| Stocks and Godfrey (1977) | Plethysmography | 1.05–2.66 | 2–67 days | — | 38.4 (airway) | — | — |
| | Plethysmography | 2.90–4.00 | 1–4 days | — | 27.9 (airway) | — | — |

*From Bancalari E: Pulmonary function testing and other diagnostic laboratory procedures, in Thibeault DW, Gregory GA (eds): *Neonatal Pulmonary Care*. East Norwalk, Conn, Appleton-Century-Crofts, 1986, pp 216–217. Used by permission.
†FRC = functional residual capacity.

## TABLE A–11.
Compliance and Resistance in the Infant Respiratory System*

| Compliance | L/cm $H_2O$ | L/cm $H_2O$/L Lung Volume |
|---|---|---|
| Total respiratory system | 0.0026 | 0.029 |
| Chest wall | 0.0236 | 0.262 |
| Lung tissue | 0.0050 | 0.055 |
| Resistance to Flow | cm $H_2O$/L/sec | Total Resistance, % |
| Total respiratory system | | |
| Expiratory | 97 | — |
| Inspiratory | 69 | 100 |
| Chest wall | — | 26 |
| Pulmonary | 35 | 74 |
| Expiratory | 35–70 | — |
| Inspiratory | 25–50 | — |
| Nose | 10 | 21 |
| Mouth-airway | 16 | 34 |
| Lung tissue | 9 | 19 |

| Infant Static Lung Volumes, ml/kg* | |
|---|---|
| Total lung capacity (TLC) | 63 |
| Inspiratory capacity (IC) | 33 |
| Thoracic gas volume (Vtg) | 30–36 |
| Functional residual capacity (FRC) | 30 |
| Vital capacity (VC) | 40 |
| Closing capacity (CC) | 35 |
| Tidal volume ($V_T$) | 6 |
| Expiratory reserve volume (ERV) | 7 |
| Closing volume (CV) | 12 |
| Residual volume (RV) | 23 |
| ERV/FRC | 0.23 |
| RV/TLC | 0.37 |
| FRC/TLC | 0.48 |
| $V_T$/FRC | 0.20 |

(Continued.)

## TABLE A–11 (cont.).

| Pulmonary Ventilation of Infant* | |
|---|---|
| Respiratory frequency, breaths/min | 34–45 |
| Tidal volume, ml/kg | 6–8 |
| Alveolar volume, ml/kg | 3.8–5.8 |
| Dead space volume, ml/kg | 2–2.2 |
| Minute ventilation, ml/kg/min | 200–260 |
| Alveolar ventilation, ml/kg/min | 100–150 |
| Wasted (dead space) ventilation, ml/kg/min | 77–99 |
| Dead space/tidal volume | 0.27–0.37 |
| $O_2$ consumption, ml/kg/min | 6–8 |
| Ventilation equivalent (alveolar ventilation/$O_2$ consumption) | 16–23 |
| **Pulmonary Mechanics of Infant*** | |
| Gas flow, L/sec | |
|   Inspiration | 0.048 |
|   Expiration | 0.037 |
|   Mean | 0.030–0.050 |
| Airway conductance (spec), L/sec/cm $H_2O$/L FRC | 0.28 |
| Forces opposing inspiration (quiet breathing) | |
|   Elastic recoil, cm $H_2O$ | 1.5 |
|   Flow resistance (mean/maximum), cm $H_2O$ | 0.4/1.9 |
|   Inertial | negligible |
| Time constant (resistance × compliance), $\Delta$ | 0.29 |
| Respiratory frequency, breaths/min | 40 (30–50) |
| Work of respiration | |
|   Total pulmonary, kg · cm/min | 1.5–2.0 |
|   Elastic, % of total | 50–70 |
| Mechanical efficiency, % | 4 |

*From Smith CA, Nelson NM: *Physiology of the Newborn Infant,* ed 4. Springfield, Ill, Charles C Thomas, Publisher, 1976. Used by permission.

# Flowcharts

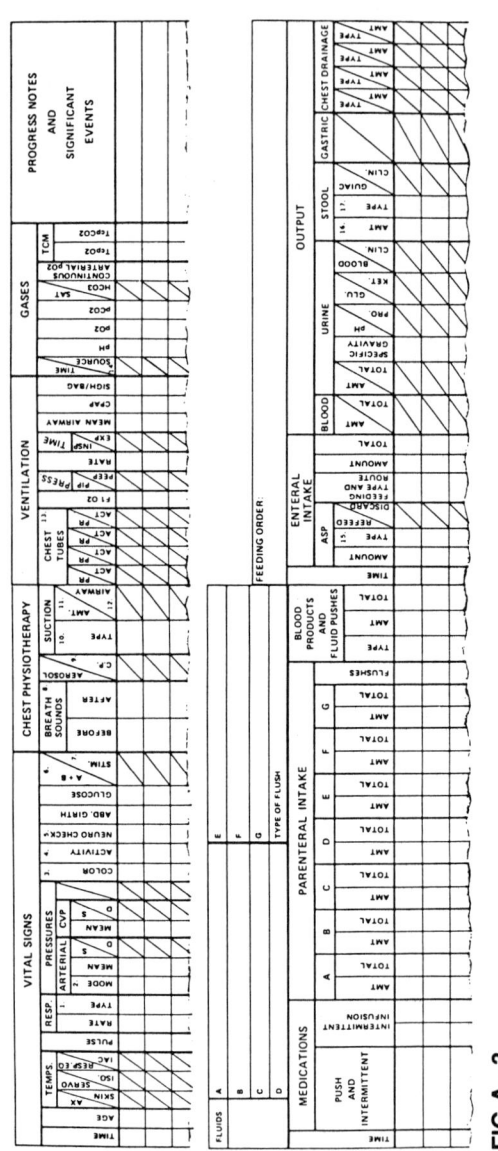

**FIG A–3.**
Neonatal intensive care flowchart. (Courtesy of Rainbow Babies and Childrens Hospital, Cleveland.)

**FIG A–4.**
Respiratory care flowchart. (Courtesy of Rainbow Babies and Childrens Hospital, Cleveland.)

# CARDIOVASCULAR SYSTEM

## Blood Pressure

**TABLE A–12.**
Blood Pressure During the First 12 Hours of Life in Normal Newborns*

| Birth Weight, gm | | Hour | | | | | | | | | | | |
|---|---|---|---|---|---|---|---|---|---|---|---|---|---|
| | | 1 | 2 | 3 | 4 | 5 | 6 | 7 | 8 | 9 | 10 | 11 | 12 |
| 1,001–2,000 | Systolic | 49 | 49 | 51 | 52 | 53 | 52 | 52 | 52 | 51 | 51 | 49 | 50 |
| | Diastolic | 26 | 27 | 28 | 29 | 31 | 31 | 31 | 31 | 31 | 30 | 29 | 30 |
| | Mean | 35 | 36 | 37 | 39 | 40 | 40 | 39 | 39 | 38 | 37 | 37 | 38 |
| 2,001–3,000 | Systolic | 59 | 57 | 60 | 60 | 61 | 58 | 64 | 60 | 63 | 61 | 60 | 59 |
| | Diastolic | 32 | 32 | 32 | 32 | 33 | 34 | 37 | 34 | 38 | 35 | 35 | 35 |
| | Mean | 43 | 41 | 43 | 43 | 44 | 43 | 45 | 43 | 44 | 44 | 43 | 42 |
| >3,000 | Systolic | 70 | 67 | 65 | 65 | 66 | 66 | 67 | 67 | 68 | 70 | 66 | 66 |
| | Diastolic | 44 | 41 | 39 | 41 | 40 | 41 | 41 | 41 | 44 | 43 | 41 | 41 |
| | Mean | 53 | 51 | 50 | 50 | 51 | 50 | 50 | 51 | 53 | 54 | 51 | 50 |

*From Kitterman JA, Tooley WH: Aortic blood pressure in normal newborn infants during the first 12 hours of life. *Pediatrics* 1969; 44:959. Used by permission.

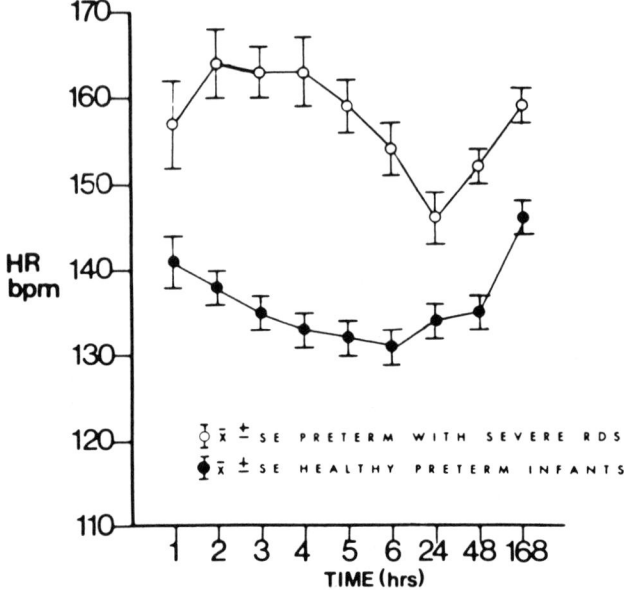

**FIG A–5.**
Effect of postnatal age on heart rate in preterm infants. RDS = respiratory distress syndrome. (From Cabal LA, Siassi B, Hodgman JE: Neonatal clinical cardiopulmonary monitoring, in Fanaroff AA, Martin RJ (eds): *Neonatal-Perinatal Medicine.* St Louis, CV Mosby Co, 1987, p 344. Used by permission.)

# GROWTH AND MATURATION
## Growth

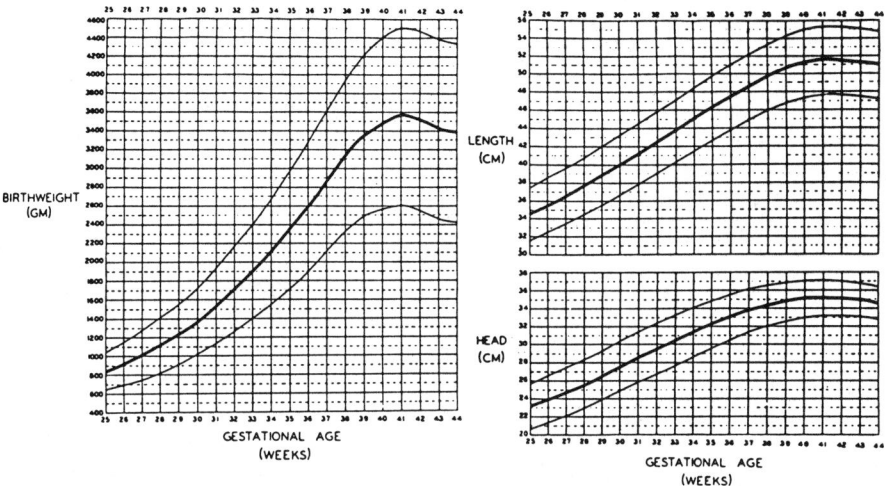

**FIG A-6.**
Intrauterine growth curves. (From Usher R, McLean F: Intrauterine growth of live-born Caucasian infants at sea level: Standards obtained from measurements in 7 dimensions of infants between 25 and 44 weeks of gestation. *J Pediatr* 1969; 74:901. Used by permission.)

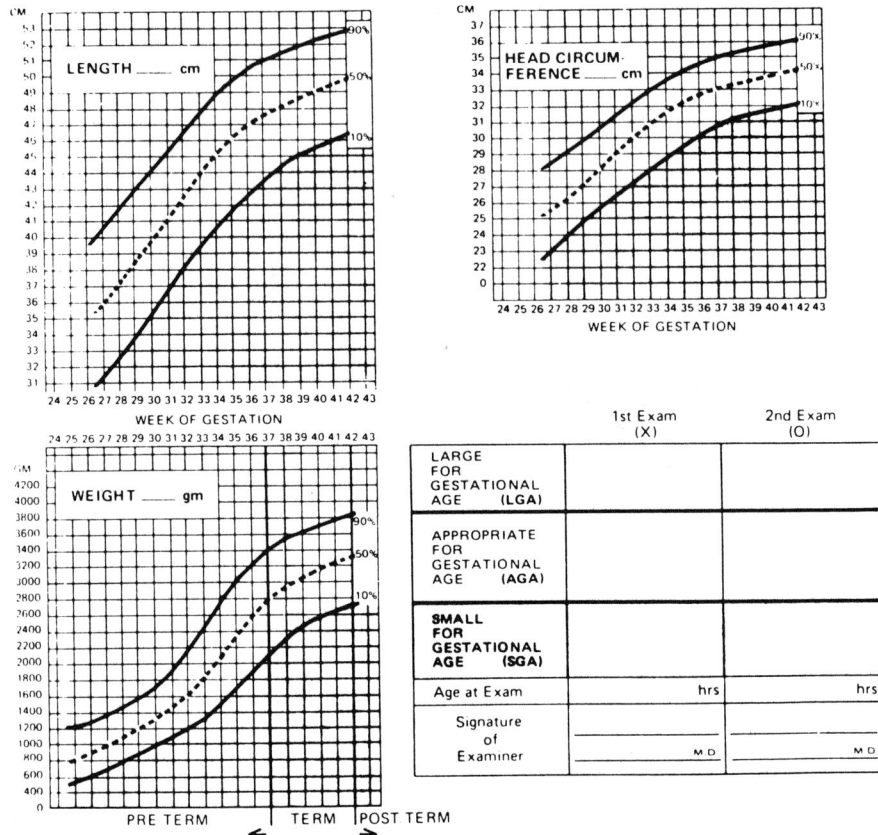

**FIG A–7.**
Classification of newborns based on maturity and intrauterine growth. (From Lubchenco LC, Hansman C, Boyd E: Intrauterine growth in length and head circumference as estimated from live births at gestational ages from 26–42 weeks. *Pediatrics* 1966; 37:403. Used by permission.)

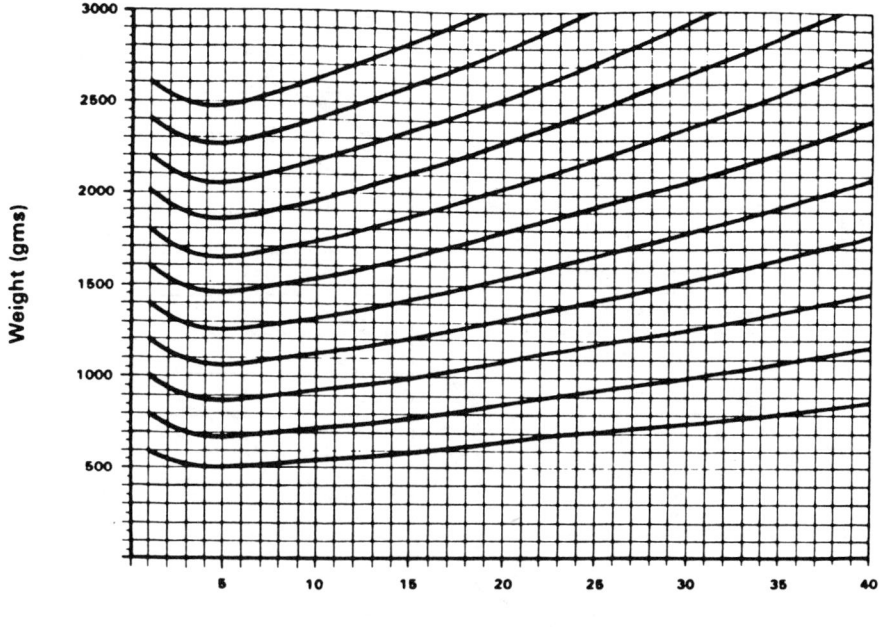

**FIG A−8.**
Extrauterine growth curves in low birth weight infants. (From Shaffer SG, Quimiro CL, Anderson JV, et al: Postnatal weight changes in low birth weight infants. *Pediatrics* 1987; 79:702. Used by permisison.)

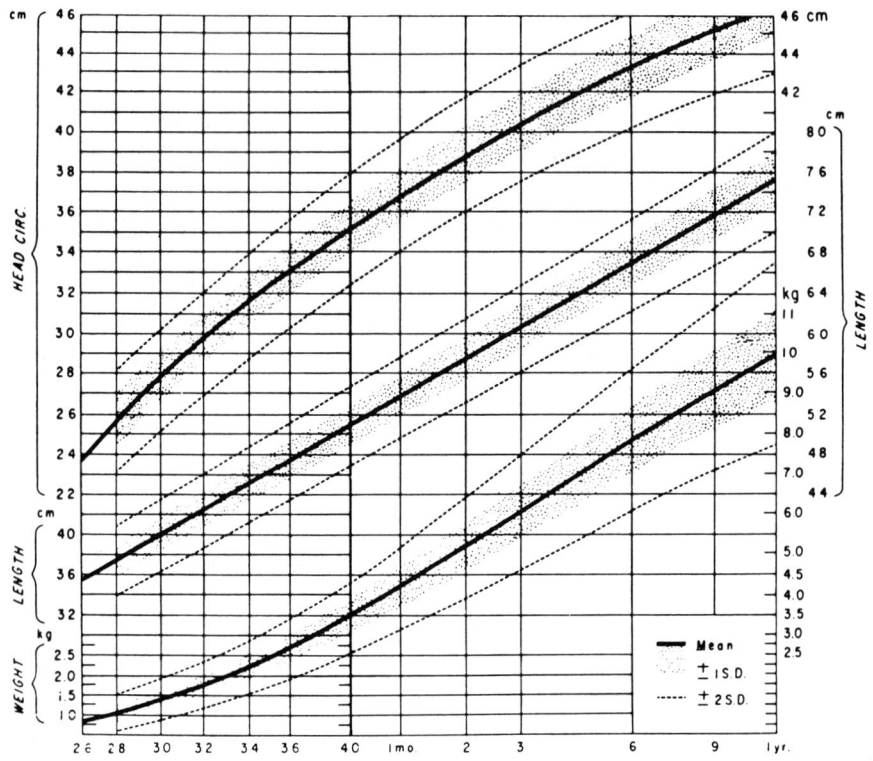

**FIG A–9.**
Extrauterine growth curves. (From Babson SG, Benda GF: Growth graphs for the clinical assessment of infants of varying gestational age. *J Pediatr* 1976; 89:814. Used by permission.)

## Maturation

### PHYSICAL MATURITY

| | 0 | 1 | 2 | 3 | 4 | 5 |
|---|---|---|---|---|---|---|
| Skin | gelatinous red, transparent | smooth pink, visible veins | superficial peeling &/or rash few veins | cracking pale area rare veins | parchment deep cracking no vessels | leathery cracked wrinkled |
| Lanugo | none | abundant | thinning | bald areas | mostly bald | |
| Plantar Creases | no crease | faint red marks | anterior transverse crease only | creases ant. 2/3 | creases cover entire sole | |
| Breast | barely percept. | flat areola no bud | stippled areola 1–2 mm bud | raised areola 3–4 mm bud | full areola 5–10 mm bud | |
| Ear | pinna flat, stays folded | sl. curved pinna; soft with slow recoil | well-curv. pinna; soft but ready recoil | formed & firm with instant recoil | thick cartilage ear stiff | |
| Genitals ♂ | scrotum empty no rugae | | testes descending, few rugae | testes down good rugae | testes pendulous deep rugae | |
| Genitals ♀ | prominent clitoris & labia minora | | majora & minora equally prominent | majora large minora small | clitoris & minora completely covered | |

### NEUROMUSCULAR MATURITY

| | 0 | 1 | 2 | 3 | 4 | 5 |
|---|---|---|---|---|---|---|
| Posture | | | | | | |
| Square Window (wrist) | 90° | 60° | 45° | 30° | 0° | |
| Arm Recoil | | 180° | 100°–180° | 90°–100° | <90° | |
| Popliteal Angle | 180° | 160° | 130° | 110° | 90° | <90° |
| Scarf Sign | | | | | | |
| Heel to Ear | | | | | | |

### MATURITY RATING

| Score | Wks |
|---|---|
| 5 | 26 |
| 10 | 28 |
| 15 | 30 |
| 20 | 32 |
| 25 | 34 |
| 30 | 36 |
| 35 | 38 |
| 40 | 40 |
| 45 | 42 |
| 50 | 44 |

**FIG A–10.**
Newborn maturity rating and classification. Add up neuromuscular and physical maturity scores. Extrapolate if necessary in the maturity rating estimation of gestational age. (From Ballard JL, Novak KZ, Driver M: A simplified score for assessment of fetal maturity of newly born infants. *J Pediatr* 1979; 95:769. Used by permission.)

# MISCELLANEOUS

## Hematologic Values

**TABLE A-13.**
Hematologic Values*†

| | | 1–3 Days | 4–7 Days | 2 Wk | 4 Wk | 6 Wk | 8 Wk |
|---|---|---|---|---|---|---|---|
| <1,200 gm birth weight | Hb, gm/dl | 15.6 | 16.4 | 15.5 | 11.3 | 8.5 | 7.8 |
| | Retic, % | 8.4 | 3.9 | 1.9 | 4.1 | 5.4 | 6.1 |
| | Plat, cells/cu mm | 148,000 ±61,000 | 163,000 ±69,000 | 162,000 | 158,000 | 210,000 | 212,000 |
| | Leuk, cells/cu mm | 14,800 ±10,200 | 12,200 ±7,000 | 15,800 | 13,200 | 10,800 | 9,900 |
| | Seg, % of total leukocytes | 46 | 32 | 41 | 28 | 23 | 23 |
| | Band, % of total leukocytes | 10.7 | 9.7 | 8.0 | 5.9 | 5.8 | 4.4 |
| | Juv, % of total leukocytes | 2.0 | 3.9 | 5.3 | 3.6 | 2.6 | 2.0 |
| | Lymph, % of total leukocytes | 32 | 43 | 39 | 55 | 61 | 65 |
| | Monos, % of total leukocytes | 5 | 7 | 5 | 4 | 6 | 3 |
| | Eos, % of total leukocytes | 0.4 | 6.2 | 1.0 | 3.7 | 2.0 | 3.8 |
| | Nucl RBC, cells/cu mm | 16.7 | 1.1 | 0.1 | 1.0 | 2.7 | 2.0 |
| >1,200–1,500 gm birth weight | Hb, gm/dl | 20.2 | 18.0 | 17.1 | 12.0 | 9.1 | 8.3 |
| | Retic, % | 2.7 | 1.2 | 0.9 | 1.0 | 2.2 | 2.7 |
| | Plat, cells/cu mm | 151,000 ±35,000 | 134,000 ±49,000 | 153,000 | 189,000 | 212,000 | 244,000 |
| | Leuk, cells/cu mm | 10,800 ±4,000 | 8,900 ±2,900 | 14,300 | 11,000 | 10,500 | 9,100 |
| | Seg, % of total leukocytes | 47 | 31 | 33 | 26 | 20 | 25 |
| | Band, % of total leukocytes | 11.9 | 10.5 | 5.9 | 3.0 | 1.4 | 2.1 |
| | Juv, % of total leukocytes | 5.1 | 2.4 | 2.7 | 1.8 | 1.7 | 1.6 |
| | Lymph, % of total leukocytes | 34 | 48 | 52 | 59 | 69 | 64 |
| | Monos, % of total leukocytes | 3 | 6 | 3 | 4 | 5 | 5 |
| | Eos, % of total leukocytes | 1.3 | 2.2 | 2.5 | 5.1 | 2.6 | 2.3 |
| | Nucl RBC, cells/cu mm | 19.8 | 0.8 | 0 | 0.4 | 1.4 | 1.0 |

*From Wolff JA, Goodfellow AM: Hematopoiesis in premature infants with special consideration of the effect of iron and of animal-protein factor. *Pediatrics* 1955; 16:753. Used by permission.

†Hb = hemoglobin; Retic = reticulocytes; Plat = platelets; Leuk = leukocytes; Seg = segmented neutrophils; Band = band neutrophils; Juv = juvenile neutrophils; Lymph = lymphocytes; Monos = monocytes; Eos = eosinophils; Nucl RBC = nucleated red blood cells.

**TABLE A-14.**
Normal Hematologic Values During the First 12 Weeks of Life*††

| Age | No. of Cases | Hb, gm % ± SD | RBC × 10⁶ ± SD | Hct, % ± SD | MCV, cu μ ± SD | MCHC, % ± SD | Retic, % ± SD |
|---|---|---|---|---|---|---|---|
| 1 Day | 19 | 19.0 ± 2.2 | 5.14 ± 0.7 | 61 ± 7.4 | 119 ± 9.4 | 31.6 ± 1.9 | 3.2 ± 1.4 |
| 2 Days | 19 | 19.0 ± 1.9 | 5.15 ± 0.8 | 60 ± 6.4 | 115 ± 7.0 | 31.6 ± 1.4 | 3.2 ± 1.3 |
| 3 Days | 19 | 18.7 ± 3.4 | 5.11 ± 0.7 | 62 ± 9.3 | 116 ± 5.3 | 31.1 ± 2.8 | 2.8 ± 1.7 |
| 4 Days | 10 | 18.6 ± 2.1 | 5.00 ± 0.6 | 57 ± 8.1 | 114 ± 7.5 | 32.6 ± 1.5 | 1.8 ± 1.1 |
| 5 Days | 12 | 17.6 ± 1.1 | 4.97 ± 0.4 | 57 ± 7.3 | 114 ± 8.9 | 30.9 ± 2.2 | 1.2 ± 0.2 |
| 6 Days | 15 | 17.4 ± 2.2 | 5.00 ± 0.7 | 54 ± 7.2 | 113 ± 10.0 | 32.2 ± 1.6 | 0.6 ± 0.2 |
| 7 Days | 12 | 17.9 ± 2.5 | 4.86 ± 0.6 | 56 ± 9.4 | 118 ± 11.2 | 32.0 ± 1.6 | 0.5 ± 0.4 |
| 1–2 wk | 32 | 17.3 ± 2.3 | 4.80 ± 0.8 | 54 ± 8.3 | 112 ± 19.0 | 32.1 ± 2.9 | 0.5 ± 0.3 |
| 2–3 wk | 11 | 15.6 ± 2.6 | 4.20 ± 0.6 | 46 ± 7.3 | 111 ± 8.2 | 33.9 ± 1.9 | 0.8 ± 0.6 |
| 3–4 wk | 17 | 14.2 ± 2.1 | 4.00 ± 0.6 | 43 ± 5.7 | 105 ± 7.5 | 33.5 ± 1.6 | 0.6 ± 0.3 |
| 4–5 wk | 15 | 12.7 ± 1.6 | 3.60 ± 0.4 | 36 ± 4.8 | 101 ± 8.1 | 34.9 ± 1.6 | 0.9 ± 0.8 |
| 5–6 wk | 10 | 11.9 ± 1.5 | 3.55 ± 0.2 | 36 ± 6.2 | 102 ± 10.2 | 34.1 ± 2.9 | 1.0 ± 0.7 |
| 6–7 wk | 10 | 12.0 ± 1.5 | 3.40 ± 0.4 | 36 ± 4.8 | 105 ± 12.0 | 33.8 ± 2.3 | 1.2 ± 0.7 |
| 7–8 wk | 17 | 11.1 ± 1.1 | 3.40 ± 0.4 | 33 ± 3.7 | 100 ± 13.0 | 33.7 ± 2.6 | 1.5 ± 0.7 |
| 8–9 wk | 13 | 10.7 ± 0.9 | 3.40 ± 0.5 | 31 ± 2.5 | 93 ± 12.0 | 34.1 ± 2.2 | 1.8 ± 1.0 |
| 9–10 wk | 12 | 11.2 ± 0.9 | 3.60 ± 0.3 | 32 ± 2.7 | 91 ± 9.3 | 34.3 ± 2.9 | 1.2 ± 0.6 |
| 10–11 wk | 11 | 11.4 ± 0.9 | 3.70 ± 0.4 | 34 ± 2.1 | 91 ± 7.7 | 33.2 ± 2.4 | 1.2 ± 0.7 |
| 11–12 wk | 13 | 11.3 ± 0.9 | 3.70 ± 0.3 | 33 ± 3.3 | 88 ± 7.9 | 34.8 ± 2.2 | 0.7 ± 0.3 |

*From Matoth Y, Zaizov R, Varsano I: Postnatal changes in some red cell parameters. *Acta Paediatr Scand* 1971; 60:317. Used by permission.
†In the term infant as determined by an electronic cell counter.
‡Hb = hemoglobin; RBC = red blood cell; Hct = hematocrit; MCV = mean corpuscular volume; MCHC = mean corpuscular hemoglobin concentration; Retic = reticulocytes.

**TABLE A–15.**
White Blood Cell Count During the First 2 Weeks*

| Age | Leukocytes | Neutrophils Total | Neutrophils Segmented | Band | Eosinophils | Basophils | Lymphocytes | Monocytes |
|---|---|---|---|---|---|---|---|---|
| **Birth** | | | | | | | | |
| Mean[†] | 18,100 | 11,000 | 9400 | 1600 | 400 | 100 | 5500 | 1050 |
| Range[‡] | 9.0—30.0 | 6.0—26 | | | 20—850 | 0—640 | 2.0—11.0 | 0.4—3.1 |
| Mean, % | — | 61 | 52 | 9 | 2.2 | 0.6 | 31 | 5.8 |
| **7 Days** | | | | | | | | |
| Mean[†] | 12,200 | 5500 | 4700 | 830 | 500 | 50 | 5000 | 1100 |
| Range[‡] | 5.0—21.0 | 1.5—10.0 | | | 70—1100 | 0—250 | 2.0—17.0 | 0.3—2.7 |
| Mean, % | — | 45 | 39 | 6 | 4.1 | 0.4 | 41 | 9.1 |
| **14 Days** | | | | | | | | |
| Mean[†] | 11,400 | 4500 | 3900 | 630 | 350 | 50 | 5500 | 1000 |
| Range[‡] | 5.0—20.0 | 1.0—9.5 | | | 70—1000 | 0—230 | 2.0—17.0 | 0.2—2.4 |
| Mean, % | — | 40 | 34 | 5.5 | 3.1 | 0.4 | 48 | 8.8 |

*From Avery GB: *Neonatology*. Philadelphia, JB Lippincott Co, 1987, p 1359. Used by permission.
[†]Count/cu mm.
[‡]Count × 10⁹/cu mm.

**TABLE A-16A.**
Platelets—Venous Platelet Counts in Normal Low Birth Weight Infants*

| Day | No. of Infants | Mean, cu mm | Range, 1,000s |
|---|---|---|---|
| 0 | 60 | 203,000 | 80–356 |
| 3 | 47 | 207,000 | 61–335 |
| 5 | 14 | 233,000 | 100–502 |
| 7 | 52 | 319,000 | 124–678 |
| 10 | 40 | 399,000 | 172–680 |
| 14 | 50 | 386,000 | 147–670 |
| 21 | 47 | 388,000 | 201–720 |
| 28 | 40 | 384,000 | 212–625 |

*From Appleyard WJ, Brinton A: Venous platelet counts in low birth weight infants. *Biol Neonate* 1971; 17:30. Used by permission.

**TABLE A-16B.**
Platelets—Platelet Counts in Full-term Infants*

| Day | Mean | Range |
|---|---|---|
| Cord | 200,000 | 100,000–280,000 |
| 1 | 192,000 | 100,000–260,000 |
| 3 | 213,000 | 80,000–320,000 |
| 7 | 248,000 | 100,000–300,000 |
| 14 | 252,000 | |

*From Blumenfeld TA: Tables of normal values, in Fanaroff AA, Martin RJ (eds): *Behrman's Neonatal-Perinatal Medicine,* ed 3. St Louis, CV Mosby Co, 1983, p 1112. Used by permission.

**TABLE A–17.**
Coagulation

|  | Normal | Term Infant (Cord Blood) | Premature Infant (Cord Blood) |
|---|---|---|---|
| Fibrinogen, mg % | 200–400 | 200–250 | 200–250 |
| Factor II, % | 50–150 | 40 | 25 |
| Factor V, % | 75–125 | 90 | 60–75 |
| Factor VII, % | 75–125 | 50 | 35 |
| Factor VIII, % | 50–150 | 100 | 80–100 |
| Factor IX, % | 50–150 | 25–40 | 25–40 |
| Factor X, % | 50–150 | 50–60 | 25–40 |
| Factor XI, % | 75–125 | 30–40 | — |
| Factor XII, % | 75–125 | 50–100 | 50–100 |
| Factor XIII, titer | 1:16 | 1:8 | 1:8 |
| Partial thromboplastin time, sec | 30–50 | 70 | 80–90 |
| Prothrombin time, sec | 10–12 | 12–18 | 14–20 |
| Thrombin time, sec | 10–12 | 12–16 | 13–20 |

*From Oski FA: Hematologic problems, in Avery GB (ed): *Neonatology*. Philadelphia, JB Lippincott Co, 1975, p 1057. Used by permission.

# Chemistry Values

**TABLE A–18.**
Normal Blood Chemistry Values, Term Infants*

| Determination | Sample Source | Cord | 1–12 hr | 12–24 hr | 24–48 hr | 48–72 hr |
|---|---|---|---|---|---|---|
| Sodium, mEq/L | Capillary | 147 (126–166) | 143 (124–156) | 145 (132–159) | 148 (134–160) | 149 (139–162) |
| Potassium, mEq/L | | 7.8 (5.6–12) | 6.4 (5.3–7.3) | 6.3 (5.3–8.9) | 6.0 (5.2–7.3) | 5.9 (5.0–7.7) |
| Chloride, mEq/L | | 103 (98–110) | 100.7 (90–111) | 103 (87–114) | 102 (92–114) | 103 (93–112) |
| Calcium, mg/100 ml | | 9.3 (8.2–11.1) | 8.4 (7.3–9.2) | 7.8 (6.9–9.4) | 8.0 (6.1–9.9) | 7.9 (5.9–9.7) |
| Phosphorus, mg/100 ml | | 5.6 (3.7–8.1) | 6.1 (3.5–8.6) | 5.7 (2.9–8.1) | 5.9 (3.0–8.7) | 5.8 (2.8–7.6) |
| Blood urea, mg/100 ml | | 29 (21–40) | 27 (8–34) | 33 (9–63) | 32 (13–77) | 31 (13–68) |
| Total protein, gm/100 ml | | 6.1 (4.8–7.3) | 6.6 (5.6–8.5) | 6.6 (5.8–8.2) | 6.9 (5.9–8.2) | 7.2 (6.0–8.5) |
| Blood sugar, mg/100 ml | | 73 (45–96) | 63 (40–97) | 63 (42–104) | 56 (30–91) | 59 (40–90) |
| Lactic acid, mg/100 ml | | 19.5 | 14.6 | 14.0 | 14.3 | 13.5 |

*From Acharya PT, Payne WW: Blood chemistry of normal full-term infants in the first 48 hours of life. Arch Dis Child 1965; 40:430. Used by permission.

**TABLE A–19.**
Normal Blood Chemistry Values, Low Birth Weight Infants, Capillary Blood, First Day*

| Determination | <1000 gm | 1001–1500 gm | 1501–2000 gm | 2001–2500 gm |
|---|---|---|---|---|
| Sodium, mEq/L | 138 | 133 | 135 | 134 |
| Potassium, mEq/L | 6.4 | 6.0 | 5.4 | 5.6 |
| Chloride, mEq/L | 100 | 101 | 105 | 104 |
| Total $CO_2$, mEq/L | 19 | 20 | 20 | 20 |
| Urea, mg/100 ml | 22 | 21 | 16 | 16 |
| TSP, gm/100 ml† | 4.8 | 4.8 | 5.2 | 5.3 |

*From Pincus JB, Gittleman IF, Saito M, et al: A study of plasma values of sodium, potassium, chloride, $CO_2$, $CO_2$ tension, sugar, urea and the protein base-binding power, pH and hematocrit in prematures on the first day of life. *Pediatrics* 1956; 18:39. Used by permission.
†TSP = total serum protein.

**TABLE A–20.**
Estimated Daily Requirements of Premature Infants[*][†]

| | Growth and Nongrowth Body Weight Intervals, gm | | | | | | | | | |
|---|---|---|---|---|---|---|---|---|---|---|
| | 750–1000 | 1000–1250 | 1250–1500 | 1500–1750 | 1750–2000 | 2000–2250 | 2250–2500 | 2500–2750 | 2750–3000 |
| **Energy** | | | | | | | | | |
| Growth, calories | 21 | 46 | 68 | 79 | 93 | 104 | 114 | 111 | 108 |
| Nongrowth, kcal | 71 | 94 | 117 | 133 | 156 | 180 | 204 | 215 | 239 |
| Total, calories/kg | 105 | 124 | 127 | 130 | 133 | 133 | 134 | 124 | 121 |
| **Protein** | | | | | | | | | |
| Growth, gm | 1.78 | 3.45 | 4.44 | 4.79 | 4.85 | 4.90 | 4.68 | 4.27 | 3.77 |
| Nongrowth, gm | 0.87 | 1.12 | 1.37 | 1.62 | 1.87 | 2.12 | 2.37 | 2.62 | 2.87 |
| Total, gm/kg[‡] | 3.02 | 4.06 | 4.22 | 3.94 | 3.58 | 3.30 | 2.96 | 2.62 | 2.30 |
| **Sodium** | | | | | | | | | |
| Growth, mEq | 0.95 | 1.68 | 2.10 | 2.21 | 2.21 | 2.21 | 2.10 | 1.89 | 1.57 |
| Nongrowth, mEq | 0.18 | 0.23 | 0.28 | 0.34 | 0.39 | 0.44 | 0.49 | 0.55 | 0.60 |
| Total, mEq/kg | 1.29 | 1.69 | 1.73 | 1.56 | 1.38 | 1.24 | 1.09 | 0.92 | 0.75 |
| **Potassium** | | | | | | | | | |
| Growth, mEq | 0.31 | 0.73 | 1.05 | 1.15 | 1.26 | 1.36 | 1.36 | 1.36 | 1.15 |
| Nongrowth, mEq | 0.20 | 0.26 | 0.32 | 0.38 | 0.43 | 0.49 | 0.55 | 0.61 | 0.66 |
| Total, mEq/kg | 0.58 | 0.88 | 0.99 | 0.94 | 0.90 | 0.87 | 0.80 | 0.75 | 0.63 |
| **Calcium** | | | | | | | | | |
| Growth, mg | 148 | 317 | 442 | 530 | 592 | 632 | 660 | 627 | 592 |
| Nongrowth, mg | — | — | — | — | — | — | — | — | — |
| Total, mg/kg | 169 | 282 | 321 | 326 | 316 | 300 | 278 | 239 | 206 |
| **Phosphorus** | | | | | | | | | |
| Growth, mg | 49 | 110 | 148 | 172 | 188 | 197 | 202 | 194 | 177 |
| Nongrowth, mg | 12 | 27 | 37 | 43 | 47 | 49 | 50 | 49 | 44 |
| Total, mg/kg | 70 | 121 | 135 | 132 | 125 | 116 | 106 | 93 | 77 |
| **Magnesium** | | | | | | | | | |
| Growth, mg | 9.0 | 18.5 | 25.2 | 30.0 | 33.5 | 35.5 | 37.0 | 35.5 | 32.5 |
| Nongrowth, mg | — | — | — | — | — | — | — | — | — |
| Total, mg/kg | 10.3 | 16.4 | 18.6 | 18.5 | 17.8 | 16.7 | 15.6 | 13.5 | 11.3 |

*From Avery ME, Taeusch HW: Schaffer's Diseases of the Newborn. New York, WB Saunders Co, 1984, p 1980.
†Assuming extent of intestinal absorption as follows: energy: 75% absorption for infants weighing 750 to 1,500 gm, 80% for those weighing 1,500 to 2,500 gm, and 85% for those weighing more than 2,500 gm; protein: 75% absorption at 750 to 1,250 gm, 77% at 1,250 to 1,500 gm, 80% at 1,500 to 2,250 gm, 83% at 2,250 to 2,500 gm, and 85% above 2,500 gm; sodium and potassium: 95% absorption throughout; calcium: 40% throughout; phosphorus: 80% throughout; magnesium: 20% throughout.
‡Based on arithmetic mean weight for the weight interval.

# Index

## A

Abdomen
  distention of, 282
  paracentesis and, 146
  radiography and, 293
  skin care and, 205
Abductor paralysis, 100
Acceleration, fetal heart rate, 64
Acid-base balance
  normal values for, 427
  physiology of, 49–59
Acidosis
  delivery room and, 147
  metabolic, 51–52
  respiratory, 50–51
Acinus, 7
Activity level, assessment of, 156
Adsorption, drug, 240–242
Adult respiratory distress syndrome, 382; see also Respiratory distress syndrome
Aeration, assessment of, 158–162
Afterload, ventricular, 168
Age
  drug metabolism and, 243
  lung size and, 425
Agenesis of lung, 4
Aircraft transport, 109
Air embolism
  pulmonary venous, 348
  radiography and, 310
Air leaks
  as complication, 348–352
  high-frequency ventilation and, 380
  radiography and, 305–310
  respiratory distress and, 274–275
Air, swallowing of
  continuous positive pressure airway pressure and, 198
  respiratory distress and, 195
Airway, 91–106
  anatomy of, 91–92
  bronchoscopy, 103–105
  care of, 92–97
  congenital abnormalities of, 98–102
  dimensions of, 425
  laryngoscopy, 103–105
  nursing assessment and, 160–161
  obstruction and, 431
Algorithm for ventilatory management, 337–343
Alimentation
  intravenous, 177–178
  parenteral, 193–194
Alkalosis
  metabolic, 52
  respiratory, 51
Altitude, 111
Alveolar-capillary membrane, 45
Alveolar ventilation, 324–325
  air leak and, 348
  hyperventilation and, 431
Alveolus
  carbon dioxide tension in, 47–48
  development of, 6, 14–15
  dimensions of, 425
  oxygen tension in, 42–43
Ambulance, 109

Amikacin
　dosage of, 245
　recommended dilution of, 172
Aminoglycoside, 245
Aminophylline
　apnea and, 160
　recommended dilution of, 172
Amniotic fluid
　fetal lung fluid and, 31
　radiography and, 303–304
Ampicillin
　dosage of, 245
　recommended dilution of, 172
Anemia, 282
Animal models
　continuous-flow apneic ventilation and, 411–412
　high-frequency ventilation and, 379–380
Anomalous pulmonary venous return, 315
Anomaly, congenital; see Congenital malformation
　delivery room assessment and, 148
　parental support and, 231–234
　radiography and, 303–305
Antepartum monitoring, 66
Antiarrhythmic agent, 247–248
Antibiotic, 244–245
　intravenous, 169–170
Anticholinergic agent, 247
Apgar score, 137
Apnea, 284–285
　assisted ventilation and, 344
　monitor and, 73
　nursing assessment and, 160–161
Apneic ventilation, continuous flow, 409–417
Apoprotein, 26, 27
Appearance, assessment of, 155–157
Arrhythmia
　nursing assessment and, 167
　respiratory distress and, 283
　in utero drug therapy and, 238–239
Arterial blood sampling, 125; see Blood sampling
Arterial catheterization, umbilical
　radiography and, 291–292
　technique of, 121–124

Arterial oxygen delivery, 161–162
Arterial partial pressure of oxygen; see also Oxygen partial pressure
　birth and, 134
　reduced, 430
Artery, development of, 16–17; see also specific artery
Artificial airway, 93–95
Arytenoid cartilage
　anatomy of, 91
　large, 99
Asphyxiation
　assisted ventilation and, 140–142
　drying and stabilization and, 138–140
　external cardiac massage and, 143–144
　medications and, 144–145
　pathophysiology of, 135–136
　respiratory distress and, 277–278
　risk of, 131
　seizure and, 147–148
　vascular access and, 142–143
Aspiration
　meconium, 146
　　blood gas changes in, 431
　　differential diagnosis and, 268
　　radiography and, 298–299
　　respiratory distress and, 272–273
　milk, 269
Assessment
　of neonatal well-being, 137–138
　nursing; see Nursing care, assessment and
Assisted ventilation, 320–346
　air leak and, 348, 350
　apnea and, 344
　bronchopulmonary dysplasia and, 360–362
　complications of, 352–353
　delivery room and, 140–142
　gas exchange and, 324–327
　high-frequency; see High-frequency ventilation
　methods for, 327–335
　persistent fetal circulation and, 276, 343–344
　pulmonary mechanics and, 321–324

Assisted ventilation (cont.)
  respiratory distress and, 267, 335–343
Asthma, 363
Atelectasis, postextubation, 352–353
Atresia, choanal, 98
Atrial pacing, 168
Atropine, 247, 249

## B

Bacterial infection
  congenital pneumonia and, 273
  delivery room assessment and, 148
Bag-and-mask system, 113–114, 140–142, 328
Barotrauma, 358
Bicarbonate
  asphyxiation and, 143
  delivery room resuscitation and, 145
  Henderson-Hasselbalch equation, 49–50
  persistent fetal circulation and, 276
  respiratory distress and, 271
  resuscitation and, 249
Biochemistry, fetal, 25–35
Biophysical profile, fetal, 69–70
Biotransformation, drug, 243
Birth
  circulation and, 24–25
  nervous system injury and, 148–149
Bladder-box assembly, 401
Blood; see also Blood gas; Blood sampling
  normal values for, 446–452
  respiratory distress and, 282–283
Blood flow; see Circulation
Blood gas
  assisted ventilation and, 336
  carbon dioxide tension and; see Carbon dioxide
  classification of disorders of, 50, 52–55
  full-term infant and, 427
  interpretation of, 55
  map and, 55, 57–58
  monitoring of; see also Blood sampling
  noninvasive, 195–196
  continuous, 126–128
  oxygen tension and; see Oxygen partial pressure
  premature infant and, 428
  respiratory distress and, 266–267
Blood pH, 49–59
  umbilical cord, 137–138
Blood pressure
  delivery room assessment and, 147
  drug therapy and, 248
  monitoring and, 74–75
  normal values for, 439
  nursing assessment and, 157
Blood sampling
  capillary, 125–126
  fetal scalp, 65–66
  indwelling line and, 187
  intermittent arterial, 125
Blood sugar, 451
Blood urea nitrogen, 451
Blood vessels
  development of, 15–18
  radiography and, 293
Body weight, 186
Bonding, 212, 216–222
Bony dysplasia, 305
Botulism, infantile, 280
Brachial plexus injury, 148–149, 281
Bradycardia
  critically ill neonate and, 157
  delivery room assessment and, 140
  feeding and, 192
  fetal, 61
  monitor and, 73
  ventilation and, 168
Brain; see also Central nervous system
  damage to, 230
  functional assessment and, 162–165
Branching of airways, abnormal, 101–102
Breath sounds, 194
Breathing
  initiation of, 132
  fetal, 32–35
  pattern of, 72–73
Bretylium, 249

Bronchiole
 barotrauma and, 419
 bronchopulmonary dysplasia, 363
 development of, 11–12
Bronchodilator, 161
Bronchopleural fistula, 380
Bronchopulmonary dysplasia, 355–362
 differential diagnosis and, 269
 radiography and, 299–301
Bronchoscopy, 103–105
 high-frequency ventilation and, 382
Bronchospasm, 362
Bronchus
 anatomy of, 92
 arteries of, 18
 congenital cyst and, 4
 development of, 11–13
 right main-stem, intubation of, 201, 352
Brown fat, 178, 179
Buccopharyngeal membrane, 4
Bud, lung, 9–10
Bumetanide, 254–255

## C

Caffeine, 249–251
 recommended dilution of, 172
Calcium
 blood chemistry and, 451
 nursing assessment and, 171
 resuscitation and, 249
Calibration of flow signal, 80
Canal, pericardioperitoneal, 18–19
Canalicular stage of lung development, 8
*Candida albicans*, 273
Cannula
 extracorporeal membrane oxygenation and, 400
 nasal, 113
  nursing care and, 197–198
Capillary blood sampling, 125–126
Capnograph, 73
Carbenicillin, 172
Carbon dioxide
 assisted ventilation and, 324–325
 high-frequency ventilation and, 374–375

 monitoring and, 73
 partial pressure of, 46–47
 placental circulation and, 21
 transcutaneous monitoring and, 78, 127
 transport and, 46–49
Cardiac compression/massage
 delivery room resuscitation and, 143–144
 heart rate and, 168
 technique of, 120–121
Cardiac glycoside, 251, 252
Cardiomegaly, 313
Cardiopulmonary resuscitation; see Resuscitation
Cardiopulmonary system; see *also* Cardiovascular system; Heart
 birth and, 132–134
 monitor and, 73
Cardiothymic silhouette, 292
Cardiovascular system; see *also* Heart
 delivery room assessment and, 147
 drug therapy and, 246–249
 high-frequency ventilation and, 381
 nursing assessment and, 165–169
 respiratory distress and, 283
Carina, 92
Cartilage
 anatomy of, 91–92
 arytenoid, 99
 bronchial, 13
Catecholamine, 246–247
Catheter
 arterial, 121–124
 esophageal pacing, 168
 extracorporeal membrane oxygenation and, 399, 400
 feeding, 194
 radiography and, 291–292
 suction, 201
 umbilical vein, 142
 venous, 125
Cavity, pleural, 18–20
Cefazolin, 172
Cefotaxime, 245
Ceftazidime, 245
Ceftriaxone, 245
Central line infusion, 169

Central nervous system
  birth injury to, 149
  nursing assessment and, 162–165
  respiratory distress and, 277–279
Cephalohematoma, 149
Cephalothin, 172
Chest
  mechanical ventilation and, 201
  physiotherapy and, 118–120, 195
  radiography of; see Radiography
  transillumination of, 350
Chest wall
  compliance and, 81
  nursing assessment and, 158–159
Childbirth class, 223–224
Chloral hydrate, 172
Chloramphenicol, 245
Chloride, 451
Choanal atresia, 98
Chylothorax, 297–298
Circulation
  nursing assessment and, 165–169
  persistent fetal; see Persistent fetal circulation
  transitional, 20–25
Clamping of umbilical cord, 135
*Clostridium botulinum*, 280
CNP; see Continuous negative pressure
Coagulation, 450
Cold stress; see Hypothermia
Collagen, 13
Color
  feeding and, 192
  nursing assessment of, 155–157
  respiratory distress and, 194
Compliance, 81–87
  assisted ventilation and, 321
  terminal bronchiole and, 419
  time constant and, 322
  values for, 435, 436
Complications, 347–365
  air leaks and, 348–352
  bronchopulmonary dysplasia and, 355–362
  endotracheal tube and, 352–353
  extracorporeal membrane oxygenation, 403–404
  infection and, 353–354
  intracranial hemorrhage and, 354

  patent ductus arteriosus and, 354–355
Compression
  cardiac
    delivery room resuscitation and, 143–144
    heart rate and, 168
    technique of, 120–121
  intrathoracic, 304–305
  trachea and bronchi and, 101
Conduction heat loss, 183
Congenital disease; see also Congenital malformation
  heart; see Heart
  myasthenia gravis and, 280
  pneumonia and
    differential diagnosis and, 268
    respiratory distress and, 273
Congenital malformation
  delivery room assessment and, 148
  lower respiratory tract, 3–4
  parental support and, 231–234
  radiography and, 303–305
  subglottic stenosis and, 100
Congestive heart failure; see Heart failure
Connective tissue, 13
Continuous blood gas monitoring, 126–128
Continuous distending pressure, 328–331
Continuous-flow apneic ventilation, 409–417
Continuous negative pressure, 328–329
Continuous positive airway pressure, 329–331
  nursing care and, 197
  weaning and, 336
Contractility, cardiac, 168
Contraction stress test, 66–69
Convection heat loss, 183–184
Cor pulmonale, 361
Cord
  umbilical
    blood pH and, 137–138
    clamping of, 135
    cutting of, 134
  vocal

Cord (cont.)
    anatomy of, 91
    paralysis of, 100
Cranial nerve injury, 148–149
Cricoid cartilage, 91–92
Curve
    growth, 441–444
    oxyhemoglobin dissociation, 44–45
    pressure-volume, 81
Cyanosis
    heart failure and, 431
    respiratory distress and, 261–262
Cyst
    bronchial, 4
    laryngeal, 100
    thyroglossal duct, 98–99
Cystic hygroma, 98
Cytidine, 27

## D

Deafness, 276
Decannulation, 97
Deceleration, fetal heart
    early, 62
    late, 63–64
    variable, 64
Delivery room management, 130–153
    asphyxia and, 135–145
    depression and, 136–137
    evaluation of treatment and, 147–148
    interventions in, 145–146
    neonatal assessment and, 137–138
    nervous system injury and, 148–149
    resuscitation errors and, 150–151
    transitional physiology and, 131–135
Depression
    blood gas changes in, 431
    causes of, 136–137
    central nervous system, 278
Dexamethasone
    bronchopulmonary dysplasia and, 362
    in utero drug therapy and, 239
    recommended dilution of, 172

Dextrose, 145
Diaphragm
    development of, 18–20
    disorder of, 281–282
    hernia and, 148
    radiography and, 293, 311–312
Diazepam, 173
Diffusion
    drug and, 237, 240–241
    gas, 21
Digitalis, 169
Digoxin, 251, 252
    recommended dilution of, 173
1,2–Dipalmitoyl-sn-glycero-3–phosphatidylcholine, 26, 27
Diuretics, 253–255
    furosemide and, 176
Dobutamine, 249
Dopamine, 249
DPPC; see 1,2–Dipalmitoyl-sn-glycero-3–phosphatidylcholine
Drip therapy, 169
Drug therapy, 236–259; see also individual drug
    antibiotics and, 244–245
    cardiovascular system and, 246–249
    delivery room resuscitation and, 144–145
    digoxin and, 251, 252
    diuretics and, 253–255
    indomethacin and, 252–253
    methylxanthines and, 249–251
    nursing care and, 169
    placenta and, 237–240
    principles of, 240–244
Drying of infant, 138–139
Duchenne-Erb paralysis, 148, 149
Duct cysts, thyroglossal, 98–99
Ductus arteriosus
    birth and, 25
    patent, 354–355
        indomethacin and, 252–253
        persistent fetal circulation and, 275
        respiratory distress and, 270–271, 283
Dysplasia
    bony, 305
    bronchopulmonary, 355–362

Dysplasia (cont.)
  differential diagnosis and, 269
  radiography and, 299–301
Dystrophy, myotonic, 280–281

**E**

Echocardiography, 275
Ectoderm, 2
Edema
  pulmonary
    bronchopulmonary dysplasia and, 361
    nursing assessment and, 159
    radiography and, 313
  total body, 146
Effusion, pleural, 297–298
Eight-point check, 158–179; see also Nursing care, assessment and
Elastin, 16–17
Electrode
  attachment of, 205
  carbon dioxide, 78
  oxygen, 77
Electrolyte, 170–171, 176
Embolism
  air, 310
  pulmonary venous air, 348
Embryological germ cell layers, 2
Embryonic period of lung development, 7–9
  blood vessels and, 15–16
  bronchial arteries, 18
Emergency equipment, 160
Emphysema
  interstitial, 274–275, 348, 351–352
  radiography and, 308–309
Endocardial fibroelastosis, 283
Endoderm, 2
Endotracheal intubation, 93–95
  complications of, 103, 352–353
  delivery room and, 141
  mechanical ventilation and, 200–202
  suctioning of, 120
  technique of, 114–118
Enterocolitis, necrotizing, 178
Epiglottis
  anatomy of, 91–92
  laryngomalacia, 99

Epinephrine
  bradycardia and, 143
  delivery room resuscitation and, 145
  resuscitation and, 249
Epiphysis, humeral, 316–317
Epithelium, 12–13
Esophageal pacing catheter, 168
Esophageal vascular ring, 101
Ethacrynic acid, 254–255
Evaporation, 182–183
Exchanger, heat, 401–402
Excretion, drug, 243–244
Expiration, forced, 86–87
External cardiac massage
  delivery room resuscitation and, 143–144
  heart rate and, 168
  technique of, 120–121
Extracorporeal membrane oxygenation, 394–408
  circuit components and, 400–402
  clinical applications of, 397
  development of, 394–395
  indications for, 395–397
  management and, 402–407
  perfusion techniques and, 398–399
Extrauterine growth curve, 443, 444
Extremity transillumination, 124
Extubation
  accidental, 352
  problems with, 95
Eye-to-eye contact, parent-infant, 220

**F**

Facial nerve paresis, 149
Fat, brown, 178, 179
FBM; see Fetal breathing movements
Feeding
  monitoring of, 178
  nursing assessment and, 157
  nursing care and, 187–194
  respiratory distress and, 195
Femoral ossification center, 316
Fetal breathing movements, 32–35
Fetal circulation, 21–24
  assisted ventilation and, 343–344
  blood gas changes and, 431
  differential diagnosis and, 268

Fetal circulation (cont.)
  respiratory distress and, 275–277
  persistent; see Persistent fetal circulation
Fetus
  biochemistry, 25–35
  circulation of; see Fetal circulation
  heart and, 23
  heart rate monitoring and, 61–65
  lung and, 8–9
    fluid in, 31–32, 132–134
  physiology, 25–35
  placental circulation and, 20
  as separate individual, 213–215
  scalp blood sampling and, 65–66
  in utero drug therapy and, 238–239
Fever, 185
Fiberoptic instrument, 104
Fibroplasia, retrolental, 363–364
Fibrosis, interstitial, 356
$FI_{O_2}$; see Fraction of oxygen
Fistula
  bronchopleural, 380
  tracheoesophageal, 3, 101
    delivery room assessment and, 148
Fixed-wing aircraft transport, 109
Flaring, nasal, 263
Flexible fiberoptic instrument, 104
Flexor tone, 156
Flow interrupter, 378
Flowchart, 438
Fluid
  bronchopulmonary dysplasia and, 359
  fetal lung, 31–32, 132–134
  heart failure and, 169
  increased intracranial pressure and, 164–165
  nursing assessment and, 176–177
  nursing care and, 184–195
  resuscitation and, 249
Fluoroscopy, 317
Foramen ovale, 275
Forced expiration, 86–87
Fraction of oxygen, 41
  transcutaneous oxygen tension and, 76

Fracture, skull, 148
Fungal infection
  bronchopulmonary dysplasia and, 361
  radiography and, 296
Furosemide, 254–255
  deafness and, 276
  nursing care and, 176
  recommended dilution of, 173

## G

Gas diffusion, 21
Gas exchange
  assessment of, 40–60
  assisted ventilation and, 324
    high-frequency, 372–375
Gas pressure monitoring, transcutaneous, 76–78
Gas trapping, 385–387
Gastric pH, 241
Gastrointestinal function, 177–178
Genitourinary function, 177–178
Gentamicin
  dosage of, 245
  recommended dilution of, 173
Germ cell layers, 2
GFR; see Glomerular filtration rate
Glomerular filtration rate, 244
Glottis, 99
Glucose
  blood, 451
  nursing assessment and, 170
  resuscitation and, 248, 249
Glycerophospholipid, 26
Glycogen
  nursing assessment and, 170
  surfactant and, 26
Glycogen storage disease, 283
Glycoside, cardiac, 251, 252
Granulation tissue, 103
Grief, 232
Groove
  laryngotracheal, 5
  palatal, 353
Growth
  respiratory system dimensions with, 424
  retardation of, 316
Growth curves, 441–444
Grunting, 263

## H

Head
  circumference of, 163
  heat loss and, 182
Head hood, 197
Heart; see also Heart failure; Heart rate
  cardiothymic silhouette and, 292
  congenital disease of
    blood gas changes in, 431
    radiography and, 313–315
  fetal development of, 23
  innervation to, 165
Heart block, 283
Heart failure
  bronchopulmonary dysplasia and, 361
  patent ductus arteriosus and, 354–355
  radiography and, 314, 315–316
  respiratory distress and, 283
  signs of, 167
  treatment of, 168–169
Heart rate
  age and, 440
  delivery room assessment and, 140
  drug therapy and, 248
  monitoring and, 61–65, 71–74
  normal, 165
  nursing assessment and, 157, 167
  respiratory distress and, 194
  support of, 168
Heat
  birth and, 134
  high-frequency ventilation and, 382–383
  incubator and, 111–112
  loss of
    mechanisms of, 179–180
    monitoring and, 75–76
    oxygen and, 136
    protection from, 139–140, 179–185
    treatment of, 184
  nursing assessment and, 178–179
  thermogenesis and, 134–135, 178, 179
Heat exchanger, 401–402
Heel-stick glucose concentration
  feeding and, 192
  nursing care and, 170–171
  parenteral alimentation and, 193
Helicopter, 109
Hemangioma
  laryngeal, 99–100
  pharynx and, 98
  radiography and, 317
Hematocrit, 282
Hematologic system
  normal values for, 446–452
  respiratory distress and, 282–283
Hematoma, subdural, 149
Hemorrhage
  intracranial, 277
  intraventricular
    nursing assessment and, 163–164
    pneumothorax and, 351
  pulmonary, 313
  subarachnoid, 149
Henderson-Hasselbalch equation, 49–50, 52–53
Hering-Breuer reflex, 83
Hernia, diaphragmatic, 148
  radiography and, 311–312
HFFI; see High-frequency flow interruption
HFJV; see High-frequency ventilation, jet
HFOV; see High-frequency oscillatory ventilation
HFPPV; see Positive-pressure ventilation, high-frequency
High-frequency flow interruption, 370
High-frequency oscillatory ventilation, 370–372
High-frequency ventilation, 366–393
  classification of, 367–372
  clinical applications of, 375–382
  gas exchange during, 372–375
  history of, 367
  jet, 369–370, 376–378
  persistent fetal circulation and, 276
  problems during, 382–388
Home management, 362
Hood, oxygen, 113, 197
Hormonal effect, surfactant and, 29–30

Humeral epiphysis, 316–317
Humidification, 382–383
Humidified oxygen, 198
Hyaline membrane disease, 431
Hydration, 186
Hydrops fetalis, 146
Hygroma, cystic, 98
Hyperbilirubinemia, 155–156
Hypercapnia, 32
Hyperthermia, 185
Hypertrophy, muscular, 356
Hyperventilation
  alveolar, 431
  deafness and, 276
Hypocalcemia, 171
Hypoglycemia, 147
  delivery room assessment and, 147
  prevention of, 170–171
  resuscitation and, 248
Hyponatremia, 171
Hypoplasia
  left heart, 314
  lung, 4, 304–305
Hypothermia
  incubator and, 111–112
  nursing assessment and, 178–179
  oxygen and, 136
  protection from, 139–140, 179–185
  treatment of, 184
Hypovolemia, 145–146
Hypoxemia, 203

## I

Incubator
  oxygen therapy and, 197
  radiography and, 290
  thermoregulation and, 111–112, 184
Indomethacin, 252–253
  oliguria and, 178
  patent ductus arteriosus and, 355
  recommended dilution of, 174
Indwelling line, 187
Infantile botulism, 280
Infection, 353–354
  bronchopulmonary dysplasia and, 359, 361, 363
  parenteral alimentation and, 193–194
  pneumonia and; see Pneumonia
Inflammation, peribronchiolar, 356
Infusion
  central line, 169
  intravenous, 142–143
Infusion pump, 402
Insensible water loss, 177
Inspiratory pressure
  bronchopulmonary dysplasia and, 358–359
  delivery and, 140–141
Inspiratory to expiratory ratio, 333–334
Inspired carbon dioxide, 48–49
Inspired oxygen, 41–42, 334
Intermittent arterial blood sampling, 125
Intermittent mandatory ventilation, 360
Intermittent respiratory movements, fetal, 132
Interstitial emphysema, 274–275, 348, 351–352
  radiography and, 308–309
Interstitial fibrosis, 356
Intra-arterial oxygen tension, 128
Intracranial hemorrhage, 354
  respiratory distress and, 277
Intracranial pressure, 164–165
Intramuscular administration, 241–242
Intrapulmonary artery, 16–17
Intrathoracic compression, 304–305
Intrauterine growth
  retardation and, 316
  growth curve for, 441, 442
  lung and, 8–9
Intravenous alimentation, 177–178
Intravenous infusion, 142–143
Intraventricular hemorrhage, 354
  nursing assessment and, 163–164
  pneumothorax and, 351
Intubation, 93–95
  complications of, 352–353
  delivery room and, 141
  endotracheal; see Endotracheal intubation
  mechanical ventilation and, 200–202

Intubation (cont.)
  nursing care and, 161
  pulmonary mechanics in, 82
In utero drug therapy, 238–239
Isoproterenol, 249

## J

Jaundice, 155–156
Jet ventilation, high-frequency, 369–370
  clinical applications of, 376–378
Jitteriness, 164

## K

Kanamycin, 245
Kidney
  drug metabolism and, 243
  fluid and, 185
  indomethacin and, 253
Klumpke's paralysis, 149

## L

L:S ratio; see Lecithin to sphingomyelin ratio
Labor
  blood sampling in, 65–66
  psychologic aspects of, 215–216
Lactic acid, 451
Laryngomalacia, 99
Laryngoscopy, 103–105
Laryngotracheal groove, 5
Larynx
  acquired abnormality of, 102–103
  anatomy of, 91–92
  congenital abnormality of, 99–100
  web and, 3
Lavage, lung, 30
Lecithin, 26
Lecithin to sphingomyelin ratio, 31
  respiratory distress and, 266
Left-to-right shunt
  radiography and, 314
  respiratory distress and, 283
Lidocaine
  arrhythmia and, 247–248
  resuscitation and, 249
Lipid, 26

Liquid ventilation, 419–423
*Listeria monocytogenes*, 273
Lobe, lung, 7
Lobule, 7
Loop diuretics, 254–255
Lower motor neuron disease, 279
Lower respiratory tract
  acquired lesions of, 103
  bronchopulmonary dysplasia, 363
  congenital abnormality of, 3–4, 100–102
  development of, 6–20
Lung
  agenesis of, 4
  development of, 7–9
    biochemical aspects of, 25–30
  fetal, 132–134
  hypoplasia and, 4, 304–305
  infection and, 353
  lavage and, 30
  maturation and, 31
  nursing assessment and, 159
  radiography and, 292–293
  size of, with age, 425
  in utero drug therapy and, 239
Lung bud, 9–10
Lung volume, 433, 434
Lymphangioma, 317

## M

Magnesium sulfate, 278
Main-stem bronchus, right, 201, 352
Malformation, congenital; see Congential malformation
Mandatory ventilation, intermittent, 360
Map, blood gas, 55, 57–58
Massage, cardiac; see Cardiac compression/massage
Mass spectrometer, 73
Maternal placental circulation, 20–21
Maternal sensitive period, 216–219
Maternal sleep-wake cycle, 34
Maturation
  lung, 31
  radiographic evidence of, 316–317
  rating of, 445
Mechanical ventilation, 200–205
Meconium aspiration, 146

Meconium aspiration (cont.)
  blood gas changes in, 431
  differential diagnosis and, 268
  radiography and, 298–299
  respiratory distress and, 272–273
Meconium-stained infant, 140
Membrane
  alveolar-capillary, 45
  pleuropericardial, 19
  pleuroperitoneal, 20
Meperidine, 174
Mesenchyme, 10
Mesoderm, 2
Metabolic acidosis, 51–52
  delivery room and, 147
Metabolic alkalosis, 52
Metabolism, drug, 243–244
Methemoglobinemia, 282–283
Methicillin, 174
Methylene blue, 282–283
Methylxanthines, 249–251
Milk aspiration pneumonia, 269
Monitoring
  antepartum, 66
  blood gas; see Blood gas; Blood sampling
  neonatal, 70–79
  prenatal, 61–70
Motor neuron disease, 279
Mourning, 232
Mucous gland, 12
Mucous plugs, 103
Muscle
  disorder of, 280–281
  nursing assessment and, 156
  respiratory
    hypertrophy and 356
    nursing assessment and, 159
  smooth, 13
Myasthenia gravis, congenital, 280
Myocardial innervation, 165
Myocarditis, 283
Myoinositol, 28–29
Myopathy, 280–281
Myotonic dystrophy, 280–281

N

Nafcillin
  dosage of, 245
  recommended dilution of, 174
Naloxone
  apnea and, 160
  delivery room resuscitation and, 145
  recommended dilution of, 174
  respiratory distress and, 278
Nasal cannula, 113
  nursing care and, 197–198
Nasal flaring, 263
Nasogastric feeding, 189–191
  monitoring of, 178
Nasopharynx
  congenital abnormality of, 98–102
  radiologic evaluation of, 317
Nasotracheal intubation, 93
  technique of, 117–118
NEC; see Necrotizing enterocolitis
Necrotizing enterocolitis, 178
Necrotizing tracheobronchitis, 353
  high-frequency ventilation and, 383–384
Negative pressure, continuous, 328–329
Neonatal circulation, 24–25
Neonatal gas exchange
  acid-base physiology, 49–59
  assessment of, 40–60
  physiology, 40–49
Neonatal monitoring, 70–79
Nerve injury, 148–149
Nervous system; see Central nervous system
Neurologic function
  long-term respiratory care and 362–364
  nursing assessment and, 162–165
Neuromuscular junction, 280
Neuron, 279
Neutral thermal environment, 180–181
  respiratory distress and, 271
Nitrogen, blood urea, 451
Nitroglycerin
  resuscitation and, 248, 249
Nitroprusside
  persistent fetal circulation and, 276
  resuscitation and, 248, 249
Nomogram, Siggaard-Andersen, 429
Noninvasive blood gas monitoring, 195–196

Nonshivering thermogenesis, 134–135, 178, 179
Nonsteroidal anti-inflammatory agent, 252–253
Nonstress test, 66
Norepinephrine, 249
Nose, 5
Nursing care, 154–211
  assessment and, 155–179
    aeration and, 158–162
    brain function and, 162–165
    circulation and, 165–169
    drug therapy and, 169–170, 172–175
    electrolytes and, 170, 176
    fluid therapy and, 176–177
    gastrointestinal function and, 177–178
    general appearance and, 155–157
    thermoregulation and, 178–179
  fluid therapy and, 185–194
  mechanical ventilation and, 200–205
  oxygen therapy and, 194–200
  psychosocial support and, 206–208
  skin care and, 205–206
  thermoregulation and, 179–185
Nursing staff, 208
Nutrition
  bronchopulmonary dysplasia and, 361
  daily requirement, 453
  nursing care and, 187–194

## O

Obstruction, airway
  blood gas changes in, 431
  bronchopulmonary dysplasia, 363
Oligohydramnios, 303–304
Oliguria, 178
Opiate, 278
Oral feedings, 188–189
Orogastric feeding, 189–191
Orogastric tube, 195
Orojejunal feeding, 191
Oropharynx, 4
Orotracheal intubation, 93
  delivery room resuscitation and, 141
  palatal groove and, 353
  technique of, 114–117
Oscillatory ventilation, high-frequency, 370–372
  clinical applications of, 378
Ossification center, 316–317
Overbed radiant warmer, 181
Oximetry, 127–128
  pulse, 79, 196
Oxygen
  altitude and, 111
  assisted ventilation and, 326–327
  delivery of, 112–114
  hypothermia and, 136
  inspired concentration of, 334
  nursing assessment and, 160
  nursing care and, 161–162, 194–200
  partial pressure of; see Oxygen partial pressure
  placental circulation and, 21
  resuscitation and, 246, 249
  toxicity and, 359
  transcutaneous blood gas monitoring, 126–127
  transport of, 40–46
Oxygenation
  assessment of, 58–59
  extracorporeal membrane; see Extracorporeal membrane oxygenation
  fetal, 22
  persistent fetal circulation and, 276
Oxygen electrode, 77
Oxygen partial pressure
  alveolar, 42–43
  arterial
    birth and, 134
    reduced, 430
  blood, 43–45
    fetal, 22, 24
  intra-arterial, 128
  pulse oximetry and, 79
  tissue, 45–46
  transcutaneous, 76–78
  transitional period and, 131
Oxyhemoglobin dissociation curve, 44–45

## P

Pacifier, 198
Pacing, atrial, 168
Palatal groove, 353
Pallor, 155
Pancuronium, 174
Pa$_{O_2}$; see Oxygen partial pressure
Paracentesis, abdominal, 146
Paralysis
   Duchenne-Erb, 148
   Klumpke's, 149
   vocal cord, 100
Parasympathetic nervous system, 165
Parenteral alimentation, 193-194
Parents, care of, 212-235
   bonding and, 216-222
   childbirth classes and, 223-224
   congenital malformation and, 231-234
   labor and delivery and, 215-216, 224-225
   pregnancy and, 213-215
   premature or sick infant and, 225-231
   psychosocial, 207
Paresis, 149
Partial pressure
   carbon dioxide, 46-47
   oxygen; see Oxygen partial pressure
Patent ductus arteriosus; see Ductus arteriosus
PDA; see Ductus arteriosus
Peak inspiratory pressure, 331-332
   bronchopulmonary dysplasia and, 358-359
Penicillin, 245
Percussion, 118
   chest physiotherapy and, 195
Percutaneous absorption, 242
Perfusion, systemic
   nursing assessment and, 165-169
   respiratory distress and, 194
Peribronchiolar inflammation, 356
Pericardial cavity, 19
Pericardioperitoneal canal, 18-19
Peripheral artery catheterization, 124
Peripheral nervous system, 148-149
Peripheral vein, 143
Persistent fetal circulation
   blood gas changes in, 431
   differential diagnosis and, 268
   respiratory distress and, 275-277
PFC; see Persistent fetal circulation
PG; see Phosphatidylglycerol
pH
   assisted ventilation and, 336
   gastric, 241
   umbilical cord blood, 137-138
Pharmacology; see Drug therapy
Pharynx, 4, 6
Phenobarbital
   intraventricular hemorrhage and, 354
   recommended dilution of, 175
   seizure and, 164
Phenytoin
   recommended dilution of, 175
   resuscitation and, 249
Phosphatidylcholine, 29
Phosphatidylglycerol
   biosynthesis of, 29
   surfactant and, 26, 27
Phosphatidylinositol
   biosynthesis of, 29
   surfactant and, 26, 27
Phosphorus, 451
Phrenic nerve injury, 149-150, 281
Physiology
   fetal, 25-35
   neonatal gas exchange, 40-49
Physiotherapy, chest, 118-120, 195
PI; see Phosphatidylinositol
Placenta
   circulation and, 20-21
   drug therapy and, 237-239
Plasma, 145
Platelet count, 449
Plethora, 155
Pleural cavity, 18-20
Pleural effusion, 297-298
Pleuropericardial membrane, 19
Pleuroperitoneal membrane, 20
Plexiglas
   heat and, 181-182
   shield and, 184
Plug, mucous, 103

Pneumocardiogram, 73
Pneumomediastinum, 274–275
  radiography and, 307–308
Pneumonia
  blood gas changes in, 431
  congenital
    differential diagnosis and, 268
    respiratory distress and, 273
  milk aspiration, 269
  radiography and, 295–296
Pneumonitis, 272
Pneumopericardium, 348
  radiography and, 308
Pneumoperitoneum, 310, 311
Pneumotachograph, 80–81
Pneumothorax, 348
  differential diagnosis and, 268
  high-frequency ventilation and, 380
  radiography and, 305–307
  respiratory distress and, 274–275
  tube displacement and, 352
$PO_2$; see Oxygen partial pressure
Poliomyelitis, 279
Polycythemia, 282
Polyhydramnios, 280
Pompe's disease, 279
Position
  nursing assessment and, 156
  radiography and, 291
  respiratory distress and, 194
  Trendelenburg, 195
Positive airway pressure, continuous, 197
Positive end-expiratory pressure, 332
Positive-pressure ventilation, high-frequency, 368–369
  assessment of, 204–205
  clinical applications of, 375–376
Postextubation atelectasis, 352–353
Potassium
  blood chemistry and, 451
  nursing assessment and, 171, 176
Potter's syndrome, 304
Povidone-iodine, 205
Preconfigured monitors, 71
Pregnancy, 213
Preload, ventricular, 168
Premature infant
  apnea and, 285
  blood gas values and, 428
  compliance and resistance values for, 435
  daily nutritional requirement and, 453
  heart rate and, 440
  parents of, 225–231
  pulmonary insufficiency of, 302
  respiratory distress and, 265
  retinopathy and, 363–364
Prenatal monitoring, 61–70
Pressure
  continuous distending, 328–331
  initial inspiratory positive, 140–141
  high-frequency ventilation and, 384–385
  intracranial, 164–165
  partial, of oxygen; see Oxygen partial pressure
  peak inspiratory, 331–332
    bronchopulmonary dysplasia and, 358–359
  positive end-expiratory, 332
Pressure ventilator, 334
Pressure-volume curve, 81
Prong, nasal, 197–198
Prostaglandin
  birth and, 134
  recommended dilution of, 175
Protein
  blood chemistry and, 451
  surfactant and, 26, 27
Pseudoglandular stage of lung development, 8
*Pseudomonas aeruginosa*, 273
Psychosocial support, 206–208
Pulmonary edema
  bronchopulmonary dysplasia and, 361
  nursing assessment and, 159
  radiography and, 313
Pulmonary function
  bronchopulmonary dysplasia and, 357
  mechanics of
    assisted ventilation and, 321–324
    values for, 435–437
  nursing assessment and, 158–162

Pulmonary function (cont.)
  testing of, 79–87
Pulmonary hemorrhage, 313
Pulmonary insufficiency of premature infant, 302
Pulmonary interstitial emphysema, 274–275, 348, 351–352
  radiography and, 308–309
Pulmonary vessel
  air embolism and, 348
  development of, 16
  radiography and, 293
  total anomalous venous return and, 315
  vascular resistance and
    birth and, 132
    nursing assessment and, 165–166
Pulse oximetry, 79
  nursing care and, 196
Pump, infusion, 402

## Q

Quality control, 70

## R

Radiant warmer, 112
Radiation heat loss, 181–182
Radiography, 289–319
  air leak syndromes and, 305–310
  basic concepts of, 289–290
  bronchopulmonary dysplasia and, 299–301
  congenital malformation and, 303–305
    cardiac, 313–315
  congestive heart failure and, 315–316
  diaphragmatic hernia and, 311–313
  hemorrhage and, 313
  maturation and, 316–317
  meconium aspiration and, 298–299
  normal, 291–293
  pleural effusion and, 297–298
  pneumonia and, 295–296
  pneumothorax and, 350

pulmonary edema and, 313
pulmonary insufficiency of premature infant and, 302
respiratory distress and, 264, 267, 292–295
transient tachypnea of newborn and, 295
upper airway and, 317
Wilson-Mikity syndrome and, 301–302
Ratio
  inspiratory to expiratory, 333–334
  lecithin to sphingomyelin, 31, 266
Red blood cell transfusion, 271
Regionalization of perinatal care, 107
Renal function, 253
Resistance, vascular
  assisted ventilation and, 322
  birth and, 132, 134
  compliance and, 85–86
  values for, 435, 436
Respiratory distress syndrome, 264–271, 293–295
  adult, 382
  air leak and, 348
  algorithm for ventilatory management of, 337–343
  assisted ventilation and, 335–343
  differential diagnosis and, 268
  feeding and, 192
  high-frequency ventilation and, 382
  respiratory rate and, 194
  in utero drug therapy and, 239
Respiratory system, 1–39, 260–288; see also Respiratory distress syndrome
  acidosis and, 50–51
  air leak syndromes and, 274–275, 348
  airway disorder and, 281–282
  alkalosis and, 51
  apnea and, 284–285
  cardiovascular disorder and, 283
  central nervous system disorder and, 277–278
  congenital pneumonia and, 273
  development of, 2–20
  embryological germ cell layers, 2
  fetal

Respiratory system (cont.)
    biochemistry and, 25–35
    intermittent respiratory movement and, 132
    physiology and, 25–35
    transitional circulation and, 20–25
    muscles of, 159
    nursing assessment and, 159–160
    hematologic disorders and, 282–283
    history and, 260
    laboratory data and, 264
    lower motor neuron disease and, 279
    meconium aspiration and, 272–273; see also Meconium aspiration
    muscle disorder and, 280–281
    neuromuscular junction disorder and, 280
    nursing care and, 161
    persistent fetal circulation; see Persistent fetal circulation
    physical examination and, 261–264
    spinal cord disease and, 279
    transient tachypnea of newborn, 271
Resuscitation
    delivery room; see Delivery room management
    drug therapy and, 246–249
    errors to avoid in, 150–151
    evaluation of treatment and, 147–148
Retardation, growth, 316
Retinopathy of prematurity, 363–364
Retraction, 262–263
Retrolental fibroplasia, 363–364
Rewarming, 184
Rib cage abnormality, 281
Right main-stem bronchus, 201, 352
Right-to-left shunt, 275

## S

Saccular stage of lung development, 8–9
Saturation, oxygen; see Oxygen partial pressure

Segment, lung, 7
Seizure
    delivery room assessment and, 147–148
    nursing assessment and, 164
Self-inflating bag, 114
Sepsis, 353; see also Infection
    delivery room assessment and, 148
    fungal, 361
Septal defect, ventricular, 283
Septum transversum, 19
Servocontrol system, temperature, 75–76
Shunt
    left-to-right
        radiography and, 314
        respiratory distress and, 283
    right-to-left, 275
Shunt fraction, 58–59
Siggaard-Andersen nomogram, 429
Single-walled incubator, 111–112
Skin
    drug absorption and, 242
    nursing care and, 205–206
    partial pressure of oxygen and, 77
    temperature and, 76
Skull fracture, 149
Sleep-wake cycle, maternal, 34
Smooth muscle, 13
Sodium
    blood chemistry and, 451
    nursing assessment and, 171
Sodium bicarbonate; see Bicarbonate
Sodium nitroprusside
    persistent fetal circulation and, 276
    resuscitation and, 248, 249
Spectrometer, mass, 73
Spinal cord disease, 279
Stabilization, 138–139
Stenosis
    choanal, 98
    laryngeal, 102
    subglottic
        acquired, 102–103
        congenital, 100
        endotracheal tube and, 353
    tracheal, 101
Steroid; see Dexamethasone

Stool
  assessment of, 178
  feeding and, 192
Streptococcal pneumonia, 273
  radiography and, 295–296
Stress, cold; see Hypothermia
Stress test, contraction, 66–69
Stridor, 99
Stroke volume, 165
Subarachnoid hemorrhage, 149
Subcutaneous air, 309
Subdural hematoma, 149
Subependymal hemorrhage, 354
Subglottic space, 91
Subglottic stenosis
  congenital, 100
  endotracheal tube and, 353
Sucking
  continuous positive airway pressure and, 198
  nursing assessment and, 178
Suctioning
  bronchoscopy versus, 105
  complication of, 103
  endotracheal tube and, 94–95
  increased intracranial pressure and, 164
  mechanical ventilation and, 201, 202–204
  nursing care and, 161
  technique of, 120
Sudden infant death syndrome, 73
Supernumerary arteries, 16
Supraventricular tachycardia
  nursing assessment and, 167, 168
  respiratory distress and, 283
  in utero drug therapy and, 238–239
Surfactant
  fetus and, 25–30
  respiratory distress and, 266, 267, 270
Surveillance, 70
SVT; see Supraventricular tachycardia
Swallowing
  of air
    continuous positive airway pressure and, 198
    respiratory distress and, 195

nursing assessment and, 178
Sympathetic nervous system, 165
Systemic perfusion, 165–169, 194
Systems assessment, 158–179; see also Nursing care, assessment and

## T

Tachycardia
  critically ill neonate and, 157
  fetal, 61
  supraventricular
    in utero drug therapy and, 238–239
    nursing assessment and, 167, 168
    respiratory distress and, 283
  systemic perfusion and, 167
Tachypnea
  critically ill neonate and, 157
  respiratory distress and, 262
  transient, 271
    differential diagnosis and, 268
    radiography and, 295
Tape
  abdomen and, 205
  endotracheal tube and, 202
$TcPO_2$; see Transcutaneous blood gas monitoring
Temperature monitoring, 75–76; see also Heat; Thermogenesis
Tension; see Oxygen partial pressure
Tension pneumothorax, 305
Terminal bronchiole, 419
Theophylline, 249–251
  apnea and, 285
  bronchopulmonary dysplasia and, 362
Thermal environment, neutral, 180–181
  respiratory distress and, 271
Thermistors, 75
Thermogenesis, nonshivering, 134–135, 178, 179
Thermoregulation, 111–112
  nursing assessment and, 178–179
  nursing care and, 179–185
Thiocyanate, 248
Thoracentesis, 146

Thoracostomy tube
  placement of, 128–129
  pneumothorax and, 305
Thorax
  surgery and, 382
  transillumination of, 128
Thymus
  cardiothymic silhouette and, 292
  pneumomediastinum and, 307
Thyroglossal duct cysts, 98–99
Thyroid cartilage, 91
Ticarcillin
  dosage of, 245
  recommended dilution of, 175
Tidal volume, 79–81
  carbon dioxide elimination and, 324
  compliance and, 83–84
  peak inspiratory pressure and, 331–332
Time constant, 322–324
Time-cycled ventilator, 334
Tissue
  carbon dioxide tension of, 46
  oxygen tension of, 45–46
Tobramycin, 245
Tolazoline
  persistent fetal circulation and, 276
  recommended dilution of, 175
Tone, muscle, 156
Total anomalous pulmonary venous return, 315
Trachea
  acquired lesion of, 103
  anatomy of, 92
  atresia and, 3
  congenital abnormality of, 100–101
  development of, 9–10
  inflammation of, 353
  stenosis and, 3
Tracheobronchitis, necrotizing, 353, 383–384
Tracheoesophageal fistula, 3, 101
  delivery room assessment and, 148
Tracheomalacia, 100–101
Tracheostomy, 96–97
Transcutaneous blood gas monitoring, 76–78, 195–196
  technique of, 126–127
  carbon dioxide tension, 78
Transfusion, red blood cell, 271
Transient tachypnea of newborn, 271
  differential diagnosis and, 268
  radiography and, 295
Transillumination
  of chest, 350
  of extremities, 124
  of thorax, 128
Transitional period
  circulation and, 24–25
  physiology and, 131–135
Transport
  oxygen, 40–46
  regionalization and, 107–110
Transpyloric feeding, 191
Trapping, air/gas
  air leak and, 348
  high-frequency ventilation and, 385–387
Trendelenburg position, 195
TTN; see Transient tachypnea of newborn
Tube; see also Endotracheal intubation; Intubation
  extracorporeal membrane oxygenation and, 401
  feeding, 189–191
  radiography and, 291–292
  thoracostomy
    placement of, 128–129
    pneumothorax and, 305
  tracheostomy, 96–97
  types of, 93
Tumor, oropharyngeal, 99
Twins, 265

## U

Ultrasound, 317–318
Ultrathin bronchoscope, 104
Umbilical artery catheterization
  radiography and, 291–292
  technique of, 121–124
Umbilical cord
  blood pH and, 137–138
  clamping of, 135
  cutting of, 134
Umbilical vein, 142
  blood in, 22, 24

Umbilical vein (cont.)
  catheterization and, 125
Upper respiratory tract
  development of, 4–6
  radiologic evaluation of, 317
Urine
  collection of, 187
  decrease in, 178
  nursing assessment and, 166–167

## V

Vancomycin, 245
Vascular access, 142–143
Vascular resistance; see Resistance, vascular
Vascular ring, 101
Vasoactive drug, 248
  nursing care and, 169
  persistent fetal circulation and, 276
Vehicle, transport, 109
Vein
  oxygen tension and, 131
  pulmonary
    air embolism and, 348
    development of, 16
    total anomalous return and, 315
  umbilical, 142
    blood in, 22, 24
    catheterization and, 125
Vena cava, fetal, 22
Venoarterial extracorporeal membrane oxygenation, 398
Venovenous extracorporeal membrane oxygenation, 398–399
Ventilation
  assessment of, 159–160
  assisted, 320–346; see also Assisted ventilation
  barotrauma, 419
  high-frequency; see High-frequency ventilation
  liquid, 419–423
  mandatory intermittent, 360
  normal values in,, 432
  nursing care and, 200–205
Ventricular afterload, 168
Ventricular preload, 168
Ventricular septal defect, 283
Vibration, 118, 120
Viral pneumonia, 273
Vital signs, 157
Vocal cord
  anatomy of, 91
  paralysis, 100
Volume, lung, 433, 434
Volume ventilator, 334
VSD; see Ventricular septal defect
$V_T$; see Tidal volume

## W

Wall, chest
  compliance and, 81
  nursing assessment and, 158–159
Warmer
  overbed radiant, 181
  radiant, 112
Water loss; see Fluid
Weaning
  bronchopulmonary dysplasia and, 361
  continuous positive airway pressure and, 336
  extracorporeal membrane oxygenation, 403
Web, laryngeal, 100
Well-being, assessment of, 137–138
Wernig-Hoffmann disease, 279
White blood cell count, 448
Wilson-Mikity syndrome
  differential diagnosis and, 269
  radiography and, 301–302

NO LONGER THE PROPERTY
OF THE
UNIVERSITY OF R.I. LIBRARY